MORAL
PROBLEMS
IN
MEDICINE

edited, with introductions, by

SAMUEL GOROVITZ

Senior Editor
Department of Philosophy
University of Maryland, College Park

ANDREW L. JAMETON

Department of Philosophy
State University of New York at Binghamton

RUTH MACKLIN

Department of Philosophy
Case Western Reserve University

JOHN M. O'CONNOR

Department of Philosophy
Case Western Reserve University

EUGENE V. PERRIN, M.D.

Department of Pathology
Children's Hospital of Michigan

BEVERLY PAGE ST. CLAIR

School of Medicine
Case Western Reserve University

SUSAN SHERWIN

Department of Philosophy
Dalhousie University

MORAL
PROBLEMS
IN
MEDICINE

PRENTICE-HALL, INC., *Englewood Cliffs, New Jersey*

Library of Congress Cataloging in Publication Data
Main entry under title:

Moral problems in medicine.

    Bibliography: p.
    Includes index.
    1. Medical ethics—Addresses, essays, lectures.
I. Gorovitz, Samuel. [DNLM: 1. Philosophy,
Medical—Collected works. 2. Ethics, Medical—
Collected works. W50 M822]
R724.M82   174'.2'08   75-42150
ISBN 0-13-600817-8

MORAL PROBLEMS IN MEDICINE
edited by Samuel Gorovitz *et al*

© 1976 by Prentice-Hall, Inc.,
Englewood Cliffs, New Jersey

Printed in the United States of America

10 9 8 7 6 5 4 3 2 1

Prentice-Hall International, Inc., *London*
Prentice-Hall of Australia Pty. Limited, *Sydney*
Prentice-Hall of Canada, Ltd., *Toronto*
Prentice-Hall of India Private Limited, *New Delhi*
Prentice-Hall of Japan, Inc., *Tokyo*
Prentice-Hall of Southeast Asia Pte. Ltd., *Singapore*

CONTENTS

PATERNALISM   *182*

Chapter 3
MORAL PROBLEMS
CONCERNING LIFE AND DEATH   *242*

INTRODUCTION   *242*

KILLING AND LETTING DIE   *249*

Chapter 4
MORAL PROBLEMS ON A SOCIAL SCALE *422*

THE NATURE OF SOCIAL JUSTICE *430*

THE RIGHT TO HEALTH CARE *454*

MEDICAL RESOURCES AS COMMODITIES *500*

ALLOCATION OF SCARCE MEDICAL RESOURCES *522*

APPENDIX A, PEDAGOGICAL POSTSCRIPT *540*

APPENDIX B, MORAL PRECEPTS IN MEDICINE *546*

INDEX *547*

PREFACE

This book is designed primarily to provide readings for a consideration of the moral issues in medicine from a philosophical point of view. The included material should be of value both to students training for the health-care professions and to those studying the humanities. Further, we hope that the book will be of interest to individuals of whatever professional or academic affiliation who are concerned with the evaluative aspects of the decisions forced upon us by modern medicine.

The notion of preparing such a book arose during the second year of the Moral Problems in Medicine Project at Case Western Reserve University. This was a joint undertaking of the Philosophy Department and the School of Medicine. Under the auspices of that project, a seminar concerning moral problems in medicine had been developed for undergraduate, graduate, and professional school students. Two aspects of our experience combined to prompt this undertaking.

First, we found it difficult to develop the curriculum. We were continually taxed to find a mixture of philosophical and medical materials that would enable us to pursue the chosen topics advantageously, and the heterogeneous composition of the class intensified the problem. We resisted the philosopher's inclination to start from a particular case and venture on a one-way journey to principles, justifications, and meta-ethics. Similarly, we resisted the medical student's proclivity to dwell on the particulars of a case without considering questions of generalization, consistency, or conflict of values. In the end, we agreed that our purposes would require both philosophical and medical materials, and a substantial amount of pedagogical caution and determination as well. To our distress, no suitable materials were readily available. Before attempting to weave the fabric, we had to find the threads one by one.

Second, we gradually came to view our pedagogical efforts as successful. We had sought to promote an increased awareness of the moral dimensions of decision-making in medical contexts and of the importance of the conceptual uncertainties that underlie some of the conventions and practices in health-related areas. While not attempting to take substantive positions on the moral problems at issue, we had sought to increase the competence with which students recognized, integrated, and reconciled the various considerations relevant to making such decisions. The response from students, and the quality of work that they produced, solidified our belief that we were learning how to achieve such objectives.

We believe that the philosophical perspective is an essential ingredient in the multidisciplinary approach that is required by moral problems in medicine. This perspective is a distinctive one, demonstrably different from those offered by law, sociology, theology, anthropology, and the rest. For it to interact optimally with the others, it must develop along with them. This book does not itself represent such development; rather, we hope the book will help catalyze the kind of activity that will constitute such development.

There are two basic alternatives in structuring a philosophical course in medical ethics. One is to divide the course according to medically conceived topics such as organ transplantation, genetic engineering, euthanasia, etc. Such an approach is wholly viable, but we have preferred not to adopt it here. Rather, we have organized the book primarily on the basis of more philosophically inspired categories. Thus, our headings invoke such notions as paternalism, truth, social justice, etc.

No issue discussed here is treated in a complete or thorough way. Further, we do not pretend to have included every important topic or point of view. Instead, we have sought simply to provide sufficient self-contained material of good quality to sustain intensive, well-informed discussion of issues of fundamental importance. Severe limitations of space constrained us to omit further treatment of the issues covered, and to leave out entirely many important topics we would have liked to cover—including, for example, such topics as psychosurgery and behavior control, definitions of health and the medical model, population and birth control, malpractice and iatrogenic injury, issues in pharmacology, and the federal regulatory role in health care research.

A number of the articles included herein contained extensive footnotes and bibliographical references when first published. We have deleted many of these notes in order to make possible the inclusion of several more articles. For those who might wish to use this volume in the classroom, we have appended a pedagogical postscript, including a list of bibliographies.

Several articles appear here for the first time. These include the essays by Bellin, Hare, Metzler, Parfit, and Perrin et al. We are grateful to these authors for making their work available to us. We are particularly indebted to Willard Gaylin, who has done much to bring about public awareness of the moral issues in medicine, for supplying us with the foreword. We are, of course, grateful to the many authors and publishers who provided permission for the inclusion of works in this book.

We have been aided in various ways in the preparation of this manuscript by Professor Herbert Long, John Merritt, Pat Merritt, Donna Moss, and Gary Schwartz. Our students over the last three years have inspired us and influenced us, and we are grateful to them for that. Rachelle Hollander has played a particularly helpful role in final editorial preparation of the manuscript and in her able handling of the complex and sometimes frustrating process of arranging for all necessary permissions.

Although no grant was made specifically to support the preparation of this manuscript, the book would not have been possible without the activities undertaken in the Moral Problems in Medicine project at Case Western Reserve, supported by the National Endowment for the Humanities under Grant EH–6028–72–111 and by the Exxon Education Foundation, and the Moral Problems in Medicine Institute sponsored by the Council for Philosophical Studies in the Summer of 1974 with the support of the Rockefeller Brothers Fund. Each of these three foundations, by its material support of our participation in directly related projects, has fair claim to view this volume as a partial consequence of that support. Finally, we are grateful to our colleagues at Prentice-Hall for the confidence they expressed in undertaking to publish the volume, for the good advice they have provided along the way, and for the spirit of congeniality with which they have dealt with us—including those inevitable battles about length.

S.G.

FOREWORD

We tend to become most interested in ethical issues when we are unsure of the direction in which we are heading. Philosophy thrives on self-doubt and self-doubt is a point every sensitive person will reach somewhere along that road from aspiration to fulfillment. When we are young and only aspiring we do not need doubts; we will shape our fantasies in perfect harmony. It is only after we begin to achieve our ends—when we realize that achievement and fulfillment are not necessarily congruent—that we must redefine our goals, guided by our doubts.

Perhaps I am merely saying that success leads to power, and power brings responsibility, and responsibility to a decent human being inevitably leads to anxiety. The urgent interest in medical ethics at this time is a symptom of the success of medicine.

It was not always this way. I look back somewhat enviously at the scientist of the late nineteenth century when medicine was, indeed, all promise and aspiration—when it seemed that science was on the threshhold of achieving all the solutions to man's needs.

This attitude persevered well into the present century, symbolized to me by a particular memory. When I first came to college, I was impressed by an unusual archeological detail: a small Victorian building of great charm, albeit somewhat run-down and decrepit, was almost completely surrounded by a functional, massive, ugly-modern building—red brick, as I remember it. The Victorian building, I was later to find out, was the divinity school, and the red brick building was the department of biology. It was a symbol of the state of things then. Biology was about to swallow up theology.

But "swallowing up" is not necessarily destroying. The psychoanalytic concept of introjection describes how that which we devour to destroy, with poetic irony, may become a part of us. To absorb something, to take it into you, may also mean that you have unwillingly undertaken its burdens. I think that *has* happened. The scientist, particularly after Hiroshima, has often been the conscience of the nation—what little conscience there has been.

I used to start my lectures in medical ethics to medical students by telling them how funny the subject was twenty years ago when I was in medical school. I could remember only a couple of examples, both of them in retrospect seeming appalling. One had to do with the crisis that might occur if, on the way to the golf course on Sunday morning, you stumbled over a child bleeding to death—the question being whether you were under any obligation to hold up your foursome by stopping to stem the flow of blood. You will be relieved to know that, at least in Ohio twenty years ago, you were under no such obligation.

The other set of problems had to deal with promotion and advertising —the size of the sign you were allowed to have in your window, etc. I remember specifically in Ohio we were not allowed to list our specialties after our names in the Yellow Pages, which fact was told to us with an air of great moral superiority, because certain states permitted such "advertising."

In retrospect, I realize that both of those issues derived from serious ethical conflicts. They arise from the ambiguities of being a man who is at the same time a healer-comforter and a man of commerce. They represent some of the conflict in the individual who has to balance those two roles.

Now, after twenty years, I am in a medical school, this time as a teacher, and the same confusions persist even in understanding the definition and nature of ethics. Two examples may illustrate. At a recent discussion, a group of ward administrators insisted that medical ethics were not neglected at all, at least not on their wards; that they indeed "spent more time on ethical issues than they did on medical issues." I thought this amazing; this was, after all, a general medical ward, and not the chaplain's office. When they explained, however, it became apparent that they were alluding to sociological issues—e.g., the mechanical problems of placing people in nursing homes, clearing the wards of "chronics," etc., and not to ethical dilemmas. This delineated their concept of the ethical issues.

The other example involves a distinguished senior physician attending on a medical ward. He felt that on the whole, ethical questions were indeed, generally neglected—but not on his ward. Here there was no problem. His statement was: "Just as I feel that I have the ultimate responsibility for making all medical decisions, I feel that I must bear the ultimate responsibility for making all ethical decisions." It was said in good faith, and it was not for me to point out to him that there is a fine line between "assumption of responsibility" and arrogation of power. He is, indisputably, an expert on medical decisions, but he is not an expert on ethical decisions. I am not sure whether there are experts in these decisions. The question is: *Should* he be the final arbiter of these decisions any more than the medical student, the nurse, the cleaning lady, or any *one* individual besides himself?

Clearly there persists a confusion about the nature of the problem that is necessary to explore. One has to know the questions before one seeks the answers. To that end I would like to refer briefly to some traditional areas of ethical dilemmas, which will be discussed in greater detail in this book, hoping to indicate how the success of medicine has added urgency to the old problems, has recast them, or has created new problems.

One of the traditional concerns of medical ethics is research on human subjects. Professor Henry Beecher has pioneered in this area. Early work rightly focused on exposing clearly unethical research; it was muckraking in the best sense. There is still, unfortunately, a place for muckraking today.

Beyond this, the rapid development of technology, permitting procedures once never contemplated, is now raising ethical problems of a more complex nature—and confusing some previously settled areas. For example, there has traditionally been a clear separation between standards of "experimental" and "therapeutic" procedure. Consider the recent discussions concerning surgery for revascularization of the heart. This is a difficult procedure used generally in patients crippled with severe angina—with the hope that it also might deter future infarctions. When originally done, it carried a high mortality rate. I needn't tell you that it had a 100 percent morbidity rate, since that is the nature of surgery. It was seen by all as an experimental procedure. However, certain surgical teams have perfected the techniques to a point where the mortality rate in this group is now less then 10 percent. With such dramatic improvements the process is now considered a standard therapeutic option. Compare now how different our attitude would be if we were discussing a drug therapy. If I suggested to you that I had a drug that would relieve the symptoms of angina, with some promise, but no evidence, that it might deter future infarction, would you be reassured by the fact that it caused 100 percent morbidity and 10 percent mortality? Would I even be permitted to market the drug? The operative procedure is not considered experimental because our whole bias toward surgery is different from what it is toward drugs, and for very obvious reasons.

Before the modern era a control mechanism over surgery analogous to drugs would have been unnecessary and foolish. Surgery was a theory of last resort—often more dreaded than the disease to which it was directed. If the pain and shock of the operation didn't kill you, the post-operative sepsis was likely to. The terror of the patient was sufficient control over the procedure. Now with the advent of sophisticated anesthesia, antisepsis, and antibiotics, serious surgical intervention (e.g., prefrontal lobotomy) can be a routine procedure.

In almost every area considered in this book, it is our success that confounds us. Examine a few. At one time there was no medical need for the physician to consider the *concept* of death. This was because the *fact* of death was generally congruent with the cessation of personhood. We are so built that when we lose those functions which make us human beings by even the crudest definitions, we generally die. With the advent of new techniques in medicine that congruence has been destroyed. So it is now quite possible to sustain life, or to sustain living matter, or to sustain a person beyond the point of previous contemplation. When this happens we are forced to consider the distinctions between human life, living matter, and persons. And so now, we find medical people facing the problems of defining personhood. These philosophical problems have equal urgency in the medical dilemmas at the beginnings of life.

But the recognition of the complexity of problems in these areas becomes most apparent when most specific. At the Columbia Law School as part of curricular development in teaching bioethics, a course was created in which law students, medical students, and seminarians were joined together. They were divided into small research groups of "lawyers," "physicians," and philosopher-theologians. They were charged to design legislation for specific problems of the biological revolution, or to present a convincing rationale as to why their subject should be excluded from the legislative area.

It has been extremely fascinating to see the impact of the medical mind, the legal mind, and the theological mind on one another; to see the differences but also to see the accommodation and growth over a semester. They were instructed to be as futuristic or as present-day oriented as they wished—and the proposals were often startling when cast with the specificity that legislation requires. For example, a contract was written for the hiring of a surrogate mother (i.e., planting a fertilized egg of one couple in the uterus of another woman to bear for nine months). The Surrogate Mother contract is in the service of an honorable old medical tradition, facilitating the desire of parents to have their own "natural" (genetic) child. But when the details are spelled out in the language of contracts the results are unnerving. The surrogate mother should have "rights of first refusal" in case the natural parents decide that they wish to abort. The surrogate mother must fulfill obligatory dietary commitments and interdictions during the gestation period. It is difficult for this to avoid sounding funny, yet renting womb space can be conceived as a respectable alternative, probably preferable to an artificial placenta, for solving the not uncommon problem of a woman who has had her uterus removed, has perfectly functioning ovaries, produces ova, and wants a "natural" child.

There were other issues considered that were much more of the present. There already exist incorporated, profit-making sperm banks. Artificial insemination with donor sperm is an accepted institution of medicine. Some very simple questions arise. Wouldn't a sperm bank with massive selection and computerized data represent a superior method of donor selection to the current technique of collaring a convenient medical student or intern who needs the money and finds the donation of sperm a more amiable procedure than the donation of blood? What then of criteria and controls? Should there be a free choice of the nature of the donor, and who should make the choice? In the past we have implicitly assumed our task as an imitation of the natural process, and we have attempted to replicate as closely as possible the natural inheritance. The obstetrician does little scientific screening. The traditional donor is, therefore, a poorish (needs the money) medical student (available) healthy and intelligent enough to have survived until, if not through, graduate education, who looks something like the father who is to raise the child (satisfy paternal wants, maintain deception, quiet gossipy speculation).

Appalling as it may seem, this represents the traditional and typical at the current time. One would think that common sense might indicate simple correctives. Why a student? A 60-year-old grandfather who has proved to be a successful sire would seem more logical. Certain late developing diseases with hereditary tendencies could be eliminated (for example, diabetes, arteriosclerotic conditions, etc.). This then introduces some aspects of positive engineering. We are moving from the "having a child" problem to the "having a special child" problem. Should such genetic variables as sex, size, IQ, or race be options? Or should they be left to chance? The student legislators mandated matching two variables to the natural parental traits, IQ and size—IQ under the assumption that a child with a high IQ might be disadvantaged with parents of low IQ, and size presumably to protect a small mother from a giant fetus. The question of race selection, beyond psychological and sociological consideration, raises problems of constitutional law.

Genetic engineering raises the kind of speculations and choices that boggle the mind and titillate the imagination. But even the less dramatic area of genetic counseling raises distressing dilemmas. Genetic counselors are now adopting the posture that psychiatrists once assumed. They presume to present the facts, eschewing value judgment. Genetic counselors, at this point in time, are geneticists first and counselors second, if at all. The sophisticated psychiatric counselor has abandoned the delusion of objectivity. He is aware that all counseling involves the conscious and unconscious intrusions of the values of the advisor. Because I have yet to meet a value-free psychiatrist, I am skeptical of the genetic counselor's comfort in "only presenting the facts."

The control of behavior is another major area to which this volume devotes substantial attention. Obviously there is a difference now that we have the capacity for mechanical and electronic control of behavior. Also, the specialization of drugs so that they now control specific modalities rather than just ups and downs adds a new dimension to mood modification. We must now ask what, if anything, is the essential ethical difference between injection of a drug, the implantation of an electrode, or the use of normal sensory inputs. The Behavior Control Research Group of the Institute of Society, Ethics and the Life Sciences has been considering this, and my comfortable and comforting biases have already been badly shaken. I started with the usual healthy revulsion against surgically messing with the brain. My emotional aversions gradually were attacked until the only remaining objection I could cling to was the recognition of the irreversibility of surgical destruction. But to a psychiatrist, certain sensory inputs, particularly if initiated early in life, carry the fixity of organic change. If there is a difference between implanting an electrode and implanting an idea, it will require more elegant intellectual attention than it has as yet received.

Finally, the question of transplants and artificial organs really does represent a new field and new conditions under which to consider traditional moral problems. The drama of the new helps illuminate vital old problems which had been relegated to back closets of medical consideration. The problem of priorities is just such an issue, which lay neglected until the transplants highlighted the less glamorous, but urgent areas. It returns us to the example that I offered from my medical school days, and raises the whole question of the marketplace mentality of medicine. There is something distasteful about the concept of selling human life. We have sold chance; we know that. We sell high risk. We will pay someone to work in a submarine. We will pay someone to build a bridge with the sure knowledge that the building of it will take a certain number of lives. But we have not yet arrived at the point where we have allowed the selling of seats in a lifeboat of a sinking ship. Or have we? When we see the posters of the American Hemophilia Society—an authentic, legitimate medical group—presenting the pictures of two young boys, and announcing that one will live a normal life because his father can afford $22,000 a year for treatment and the other one is not going to live because his father cannot afford this, I wonder. I also wonder about the sensitivity of people who would advertise the fact. If it were indeed a fact of necessity that one had no choice but to distribute a life-saving commodity by auction, I might have to live with it, but I wouldn't want to advertise it.

There are, again, no easy answers to the establishment of medical priorities. One seductive solution is to suggest the elimination of them by utilizing chance alone in the form of lotteries. This was suggested by that group of medical, theological, and law students in that experimental course at Columbia Law School. The students felt scarce resources—body parts, for example—ought to be allocated, once medical determinants were the same, by fishbowl lottery with no moral or sociological evaluations. Then, however, they were given the specific case of parents with a six-months' premature baby and their own 6-year-old daughter, and a limited facility needed for survival by both, and asked whether they would want those two names thrown into a fishbowl. The example served to unsettle the majority and to illustrate the difficulty of assuming that chance guarantees equity.

Returning to the question of medical priorities, let us take another undramatic example. Research has always been the most hallowed area of medicine—so much so that a contempt for the general practitioner was commonplace in medical schools. Because the researchers for the most part were running the medical schools, references to the LMD (local medical doctor) carried the tone and implications associated with mention of the village idiot. Nowadays, we are beginning to raise questions, even here, about our priorities. We question whether research in certain life-sustaining areas is justified when that same amount of money might be applied to the distribution of the fruits of research that has already been done. And so we have a conflict. For the first time, to my knowledge, research, which has in general (as distinguished from specific pieces of research) always been treated with the greatest respect, is now being attacked as an elitist phenomenon and, as such, as immoral or unethical.

This, too, is but one part of the larger problem of a redefinition of the physician's role, the physician-patient relationship, the social role of medicine, and, most important, the ethical and political implications of the concept of health.

I would now like to show how such problems evolve, and to indicate some of the social complications of certain "medical" developments. In doing so, it will be necessary to consider three closely related areas. One is the definition of normal; the second is the power of the medical model; and the third is the expansion of individual treatment into social engineering. These are all drawn from the field of psychiatry, but I think they have a validity for the kind of ethical questions that arise in other areas of medicine

—they deal, after all, with fundamental problems: freedom and coercion, individual and society, rights versus privileges, definitions of good, etc.

The definition of normalcy has caused particular mischief in the area of mental health, where it is compounded by incorporation into the medical-therapeutic model.

Psychoanalysis liberated whole areas of behavior from the domain of religion and morality, and redefined them in medical terms. A piece of behavior, like a blood-pressure reading or respiratory rate, could now be seen as sick or healthy, neither more nor less. The implication of this was not immediately apparent. To some, this was seen as purely a semantic shift. What was sinful sixty years ago became immoral thirty years ago, and today is merely called sick or immature. To some this was a minor change. We had only changed the name of the game. Health had simply become a new morality. But this is a dangerous underestimation, because in changing the name we changed much more. The changing of the frame of reference to a medical or scientific one had a profound impact on controlling individual action.

The unparalleled power that we place in the hands of the medical man stems directly from the existential fear of death that we all share. The preserver of life has often been exempted from normal limits of behavior. This is true whether he is called a priest or physician, and there have been times when both have literally gotten away with murder. Democratic society prides itself on its toleration of differences in values. However, there are certain areas where one approaches absolutism. Health and sickness is such a polarity. No person aspires to sickness (at least no "healthy" person). We are frightened of sickness because it is the prelude to death. That is why we listen to our lawyer's "advice" but we follow a doctor's "orders." By defining behavior as either healthy or sick the psychiatrist has a profound effect in directing the course of behavior while, with an unbelievable conceit, claiming a neutral stand in the field of morals.

Let me restate what I believe has happened. If a piece of behavior is defined as immoral by a religious authority, the individual still feels free to accept or reject that definition, particularly in our society, which endows religious or moral leaders with little authority or punitive power. It is often easier to change one's religion than to abandon a condemned but desired activity. If, however, you define the very same piece of behavior as "abnormal" or sick, and if the individual can be convinced of your expertise in matters of health, he will often be forced by fear to abandon that activity. He will in addition not feel forced. He will wish to do that which you wish. The universal terror of illness, operating under the imprimatur of the medical establishment, makes coercion in the traditional sense unnecessary. This is a potent force in behavior control which has not been nearly sufficiently analyzed, evaluated, or supervised.

What I am saying is that by changing the frame of reference, we have created a potentially explosive and sociologically significant change. We live in a culture that has always, at least theoretically, respected diversity in moral and religious areas. But we live in a culture in which medicine has always been seen as having certain rights to coercion. In other words, we have resisted coercing people on grounds of their moral right or religious right in recent times, but we have *not* in terms of medical rights. By redefining morality and values into medical terms, we are expanding the mechanism for controlling human behavior. By redefining a piece of behavior as abnormal, rather than immoral, you are subjecting it to the coercive aspects of law. But even without that, you will have the coercive aspects of anxiety in operation.

Even when an organized attempt to avoid the intrusion of values is made, it can never be successful. Psychoanalysis has for years operated with the conceit of a value-free system. Yet time and time again the imposition of values has been demonstrated.

Some unique aspects of the power of the medical model became apparent during meetings of the Behavior Control Research Group evaluating psychosurgery and psychotropic drugs as means of modifying behavior. Much of the discussion of the first conference was on control of violence related to temporal lobe epilepsy. It was interesting to observe the consistency of response in a mixed disciplinary group when confronted by the technologies of those neurosurgeons who went into the brain with scalpels, probes, and electrodes. The general conclusion and feeling of the group seemed to be that if a man is susceptible to rages that have nothing to do with electroencephalographic changes, you have absolutely no right to go in and disturb his brain—even if you can get rid of his rages. However, if there *is* a temporal lobe focus and you can establish that there is a relationship between the focus and the rage, then you *do* have a right to go in and remove the anterior part of the temporal lobe.

This is an interesting concept. I wonder why we are happier and more satisfied with that medical model. I submit that what we are treating anyway is not the focus or EEG change, but the behavior. After surgery, the patient will have, if we are speaking anatomically rather than functionally, a more damaged brain. He may even have greater functional loss—but of a personal rather than interpersonal significance.

Imagine for a moment an EEG change correlated with increased intelligence, creativity, or sensitivity. We are not going to encourage operation on the "abnormality." No, what we want to change is a piece of behavior that we have decided is undesirable. But we all feel uncomfortable in doing it just as a direct matter of behavior control. If we can link it to epilepsy, if we can link it to the epileptic model, even if the only signs of epilepsy are the electroencephalographic changes (and the rages), we feel more secure. There is an illogicality here. If the rages are destructive, if the only way to control them is by surgery, and if we feel that it is legitimate to help a man to facilitate his life by operating on his brain, why not go ahead and do it? We traditionally destroy healthy tissue surgically to enhance life adjustment. Yet few present at the Institute's discussion were prepared to do it when social behavior was involved, unless they had the comfort of the medical model—although the distinction logically pursued may be elusive, arbitrary, capricious, or even nonexistent.

We are happier in the justification of changing behavior when we can utilize a medical model. There are illogicalities, and inequities, here—but the alternatives, as yet not adequately explored, may be even more troublesome. This leads inevitably into the discussion of social engineering and how one may be projected into this area—even when reluctant and resistant. In the nineteenth century, psychiatry and physical medicine were fairly parallel in their views of human pathology. They both saw disease as something imposed on the person from the outside, an invasion, if you will. And they both saw pathology in terms of organ deterioration. If you recall the fact that in the late nineteenth century the majority of patients admitted to psychiatric hospitals were suffering from tertiary syphilis, they weren't too far wrong. The disease then was something external, gross, and bizarre occupying and reducing the individual. The treatment for it became obvious —repel the invader. And you need not worry about definitions of normalcy. The pathological condition was so eccentric that merely removing the eccentricity was presumed to reinstate implicitly the state of normalcy. If someone comes to a doctor with a turnip growing out of his ear, he knows he has to remove the thing, and knows that what remains after the operation is a normal individual, turnipless ears being an implicit part of our definition of normalcy.

Then came the revolution in psychodynamics introduced by Freud. We began to see that people didn't have to be all crazy but only partially so. Healthy, nice, decent people like psychiatrists and judges could be normal in the traditional sense yet have isolated pieces of behavior that were aberrant—phobias, compulsions, etc. The next stage beyond this was the defining of character neuroses. That meant that nothing need necessarily be "crazy" to warrant a classification as abnormal. One could be defined as neurotic on the basis of a constricted character structure. If the personality didn't add up to a productive, happy, or self-fulfilled individual this could be seen as a form of mental illness.

Finally, psychiatry began to conceive of illness in terms of significant behavioral omissions. We decided that there are certain pieces of behavior that *ought* to be present, that *should* be present, that were *normal* to be there. Their absence, therefore, was taken as a sign of neuroses. Now when you begin to raise "ought" questions, of course, you are on that fine borderline between medicine and ethics. This progression into values received added impetus, because simultaneously there was a different model evolving in medicine in general. The therapeutic goal was being replaced by a prophylactic one. When you deal with disease, regardless of how rampant an epidemic, you are dealing with 15, 20, 30 percent of the population. When you're dealing with preventive medicine, you're dealing with 100 percent of the population.

The results of those progressions were inevitable. As psychiatry reduced the criteria for mental illness, it expanded the number of the mentally ill. By requiring less and less to define mental illness, you place larger and larger percentages of the population into the category of the mentally ill. When you then introduce a prophylactic model, you give the privilege of social control of the total population to the physician. This is then added to the considerable powers society has already granted him: the moral imprimatur of the healer, and the coercive privileges of law.

It is now easy to see how we have traveled unwittingly from the safe role of comforter to the sick to the uneasy position of political advocate and social engineer. Yet here we are. The issues are fused and cannot be avoided. Nor should they be. Even if the power of decision is shared, the physician will always be an inevitable and important co-participant. It is an authentic part of his role, and he must be trained for it. He is a value-maker, ethicist, social force, and political influence in the lives of his patient and beyond. He is, whether he wishes to be or not. There is no such thing as a value-free medicine, nor has there ever been. To accept this as a fact of professional life is not arrogance but honesty, and the first step toward that redefinition of the physician's role that is necessitated by the coming of age of medicine. It is our success that demands a new sensitivity, a new humility, and a new training.

WILLARD GAYLIN

INTRODUCTION

THE TRADITIONAL TAXONOMY

Our objective in this book is critically to examine the moral dimensions of decision-making in medical contexts and in contexts involving the biological sciences. By "medical contexts" we refer to the full spectrum of activities pertaining to the provision of health care. These include specific clinical interactions between a physician or other health care provider and patient, and social policy decisions about the allocation of resources as between preventive and curative medicine, therapeutic medicine and medical research, and between health-related expenditures and other kinds of social programs. We also include such conceptual issues as clarification of the concept of health and identification of what kinds of physiological, psychological, or sociological states justify medical intervention. By "the biological sciences" we refer to scientific inquiries into organic and biochemical processes—including both the results of such inquiries and the protocols by which such inquiries are advanced.

The moral problems in medicine have received a great deal of attention in recent years. That attention, however, has not included any systematic attempt to address those problems from the point of view of contemporary analytic philosophy. The problems themselves have been characterized in a taxonomy that is primarily medical and biological in conception, but we shall argue here for the value of a philosophically inspired taxonomy of problems as a valuable new perspective in terms of which familiar problems can be more fruitfully addressed.

We begin by reviewing the traditional way of describing the moral problems in medicine. We cannot here provide any exhaustive account of those problems, but a sense of the subject as it is typically conceived can be conveyed by the brief citation of several general areas, along with a specific illustrative problem within each area. These citations are neither exhaustive nor mutually exclusive.

The allocation of limited resources. At every level, from the individual practitioner to the federal government, needs outstrip resources, and the resulting conflicts about priorities are laden with evaluative questions.

1

Illustration: Given limited governmental capacity to finance health-related endeavors, how much of the available resources should be allocated to improving future health care through basic research, and how much to improving the quality of present health care through support for rural clinics, new medical schools, etc?

The regulation of health care.   Medical practice has been largely regulated by the medical profession, but there is a growing sense that it is too important for that. Yet the proper locus and limits of external regulation can only be determined in light of a viewpoint about social and political organization, and the nature of the conflict between social needs and individual rights. Illustration: Under what conditions and for what reasons should mass screening for heritable diseases or severe birth defects via amniocentesis (examination of fetal cells drawn from the amniotic fluid) or other means be required or encouraged as a matter of public policy?

The use of human subjects in experimentation.   Although this issue has received wide attention within the scientific community, with certain codes of conduct having gained acceptance, there are still questions that are vigorously disputed. Illustration: What, precisely, is the nature of informed consent to participation as a subject in an experiment on the part of persons who are disadvantaged with respect to making autonomous decisions—e.g., infants, the mentally retarded, or those who are involuntarily confined?

The scope of medical prerogative.   It has been largely conceded that medical decisions should be made by medical professionals, but it is a matter of some dispute what constitutes a medical decision. Illustration: Are these strictly medical questions, and if not, what sort are they—whether a diabetic should be treated with insulin, whether a kidney patient should receive renal dialysis, whether a woman should have an abortion, whether a homosexual or drug user is sick, whether a new drug or surgical procedure is suitable for general use.

Constraint of research objectives.   Here the issues go beyond the mores of using human subjects to the question of the fundamental purposes and possible effects of research. Illustration: Should experimentation that may lead to the raising of experimental subjects in vitro, via nuclear implantation from human genetic material, be permitted or regulated?

Responsibility for dependent persons.   Many people deviate from what may be considered normal in the functional capacity of a human being, the reasons for such diminished capacity including retardation, congenital deformity, blindness, severe illness, injury, advanced age, and the like. Medical practice is closely involved in the plight of such persons. But it is not clear what the nature and locus of responsibility are for those who, for whatever reason, are unable to function independently. Illustration: If social policy or law prohibits infanticide in cases of radical deformity or readily demonstrable severe retardation, is there also a communal responsibility to provide resources and facilities for the care of such individuals? Are the problems, principles, and responsibilities different in cases of severe senility or other geriatric infirmity?

Death and dying. New criteria of death are being shaped, used as guidelines, and affirmed in the courts. But questions remain concerning policy toward the terminally ill. Illustration: What principles should govern decisions concerning euthanasia, withdrawal of costly or scarce life-support systems, determination of narcotic dosages, aggressiveness of treatment of life-threatening infections, and the like, in the terminally ill patient; and what is the relevance, if any, of the patient's age, economic status, or choice?

Commitments of the medical profession. The physician's classical commitment to prolong life and relieve suffering places him in conflict situations where adherence to one value requires violation of the other. This is merely a special case of the conflicts inherent in the physician's multiple commitments to his patient, his profession, his own monetary or other career-related interests, the medical profession generally, his community, and his own value structure. Illustration: A physician treating a neighbor's 22-year-old son on an emergency basis for an injury discovers a large quantity of illegal narcotics in the son's possession. What should the physician's response be to the patient, the neighbor, and the police? Does it matter whether or not the physician is personally an advocate of strict law enforcement with respect to narcotics?

The physician-patient relationship. Physicians have a uniquely privileged and powerful position with regard to their patients, and the nature of the actual and optimal relationship between physician and patient is thus a highly charged question for both. Illustration: When a physician discovers an infant to have a heritable disease, and upon testing the ostensible parents discovers that neither is the carrier, what should he tell to whom, and why?

Control of behavior. The increasing prominence of psychopharmaceutical techniques of behavior control, psychosurgery, behavior modification by aversive conditioning, and the conjectured prospects for intervention via electrode implantation, have all received a good deal of public attention as issues raising moral dilemmas. Confronted by the power of such techniques, one can hardly help but ask what sorts of behavior may justifiably be controlled, by whom, in what ways, for what purposes, in accordance with what values. But less obvious issues also need to be brought to the surface. Illustration: The "medical model" has been debated at length with regard to its appropriateness for conceptualization in mental health or behavior problem areas. But as Willard Gaylin has pointed out, in some ways the medical model itself, with its classification of people by experts into categories of normal or deviant functioning, is an ominously powerful force in general. Given the influence that medical judgments have on attitudes and behavior—what Gaylin calls the physician's special "rights to coercion" —should the concepts of normality that underlie medical practices and public health policy be subjected to greater critical scrutiny from outside the medical profession? Just what are those concepts of normality—how do they limit or influence therapeutic intervention? Are there credible alternatives to them—and if so, how ought differing models of normality be evaluated?

THE PHILOSOPHICAL TAXONOMY

In an earlier era, the phrase "medical ethics" was frequently taken to refer to a variety of issues concerning the conventions of medical practice. This tradition is reflected even today in the views of the Judicial Council of the American Medical Association, which, in its statement on the principles of medical ethics, addresses attention to such questions as whether physicians may advertise, collect referral commissions, lecture to groups of chiropractors, etc., as well as to questions of social responsibility, confidentiality, and the like, in the interest of rendering "service to humanity with full respect for the dignity of man."

More recently, medical ethics has come to be taken as referring to problems of the sort exemplified in the illustrations above, characterized in terms that are essentially medical or biological. Thus, the focus has shifted to problems of abortion, birth defects, confidentiality in the physician-patient relationship, dying, euthanasia, financing of health care, genetic counseling, human subjects in experimentation, involuntary confinement, etc. This taxonomy persists as the most prominent interpretation of the moral problems in medicine. It is legitimate and useful; the problems thus described are real and important. However, I wish to argue for the concomitant importance of a different taxonomy.

Inquiry into many of the medical contexts that generate moral dilemmas reveals certain common threads of philosophical puzzlement. For example, questions about the right to suicide, about the right of an individual who has committed no crime to be free from involuntary confinement, about a religious group's right to refuse blood transfusions, and about whether the adolescent patient should have access to medical treatment in confidence from parents (who perhaps directly or indirectly cover its costs), all involve issues of personal autonomy and the justifiability of paternalistic intervention. Similarly, questions about responsibility to sustain the lives of seriously deformed newborn infants, like questions about responsibility to sustain the lives of severely deteriorated, terminally ill victims of injury, illness, or advanced age, raise questions about the value of life and the relevance of considerations of quality of life to the assessment of value of life. *Only a consistent point of view about personal autonomy, the justifiability of paternalistic intervention, and the considerations that are relevant to determining the value of life in general or a given life in particular, can allow one to develop a consistent perspective on the various different moral problems in medicine that are reflected in a medically inspired taxonomy.*

There is thus a taxonomy of topics, fundamentally philosophical in conception, that must be addressed as a part of the process of dealing with the moral problems in medicine characterized medically or biologically. These philosophical topics are not new. What is perhaps new is the extent to which clarity about them is demanded for the resolution of pressing problems that arise elsewhere. Typical of such topics are the following:

Autonomy. To what extent is it morally required to allow individuals to act in pursuit of their own aspirations? Does an individual with self-destructive aspirations thereby lose the right to autonomy generally enjoyed by others? Should freedom to act include freedom to follow a foolish or tragic (e.g., suicidal) course of events, or is it justifiable to override another's autonomy paternalistically, as well as for reasons of social benefit? Does respect for a patient's autonomy require honesty on the part of the physician, even when deception seems medically prudent?

Coercion. When is an act voluntary? What conditions must be met for an experimental subject to have volunteered? Do federal programs related to public health or population planning become coercive if they are based on the provision of powerful incentives? Under what conditions is coercion justified in medical contexts?

Normality. Does it make any sense to try to characterize health or illness in terms of a notion of normality? What are the criteria for distinguishing between desirable and undesirable deviations from physiological or psychological normality for health-related purposes, assuming that the notion of normality is useful?

Naturalness. Can the familiar case be sustained that it is sometimes right to prolong life using natural means but wrong to sustain it by artificial means? Is the distinction between artificial and natural means an intelligible one? Is "exotic" life-saving therapy any less natural than routine abdominal surgery or the use of antibiotics?

Rights. Much of the talk about ethical issues in medicine invokes the notion of rights. Is there a right of a fetus to be born, of a patient to have access to his medical record, of a sick person to receive medical treatment, or of a physician to practice where he pleases? Insofar as claims about rights and the resolution of conflicts of rights are obscure, so too are the arguments that involve such claims.

Dependency. Is there a sense in which some individuals can be identified as dependent persons in medically relevant ways? Is anyone genuinely independent? If the notion of dependency is a medically legitimate one, what consequence does a person's being dependent have for the justifiability of paternalistic intervention in his life?

Justice. Is it unjust to distribute health care as a free market commodity, or to consider the social utility of patients in distributing scarce medical resources? Should disputes about damages for medically caused injury be handled by the judicial system or by a special system? Are there unique features of medical situations that raise idiosyncratic problems of justice, or do general considerations of justice apply unaltered in medical contexts?

Needs and Wants. Even granting that one's health-related needs should be met, how are needs to be distinguished from wants that would justify a lesser claim on the benefits of social organization? Insofar as it makes sense to speak of a right to health care, is there a distinction between the need for antibiotic intervention to combat a life threatening infection on the one hand and the desire for cosmetic surgery to alleviate the evidence of aging on the other?

Responsibility.   If there can be said to be a right to health care—in the sense that the body politic must make treatment available to individuals suffering from specific diseases the treatments for which are known—is this right to be limited in any way by considerations of personal responsibility? For example, under a system of federally financed free medical care, should the individual whose chronic smoking results in respiratory disease or who is seriously injured because he refused to wear a helmet when riding his motorcycle, be entitled to treatment at public expense, when his imprudent behavior took place in the face of warnings in virtue of which his illness or injury can be viewed to some extent as voluntary?

Personhood.   Under what conditions is it appropriate to consider an organism to be a person? What is the relationship between this issue and questions of abortion, the use of fetal tissue in research, and the withdrawal of life support systems from an irreversibly comatose patient?

One could go on at length. The point is merely to show that many familiar philosophical topics are centrally important to the illumination of moral problems in medicine—and, more importantly, that each such philosophical topic cuts across a variety of such problems. Thus, a philosophical inquiry into medical ethics might well focus, say, on the notion of *paternalism,* and investigate the variety of medical and scientific contexts in which that issue arises; likewise for each of the other entries in the philosophical taxonomy. One of the virtues of such an approach is that it enables the philosopher to concentrate on new problems in a way that is familiar and in the use of which he has substantial expertise. An additional virtue of this approach is that it helps those outside philosophy to see connections among medical and scientific problems that are not so easily seen otherwise, and it thereby exhibits more plainly the importance of philosophical inquiry to the resolution of problems of broad social interest.

OLD PROBLEMS AND NEW PROBLEMS

The question of whether death is always and everywhere an evil, whether one has a right willingly to embrace it, and whether life has value independently of the experiences for which it is a precondition, are ancient questions. So too are a number of questions pertaining to the responsibilities of the physician in regard to his patient. Other problems, which seem to arise out of new developments in biomedical research, are largely old problems given new force by recent developments. But there are genuinely new problems as well.

Among the old problems given new force by recent developments are many of those arising in clinical medicine. For example, it is not a new puzzlement to wonder about the appropriate societal constraints on parental reactions to newborn infants who are undesirable by virtue of having certain unanticipated and repugnant characteristics. What is new is the power of the medical profession to save malformed infants who would have died under earlier circumstances. Similarly, what gives deliberations about euthanasia a new urgency is our increased capacity to sustain life beyond reasonable hope of recovery. How one ought to die, and the extent to which one ought to be able to influence or determine the manner and mode of one's death, are old questions. What is new is the power of medical technology to intervene in what were previously dramas that played out largely in their own way.

Our new abilities to gain information also intensify old conflicts. For example, that we can learn via amniocentesis that a fetus is defective sharpens the debate about abortion. We can now identify certain individuals as defective (sometimes grievously) before birth, and hence can circumvent the question of infanticide by advocating early abortion in such instances. Debate about the justifiability of abortion is not new; what is new is our power to perform safe abortions, and the quality of the information that we can bring to bear in some instances in stating the case for abortion.

The genuinely new problems arising from technical developments can be divided into those that arise from developments in health-care technology and those that stem from developments of other sorts. Among the most important developments in health care technology that generate new moral problems are these:

> The ability to separate sexual and reproductive activity.
>
> New techniques for obtaining and handling information, including (1) specific testing procedures such as amniocentesis, (2) an understanding of statistical phenomena such as are considered in epidemiology, and (3) the powers of information-handling provided by computerization.
>
> Increased understanding of both the physiological and psychological dimensions of a person—each as a complex set of interrelated systems that can to some extent be separated and acted on independently—e.g., as respiration can be sustained despite renal failure.
>
> The development of psychopharmaceuticals and other technological methods of influencing or controlling behavior.
>
> The ability to conduct research or intervene therapeutically in a way that involves manipulation of human development.

Among the technical developments not directly related to health care, but with substantial impact on questions of health, are the developments in food technology, including the widespread use of chemical food additives, and industrialization, with its attendant pollution of the environment with substances directly related to the pathogenesis of a large variety of diseases.

Each of these areas of technical progress generates or intensifies a cluster of ethically troubling issues. It is hard to overestimate the extent to which our social customs and moral traditions reflect the belief that sexual and reproductive behavior, though distinguishable, are not separable. Now, relatively suddenly, they are quite separable as a result of technical developments. The ramifications of this fact for family structure, educational policy, child-rearing, population planning, and even such a fundamental issue as the right to reproduce, are hardly fathomable at this point. One ramification, however, seems clear: questions must now be answered that previously were not even raised.

Our understanding of epidemiology raises some fundamental questions about the competing claims of curative and preventive medicine. It is justifiable as social policy, for example, that we have allocated $600 million in quest of cures for malignant diseases, and only $30 million to exploration of the carcinogenic effects of environmental pollutants, when there seems to be increasing evidence that a large percentage of malignant disease arises from the presence in the environment of substances that could be regulated? To be sure, curing disease is more dramatic than preventing it, and hence has more appeal both politically and medically. Still, it is not implausible that reflection on the relationship between social responsibility and health would produce arguments in favor of shifting resources dramatically from curative to preventive medicine.

In older, simpler times, an individual was thought to be either alive or dead—the occasional problem being to determine which. Now that we realize that physiological systems deteriorate at different rates and in different ways, we are forced to recognize that, in some of the more difficult cases, whether we have an instance of death or not depends on decisions that we make about which systems have a fundamental importance to our conception of life. Thus, the respirating, digesting, irreversibly comatose quasi-person devoid of neocortical activity challenges us, not to discover whether death or life is present, but to decide which physiological systems are to count in what ways in our deliberations about how to behave in regard to the person or corpse at issue. It is because we understand so much better than we used to what is happening physiologically, and have so much more ability to influence it, that the definition of death is now problematic.

There is no serious question that some use of chemotherapy for psychological purposes is laudable. For example, lithium compounds can transform the lives of certain manic-depressive patients, enabling even some who had required institutionalization to lead happy, productive, stable lives. There seems little basis for dispute about the justifiability of this sort of pharmacological intervention. But the use of drugs such as ritalin as a means of controlling the behavior of inattentive and disruptive school children who lack any identifiable organic deficiency seems a highly suspect use of chemicals to control behavior. Perhaps, after all, it is the school setting that is in need of therapy. But by what principles do we condemn the latter use of drugs while lauding the former?

The horror that some express at the prospects of genetic experimentation results in part from an unwarranted extrapolation from what is presently possible, or even plausible for the foreseeable future, to a fictionalized vision of malevolent geneticists manufacturing humans and quasi-humans in inhumane ways for inhumane purposes. But some genetic research, particularly that involving recombinatory use of genetic material, raises troubling questions now. Thus, the temporary self-imposed moratorium of 1974–75 on such research, and the stringent new guidelines suggested by the research community itself for conducting such experiments safely, reflect the fact that geneticists are now able to create new forms of life with characteristics that are not fully predictable and which, while they fall far short of the fictional mass production of human beings, nevertheless could have substantial impact on the well-being of human beings. And it is explicit in the programs of some of those engaged in such research that a possible future benefit of the work is direct intervention in the genetic development of individual human beings.

Scientific inquiry is a social enterprise supported and conducted at the pleasure of the public whom it ultimately serves. Yet, like medicine, it is practised by a professional elite whose judgments are based on considerations that are essentially obscure in many ways to the public at large. Thus we find, in grappling with questions pertaining to public regulation and public accountability in regard to scientific research, that we must confront traditional questions concerning the proper scope of democratic processes and the prudence of establishing and supporting social institutions that invest power in elite groups charged to act in the interest of a comparatively benighted public.

Two additional points bear mention. First, in the medical context, issues of distributive justice and scarcity are particularly apposite. Medical science is in its infancy. Its successes, largely in the area of infectious diseases and surgical techniques, are impressive. Still, next to nothing is known about the pathogenesis of malignancies, circulatory or cardiac ailments, arthritis, degenerative neurological diseases, and many other conditions. The best and most advanced of medical care, as more and more is learned about the etiology and cure of disease, will for the foreseeable future be in scarce supply. Further, medicine in its entirety will be in competition with other socially valued enterprises for resources that are limited. It will be necessary to address these problems in terms of an unending need to allocate limited resources in the face of competing claims.

Finally, it is clear that there is an inherent conflict between epistemological and ethical aspects of experimentation. For certain kinds of experiments, to inform the subject of the nature of the experiment is to destroy the validity of the experiment at the same time. For examples, if we wish to screen newborn infants for the notorious XYY syndrome, as the first step in a longitudinal study aimed at determining whether or not such individuals are predisposed to antisocial behavior, we cannot inform the parents about the nature of our study without introducing a potentially distorting influence on the relationship between the parents and the children that might itself alter each child's propensity to engage in antisocial behavior. Yet it has been argued that no study of a child is morally permissible without the informed consent of the adults who have responsibility for the child's well-being. Other forms of experimentation that would likely contribute to the general welfare are simply morally repugnant because of their violation of individual rights. For example, we might learn a great deal about language acquisition, with a view toward improving the linguistic ability of underprivileged children, by raising a few children in total isolation from linguistic input for various periods of time—say, two or three years—before immersing them in verbal environments. There should be no question about the scientific utility of such an undertaking, nor should there be any question about its moral unacceptability.

PHILOSOPHY AND MEDICINE

These problems have a special urgency that distinguishes them from many of the issues that philosophers traditionally address. Decisions in clinical medicine do not await philosophical reflection. Nor do government agencies, in establishing regulations that can facilitate or cripple medical research, come to terms as a first step with conflicts between competing ethical theories. Nor do the courts, in ordering life-sustaining treatment of a neonatal monster, come first to some clear general view about the relationship between the value of an individual life and the characteristics of the person whose life it is. Yet these decisions do get made against a backdrop of assumptions and confusions about essentially philosophical topics. For philosophers to address themselves explicitly to those topics as they arise in medical contexts is in no way to abandon the essential character of their philosophical commitments. It is, on the contrary, to do philosophy in a particularly rewarding way, by bringing the strengths of philosophical analysis to bear on problems that engage the immediate interest of physicians, lawyers, policy-makers, legislators, patients, and all the rest of the public in its grand diversity. And for physicians and other health-care professionals to adopt the philosophical perspective is in no way to abandon their commitments to providing care. Rather, it is to broaden the context of sensitivity and understanding within which they provide it—and is thus ultimately to reflect a resolve to provide it in a more humane and enlightened way.

That science exists in the final analysis at the pleasure and for the benefit of society generally is a point to which philosophers generally accede readily. What is perhaps less often noted by them is that philosophy, too, is a social enterprise supported in the final analysis by the public to whose interest it ultimately accrues. It is entirely opportune that philosophers in increasing numbers are addressing their attention to issues with which large portions of the nonphilosophical public can readily identify. When rigorous philosophical work illuminates problems of interest to the public, it is far easier to make the case that the philosophical community, like the scientific, merits public support and respect because it, too, is prepared to respond constructively to pressing social concerns—both because of the essential philosophical interest of those concerns and out of its own sense of social responsibility.

This volume has been prepared in the conviction that both better philosophy and better health care can result from philosophical reflection on medical problems. The chapters that follow have been designed to facilitate such reflection on selected moral problems in medicine. Many moral issues are untreated here that might with equal appropriateness have been included, and even the full range of moral problems in medicine constitutes only a part of the philosophy of medicine. Epistemological issues, such as questions of evidence and predictability, and questions of conceptual clarification, for example, are also important parts of the philosophy of medicine. But the moral problems seem to have a way of commanding center stage, and it is time the philosopher's light was aimed more directly at them.

S. G.

MORAL PHILOSOPHY

Chapter 1

INTRODUCTION

In many cases we believe we know what the morally correct action is. When faced with the choice of keeping a promise or breaking it, we believe we should keep it. When faced with an opportunity to help another in need at no cost to ourselves, we believe we should help. Further, we sometimes think we can justify our actions and decisions in light of general principles. For example, we may decide to tell a dying patient that he or she is dying because we hold the general principle that the truth should always be told. Or we may refuse to experiment on a patient without having obtained that patient's informed and voluntary consent because we hold the general principle that the only one who has a right to make that decision is the potential subject himself. Some believe that such general principles can and should themselves be justified in terms of even more general principles. For example, one might believe that the reason one should always tell the truth is that to do otherwise is to treat another person as an object rather than as a being deserving of respect. Similarly, one might believe that the reason one should always obtain informed and voluntary consent is that to follow any other policy will in the long run diminish the total amount of happiness in the universe.

However, there are situations in which we do not feel confident about what course of action is morally correct. We may believe that a dying patient should be told the truth about his condition. But we may also be aware that telling a particular patient the truth may cause him great harm. If we also believe that one should never cause unnecessary harm to another person, we seem to have to violate one of our principles no matter what we do. Cases of conflict of principle force us to re-examine our moral beliefs.

Further, we may find ourselves in situations in which our moral principles do not seem clearly to apply. We may hold the principle that killing a human being is wrong. However, in the case of a proposed abortion it is a matter of dispute whether the fetus should be counted as a human being. One way of describing the abortion issue, then, is to say that we must decide whether an already accepted principle applies in such cases.

Another problematic situation occurs when others seem to disagree with us about principles. We may believe that it is never correct to operate on a person without obtaining that person's consent. Others, however, might believe that it is morally permissible to operate on a person if such an operation will help that person. While we may refuse to listen to what others say in such situations, it seems more reasonable to examine the various proposed principles and their justifications in an attempt to reach agreement on what to do.

It is in part because of problems like these that the moral philosopher becomes interested in the general area of medical ethics. The moral philosopher wants to develop a set of principles or perhaps a single principle that will enable us to make morally correct decisions and perform morally correct actions. Ideally, such principles or principle will be comprehensive (applicable to all cases that arise), decisive (yielding an answer in all cases), and justified (defensible against other proposed principles). Further, we want the principles or principle to be specific enough to give us actual guidance in real cases. A principle such as "Do as little harm as possible" would not be specific in the relevant sense unless we had some way of determining or measuring and comparing harm. Similarly, a principle that tells us to treat persons as having dignity would require for its use that we have a clear idea of what counts as treating a person with dignity.

One further feature should be noted. Even if we develop some apparently comprehensive, decisive, justified, and specific moral principles, we must consider how the results obtained by using them coincide with our most thoughtful and deeply held moral intuitions. In many cases the actions we perform cannot be undone nor can their consequences be negated. This is why we must continually reflect upon the guidance given by our principles: Our thoughtful moral intuitions may provide a last line of defense against doing something terribly wrong. Those who "follow orders" and as a result kill many innocent persons perhaps would not have done so if they had reflected on their moral intuition about killing before they acted. However, these intuitions must not be taken as a final, automatically acceptable court of appeal. Sometimes they are based upon our own prejudices from the past, or upon a commitment to some role. It is up to us to examine our theories in light of our thoughtful intuitions and also our intuitions in light of our thoughtfully developed theories.

Concerns of moral philosophers can very roughly be divided into two sorts—normative ethical concerns and meta-ethical concerns. Normative ethics deals with developing a set of moral principles that tell us what acts are right or wrong, good or bad, obligatory, permissible, or forbidden; and also provides reasons for accepting these principles. Although this may seem to exhaust the important role of moral philosophy, it does not. For in attempting to answer such normative questions as "What actions are right?" or "What things are morally good?" one must have some understanding of what it means to say that something is right or morally good, and of what morality, moral principles, and justification in ethics *are*. These questions in meta-ethics are questions about ethics, but they are not psychological questions about what values certain groups accept (though both of these areas may be of interest to moral philosophers). Rather, meta-ethical questions are conceptual questions whose answers help us to understand what we mean when we search for specific principles, and indeed what would count as answers to our normative questions. In this section the primary, though not the sole, emphasis is on normative questions.

There are two main sorts of normative ethical theories: The first is the *deontological* or *formalist* theory. Such a theory holds that the rightness or wrongness of an action is to be determined by examining the sort of action in question, or perhaps the motive with which the action is done. Common to this type of theory is the view that the rightness or wrongness of an action should not depend on what the consequences of the action are. It is what is done, the way in which it was done, or the reason behind the doing that are relevant to determining moral rightness or wrongness—not what results the action had.

The other main sort of normative theory is called *teleological* or *consequentialist*. According to such a theory, the rightness or wrongness of an action is determined by the results of the action. To determine whether or not an action is morally right we should examine the probable consequences of that action, compared with the probable consequences of other available actions, to see if the action in question would produce a greater balance of good over evil than any other action.

Briefly put, deontological theories hold that one can determine the rightness of an action independent of determining the consequences of that proposed action. Teleological theories deny this.

Perhaps the most significant deontological theory is that of Immanuel Kant. Kant begins his quest for a foundation for morality by focusing on the morally good person. Such a person has a good will. What makes a good will is not that the person who possesses it does things that have happy results. It may be that actions done from selfish motives have happy results, and we certainly should not have respect for a person from a moral point of view merely because his selfishly intended actions happen to work out well. Kant even goes so far as to say that we should not have moral respect for a person who happens to like doing things for other persons. We might like and approve of such a person, but according to Kant, it is a psychological accident that some persons happen to like helping others. Morality should not depend upon how one happens to be psychologically constructed. Rather, for Kant, from the moral point of view, one deserves respect for one's action only if the action was done for the sake of doing the moral thing—done *from* a respect for duty, not merely in accord with duty.

Kant begins to answer the question of what our duties are by noticing that humans are by nature rational and are truest to themselves when they act so as to express this nature. According to Kant, one central feature of rationality is that its principles are universal—i.e., they apply to all beings at all times and places. For example, the laws of logic are not different at different times or places. Therefore Kant proposes as the basic principle of morality a principle that combines universality with duty: Act always so that the maxim of your action can consistently be willed to be a universal law. He calls this the *categorical imperative*. This imperative gives no direct guidance as to what to do, but is nevertheless applicable in situations where we are considering what action to perform. The procedure is this: Suppose we have made a promise we would now rather not keep, perhaps because it would be inconvenient for us to keep it. We contemplate breaking it. Would this be morally acceptable? First we formulate the maxim of our action, describing what we propose to do. In this case we propose to break a promise on grounds of convenience. Now we test this maxim in terms of the categorical imperative. Can we will that such a maxim be a universal law? That is, can we, as rational persons who desire happiness, accept a state of affairs in which it is publicly acknowledged and admitted that persons may break promises whenever they find it inconvenient to keep them? Kant would say no. If such a maxim were a universal law, it would render incoherent the institution of promising. Note that Kant is not saying that if such a principle were accepted the consequences of its acceptance would be such that in time the institution of promising would no longer be of much use to people. Rather, he means that it would be irrational to have such an escape clause built into the institution. The institution would contain an incoherent set of rules.

Kant then attempts to extend a similar form of reasoning to rule out other proposed maxims. Whether and to what extent he is successful is a matter of dispute.

Of great importance is that for Kant there were other ways of formulating the categorical imperative. The most striking of these is that we should act "as to treat humanity, whether in thine own person or in that of any other, in every case as end withal, never as means only." Kant's view here is difficult to grasp fully, but part of what he has in mind is that insofar as we act, using the categorical imperative, we express our nature as rational beings. Because all persons are similar to us in this respect we are making decisions and acting, as it were, for all persons. Hence, we must recognize each person as a moral being deserving of respect and never use anyone merely as means. To put it briefly, we could never accept such treatment by others and because duty is a universal notion we cannot inflict such treatment on them.

The most common form of teleological theory is utilitarianism. Perhaps the most significant form of utilitarianism is that put forward by John Stuart Mill. Mill holds that an action is right in proportion as it tends to produce happiness and wrong as it tends to produce unhappiness. By happiness Mill means pleasure and the absence of pain and by unhappiness he means pain and the absence of pleasure. In computing the amount of pleasure and pain, Mill believes that we should count each person as one. It is not possible to prove strictly that the utilitarian principle is the correct basic moral principle. But, according to Mill, people do in fact seek happiness, and with proper upbringing they can be brought to generalize this desire to include the happiness of all persons.

Some have objected to Mill's view, saying that it demeans human beings by regarding them as no more than mere animals, because pleasure and pain are taken to be the determinants of moral rightness and wrongness. Mill argues in response to this that pleasures differ not only in quantity but also in quality. He claims that there are pleasures accessible to human beings that are higher in quality than those available to any animal. He tells us that it is better to be Socrates dissatisfied than a pig satisfied. Which pleasures are qualitatively better than others is to be determined by consulting a person of sensitivity and broad experience.

Both Kant's theory and Mill's theory seem to embody a number of central notions that we believe are important to morality. Kant's notion of treating others never solely as means seems to capture at least part of our idea of human dignity. Mill's concept of the greatest happiness of the greatest number seems both humane and perhaps realistic when we face moral issues as they arise in society. On one view or the other we may be able to come to some decision concerning the legitimacy of prolonging the life of a suffering patient or of experimenting on persons. Still, the views seem to issue conflicting directives in some particular cases. One might argue, for example, that according to Kant it would always be wrong to experiment on a person without his consent, for this would be treating him as a means only and, hence, would undermine his dignity. On the other hand, if such experimentation would yield a cure for disease it might, on Mill's theory, be justified on the grounds of its social utility. Perhaps the Kantian could reformulate a maxim so that in some cases such experimentation would be acceptable. Or perhaps one could show that undermining a person's dignity would in the long run produce more unhappiness than happiness for society. That is, more thinking might enable us to use the two theories or variants of them to arrive at a justified and acceptable set of principles. Some philosophers who are sympathetic to utilitarianism believe that it needs supplementation by a Kantian-like theory. In particular, while utilitarianism directs us to maximize happiness, it gives no clear guidance as to how to distribute happiness. For example, a world of one thousand people in which one person has one million units of happiness while the other people have none is equal in total amount of happiness to a world in which each of the thousand people has a thousand units of happiness, and yet the world with equal distribution seems morally superior. A principle that tells us merely that we should maximize total happiness would, it seems, give us no moral grounds for preferring the world with equal distribution. Some philosophers believe that a Kantian sort of theory embodying the notion of justice is a necessary component of an adequate moral theory, because it sets limits to the morally acceptable ways of maximizing happiness. The utilitarian and Kantian views are included, then, not so that one might have an automatic way of deciding moral problems; rather, they are included because they represent the most significant theories developed by persons trying to face the problem of living morally. But neither theory can relieve one from the burden of moral responsibility.

The last point can be seen in the challenge presented by Sartre. Central in his short essay is his idea that even if a person accepts some moral theory, he does not thereby exempt himself from moral responsibility for his actions. Should a person upon reflection decide that, for example, utilitarianism is the correct theory and go on to make decisions and perform actions as such a theory would favor, he still must realize that he is the actor and that he is responsible. After all, he chose the theory, and is free to revise or reject it at any time.

However, some persons who agree with this go on to claim that because morality is a matter of being responsible for our choices, it makes no difference what we choose to do as long as we are sincere. Others point out that we are not fair to ourselves if we replace the search for principles with the idea that being sincere is enough. That is, if we act as we feel, and refuse to reflect upon our actions in light of some principles, then we in effect have surrendered what makes us distinctively persons. If we can be said to be doomed to be responsible for our actions, so it might be said that we are doomed to have principles, for even one who claims not to have any moral principles is in effect adopting a principle—the principle that actions may rightly follow inclination. Once we realize this then we must go on to ask whether that principle is the best one. At this point we are already engaged in thinking seriously about our most basic principles. That is, perhaps in spite of ourselves, we are unavoidably involved in moral philosophy.

The following selections represent some of the most significant attempts to come to grips with the basic issues in this area.

J.O'C.

SOME EXAMPLES OF MAJOR ETHICAL THEORIES

From "Fundamental Principles of the Metaphysics of Morals"

Immanuel Kant

Nothing can possibly be conceived in the world, or even out of it, which can be called good without qualification, except a *good will.* Intelligence, wit, judgment, and the other *talents* of the mind, however they may be named, or courage, resolution, perseverance, as qualities of temperament, are undoubtedly good and desirable in many respects; but these gifts of nature may also become extremely bad and mischievous if the will which is to make use of them, and which, therefore, constitutes what is called *character,* is not good. It is the same with the *gifts of fortune.* Power, riches, honor, even health, and the general well-being and contentment with one's condition which is called *happiness,* inspire pride, and often presumption, if there is not a good will to correct the influence of these on the mind, and with this also

Reprinted, with deletions, from Immanuel Kant, *Fundamental Principles of the Metaphysics of Morals,* in Kant's *Critique of Practical Reason and Other Works on the Theory of Ethics,* 1898, translated by Thomas K. Abbott.

to rectify the whole principle of acting, and adapt it to its end. The sight of a being who is not adorned with a single feature of a pure and good will, enjoying unbroken prosperity, can never give pleasure to an impartial rational spectator. Thus a good will appears to constitute the indispensable condition even of being worthy of happiness.

There are even some qualities which are of service to this good will itself, and may facilitate its action, yet which have no intrinsic unconditional value, but always presuppose a good will, and this qualifies the esteem that we justly have for them, and does not permit us to regard them as absolutely good. Moderation in the affections and passions, self-control, and calm deliberation are not only good in many respects, but even seem to constitute part of the intrinsic worth of the person; but they are far from deserving to be called good without qualification, although they have been so unconditionally praised by the ancients. For without the principles of a good will, they may become extremely bad; and the coolness of a villain not only makes him far more dangerous, but also directly makes him more abominable in our eyes than he would have been without it.

A good will is good not because of what it performs or effects, not by its aptness for the attainment of some proposed end, but simply by virtue of the volition—that is, it is good in itself, and considered by itself is to be esteemed much higher than all that can be brought about by it in favor of any inclination, nay, even of the sum-total of all inclinations. Even if it should happen that, owing to special disfavor of fortune, or the niggardly provision of a step-motherly nature, this will should wholly lack power to accomplish its purpose, if with its greatest efforts it should yet achieve nothing, and there should remain only the good will (not, to be sure, a mere wish, but the summoning of all means in our power), then, like a jewel, it would still shine by its own light, as a thing which has its whole value in itself. Its usefulness or fruitlessness can neither add to nor take away anything from this value. It would be, as it were, only the setting to enable us to handle it the more conveniently in common commerce, or to attract to it the attention of those who are not yet connoisseurs, but not to recommend it to true connoisseurs, or to determine its value.

There is, however, something so strange in this idea of the absolute value of the mere will, in which no account is taken of its utility, that notwithstanding the thorough assent of even common reason to the idea, yet a suspicion must arise that it may perhaps really be the product of mere high-flown fancy, and that we may have misunderstood the purpose of nature in assigning reason as the governor of our will. Therefore we will examine this idea from this point of view.

In the physical constitution of an organized being, that is, a being adapted suitably to the purposes of life, we assume it as a fundamental principle that no organ for any purpose will be found but what is also the fittest and best adapted for that purpose. Now in a being which has reason and a will, if the proper object of nature were its *conservation*, its *welfare*, in a word, its *happiness*, then nature would have hit upon a very bad arrangement in selecting the reason of the creature to carry out this purpose. For all the actions which the creature has to perform with a view to this purpose, and the whole rule of its conduct, would be far more surely prescribed to it by instinct, and that end would have been attained thereby much more certainly than it ever can be by reason. Should reason have been communicated to this favored creature over and above, it must only have served it to contemplate the happy constitution of its nature, to admire it, to congratulate itself thereon, and to feel thankful for it to the beneficent cause, but not that it should subject its desires to that weak and delusive guidance, and meddle bunglingly with the purpose of nature. In a word, nature would have taken care that reason should not break forth into *practical exercise,* nor have the presumption, with its weak insight, to think out for itself the plan of happiness and of the means of attaining it. Nature would not only have taken on herself the choice of the ends but also of the means, and with wise foresight would have entrusted both to instinct.

And, in fact, we find that the more a cultivated reason applies itself with deliberate purpose to the enjoyment of life and happiness, so much the more does the man fail of true satisfaction. And from this circumstance there arises in many, if they are candid enough to confess it, a certain degree of *misology,* that is, hatred of reason, especially in the case of those who are most experienced in the use of it, because after calculating all the advantages they derive—I do not say from the invention of all the arts of common luxury, but even from the sciences (which seem to them to be after all only a luxury of the understanding)—they find that they have, in fact, only brought more trouble on their shoulders rather than gained in happiness; and they end by envying rather than despising the more common stamp of men who keep closer to the guidance of mere instinct, and do not allow their reason much influence on their conduct. And this we must admit, that the judgment of those who would very much lower the lofty eulogies of the advantages which reason gives us in regard to the happiness and satisfaction of life, or who would even reduce them below zero, is by no means morose or ungrateful to the goodness with which the world is governed, but that there lies at the root of these judgments the idea that our existence has a different and far nobler end, for which, and not for happiness, reason is properly intended, and which must, therefore, be regarded as the supreme condition to which the private ends of man must, for the most part, be postponed.

For as reason is not competent to guide the will with certainty in regard to its objects and the satisfaction of all our wants (which it to some extent even multiplies), this being an end to which an implanted instinct would have led with much greater certainty; and since, nevertheless, reason is imparted to us as a practical faculty, that is, as one which is to have influence on the *will,* therefore, admitting that nature generally in the distribution of her capacities has adapted the means to the end, its true destination must be to produce a *will,* not merely good as a *means* to something else, but *good in itself,* for which reason was absolutely necessary. This will then, though not indeed the sole and complete good, must be the supreme good and the condition of every other, even of the desire of happiness. Under these circumstances, there is nothing inconsistent with the wisdom of nature in the fact that the cultivation of the reason, which is requisite for the first and unconditional purpose, does in many ways interfere, at least in this life, with the attainment of the second, which is always conditional—namely, happiness. Nay, it may even reduce it to nothing, without nature thereby failing of her purpose. For reason recognizes the establishment of a good will as its practical destination, and in attaining this purpose is capable only of a satisfaction of its own proper kind, namely, that from the attainment of an end, which end again is determined by reason only, notwithstanding that this may involve many a disappointment to the ends of inclination.

We have then to develop the notion of a will which deserves to be highly esteemed for itself, and is good without a view to anything further, a notion which exists already in the sound natural understanding, requiring rather to be cleared up than to be taught, and which in estimating the value of our actions always takes the first place and constitutes the condition of all the rest. In order to do this, we will take the notion of duty, which includes that of a good will, although implying certain subjective restrictions and hindrances. These, however, far from concealing it or rendering it unrecognizable, rather bring it out by contrast and make it shine forth so much the brighter.

I omit here all actions which are already recognized as inconsistent with duty, although they may be useful for this or that purpose, for with these the question whether they are done *from duty* cannot arise at all, since they even conflict with it. I also set aside those actions which really conform to duty, but to which men have *no* direct *inclination,* performing them because they are impelled thereto by some other inclination. For in this case we can readily distinguish whether the action which agrees with duty is done *from duty* or from a selfish view. It is much harder to make this distinction when the action accords with duty, and the subject has besides a *direct* inclination to it. For example, it is always a matter of duty that a dealer should not overcharge an inexperienced purchaser; and wherever there is much commerce the prudent tradesman does not overcharge, but keeps a fixed price for everyone, so that a child buys of him as well as any other. Men are thus *honestly* served; but this is not enough to make us believe that the tradesman has so acted from duty and from principles of honesty; his own advantage required it; it is out of the question in this case to suppose that he might besides have a direct inclination in favor of the buyers, so that, as it were, from love he should give no advantage to one over another. Accordingly the action was done neither from duty nor from direct inclination, but merely with a selfish view.

On the other hand, it is a duty to maintain one's life; and, in addition, everyone has also a direct inclination to do so. But on this account the often anxious care which most men take for it has no intrinsic worth, and their maxim has no moral import. They preserve their life *as duty requires,* no doubt, but not *because duty requires.* On the other hand, if adversity and hopeless sorrow have completely taken away the relish for life, if the unfortunate one, strong in mind, indignant at his fate rather than desponding or dejected, wishes for death, and yet preserves his life without loving it— not from inclination or fear, but from duty—then his maxim has a moral worth.

To be beneficent when we can is a duty; and besides this, there are many minds so sympathetically constituted that, without any other motive of vanity or self-interest, they find a pleasure in spreading joy around them, and can take delight in the satisfaction of others so far as it is their own work. But I maintain that in such a case an action of this kind, however proper, however amiable it may be, has nevertheless no true moral worth, but is on a level with other inclinations, for example, the inclination to honor, which, if it is happily directed to that which is in fact of public utility and accordant with duty, and consequently honorable, deserves praise and encouragement, but not esteem. For the maxim lacks the moral import, namely, that such actions be done *from duty,* not from inclination. Put the case that the mind of that philanthropist was clouded by sorrow of his own, extinguishing all sympathy with the lot of others, and that while he still has the power to benefit others in distress, he is not touched by their trouble because he is absorbed with his own; and now suppose that he tears himself out of this dead insensibility and performs the action without any inclination to it, but simply from duty, then first has his action its genuine moral worth. Further still, if nature has put little sympathy in the heart of this or that man, if he, supposed to be an upright man, is by temperament cold and indifferent to the sufferings of others, perhaps because in respect of his own he is provided with the special gift of patience and fortitude, and supposes, or even requires, that others should have the same—and such a man would certainly not be the meanest product of nature—but if nature had not specially framed him for a philanthropist, would he not still find in himself a source from whence to give himself a far higher worth than that of a good-natured temperament could be? Unquestionably. It is just in this that the moral worth of the character is brought out which is incomparably the highest of all, namely, that he is beneficent, not from inclination, but from duty.

To secure one's own happiness is a duty, at least indirectly; for discontent with one's condition, under a pressure of many anxieties and amidst unsatisfied wants, might easily become a great *temptation to transgression of duty.* But here again, without looking to duty, all men have already the strongest and most intimate inclination to happiness, because it is just in this idea that all inclinations are combined in one total. But the precept of happiness is often of such a sort that it greatly interferes with some inclinations, and yet a man cannot form any definite and certain conception of the sum of satisfaction of all of them which is called happiness. It is not then to be wondered at that a single inclination, definite both as to what it promises and as to the time within which it can be gratified, is often able to overcome such a fluctuating idea, and that a gouty patient, for instance, can choose to enjoy what he likes, and to suffer what he may, since, according to his calculation, on this occasion at least, he has [only] not sacrificed the enjoyment of the present moment to a possibly mistaken expectation of a happiness which is supposed to be found in health. But even in this case, if the general desire for happiness did not influence his will, and supposing that in his particular case health was not a necessary element in this calculation, there yet remains in this, as in all other cases, this law—namely, that he should promote his happiness not from inclination but from duty, and by this would his conduct first acquire true moral worth.

It is in this manner, undoubtedly, that we are to understand those passages of Scripture also in which we are commanded to love our neighbor, even our enemy. For love, as an affection, cannot be commanded, but beneficence for duty's sake may, even though we are not impelled to it by any inclination—nay, are even repelled by a natural and unconquerable aversion. This is *practical* love, and not *pathological*—a love which is seated in the will, and not in the propensions of sense—in principles of action and not of tender sympathy; and it is this love alone which can be commanded.

The second proposition is: That an action done from duty derives its moral worth, *not from the purpose* which is to be attained by it, but from the maxim by which it is determined, and therefore does not depend on the realization of the object of the action, but merely on the *principle of volition* by which the action has taken place, without regard to any object of desire. It is clear from what precedes that the purposes which we may have in view in our actions, or their effects regarded as ends and springs of the will, cannot give to actions any unconditional or moral worth. In what, then, can their worth lie if it is not to consist in the will and in reference to its expected effect? It cannot lie anywhere but in the *principle of the will* without regard to the ends which can be attained by the action. For the will stands between its *a priori* principle, which is formal, and its *a posteriori* spring, which is material, as between two roads, and as it must be determined by something, it follows that it must be determined by the formal principle of volition when an action is done from duty, in which case every material principle has been withdrawn from it.

The third proposition, which is a consequence of the two preceding, I would express thus: *Duty is the necessity of acting from respect for the law.* I may have *inclination* for an object as the effect of my proposed action, but I cannot have *respect* for it just for this reason that it is an effect and not an energy of will. Similarly, I cannot have respect for inclination, whether my own or another's; I can at most, if my own, approve it; if another's, sometimes even love it, that is, look on it as favorable to my own interest. It is only what is connected with my will as a principle, by no means as an effect —what does not subserve my inclination, but overpowers it, or at least in case of choice excludes it from its calculation—in other words, simply the law of itself, which can be an object of respect, and hence a command. Now an action done from duty must wholly exclude the influence of inclination, and with it every object of the will, so that nothing remains which can determine the will except objectively the *law*, and subjectively *pure respect* for this practical law, and consequently the maxim[1] that I should follow this law even to the thwarting of all my inclinations.

Thus the moral worth of an action does not lie in the effect expected from it, nor in any principle of action which requires to borrow its motive from this expected effect. For all these effects—agreeableness of one's condition, and even the promotion of the happiness of others—could have been also brought about by other causes, so that for this there would have been

---

[1]A *maxim* is the subjective principle of volition. The objective principle (*i.e.*, that which would also serve subjectively as a practical principle to all rational beings if reason had full power over the faculty of desire) is the practical *law*.

no need of the will of a rational being; whereas it is in this alone that the supreme and unconditional good can be found. The preeminent good which we call moral can therefore consist in nothing else than *the conception of law* in itself, *which certainly is only possible in a rational being,* in so far as this conception, and not the expected effect, determines the will. This is a good which is already present in the person who acts accordingly, and we have not to wait for it to appear first in the result.[2]

But what sort of law can that be the conception of which must determine the will, even without paying any regard to the effect expected from it, in order that this will may be called good absolutely and without qualification? As I have deprived the will of every impulse which could arise to it from obedience to any law, there remains nothing but the universal conformity of its actions to law in general, which alone is to serve the will as a principle, that is, I am never to act otherwise than so *that I could also will that my maxim should become a universal law.* Here, now, it is the simple conformity to law in general, without assuming any particular law applicable to certain actions, that serves the will as its principle, and must so serve it if duty is not to be a vain delusion and a chimerical notion. The common reason of men in its practical judgments perfectly coincides with this, and always has in view the principle here suggested. Let the question be, for example: May I when in distress make a promise with the intention not to keep it? I readily distinguish here between the two significations which the question may have: whether it is prudent or whether it is right to make a false promise? The former may undoubtedly often be the case. I see clearly indeed that it is not enough to extricate myself from a present difficulty by means of this subterfuge, but it must be well considered whether there may not hereafter spring from this lie much greater inconvenience than that from which I now free myself, and as, with all my supposed *cunning,* the consequences cannot be so easily foreseen but that credit once lost may be much more injurious to me than any mischief which I seek to avoid at present, it should be considered whether it would not be more *prudent* to act herein according to a

---

[2]It might be here objected to me that I take refuge behind the word *respect* in an obscure feeling, instead of giving a distinct solution of the question by a concept of the reason. But although respect is a feeling, it is not a feeling *received* through influence, but is *self-wrought* by a rational concept, and, therefore, is specifically distinct from all feelings of the former kind, which may be referred either to inclination·or fear. What I recognize immediately as a law for me, I recognize with respect. This merely signifies the consciousness that my will is *subordinate* to a law, without the intervention of other influences on my sense. The immediate determination of the will by the law, and the consciousness of this, is called *respect,* so that this is regarded as an *effect* of the law on the subject, and not as the *cause* of it. Respect is properly the conception of a worth which thwarts my self-love. Accordingly it is something which is considered neither as an object of inclination nor of fear, although it has something analogous to both. The *object* of respect is the *law* only, that is, the law which we impose on *ourselves,* and yet recognize as necessary in itself. As a law, we are subjected to it without consulting self-love; as imposed by us on ourselves, it is a result of our will. In the former aspect it has an analogy to fear, in the latter to inclination. Respect for a person is properly only respect for the law (of honesty, etc.) of which he gives us an example. Since we also look on the improvement of our talents as a duty, we consider that we see in a person of talents, as it were, the *example of a law* (viz, to become like him in this by exercise), and this constitutes our respect. All so-called moral *interest* consists simply in *respect* for the law.

universal maxim, and to make it a habit to promise nothing except with the intention of keeping it. But it is soon clear to me that such a maxim will still only be based on the fear of consequences. Now it is a wholly different thing to be truthful from duty, and to be so from apprehension of injurious consequences. In the first case, the very notion of the action already implies a law for me; in the second case, I must first look about elsewhere to see what results may be combined with it which would affect myself. For to deviate from the principle of duty is beyond all doubt wicked; but to be unfaithful to my maxim of prudence may often be very advantageous to me, although to abide by it is certainly safe. The shortest way, however, and an unerring one, to discover the answer to this question whether a lying promise is consistent with duty, is to ask myself, Should I be content that my maxim (to extricate myself from difficulty by a false promise) should hold good as a universal law, for myself as well as for others; and should I be able to say to myself, "Every one may make a deceitful promise when he finds himself in a difficulty from which he cannot otherwise extricate himself"? Then I presently become aware that, while I can will the lie, I can by no means will that lying should be a universal law. For with such a law there would be no promises at all, since it would be in vain to allege my intention in regard to my future actions to those who would not believe this allegation, or if they over-hastily did so, would pay me back in my own coin. Hence my maxim, as soon as it should be made a universal law, would necessarily destroy itself.

I do not, therefore, need any far-reaching penetration to discern what I have to do in order that my will may be morally good. Inexperienced in the course of the world, incapable of being prepared for all its contingencies, I only ask myself: Canst thou also will that thy maxim should be a universal law? If not, then it must be rejected, and that not because of a disadvantage accruing from it to myself or even to others, but because it cannot enter as a principle into a possible universal legislation, and reason extorts from me immediate respect for such legislation. I do not indeed as yet *discern* on what this respect is based (this the philosopher may inquire), but at least I understand this—that it is an estimation of the worth which far outweighs all worth of what is recommended by inclination, and that the necessity of acting from *pure* respect for the practical law is what constitutes duty, to which every other motive must give place because it is the condition of a will being good *in itself,* and the worth of such a will is above everything.

Thus, then, without quitting the moral knowledge of common human reason, we have arrived at its principle. And although, no doubt, common men do not conceive it in such an abstract and universal form, yet they always have it really before their eyes and use it as the standard of their decision. Here it would be easy to show how, with this compass in hand, men are well able to distinguish, in every case that occurs, what is good, what bad, conformably to duty or inconsistent with it, if, without in the least teaching them anything new, we only, like Socrates, direct their attention to the principle they themselves employ; and that, therefore, we do not need science and philosophy to know what we should do to be honest and good, yea, even wise and virtuous. Indeed we might well have conjectured beforehand that the knowledge of what every man is bound to do, and therefore also to know, would be within the reach of every man, even the commonest. Here we cannot forbear admiration when we see how great an advantage the practical judgment has over the theoretical in the common understanding of men. In the latter, if common reason ventures to depart from the laws of experience and from the perceptions of the senses, it falls into mere inconceivabilities and self-contraditions, at least into a chaos of uncertainty, obscurity, and instability. But in the practical sphere it is just when the common understanding excludes all sensible springs from practical laws that its power of judgment begins to show itself to advantage. It then becomes even subtle, whether it be that it chicanes with its own conscience or with other claims respecting what is to be called right, or whether it desires for its own instruction to determine honestly the worth of actions; and, in the latter case, it may even have as good a hope of hitting the mark as any philosopher whatever can promise himself. Nay, it is almost more sure of doing so, because the philosopher cannot have any other principle, while he may easily perplex his judgment by a multitude of considerations foreign to the matter, and so turn aside from the right way. Would it not therefore be wiser in moral concerns to acquiesce in the judgment of common reason, or at most only to call in philosophy for the purpose of rendering the system of morals more complete and intelligible, and its rules more convenient for use (especially for disputation), but not so as to draw off the common understanding from its happy simplicity, or to bring it by means of philosophy into a new path of inquiry and instruction?

Innocence is indeed a glorious thing; only, on the other hand, it is very sad that it cannot well maintain itself, and is easily seduced. On this account even wisdom—which otherwise consists more in conduct than in knowledge —yet has need of science, not in order to learn from it, but to secure for its precepts admission and permanence. Against all the commands of duty which reason represents to man as so deserving of respect, he feels in himself a powerful counterpoise in his wants and inclinations, the entire satisfaction of which he sums up under the name of happiness. Now reason issues its commands unyieldingly, without promising anything to the inclinations, and, as it were, with disregard and contempt for these claims, which are so impetuous and at the same time so plausible, and which will not allow themselves to be suppressed by any command. Hence there arises a natural *dialectic,* that is, a disposition to argue against these strict laws of duty and to question their validity, or at least their purity and strictness; and, if possible, to make them more accordant with our wishes and inclinations, that is to say, to corrupt them at their very source and entirely to destroy their worth—a thing which even common practical reason cannot ultimately call good. . . .

Everything in nature works according to laws. Rational beings alone have the faculty of acting according *to the conception* of laws—that is, according to principles, that is, have a *will.* Since the deduction of actions from principles requires *reason,* the will is nothing but practical reason. If reason infallibly determines the will, then the actions of such a being which are recognized as objectively necessary are subjectively necessary also, that is, the will is a faculty to choose *that only* which reason independent of inclination recognizes as practically necessary, that is, as good. But if reason of itself does not sufficiently determine the will, if the latter is subject also to subjective conditions (particular impulses) which do not always coincide with the objective conditions, in a word, if the will does not *in itself* completely accord with reason (which is actually the case with men), then the actions which objectively are recognized as necessary are subjectively contingent, and the determination of such a will according to objective laws is *obligation,* that is to say, the relation of the objective laws to a will that is not thoroughly good is conceived as the determination of the will of a rational being by principles of reason, but which the will from its nature does not of necessity follow.

The conception of an objective principle, in so far as it is obligatory for a will, is called a command (of reason), and the formula of the command is called an Imperative.

All imperatives are expressed by the word *ought* [or *shall*], and thereby indicate the relation of an objective law of reason to a will which from its subjective constitution is not necessarily determined by it (an obligation). They say that something would be good to do or to forbear, but they say it to a will which does not always do a thing because it is conceived to be good to do it. That is practically *good,* however, which determines the will by means of the conceptions of reason, and consequently not from subjective causes, but objectively, that is, on principles which are valid for every rational being as such. It is distinguished from the *pleasant* as that which influences the will only by means of sensation from merely subjective causes, valid only for the sense of this or that one, and not as a principle of reason which holds for every one.[3]

A perfectly good will would therefore be equally subject to objective laws (viz., laws of good), but could not be conceived as *obliged* thereby to act lawfully, because of itself from its subjective constitution it can only be determined by the conception of good. Therefore no imperatives hold for the Divine will, or in general for a *holy* will; *ought* is here out of place because the volition is already of itself necessarily in unison with the law. Therefore imperatives are only formulae to express the relation of objective laws of all volition to the subjective imperfection of the will of this or that rational being, for example, the human will.

---

[3]The dependence of the desires on sensations is called inclination, and this accordingly always indicates a *want.* The dependence of a contingently determinable will on principles of reason is called an *interest.* This, therefore, is found only in the case of a dependent will which does not always of itself conform to reason; in the Divine will we cannot conceive any interest. But the human will can also *take an interest* in a thing without therefore acting *from interest.* The former signifies the *practical* interest in the action, the latter the *pathological* in the object of the action. The former indicates only dependence of the will on principles of reason in themselves; the second, dependence on principles of reason for the sake of inclination, reason supplying only the practical rules how the requirement of the inclination may be satisfied. In the first case the action interests me; in the second the object of the action (because it is pleasant to me). We have seen in the first section that in an action done from duty we must look not to the interest in the object, but only to that in the action itself, and in its rational principle (viz., the law).

Now all *imperatives* command either *hypothetically* or *categorically*. The former represent the practical necessity of a possible action as means to something else that is willed (or at least which one might possibly will). The categorical imperative would be that which represented an action as necessary of itself without reference to another end, that is, as objectively necessary.

Since every practical law represents a possible action as good, and on this account, for a subject who is practically determinable by reason as necessary, all imperatives are formulae determining an action which is necessary according to the principle of a will good in some respects. If now the action is good only as a means *to something else*, then the imperative is *hypothetical;* if it is conceived of as good *in itself* and consequently as being necessarily the principle of a will which of itself conforms to reason, then it is *categorical.*

Thus the imperative declares what action possible by me would be good, and presents the practical rule in relation to a will which does not forthwith perform an action simply because it is good, whether because the subject does not always know that it is good, or because, even if it knows this, yet its maxims might be opposed to the objective principle of practical reason.

Accordingly the hypothetical imperative only says that the action is good for some purpose, *possible* or *actual.* In the first case it is a *problematical,* in the second an *assertorial* practical principle. The categorical imperative which declares an action to be objectively necessary in itself without reference to any purpose, that is, without any other end, is valid as an *apodictic* (practical) principle.

Whatever is possible only by the power of some rational being may also be conceived as a possible purpose of some will; and therefore the principles of action as regards the means necessary to attain some possible purpose are in fact infinitely numerous. All sciences have a practical part consisting of problems expressing that some end is possible for us, and of imperatives directing how it may be attained. These may, therefore, be called in general imperatives of *skill.* Here there is no question whether the end is rational and good, but only what one must do in order to attain it. The precepts for the physician to make his patient thoroughly healthy, and for a poisoner to ensure certain death, are of equal value in this respect, that each serves to effect its purpose perfectly. Since in early youth it cannot be known what ends are likely to occur to us in the course of life, parents seek to have their children taught a *great many things,* and provide for their *skill* in the use of means for all sorts of arbitrary ends, of none of which can they determine whether it may not perhaps hereafter be an object to their pupil, but which it is at all events *possible* that he might aim at; and this anxiety is so great that they commonly neglect to form and correct their judgment on the value of the things which may be chosen as ends.

There is *one* end, however, which may be assumed to be actually such to all rational beings (so far as imperatives apply to them, viz., as dependent beings), and, therefore, one purpose which they not merely *may* have, but which we may with certainty assume that they all actually *have* by a natural necessity, and this is *happiness*. The hypothetical imperative which expresses the practical necessity of an action as means to the advancement of happiness is *assertorial*. We are not to present it as necessary for an uncertain and merely possible purpose, but for a purpose which we may presuppose with certainty and *a priori* in every man, because it belongs to his being. Now skill in the choice of means to his own greatest well-being may be called *prudence*, [4] in the narrowest sense. And thus the imperative which refers to the choice of means to one's own happiness, that is, the precept of prudence, is still always *hypothetical;* the action is not commanded absolutely, but only a means to another purpose.

Finally, there is an imperative which commands a certain conduct immediately, without having as its condition any other purpose to be attained by it. This imperative is *categorical*. It concerns not the matter of the action, or its intended result, but its form and the principle of which it is itself a result; and what is essentially good in it consists in the mental disposition, let the consequence be what it may. This imperative may be called that of *morality*.

There is a marked distinction also between the volitions on these three sorts of principles in the *dissimilarity* of the obligation of the will. In order to mark this difference more clearly, I think they would be most suitably named in their order if we said they are either *rules* of skill, or *counsels* of prudence, or *commands* (*laws*) of morality. For it is *law* only that involves the conception of an *unconditional* and objective necessity, which is consequently universally valid; and commands are laws which must be obeyed, that is, must be followed, even in opposition to inclination. *Counsels*, indeed, involve necessity but one which can only hold under a contingent subjective condition, viz., they depend on whether this or that man reckons this or that as part of his happiness; the categorical imperative, on the contrary, is not limited by any condition, and as being absolutely, although practically, necessary may be quite properly called a command. We might also call the first kind of imperatives *technical* (belonging to art), the second *pragmatic*[5] (belonging to welfare), the third *moral* (belonging to free conduct generally, that is, to morals). . . .

When I conceive a hypothetical imperative, in general I do not know beforehand what it will contain until I am given the condition. But when I conceive a categorical imperative, I know at once what it contains. For as the

---

[4]The word *prudence* is taken in two senses: in the one it may bear the name of knowledge of the world, in the other that of private prudence. The former is a man's ability to influence others so as to use them for his own purposes. The latter is the sagacity to combine all these purposes for his own lasting benefit. This latter is properly that to which the value even of the former is reduced, and when a man is prudent in the former sense, but not in the latter, we might better say of him that he is clever and cunning, but, on the whole, imprudent.

[5]It seems to me that the proper signification of the word *pragmatic* may be most accurately defined in this way. For *sanctions* are called pragmatic which flow properly, not from the law of the states as necessary enactments, but from *precaution* for the general welfare. A history is composed pragmatically when it teaches *prudence*, that is, instructs the world how it can provide for its interests better, or at least as well as the men of former time.

imperative contains besides the law only the necessity that the maxims[6] shall conform to this law, while the law contains no conditions restricting it, there remains nothing but the general statement that the maxim of the action should conform to a universal law, and it is this conformity alone that the imperative properly represents as necessary.

There is therefore but one categorical imperative, namely, this: *Act only on that maxim whereby thou canst at the same time will that it should become a universal law.*

Now if all imperatives of duty can be deduced from this one imperative as from their principle, then, although it should remain undecided whether what is called duty is not merely a vain notion, yet at least we shall be able to show what we understand by it and what this notion means.

Since the universality of the law according to which effects are produced constitutes what is properly called *nature* in the most general sense (as to form)—that is, the existence of things so far as it is determined by general laws—the imperative of duty may be expressed thus: *Act as if the maxim of thy action were to become by thy will a universal law of nature.*

We will now enumerate a few duties, adopting the usual division of them into duties to ourselves and to others, and into perfect and imperfect duties.[7]

1.   A man reduced to despair by a series of misfortunes feels wearied of life, but is still so far in possession of his reason that he can ask himself whether it would not be contrary to his duty to himself to take his own life. Now he inquires whether the maxim of his action could become a universal law of nature. His maxim is: From self-love I adopt it as a principle to shorten my life when its longer duration is likely to bring more evil than satisfaction. It is asked then simply whether this principle founded on self-love can become a universal law of nature. Now we see at once that a system of nature of which it should be a law to destroy life by means of the very feeling whose special nature it is to impel to the improvement of life would contradict itself, and therefore could not exist as a system of nature; hence that maxim cannot possibly exist as a universal law of nature, and consequently would be wholly inconsistent with the supreme principle of all duty.

2.   Another finds himself forced by necessity to borrow money. He knows that he will not be able to repay it, but sees also that nothing will be lent to

---

[6]A "maxim" is a subjective principle of action, and must be distinguished from the *objective principle*, namely, practical law. The former contains the practical rule set by reason according to the conditions of the subject (often its ignorance or its inclinations), so that it is the principle on which the subject *acts;* but the law is the objective principle valid for every rational being, and is the principle on which it *ought to act*—that is an imperative.

[7]It must be noted here that I reserve the division of duties for a future *metaphysic of morals;* so that I give it here only as an arbitrary one (in order to arrange my examples). For the rest, I understand by a perfect duty one that admits no exception in favor of inclination, and then I have not merely external but also internal perfect duties. This is contrary to the use of the word adopted in the schools; but I do not intend to justify it here, as it is all one for my purpose whether it is admitted or not. [*Perfect* duties are usually understood to be those which can be enforced by external law; *imperfect*, those which cannot be enforced. They are also called respectively *determinate* and *indeterminate, officia juris* and *officia virtutis.*]

him unless he promises stoutly to repay it in a definite time. He desires to make this promise, but he has still so much conscience as to ask himself: Is it not unlawful and inconsistent with duty to get out of a difficulty in this way? Suppose, however, that he resolves to do so, then the maxim of his action would be expressed thus: When I think myself in want of money, I will borrow money and promise to repay it, although I know that I never can do so. Now this principle of self-love or of one's own advantage may perhaps be consistent with my whole future welfare; but the question now is, Is it right? I change then the suggestion of self-love into a universal law, and state the question thus: How would it be if my maxim were a universal law? Then I see at once that it could never hold as a universal law of nature, but would necessarily contradict itself. For supposing it to be a universal law that everyone when he thinks himself in a difficulty should be able to promise whatever he pleases, with the purpose of not keeping his promise, the promise itself would become impossible, as well as the end that one might have in view in it, since no one would consider that anything was promised to him, but would ridicule all such statements as vain pretenses.

3.   A third finds in himself a talent which with the help of some culture might make him a useful man in many respects. But he finds himself in comfortable circumstances and prefers to indulge in pleasure rather than to take pains in enlarging and improving his happy natural capacities. He asks, however, whether his maxim of neglect of his natural gifts, besides agreeing with his inclination to indulge, agrees also with what is called duty. He sees then that a system of nature could indeed subsist with such a universal law, although men (like the South Sea islanders) should let their talents rest and resolve to devote their lives merely to idleness, amusement, and propagation of their species—in a word, to enjoyment; but he cannot possibly *will* that this should be a universal law of nature, or be implanted in us as such by a natural instinct. For, as a rational being, he necessarily wills that his faculties be developed, since they serve him, and have been given him, for all sorts of possible purposes.

4.   A fourth, who is in prosperity, while he sees that others have to contend with great wretchedness and that he could help them, thinks: What concern is it of mine? Let everyone be as happy as Heaven pleases, or as he can make himself; I will take nothing from him nor even envy him, only I do not wish to contribute anything to his welfare or to his assistance in distress! Now no doubt, if such a mode of thinking were a universal law, the human race might very well subsist, and doubtless even better than in a state in which everyone talks of sympathy and good-will, or even takes care occasionally to put it into practice, but, on the other side, also cheats when he can, betrays the rights of men, or otherwise violates them. But although it is possible that a universal law of nature might exist in accordance with that maxim, it is impossible to *will* that such a principle should have the universal validity of a law of nature. For a will which resolved this would contradict itself, inasmuch as many cases might occur in which one would have need of the love and sympathy of others, and in which, by such a law of nature, sprung from his own will, he would deprive himself of all hope of the aid he desires.

These are a few of the many actual duties, or at least what we regard as such, which obviously fall into two classes on the one principle that we have laid down. We must be *able to will* that a maxim of our action should be a universal law. This is the canon of the moral appreciation of the action generally. Some actions are of such a character that their maxim cannot without contradiction be even *conceived* as a universal law of nature, far from it being possible that we should *will* that it *should* be so. In others, this intrinsic impossibility is not found, but still it is impossible to *will* that their maxim should be raised to the universality of a law of nature, since such a will would contradict itself. It is easily seen that the former violate strict or rigorous (inflexible) duty; the latter only laxer (meritorious) duty. Thus it has been completely shown by these examples how all duties depend as regards the nature of the obligation (not the object of the action) on the same principle.

If now we attend to ourselves on occasion of any transgression of duty, we shall find that we in fact do not will that our maxim should be a universal law, for that is impossible for us; on the contrary, we will that the opposite should remain a universal law, only we assume the liberty of making an *exception* in our own favor or (just for this time only) in favor of our inclination. Consequently, if we considered all cases from one and the same point of view, namely, that of reason, we should find a contradiction in our own will, namely, that a certain principle should be objectively necessary as a universal law, and yet subjectively should not be universal, but admit of exceptions. As, however, we at one moment regard our action from the point of view of a will wholly conformed to reason, and then again look at the same action from the point of view of a will affected by inclination, there is not really any contradiction, but an antagonism of inclination to the precept of reason, whereby the universality of the principle is changed into a mere generality, so that the practical principle of reason shall meet the maxim half way. Now, although this cannot be justified in our own impartial judgment, yet it proves that we do really recognize the validity of the categorical imperative and (with all respect for it) only allow ourselves a few exceptions which we think unimportant and forced from us.

We have thus established at least this much—that if duty is a conception which is to have any import and real legislative authority for our actions, it can only be expressed in categorical, and not at all in hypothetical, imperatives. We have also, which is of great importance, exhibited clearly and definitely for every practical application the content of the categorical imperative, which must contain the principle of all duty if there is such a thing at all. We have not yet, however, advanced so far as to prove *a priori* that there actually is such an imperative, that there is a practical law which commands absolutely of itself and without any other impulse, and that the following of this law is duty.

With the view of attaining to this it is of extreme importance to remember that we must not allow ourselves to think of deducing the reality of this principle from the *particular attributes of human nature.* For duty is to be a practical, unconditional necessity of action; it must therefore hold for all rational beings (to whom an imperative can apply at all), and for *this reason only* be also a law for all human wills. On the contrary, whatever is deduced from the particular natural characteristics of humanity, from certain feelings and propensions, nay, even, if possible, from any particular tendency proper to human reason, and which need not necessarily hold for the will of every rational being—this may indeed supply us with a maxim but not with a law; with a subjective principle on which we may have a propension and inclination to act, but not with an objective principle on which we should be *enjoined* to act, even though all our propensions, inclinations, and natural dispositions were opposed to it. In fact, the sublimity and intrinsic dignity of the command in duty are so much the more evident, the less the subjective impulses favor it and the more they oppose it, without being able in the slightest degree to weaken the obligation of the law or to diminish its validity.

Here then we see philosophy brought to a critical position, since it has to be firmly fixed, notwithstanding that it has nothing to support it in heaven or earth. Here it must show its purity as absolute director of its own laws, not the herald of those which are whispered to it by an implanted sense or who knows what tutelary nature. Although these may be better than nothing, yet they can never afford principles dictated by reason, which must have their source wholly *a priori* and thence their commanding authority, expecting everything from the supremacy of the law and the due respect for it, nothing from inclination, or else condemning the man to self-contempt and inward abhorrence.

Thus every empirical element is not only quite incapable of being an aid to the principle of morality, but is even highly prejudicial to the purity of morals; for the proper and inestimable worth of an absolutely good will consists just in this that the principle of action is free from all influence of contingent grounds, which alone experience can furnish. We cannot too much or too often repeat our warning against this lax and even mean habit of thought which seeks for its principle among empirical motives and laws; for human reason in its weariness is glad to rest on this pillow, and in a dream of sweet illusions (in which, instead of Juno, it embraces a cloud) it substitutes for morality a bastard patched up from limbs of various derivation, which looks like anything one chooses to see in it; only not like virtue to one who has once beheld her in her true form.

The question then is this: Is it a necessary law *for all rational beings* that they should always judge of their actions by maxims of which they can themselves will that they should serve as universal laws? If it is so, then it must be connected (altogether *a priori*) with the very conception of the will of a rational being generally. But in order to discover this connection we must, however reluctantly, take a step into metaphysic, although into a domain of it which is distinct from speculative philosophy—namely, the metaphysic of morals. In a practical philosophy, where it is not the reasons of what *happens* that we have to ascertain, but the laws of what *ought to happen*, even although it never does, that is, objective practical laws, there it is not necessary to inquire into the reasons why anything pleases or displeases, how the pleasure of mere sensation differs from taste, and whether the latter is distinct from a general satisfaction of reason; on what the feeling of pleasure or pain rests, and how from it desires and inclinations arise, and from these again maxims by the cooperation of reason; for all this belongs to an empirical psychology, which would constitute the second part of physics, if we regard physics as the *philosophy* of nature, so far as it is based on *empirical laws.* But here we are concerned with objective practical laws, and consequently with the relation of the will to itself so far as it is determined by reason alone, in which case whatever has reference to anything empirical is necessarily excluded; since if *reason of itself alone* determines the conduct (and it is the possibility of this that we are now investigating), it must necessarily do so *a priori.*

The will is conceived as a faculty of determining oneself to action *in accordance with the conception of certain laws.* And such a faculty can be found only in rational beings. Now that which serves the will as the objective ground of its self-determination is the *end,* and if this is assigned by reason alone, it must hold for all rational beings. On the other hand, that which merely contains the ground of possibility of the action of which the effect is the end, this is called the *means.* The subjective ground of the desire is the *spring,* the objective ground of the volition is the *motive;* hence the distinction between subjective ends which rest on springs, and objective ends which depend on motives valid for every rational being. Practical principles are *formal* when they abstract from all subjective ends; they are *material* when they assume these, and therefore particular, springs of action. The ends which a rational being proposes to himself at pleasure as *effects* of his actions (material ends) are all only relative, for it is only their relation to the particular desires of the subject that gives them their worth, which therefore cannot furnish principles universal and necessary for all rational beings and for every volition, that is to say, practical laws. Hence all these relative ends can give rise only to hypothetical imperatives.

Supposing, however, that there were something *whose existence* has *in itself* an absolute worth, something which, being *an end in itself,* could be a source of definite laws, then in this and this alone would lie the source of a possible categorical imperative, that is, a practical law.

Now I say: man and generally any rational being *exists* as an end in himself, *not merely as a means* to be arbitrarily used by this or that will, but in all his actions, whether they concern himself or other rational beings, must be always regarded at the same time as an end. All objects of the inclinations have only a conditional worth; for if the inclinations and the wants founded on them did not exist, then their object would be without value. But the inclinations themselves, being sources of want, are so far from having an absolute worth for which they should be desired that, on the contrary, it must be the universal wish of every rational being to be wholly free from them. Thus the worth of any object which is *to be acquired* by our action is always conditional. Beings whose existence depends not on our will but on nature's, have nevertheless, if they are rational beings, only a relative value as means, and are therefore called *things;* rational beings, on the contrary, are called *persons,* because their very nature points them out as ends in themselves, that is, as something which must not be used merely as means, and so far therefore restricts freedom of action (and is an object of respect). These, therefore, are not merely subjective ends whose existence has a worth *for us* as an effect of our action, but *objective ends,* that is, things whose existence is an end in itself—an end, moreover, for which no other can be substituted, which they should subserve *merely* as means, for otherwise nothing whatever would possess *absolute worth;* but if all worth were conditioned and therefore contingent, then there would be no supreme practical principle of reason whatever.

If then there is a supreme practical principle or, in respect of the human will, a categorical imperative, it must be one which, being drawn from the conception of that which is necessarily an end for everyone because it is *an end in itself,* constitutes an *objective* principle of will, and can therefore serve as a universal practical law. The foundation of this principle is: *rational nature exists as an end in itself.* Man necessarily conceives his own existence as being so; so far then this is a *subjective* principle of human actions. But every other rational being regards its existence similarly, just on the same rational principle that holds for me; so that it is at the same time an objective principle from which as a supreme practical law all laws of the will must be capable of being deduced. Accordingly the practical imperative will be as follows: *So act as to treat humanity, whether in thine own person or in that of any other, in every case as an end withal, never as means only.* We will now inquire whether this can be practically carried out.

To abide by the previous examples:

First, under the head of necessary duty to oneself: He who contemplates suicide should ask himself whether his action can be consistent with the idea of humanity *as an end in itself.* If he destroys himself in order to escape from painful circumstances, he uses a person merely as *a mean* to maintain a tolerable condition up to the end of life. But a man is not a thing, that is to say, something which can be used merely as means, but must in all his actions be always considered as an end in himself. I cannot, therefore, dispose in any way of a man in my own person so as to mutilate him, to damage or kill him. (It belongs to ethics proper to define this principle more precisely, so as to avoid all misunderstanding, for example, as to the amputation of the limbs in order to preserve myself; as to exposing my life to danger with a view to preserve it, etc. This question is therefore omitted here.)

Secondly, as regards necessary duties, or those of strict obligation, towards others: He who is thinking of making a lying promise to others will see at once that he would be using another man *merely as a mean,* without the latter containing at the same time the end in himself. For he whom I propose by such a promise to use for my own purposes cannot possibly assent to my mode of acting towards him, and therefore cannot himself contain the end of this action. This violation of the principle of humanity in other men is more obvious if we take in examples of attacks on the freedom and property of others. For then it is clear that he who transgresses the rights of men intends to use the person of others merely as means, without considering that as rational beings they ought always to be esteemed also as ends, that is, as beings who must be capable of containing in themselves the end of the very same action.

Thirdly, as regards contingent (meritorious) duties to oneself: It is not enough that the action does not violate humanity in our own person as an end in itself, it must also *harmonize with it.* Now there are in humanity capacities of greater perfection which belong to the end that nature has in view in regard to humanity in ourselves as the subject; to neglect these might perhaps be consistent with the *maintenance* of humanity as an end in itself, but not with the *advancement* of this end.

Fourthly, as regards meritorious duties towards others: The natural end which all men have is their own happiness. Now humanity might indeed subsist although no one should contribute anything to the happiness of others, provided he did not intentionally withdraw anything from it; but after all, this would only harmonize negatively, not positively, with *humanity as an end in itself,* if everyone does not also endeavor, as far as in him lies, to forward the ends of others. For the ends of any subject which is an end in himself ought as far as possible to be *my* ends also, if that conception is to have its *full* effect with me.

From *Utilitarianism*

John Stuart Mill

There are few circumstances among those which make up the present condition of human knowledge more unlike what might have been expected, or more significant of the backward state in which speculation on the most important subjects still lingers, than the little progress which has been made in the decision of the controversy regarding the criterion of right and wrong. From the dawn of philosophy, the question concerning the *summum bonum,* or, what is the same thing, concerning the foundation of morality, has been accounted the main problem in speculative thought, has occupied the most gifted intellects and divided them into sects and schools carrying on a vigorous warfare against one another. And after more than two thousand years the same discussions continue, philosophers are still ranged under the same contending banners, and neither thinkers nor mankind at large seem nearer to being unanimous on the subject than when the youth Socrates listened to the old Protagoras and asserted (if Plato's dialogue be grounded on a real conversation) the theory of utilitarianism against the popular morality of the so-called sophist.

It is true that similar confusion and uncertainty and, in some cases, similar discordance exist respecting the first principles of all the sciences, not excepting that which is deemed the most certain of them—mathematics, without much impairing, generally indeed without impairing at all, the trustworthiness of the conclusions of those sciences. An apparent anomaly, the explanation of which is that the detailed doctrines of a science are not usually deduced from, nor depend for their evidence upon, what are called

Reprinted, with deletions from text but without editors' note as it appears in *Introductory Philosophy,* edited by F. A. Tillman, B. Berofsky, and J. O'Connor (New York: Harper & Row, 1971), pp. 323–38.

its first principles. Were it not so, there would be no science more precarious, or whose conclusions were more insufficiently made out, than algebra, which derives none of its certainty from what are commonly taught to learners as its elements, since these, as laid down by some of its most eminent teachers, are as full of fictions as English law, and of mysteries as theology. The truths which are ultimately accepted as the first principles of a science are really the last results of metaphysical analysis practiced on the elementary notions with which the science is conversant; and their relation to the science is not that of foundations to an edifice, but of roots to a tree, which may perform their office equally well though they be never dug down to and exposed to light. But though in science the particular truths precede the general theory, the contrary might be expected to be the case with a practical art, such as morals or legislation. All action is for the sake of some end, and rules of action, it seems natural to suppose, must take their whole character and color from the end to which they are subservient. When we engage in a pursuit, a clear and precise conception of what we are pursuing would seem to be the first thing we need, instead of the last we are to look forward to. A test of right and wrong must be the means, one would think, of ascertaining what is right or wrong, and not a consequence of having already ascertained it.

The difficulty is not avoided by having recourse to the popular theory of a natural faculty, a sense or instinct, informing us of right and wrong. For— besides that the existence of such a moral instinct is itself one of the matters in dispute—those believers in it who have any pretensions to philosophy have been obliged to abandon the idea that it discerns what is right or wrong in the particular case in hand, as our other senses discern the sight or sound actually present. Our moral faculty, according to all those of its interpreters who are entitled to the name of thinkers, supplies us only with the general principles of moral judgments; it is a branch of our reason, not of our sensitive faculty; and must be looked to for the abstract doctrines of morality, not for perception of it in the concrete. The intuitive, no less than what may be termed the inductive, school of ethics insists on the necessity of general laws. They both agree that the morality of an individual action is not a question of direct perception, but of the application of a law to an individual case. They recognize also, to a great extent, the same moral laws, but differ as to their evidence and the source from which they derive their authority. According to the one opinion, the principles of morals are evident *a priori*, requiring nothing to command assent except that the meaning of the terms be understood. According to the other doctrine, right and wrong, as well as truth and falsehood, are questions of observation and experience. But both hold equally that morality must be deduced from principles; and the intuitive school affirm as strongly as the inductive that there is a science of morals. Yet they seldom attempt to make out a list of the *a priori* principles which are to serve as the premises of the science; still more rarely do they make any effort to reduce those various principles to one first principle or common ground of obligation. They either assume the ordinary precepts of morals as of *a priori* authority, or they lay down as the common groundwork of those maxims some generality much less obviously authoritative than the maxims themselves, and which has never succeeded in gaining popular acceptance. Yet to support their pretensions there ought either to be some one fundamental principle or law at the root of all morality, or, if there be several, there should be a determinate order of precedence among them; and the one principle, or the rule for deciding between the various principles when they conflict, ought to be self-evident.

To inquire how far the bad effects of this deficiency have been mitigated in practice, or to what extent the moral beliefs of mankind have been vitiated or made uncertain by the absence of any distinct recognition of an ultimate standard, would imply a complete survey and criticism of past and present ethical doctrine. It would, however, be easy to show that whatever steadiness or consistency these moral beliefs have attained has been mainly due to the tacit influence of a standard not recognized. Although the nonexistence of an acknowledged first principle has made ethics not so much a guide as a consecration of men's actual sentiments, still, as men's sentiments, both of favor and of aversion, are greatly influenced by what they suppose to be the effects of things upon their happiness, the principle of utility, or, as Bentham latterly called it, the greatest happiness principle, has had a large share in forming the moral doctrines even of those who most scornfully reject its authority. Nor is there any school of thought which refuses to admit that the influence of actions on happiness is a most material and even predominant consideration in many of the details of morals, however unwilling to acknowledge it as the fundamental principle of morality and the source of moral obligation. I might go much further and say that to all those *a priori* moralists who deem it necessary to argue at all, utilitarian arguments are indispensable. It is not my present purpose to criticize these thinkers; but I cannot help referring, for illustration, to a systematic treatise by one of the most illustrious of them, the *Metaphysics of Ethics* by Kant. This remarkable man, whose system of thought will long remain one of the landmarks in the history of philosophical speculation, does, in the treatise in question, lay down a universal first principle as the origin and ground of moral obligation; it is this: "So act that the rule on which thou actest would admit of being adopted as a law by all rational beings." But when he begins to deduce from this precept any of the actual duties of morality, he fails, almost grotesquely, to show that there would be any contradiction, any logical (not to say physical) impossibility, in the adoption by all rational beings of the most outrageously immoral rules of conduct. All he shows is that the *consequences* of their universal adoption would be such as no one would choose to incur.

On the present occasion, I shall, without further discussion of the other theories, attempt to contribute something towards the understanding and appreciation of the "utilitarian" or "happiness" theory, and towards such proof as it is susceptible of. It is evident that this cannot be proof in the ordinary and popular meaning of the term. Questions of ultimate ends are not amenable to direct proof. Whatever can be proved to be good must be so by being shown to be a means to something admitted to be good without proof. The medical art is proved to be good by its conducing to health; but how is it possible to prove that health is good? The art of music is good, for the reason, among others, that it produces pleasure; but what proof is it possible to give that pleasure is good? If, then, it is asserted that there is a comprehensive formula, including all things which are in themselves good, and that whatever else is good is not so as an end but as a means, the formula may be accepted or rejected, but is not a subject of what is commonly understood by proof. We are not, however, to infer that its acceptance or rejection must depend on blind impulse, or arbitrary choice. There is a larger meaning of the word "proof," in which this question is as amenable to it as any other of the disputed questions of philosophy. The subject is within the cognizance of the rational faculty; and neither does that faculty deal with it solely in the way of intuition. Considerations may be presented capable of determining the intellect either to give or withhold its assent to the doctrine; and this is equivalent to proof. . . .

The creed which accepts as the foundation of morals "utility" or the "greatest happiness principle" holds that actions are right in proportion as they tend to promote happiness; wrong as they tend to produce the reverse of happiness. By happiness is intended pleasure and the absence of pain; by unhappiness, pain and the privation of pleasure. To give a clear view of the moral standard set up by the theory, much more requires to be said; in particular, what things it includes in the ideas of pain and pleasure, and to what extent this is left an open question. But these supplementary explanations do not affect the theory of life on which this theory of morality is grounded—namely, that pleasure and freedom from pain are the only things desirable as ends; and that all desirable things (which are as numerous in the utilitarian as in any other scheme) are desirable either for the pleasure inherent in themselves or as means to the promotion of pleasure and the prevention of pain.

Now such a theory of life excites in many minds, and among them in some of the most estimable in feeling and purpose, inveterate dislike. To suppose that life has (as they express it) no higher end than pleasure—no better and nobler object of desire and pursuit—they designate as utterly mean and groveling, as a doctrine worthy only of swine, to whom the followers of Epicurus were, at a very early period, contemptuously likened; and modern holders of the doctrine are occasionally made the subject of equally polite comparisons by its German, French, and English assailants.

When thus attacked, the Epicureans have always answered that it is not they, but their accusers, who represent human nature in a degrading light, since the accusation supposes human beings to be capable of no pleasures except those of which swine are capable. If this supposition were true, the charge could not be gainsaid, but would then be no longer an imputation; for if the sources of pleasure were precisely the same to human beings and to swine, the rule of life which is good enough for the one would be good enough for the other. The comparison of the Epicurean life to that of beasts is felt as degrading, precisely because a beast's pleasures do not satisfy a human being's conceptions of happiness. Human beings have faculties more elevated than the animal appetites and, when once made conscious of them, do not regard anything as happiness which does not include their gratification. I do not, indeed, consider the Epicureans to have been by any means faultless in drawing out their scheme of consequences from the utilitarian principle. To do this in any sufficient manner, many Stoic, as well as Christian, elements require to be included. But there is no known Epicurean theory of life which does not assign to the pleasures of the intellect, of the feelings and imagination, and of the moral sentiments a much higher value as pleasures than to those of mere sensation. It must be admitted, however, that utilitarian writers in general have placed the superiority of mental over bodily pleasures chiefly in the greater permanency, safety, uncostliness, etc., of the former—that is, in their circumstantial advantages rather than in their intrinsic nature. And on all these points utilitarians have fully proved their case; but they might have taken the other and, as it may be called, higher ground with entire consistency. It is quite compatible with the principle of utility to recognize the fact that some kinds of pleasure are more desirable and more valuable than others. It would be absurd that, while in estimating all other things, quality is considered as well as quantity, the estimation of pleasures should be supposed to depend on quantity alone.

If I am asked what I mean by difference of quality in pleasures, or what makes one pleasure more valuable than another merely, as a pleasure, except its being greater in amount, there is but one possible answer. Of two pleasures, if there be one to which all or almost all who have experience of both give a decided preference, irrespective of any feeling of moral obligation to prefer it, that is the more desirable pleasure. If one of the two is, by those who are competently acquainted with both, placed so far above the other that they prefer it, even though knowing it to be attended with a greater amount of discontent, and would not resign it for any quantity of the other pleasure which their nature is capable of, we are justified in ascribing to the preferred enjoyment a superiority in quality so far outweighing quantity as to render it, in comparison, of small account.

Now it is an unquestionable fact that those who are equally acquainted with and equally capable of appreciating and enjoying both do give a most marked preference to the manner of existence which employs their higher faculties. Few human creatures would consent to be changed into any of the lower animals for a promise of the fullest allowance of a beast's pleasures; no intelligent human being would consent to be a fool, no instructed person would be an ignoramus, no person of feeling and conscience would be selfish and base, even though they should be persuaded that the fool, the dunce, or the rascal is better satisfied with his lot than they are with theirs. They would not resign what they possess more than he for the most complete satisfaction of all the desires which they have in common with him. If they ever fancy they would, it is only in cases of unhappiness so extreme that to escape from it they would exchange their lot for almost any other, however undesirable in their own eyes. A being of higher faculties requires more to make him happy, is capable probably of more acute suffering, and certainly accessible to it at more points, than one of an inferior type; but in spite of these liabilities, he can never really wish to sink into what he feels to be a lower grade of existence. We may give what explanation we please of this unwillingness; we may attribute it to pride, a name which is given indiscriminately to some of the most and to some of the least estimable feelings of which mankind are capable; we may refer it to the love of liberty and personal independence, and appeal to which was with the Stoics one of the most effective means for the inculcation of it; to the love of power or to the love of excitement, both of which do really enter into and contribute to it; but its most appropriate appellation is a sense of dignity, which all human beings possess in one form or other, and in some, though by no means in exact, proportion to their higher faculties, and which is so essential a part of the happiness of those in whom it is strong that nothing which conflicts with it could be otherwise than momentarily an object of desire to them. Whoever supposes that this preference takes place at a sacrifice of happiness—that the superior being, in anything like equal circumstances, is not happier than the inferior—confounds the two very different ideas of happiness and content. It is indisputable that the being whose capacities of enjoyment are low has the greatest chance of having them fully satisfied; and a highly endowed being will always feel that any happiness which he can look for, as the world is constituted, is imperfect. But he can learn to bear its imperfections if they are at all bearable; and they will not make him envy the being who is indeed unconscious of the imperfections, but only because he feels not at all the good which those imperfections qualify. It is better to be a human being dissatisfied than a pig satisfied; better to be Socrates dissatisfied than a fool satisfied. And if the fool, or the pig, are of a different opinion, it is because they only know their own side of the question. The other party to the comparison knows both sides. . . .

According to the greatest happiness principle, as above explained, the ultimate end, with reference to and for the sake of which all other things are desirable—whether we are considering our own good or that of other people—is an existence exempt as far as possible from pain, and as rich as possible in enjoyments, both in point of quantity and quality; the test of quality and the rule for measuring it against quantity being the preference felt by those who, in their opportunities of expereince, to which must be added their habits of self-consciousness and self-observation, are best furnished with the means of comparison. This, being according to the utilitarian opinion the end of human action, is necessarily also the standard of morality, which may accordingly be defined "the rules and precepts for human conduct," by the observance of which an existence such as has been described might be, to the greatest extent possible, secured to all mankind; and not to them only, but, so far as the nature of things admits, to the whole sentient creation.

Against this doctrine, however, arises another class of objectors who say that happiness, in any form, cannot be the rational purpose of human life and action; because, in the first place, it is unattainable; and they contemptuously ask, What right hast thou to be happy?—a question which Mr. Carlyle clinches by the addition, What right, a short time ago, hadst thou even *to be?* Next they say that men can do *without* happiness; that all noble human beings have felt this, and could not have become noble but by learning the lesson of *Entsagen*, or renunciation; which lesson, thoroughly learnt and submitted to, they affirm to be the beginning and necessary condition of all virtue.

The first of these objections would go to the root of the matter were it well founded; for if no happiness is to be had at all by human beings, the attainment of it cannot be the end of morality or of any rational conduct. Though, even in that case, something might still be said for the utilitarian theory, since utility includes not solely the pursuit of happiness, but the prevention or mitigation of unhappiness; and if the former aim be chimerical, there will be all the greater scope and more imperative need for the latter, so long at least as mankind think fit to live and do not take refuge in the simultaneous act of suicide recommended under certain conditions by Novalis. When, however, it is thus positively asserted to be impossible that human life should be happy, the assertion, if not something like a verbal quibble, is at least an exaggeration. If by happiness be meant a continuity of highly pleasurable excitement, it is evident enough that this is impossible. A state of exalted pleasure lasts only moments or in some cases, and with some intermissions, hours or days, and is the occasional brilliant flash of enjoyment, not its permanent and steady flame. Of this the philosophers who have taught that happiness is the end of life were as fully aware as those who taunt them. The happiness which they meant was not a life of rapture, but moments of such, in an existence made up of few and transitory pains, many and various pleasures, with a decided predominance of the active over the passive, and having as the foundation of the whole not to expect more from life than it is capable of bestowing. A life thus composed, to those who have been fortunate enough to obtain it, has always appeared worthy of the name of happiness. And such an existence is even now the lot of many during some considerable portion of their lives. The present wretched education and wretched social arrangements are the only real hindrance to its being attainable by almost all.

The objectors perhaps may doubt whether human beings, if taught to consider happiness as the end of life, would be satisfied with such a moderate share of it. But great numbers of mankind have been satisfied with much less. The main constituents of a satisfied life appear to be two, either of which by itself is often found sufficient for the purpose: tranquillity and excitement. With much tranquillity, many find that they can be content with very little pleasure; with much excitement, many can reconcile themselves to a considerable quantity of pain. There is assuredly no inherent impossibility of enabling even the mass of mankind to unite both, since the two are so far from being incompatible that they are in natural alliance, the prolongation of either being a preparation for, and exciting a wish for, the other. It is only those in whom indolence amounts to a vice that do not desire excitement after an interval of repose; it is only those in whom the need of excitement is a disease that feel the tranquillity which follows excitement dull and insipid, instead of pleasurable in direct proportion to the excitement which preceded it. When people who are tolerably fortunate in their outward lot do not find in life sufficient enjoyment to make it valuable to them, the cause generally is caring for nobody but themselves. To those who have neither public nor private affections, the excitements of life are much curtailed, and in any case dwindle in value as the time approaches when all selfish interests must be terminated by death; while those who leave after them objects of personal affection, and especially those who have also culti-vated a fellow feeling with the collective interests of mankind, retain as lively an interest in life on the eve of death as in the vigor of youth and health. Next to selfishness, the principal cause which makes life unsatisfactory is want of mental cultivation. A cultivated mind—I do not mean that of a philosopher, but any mind to which the fountains of knowledge have been opened, and which has been taught, in any tolerable degree, to exercise its faculties—finds sources of inexhaustible interest in all that surrounds it: in the objects of nature, the achievements of art, the imaginations of poetry, the incidents of history, the ways of mankind, past and present, and their prospects in the future. It is possible, indeed, to become indifferent to all this, and that too without having exhausted a thousandth part of it, but only when one has had from the beginning no moral or human interest in these things, and has sought in them only the gratification of curiosity.

Now there is absolutely no reason in the nature of things why an amount of mental culture sufficient to give an intelligent interest in these objects of contemplation should not be the inheritance of everyone born in a civilized country. As little is there an inherent necessity that any human being should be a selfish egotist, devoid of every feeling or care but those which center in his own miserable individuality. Something far superior to this is sufficiently common even now, to give ample earnest of what the human species may be made. Genuine private affections and a sincere inter-est in the public good are possible, though in unequal degrees, to every rightly brought up human being. In a world in which there is so much to interest, so much to enjoy, and so much also to correct and improve, every-one who has this moderate amount of moral and intellectual requisites is capable of an existence which may be called enviable; and unless such a person, through bad laws or subjection to the will of others, is denied the liberty to use the sources of happiness within his reach, he will not fail to find this enviable existence, if he escape the positive evils of life, the great sources of physical and mental suffering—such as indigence, disease, and the unkindness, worthlessness, or premature loss of objects of affection. The main stress of the problem lies, therefore, in the contest with these calamities from which it is a rare good fortune entirely to escape; which, as things now are, cannot be obviated, and often cannot be in any material degree mitigated. Yet no one whose opinion deserves a moment's consider-ation can doubt that most of the great positive evils of the world are in themselves removable, and will, if human affairs continue to improve, be in the end reduced within narrow limits. Poverty, in any sense implying suffer-ing, may be completely extinguished by the wisdom of society combined with the good sense and providence of individuals. Even that most intracta-ble of enemies, disease, may be indefinitely reduced in dimensions by good physical and moral education and proper control of noxious influences, while the progress of science holds out a promise for the future of still more direct conquests over this detestable foe. And every advance in that direction relieves us from some, not only of the chances which cut short our own lives, but, what concerns us still more, which deprive us of those in whom our happiness is wrapt up. As for vicissitudes of fortune and other disappointments connected with worldly circumstances, these are principally the effect, either of gross imprudence, of ill-regulated desires, or of bad or imperfect social institutions. All the grand sources, in short, of human suffering are in a great degree, many of them almost entirely, conquerable by human care and effort; and though their removal is grievously slow—though a long succession of generations will perish in the breach before the conquest is completed, and this world becomes all that, if will and knowledge were not wanting, it might easily be made—yet every mind sufficiently intelligent and generous to bear a part, however small and inconspicuous, in the endeavor will draw a noble enjoyment from the contest itself, which he would not for any bribe in the form of selfish indulgence consent to be without.

And this leads to the true estimation of what is said by the objectors concerning the possibility and the obligation of learning to do without happiness. Unquestionably it is possible to do without happiness; it is done involuntarily by nineteen-twentieths of mankind, even in those parts of our present world which are least deep in barbarism; and it often has to be done voluntarily by the hero or the martyr, for the sake of something which he prizes more than his individual happiness. But this something, what is it, unless the happiness of others or some of the requisites of happiness? It is noble to be capable of resigning entirely one's own portion of happiness, or chances of it; but, after all, this self-sacrifice must be for some end; it is not its own end; and if we are told that its end is not happiness but virtue, which is better than happiness, I ask, would the sacrifice be made if the hero or martyr did not believe that it would earn for others immunity from similar sacrifices? Would it be made if he thought that his renunciation of happiness for himself would produce no fruit for any of his fellow creatures, but to make their lot like his, and place them also in the condition of persons who have renounced happiness? All honor to those who can abnegate for themselves the personal enjoyment of life when by such renunciation they contribute worthily to increase the amount of happiness in the world; but he who does it or professes to do it for any other purpose is no more deserving of admiration than the ascetic mounted on his pillar. He may be an inspiriting proof of what men *can* do, but assuredly not an example of what they *should*.

Though it is only in a very imperfect state of the world's arrangements that anyone can best serve the happiness of others by the absolute sacrifice of his own, yet, so long as the world is in that imperfect state, I fully acknowledge that the readiness to make such a sacrifice is the highest virtue which can be found in man. I will add that in this condition of the world, paradoxical as the assertion may be, the conscious ability to do without happiness gives the best prospect of realizing such happiness as is attainable. For nothing except that consciousness can raise a person above the chances of life, by making him feel that, let fate and fortune do their worst, they have not power to subdue him; which, once felt, frees him from excess of anxiety concerning the evils of life, and enables him, like many a Stoic in the worst times of the Roman Empire, to cultivate in tranquillity the sources of satisfaction accessible to him, without concerning himself about the uncertainty of their duration any more than about their inevitable end.

Meanwhile, let utilitarians never cease to claim the morality of self-devotion as a possession which belongs by as good a right to them as either to the Stoic or to the Transcendentalist. The utilitarian morality does recognize in human beings the power of sacrificing their own greatest good for the good of others. It only refuses to admit that the sacrifice is itself a good. A sacrifice which does not increase or tend to increase the sum total of happiness, it considers as wasted. The only self-renunciation which it applauds is devotion to the happiness, or to some of the means of happiness, of others, either of mankind collectively or of individuals within the limits imposed by the collective interests of mankind.

I must again repeat what the assailants of utilitarianism seldom have the justice to acknowledge, that the happiness which forms the utilitarian standard of what is right in conduct is not the agent's own happiness but that of all concerned. As between his own happiness and that of others, utilitarianism requires him to be as strictly impartial as a disinterested and benevolent spectator. In the golden rule of Jesus of Nazareth, we read the complete spirit of the ethics of utility. "To do as you would be done by," and "to love your neighbor as yourself," constitute the ideal perfection of utilitarian morality. As the means of making the nearest approach to this ideal, utility would enjoin, first, that laws and social arrangements should place the happiness or (as, speaking practically, it may be called) the interest of every individual as nearly as possible in harmony with the interest of the whole; and, secondly, that education and opinion, which have so vast a power over human character, should so use that power as to establish in the mind of every individual an indissoluble association between his own happiness and the good of the whole, especially between his own happiness and the practice of such modes of conduct, negative and positive, as regard for the universal happiness prescribes; so that not only he may be unable to conceive the possibility of happiness to himself, consistently with conduct opposed to the general good, but also that a direct impulse to promote the general good may be in every individual one of the habitual motives of action, and the sentiments connected therewith may fill a large and prominent place in every human being's sentient existence. If the impugners of the utilitarian morality represented it to their own minds in this its true character, I know not what recommendation possessed by any other morality they could possibly affirm to be wanting to it; what more beautiful or more exalted developments of human nature any other ethical system can be supposed to foster, or what springs of action, not accessible to the utilitarian, such systems rely on for giving effect to their mandates.

The objectors to utilitarianism cannot always be charged with representing it in a discreditable light. On the contrary, those among them who entertain anything like a just idea of its disinterested character, sometimes find fault with its standard as being too high for humanity. They say it is exacting too much to require that people shall always act from the inducement of promoting the general interests of society. But this is to mistake the very meaning of a standard of morals, and confound the rule of action with the motive of it. It is the business of ethics to tell us what are our duties, or by what test we may know them; but no system of ethics requires that the sole motive of all we do shall be a feeling of duty; on the contrary, ninety-nine hundredths of all our actions are done from other motives, and rightly so done, if the rule of duty does not condemn them. It is the more unjust to utilitarianism that this particular misapprehension should be made a ground of objection to it, inasmuch as utilitarian moralists have gone beyond almost all others in affirming that the motive has nothing to do with the morality of the action, though much with the worth of the agent. He who saves a fellow creature from drowning does what is morally right, whether his motive be duty, or the hope of being paid for his trouble; he who betrays the friend that trusts him, is guilty of a crime, even if his object be to serve another friend to whom he is under greater obligations. But to speak only of actions done from the motive of duty, and in direct obedience to princi-ple: it is a misapprehension of the utilitarian mode of thought, to conceive it as implying that people should fix their minds upon so wide a generality as the world, or society at large. The great majority of good actions are intended not for the benefit of the world, but for that of individuals, of which the good of the world is made up; and the thoughts of the most virtuous man need not on these occasions travel beyond the particular persons con-cerned, except so far as is necessary to assure himself that in benefiting them he is not violating the rights, that is, the legitimate and authorized expecta-tions, of any one else. The multiplication of happiness is, according to the utilitarian ethics, the object of virtue: the occasions on which any person (except one in a thousand) has it in his power to do this on an extended scale, in other words to be a public benefactor, are but exceptional; and on these occasions alone is he called on to consider public utility; in every other case, private utility, the interest or happiness of some few persons, is all he has to attend to. Those alone the influence of whose actions extends to society in general, need concern themselves habitually about so large an object. In the case of abstinences indeed—of things which people forbear to do from moral considerations, though the consequences in the particular case might be beneficial—it would be unworthy of an intelligent agent not to be consciously aware that the action is of a class which, if practiced generally, would be generally injurious, and that this is the ground of the obligation to abstain from it. The amount of regard for the public interest implied in this recognition, is no greater than is demanded by every system of morals, for they all enjoin to abstain from whatever is manifestly perni-cious to society. . . .

Again, Utility is often summarily stigmatized as an immoral doctrine by giving it the name of Expediency, and taking advantage of the popular use of that term to contrast it with Principle. But the Expedient, in the sense in which it is opposed to the Right, generally means that which is expedient for the particular interest of the agent himself; as when a minister sacrifices the interests of his country to keep himself in place. When it means anything better than this, it means that which is expedient for some immediate object, some temporary purpose, but which violates a rule whose observance is expedient in a much higher degree. The Expedient, in this sense, instead of being the same thing with the useful, is a branch of the hurtful. Thus, it would often be expedient, for the purpose of getting over some momentary embarrassment, or attaining some object immediately useful to ourselves or others, to tell a lie. But inasmuch as the cultivation in ourselves of a sensitive feeling on the subject of veracity, is one of the most useful, and the enfeeblement of that feeling one of the most hurtful, things to which our conduct can be instrumental; and inasmuch as any, even unintentional, deviation from truth, does that much towards weakening the trustworthiness of human assertion, which is not only the principal support of all present social well-being, but the insufficiency of which does more than any one thing that can be named to keep back civilisation, virtue, everything on which human happiness on the largest scale depends; we feel that the violation, for a present advantage, of a rule of such transcendant expediency, is not expedient, and that he who, for the sake of a convenience to himself or to some other individual, does what depends on him to deprive mankind of the good, and inflicts upon them the evil, involved in the greater or less reliance which they can place in each other's word, acts the part of one of their worst enemies. Yet that even this rule, sacred as it is, admits of possible exceptions, is acknowledged by all moralists; the chief of which is when the withholding of some fact (as of information from a malefactor, or of bad news from a person dangerously ill) would save an individual (especially an individual other than oneself) from great and unmerited evil, and when the withholding can only be effected by denial. But in order that the exception may not extend itself beyond the need, and may have the least possible effect in weakening reliance on veracity, it ought to be recognized, and, if possible, its limits defined; and if the principle of utility is good for anything, it must be good for weighing these conflicting utilities against one another, and marking out the region within which one or the other preponderates. . . .

It has already been remarked that questions of ultimate ends do not admit of proof, in the ordinary acceptation of the term. To be incapable of proof by reasoning is common to all first principles, to the first premises of our knowledge, as well as to those of our conduct. . . .

Questions about ends are, in other words, questions about what things are desirable. The utilitarian doctrine is that happiness is desirable, and the only thing desirable as an end; all other things being only desirable as means to that end. What ought to be required of this doctrine, what conditions is it requisite that the doctrine should fulfill—to make good its claim to be believed?

The only proof capable of being given that an object is visible is that people actually see it. The only proof that a sound is audible is that people hear it; and so of the other sources of our experience. In like manner, I apprehend, the sole evidence it is possible to produce that anything is desirable is that people do actually desire it. If the end which the utilitarian doctrine proposes to itself were not, in theory and in practice, acknowledged to be an end, nothing could ever convince any person that it was so. No reason can be given why the general happiness is desirable, except that each person, so far as he believes it to be attainable, desires his own happiness. This, however, being a fact, we have not only all the proof which the case admits of, but all which it is possible to require, that happiness is a good, that each person's happiness is a good to that person, and the general happiness, therefore, a good to the aggregate of all persons. Happiness has made out its title as *one* of the ends of conduct and, consequently, one of the criteria of morality. . . .

But it has not, by this alone, proved itself to be the sole criterion. To do that, it would seem, by the same rule, necessary to show, not only that people desire happiness, but that they never desire anything else. Now it is palpable that they do desire things which, in common language, are decidedly distinguished from happiness. They desire, for example, virtue, and the absence of vice, no less really than pleasure and the absence of pain. The desire of virtue is not as universal, but it is as authentic a fact, as the desire of happiness. And hence the opponents of the utilitarian standard deem that they have a right to infer that there are other ends of human action besides happiness, and that happiness is not the standard of approbation and disapprobation.

But does the utilitarian doctrine deny that people desire virtue, or maintain that virtue is not a thing to be desired? The very reverse. It maintains not only that virtue is to be desired, but that it is to be desired disinterestedly, for itself. Whatever may be the opinion of utilitarian moralists as to the original conditions by which virtue is made virtue; however they may believe (as they do) that actions and dispositions are only virtuous because they promote another end than virtue; yet this being granted, and it having been decided, from considerations of this description, what *is* virtuous, they not only place virtue at the very head of the things which are good as means to the ultimate end, but they also recognise as a psychological fact the possibility of its being, to the individual, a good in itself, without looking to any end beyond it; and hold, that the mind is not in a right state, not in a state conformable to Utility, not in the state most conducive to the general happiness, unless it does love virtue in this manner—as a thing desirable in itself, even although, in the individual instance, it should not produce those other desirable consequences which it tends to produce, and on account of which it is held to be virtue. This opinion is not, in the smallest degree, a departure from the Happiness principle. The ingredients of happiness are very various, and each of them is desirable in itself, and not merely when considered as swelling an aggregate. The principle of utility does not mean that any given pleasure, as music, for instance, or any given exemption from pain, as for example health, is to be looked upon as means to a collective something termed happiness, and to be desired on that account. They are desired and desirable in and for themselves; besides being means, they are part of the end. Virtue, according to the utilitarian doctrine, is not naturally and originally part of the end, but it is capable of becoming so; and in those who live it disinterestedly it has become so, and is desired and cherished, not as a means to happiness, but as a part of their happiness.

To illustrate this farther, we may remember that virtue is not the only thing, originally a means, and which if it were not a means to anything else, would be and remain indifferent, but which by association with what it is a means to, comes to be desired for itself, and that too with the utmost intensity. What, for example, shall we say of the love of money? There is nothing originally more desirable about money than about any heap of glittering pebbles. Its worth is solely that of the things which it will buy; the desires for other things than itself, which it is a means of gratifying. Yet the love of money is not only one of the strongest moving forces of human life, but money is, in many cases, desired in and for itself; the desire to possess it is often stronger than the desire to use it, and goes on increasing when all the desires which point to ends beyond it, to be compassed by it, are falling off. It may, then, be said truly that money is desired not for the sake of an end, but as part of the end. From being a means to happiness, it has come to be itself a principal ingredient of the individual's conception of happiness. The same may be said of the majority of the great objects of human life—power, for example, or fame; except that to each of these there is a certain amount of immediate pleasure annexed, which has at least the semblance of being naturally inherent in them; a thing which cannot be said of money. Still, however, the strongest natural attraction, both of power and of fame, is the immense aid they give to the attainment of our other wishes; and it is the strong association thus generated between them and all our objects of desire, which gives to the direct desire of them the intensity it often assumes, so as in some characters to surpass in strength all other desires. In these cases the means have become a part of the end, and a more important part of it than any of the things which they are means to. What was once desired as an instrument for the attainment of happiness, has come to be desired for its own sake. In being desired for its own sake it is, however, desired as *part* of happiness. The person is made, or thinks he would be made, happy by its mere possession; and is made unhappy by failure to obtain it. The desire of it is not a different thing from the desire of happiness, any more than the love of music, or the desire of health. They are included in happiness. They are some of the elements of which the desire of happiness is made up. Happiness is not an abstract idea, but a concrete whole; and these are some of its parts. And the utilitarian standard sanctions and approves their being so. Life would be a poor thing, very ill provided with sources of happiness, if there were not this provision of nature, by which things originally indifferent, but conducive to, or otherwise associated with, the satisfaction of our primitive desires, become in themselves sources of pleasure more valuable than the primitive pleasures, both in permanency, in the space of human existence that they are capable of covering, and even in intensity.

Virtue, according to the utilitarian conception, is a good of this description. There was no original desire of it, or motive to it, save its conduciveness to pleasure, and especially to protection from pain. But through the association thus formed, it may be felt a good in itself, and desired as such with as great intensity as any other good; and with this difference between it and the love of money, of power, or of fame, that all of these may, and often do, render the individual noxious to the other members of the society to which he belongs, whereas there is nothing which makes him so much a blessing to them as the cultivation of the disinterested love of virtue. And consequently, the utilitarian standard, while it tolerates and approves those other acquired desires, up to the point beyond which they would be more injurious to the general happiness than promotive of it, enjoins and requires the cultivation of the love of virtue up to the greatest strength possible, as being above all things important to the general happiness.

It results from the preceding considerations, that there is in reality nothing desired except happiness. Whatever is desired otherwise than as a means to some end beyond itself, and ultimately to happiness, is desired as itself a part of happiness, and is not desired for itself until it has become so. Those who desire virtue for its own sake, desire it either because the consciousness of it is a pleasure, or because the consciousness of being without it is a pain, or for both reasons united; as in truth the pleasure and pain seldom exist separately, but almost always together, the same person feeling pleasure in the degree of virtue attained, and pain in not having attained more. If one of these gave him no pleasure, and the other no pain, he would not love or desire virtue, or would desire it only for the other benefits which it might produce to himself or to persons whom he cared for.

We have now, then, an answer to the question, of what sort of proof the principle of utility is susceptible. If the opinion which I have now stated is psychologically true—if human nature is so constituted as to desire nothing which is not either a part of happiness or a means of happiness, we can have no other proof, and we require no other, that these are the only things desirable. If so, happiness is the sole end of human action, and the promotion of it the test by which to judge of all human conduct; from whence it necessarily follows that it must be the criterion of morality, since a part is included in the whole.

And now to decide whether this is really so; whether mankind do desire nothing for itself but that which is a pleasure to them, or of which the absence is a pain; we have evidently arrived at a question of fact and experience, dependent, like all similar questions, upon evidence. It can only be determined by practiced self-consciousness and self-observation, assisted by observation of others. I believe that these sources of evidence, impartially consulted, will declare that desiring a thing and finding it pleasant, aversion to it and thinking of it as painful, are phenomena entirely inseparable, or rather two parts of the same phenomenon; in strictness of language, two different modes of naming the same psychological fact: that to think of an object as desirable (unless for the sake of its consequences), and to think of it as pleasant, are one and the same thing; and that to desire anything, except in proportion as the idea of it is pleasant, is a physical and metaphysical impossibility.

So obvious does this appear to me, that I expect it will hardly be disputed: and the objection made will be, not that desire can possibly be directed to anything ultimately except pleasure and exemption from pain, but that the will is a different thing from desire; that a person of conformed virtue, or any other person whose purposes are fixed, carries out his purposes without any thought of the pleasure he has in contemplating them, or expects to derive from their fulfillment; and persists in acting on them, even though these pleasures are much diminished, by changes in his character or decay of his passive sensibilities, or are outweighed by the pains which the pursuit of the purposes may bring upon him. All this I fully admit, and have stated it elsewhere, as positively and emphatically as any one. Will, the active phenomenon, is a different thing from desire, the state of passive sensibility, and though originally an offshoot from it, may in time take root and detach itself from the parent stock; so much so, that in the case of an habitual purpose, instead of willing the thing because we desire it, we often desire it only because we will it. This however, is but an instance of that familiar fact, the power of habit, and is nowise confined to the case of virtuous actions. Many indifferent things, which men originally did from a motive of some sort, they continue to do from habit. Sometimes this is done unconsciously, the consciousness coming only after the action: at other times with conscious volition, but volition which has become habitual, and is put in operation by the force of habit, in opposition perhaps to the deliberate preference, as often happens with those who have contracted habits of vicious or hurtful indulgence. Third and last comes the case in which the habitual act of will in the individual instance is not in contradiction to the general intention prevailing at other times, but in fulfillment of it; as in the case of the person of conformed virtue, and of all who pursue deliberately and consistently any determinate end. The distinction between will and desire thus understood is an authentic and highly important psychological fact; but the fact consists solely in this—that will, like all other parts of our constitution, is amenable to habit, and that we may will from habit what we no longer desire for itself, or desire only because we will it. It is not the less true that will, in the beginning, is entirely produced by desire; including in that term the repelling influence of pain as well as the attractive one of pleasure. Let us take into consideration, no longer the person who has a confirmed will to do right, but him in whom that virtuous will is still feeble, conquerable by temptation, and not to be fully relied on; by what means can it be strengthened? How can the will to be virtuous, where it does not exist in sufficient force, be implanted or awakened? Only by making the person *desire* virtue—by making him think of it in a pleasurable light, or of its absence in a painful one. It is by associating the doing right with pleasure, or the doing wrong with pain, or by eliciting and impressing and bringing home to the person's experience the pleasure naturally involved in the one or the pain in the other, that it is possible to call forth that will to be virtuous, which, when confirmed, acts without any thought of either pleasure or pain. Will is the child of desire, and passes out of the dominion of its parent only to come under that of habit. That which is the result of habit affords no presumption of being intrinsically good; and there would be no reason for wishing that the purpose of virtue should become independent of pleasure and pain, were it not that the influence of the pleasurable and painful associations which prompt to virtue is not sufficiently to be depended on for unerring constancy of action until it has acquired the support of habit. Both in feeling and in conduct, habit is the only thing which imparts certainty; and it is because of the importance to others of being able to rely absolutely on one's feelings and conduct, and to oneself of being able to rely on one's own, that the will to do right ought to be cultivated into this habitual independence. In other words, this state of the will is a means to good, not intrinsically a good; and does not contradict the doctrine that nothing is a good to human beings but in so far as it is either itself pleasurable, or a means of attaining pleasure or averting pain.

But if this doctrine be true, the principle of utility is proved. Whether it is so or not, must now be left to the consideration of the thoughtful reader.

From *Existentialism and Human Emotions*

Jean-Paul Sartre

If existence really does precede essence, there is no explaining things away by reference to a fixed and given human nature. In other words, there is no determinism, man is free, man is freedom. On the other hand, if God does not exist, we find no values or commands to turn to which legitimize our conduct. So, in the bright realm of values, we have no excuse behind us, nor justification before us. We are alone, with no excuses.

That is the idea I shall try to convey when I say that man is condemned to be free. Condemned, because he did not create himself, yet, in other respects is free; because, once thrown into the world, he is responsible for everything he does. The existentialist does not believe in the power of passion. He will never agree that a sweeping passion is a ravaging torrent which fatally leads a man to certain acts and is therefore an excuse. He thinks that man is responsible for his passion.

The existentialist does not think that man is going to help himself by finding in the world some omen by which to orient himself. Because he thinks that man will interpret the omen to suit himself. Therefore, he thinks that man, with no support and no aid, is condemned every moment to invent man. Ponge, in a very fine article, has said, "Man is the future of man." That's exactly it. But if it is taken to mean that this future is recorded in heaven, that God sees it, then it is false, because it would really no longer be a future. If it is taken to mean that, whatever a man may be, there is a future to be forged, a virgin future before him, then this remark is sound. But then we are forlorn.

To give you an example which will enable you to understand forlornness better, I shall cite the case of one of my students who came to see me under the following circumstances: his father was on bad terms with his mother, and, moreover, was inclined to be a collaborationist; his older brother had been killed in the German offensive of 1940, and the young

Reprinted with permission from *Existentialism and Human Emotions*, translated by Bernard Frichtman (New York: Philosophical Library, 1947).

man, with somewhat immature but generous feelings, wanted to avenge him. His mother lived alone with him, very much upset by the half-treason of her husband and the death of her older son; the boy was her only consolation.

The boy was faced with the choice of leaving for England and joining the Free French Forces—that is, leaving his mother behind—or remaining with his mother and helping her to carry on. He was fully aware that the woman lived only for him and that his going-off—and perhaps his death—would plunge her into despair. He was also aware that every act that he did for his mother's sake was a sure thing, in the sense that it was helping her to carry on, whereas every effort he made toward going off and fighting was an uncertain move which might run aground and prove completely useless; for example, on his way to England he might, while passing through Spain, be detained indefinitely in a Spanish camp; he might reach England or Algiers and be stuck in an office at a desk job. As a result, he was faced with two very different kinds of action: one, concrete, immediate, but concerning only one individual; the other concerned an incomparably vaster group, a national collectivity, but for that very reason was dubious, and might be interrupted en route. And, at the same time, he was wavering between two kinds of ethics. On the one hand, an ethics of sympathy, of personal devotion; on the other, a broader ethics, but one whose efficacy was more dubious. He had to choose between the two.

Who could help him choose? Christian doctrine? No. Christian doctrine says, "Be charitable, love your neighbor, take the more rugged path, etc., etc." But which is the more rugged path? Whom should he love as a brother? The fighting man or his mother? Which does the greater good, the vague act of fighting in a group, or the concrete one of helping a particular human being to go on living? Who can decide *a priori*? Nobody. No book of ethics can tell him. The Kantian ethics says, "Never treat any person as a means, but as an end." Very well, if I stay with my mother, I'll treat her as an end and not as a means; but by virture of this very fact, I'm running the risk of treating the people around me who are fighting, as means; and, conversely, if I go to join those who are fighting, I'll be treating them as an end, and, by doing that, I run the risk of treating my mother as a means.

If values are vague, and if they are always too broad for the concrete and specific case that we are considering, the only thing left for us is to trust our instincts. That's what this young man tried to do; and when I saw him, he said, "In the end, feeling is what counts. I ought to choose whichever pushes me in one direction. If I feel that I love my mother enough to sacrifice everything else for her—my desire for vengeance, for action, for adventure—then I'll stay with her. If, on the contrary, I feel that my love for my mother isn't enough, I'll leave."

But how is the value of a feeling determined? What gives his feeling for his mother value? Precisely the fact that he remained with her. I may say that I like so-and-so well enough to sacrifice a certain amount of money for him, but I may say so only if I've done it. I may say "I love my mother well enough to remain with her" if I have remained with her. The only way to determine the value of this affection is, precisely, to perform an act which confirms and defines it. But, since I require this affection to justify my act, I find myself caught in a vicious circle.

On the other hand, Gide has well said that a mock feeling and a true feeling are almost indistinguishable; to decide that I love my mother and will remain with her, or to remain with her by putting on an act, amount somewhat to the same thing. In other words, the feeling is formed by the acts one performs; so, I can not refer to it in order to act upon it. Which means that I can neither seek within myself the true condition which will impel me to act, nor apply to a system of ethics for concepts which will permit me to act. You will say, "At least, he did go to a teacher for advice." But if you seek advice from a priest, for example, you have chosen this priest; you already knew, more or less, just about what advice he was going to give you. In other words, choosing your adviser is involving yourself. The proof of this is that if you are a Christian, you will say, "Consult a priest." But some priests are collaborating, some are just marking time, some are resisting. Which to choose? If the young man chooses a priest who is resisting or collaborating, he has already decided on the kind of advice he's going to get. Therefore, in coming to see me he knew the answer I was going to give him, and I had only one answer to give: "You're free, choose, that is, invent." No general ethics can show you what is to be done; there are no omens in the world. The Catholics will reply, "But there are." Granted—but, in any case, I myself choose the meaning they have.

MORAL PROBLEMS IN THE PHYSICIAN-PATIENT RELATIONSHIP

Chapter 2

INTRODUCTION*

This chapter explores a variety of moral problems that pervade the physician-patient relationship—a relationship that often endures a measure of conflict. Philosophers are generally agreed that the need for a system of ethics arises out of the existence of conflict. Much of the time, discord arises among persons in their wants, desires, or interests. Sometimes a conflict is best described in terms of a clash of moral principles; these principles are of the sort that lie at the heart of our social institutions and practices, as well as reflecting our commonly held moral beliefs. If the need for having an ethical system does, indeed, occur as a result of conflicts among persons or principles, then a satisfactory ethical theory must address these various conflicts and offer a method for resolving them. In each section of this chapter, a different cluster of moral problems in medicine, arising out of conflicts of one or another sort, will be examined.

Some conflicts may emerge as a result of different perspectives that different persons have, whether these perspectives represent permanent features of their situation or temporary disparities in points of view. For example, the status of being a patient is one that confers certain properties on anyone who occupies that status. One such property is that of dependency. Especially in the case of the hospitalized patient, the personal freedom and decision-making autonomy that we normally consider to be the rights of human beings are diminished or, in some cases, even abolished. In addition to the sorts of conflicts that arise because of differing points of view, others may emerge as a result of differing *roles* or positions that persons occupy. Problems of both sorts are examined in the chapter section entitled "The Physician-Patient Relationship."

Conflict may also arise *within* a person who is faced with making a moral choice or decision. Sometimes this sort of internal dilemma occurs because of *conflicting loyalties* a person may have simultaneously: loyalty to

*Selected portions of an earlier version of this introductory chapter were recorded for the Behavioral Sciences Tape Library.

two or more persons, institutions, or groups. Most of the conflicting loyalties that fall into this class are explored in the section entitled "Confidentiality." Indeed, most situations in which the ethical issues focus on privacy, rights of privileged communication, and confidentiality are of this type.

Another way of dealing with "internal conflicts" focuses on the notion of *moral principles.* This approach is illustrated in the sections entitled "Truth-Telling," "Informed Consent and Coercion," and "Paternalism." Here we investigate the problem of a clash between two or more moral principles to which a person subscribes but which he cannot simultaneously follow because of special circumstances. Dilemmas of informed consent appear generally to be of this type, as are questions concerning the justifiability of paternalistic acts or practices whose purpose is (primarily) to benefit someone believed incapable of acting rationally in his own behalf. Attempts to resolve disputes about these matters almost always proceed by appealing to one or another moral principle, and the particular principles involved are often agreed to by the disputants as being fundamental to our moral way of life. The disagreement, in such cases, rests on a matter of priorities: which ethical principle ought one to invoke when two or more come into conflict with one another?

Let us turn now to a more detailed look at the specific types of moral problems in the physician-patient relationship, as exemplified in the readings grouped under the various sections of this chapter. In the first section of readings we see an illustration of the fact that moral issues often arise out of different perspectives or points of view—whether temporary or enduring—that people are bound to assume. Although being a patient is, for most people, a relatively temporary state, it is nonetheless significant in the emotional investment and anxiety produced, largely as a result of fear, uncertainty, and the pervasive threat to bodily integrity. One of the salient features of the life of a patient in an era of impressive medical technology and advanced therapeutic procedures is the so-called "dehumanization" a person may suffer in this context. A closely related aspect is the occurrence of diminished autonomy and freedom of choice, which can be observed, as well, in other institutionalized populations (for example, prisoners, old persons, and the retarded). Taken together, these two facets of patient life are sometimes viewed as constituting a threat to fundamental human rights.

Another sort of problem in the physician-patient relationship is the frequent failure on the part of physicians to see things from the point of view of the patient. This situation is illustrated in the selection by Dr. Oliver Cope, in which a female patient describes her physician's failure to deal with the emotional consequences of the threat involved in surgical removal of her breast.

Moreover, conflicts may arise within the physician's role itself. There may be several different ways in which this role can be construed, as Szasz and Hollender point out, and the issue is further complicated by the many aims or goals embodied in this role. The physician has a special set of duties and obligations, as well as the usual sorts of duties that all persons possess by virtue of their membership in human society; some of the issues are addressed by Robert Veatch in "Medical Ethics: Professional or Universal?"

Within the physician's role, conflicts may occur between two or more of the acknowledged goals of the medical profession—for example, the aim of alleviating the pain and suffering of the sick versus that of contributing new knowledge to medical science. This particular conflict may appear in cases in which new drugs or modes of treatment are contemplated; it is often hard to draw a clear-cut line between "pure" therapy and treatment where an element of experimentation enters in. In practice, the existence of conflicts of interest (e.g., the patient's, society's, the medical profession's), as well as the sometimes divergent goals of medicine, may cause moral dilemmas, and there is no universal ethical prescription that can provide a solution to all of these. But there are principles of varying degrees of strength that might be adopted by a physician, such as the view propounded in the selection by Hans Jonas: "In the course of treatment, the physician is obligated to the patient and to no one else. He is not the agent of society, nor of the interests of medical science, the patient's family, the patient's co-sufferers, or future sufferers from the same disease. The patient alone counts when he is under the physician's care." This principle sets up a clear order of priorities among the subgoals embodied in the physician's role; however, not everyone would agree to it; and even where agreement is secured, problematic cases may still arise that require reflective moral judgments.

The problems considered in the section entitled "Confidentiality" fall into the category of conflicting loyalties, especially in those cases involving confidentiality, privileged communication, and privacy. Should a patient's confidence ever be violated? Is medical confidentiality abused? If so, in what ways? Are there special problems that arise in this area in the case of psychotherapy? For example, if a psychiatric patient tells his therapist that he has suicidal impulses or has made a suicide attempt or is reading books about fast-acting, lethal drugs, where does the therapist's obligation lie? Ought he to maintain his patient's confidentiality and not inform anyone? Or should he alert the patient's family or even, perhaps, others, to the possibility that the person might make a suicide attempt? It goes without saying that these questions only arise as moral problems if, in the considered professional judgment of the psychiatrist, the patient is *likely* to make a successful attempt at suicide. Mere logical possibilities are not an appropriate subject for normative ethics. But how likely is likely? How high should the probability be that this patient could make a successful suicide attempt in order to justify the therapist's violating confidentiality? Can such probabilities even be meaningfully assessed? Some might claim that the principle "Always maintain confidentiality" is fully acceptable no matter what the consequences. Adherence to such dogmatic principles is rarely found in anyone, however. But most people believe that the physician's primary obligation is to his patient, rather than to any other person or group. In the example used earlier, one might argue that the moral judgment holding that the physician should tell no one about his suicidal patient follows from the principle that the physician's primary obligation is to his patient. Another might reply that taking steps to preserve his patient's life is fulfilling this obligation, and therefore, violating confidentiality is justified according to the same principle. This can now be identified as largely a dispute about the facts of a specific case, since the parties to the moral dispute appear to agree on their main ethical principle. One might argue that new value issues enter the dispute at another level, however: whether it is appropriate to place a higher priority on keeping trust or on preserving life. In this example, it is hard to imagine that anyone would value keeping trust over preserving life, but the matter is not as simple as this description implies. It is not a question here of a direct life-saving act, but rather, a small step in a chain of acts—a step that is based on a subjective judgment of probabilities by one physician. Nevertheless, it is questionable whether a closer or more detailed look at the facts of the case would provide the sort of evidence that could settle this dispute. An ethical issue like this may, in the last analysis, reduce to a question of one's ultimate value preferences.

The moral presumption seems to be on the side of *breaking* doctor-patient confidentiality in cases in which a patient shows evidence of being potentially dangerous to other persons. Here, it might reasonably be argued, the physician has an overriding moral duty to prevent harm to innocent persons and this obligation supersedes the narrower or weaker obligation to maintain confidentiality. The same type of justification is offered for a variety of coercive acts in medical contexts, a number of which are explored in the section called "Informed Consent and Coercion" (see, for example, the article by Livermore, Malmquist, and Meehl, "On the Justification for Civil Commitment"). But whether this reason is offered to justify breaking confidence or to support taking coercive measures, the strength of the position rests on the knowledge that a physician or therapist has to make judgments about the likelihood of his patient committing acts of violence or harm to others. In any case, the dilemma must be viewed as a genuine ethical conflict—one that poses two alternative courses of action, each of which has moral reasons that can be urged on its behalf.

A special set of moral problems is singled out for more detailed examination in the section entitled "Truth-Telling." These involve some sort of conflict between the precept that one ought to tell the truth and some other prominent ethical directive; here again, two generally held moral principles come into conflict and cannot both be followed simultaneously. Few, if any, moral philosophers have maintained the ethical principle enjoining truth-telling in an absolutist form—for example, "always, in all kinds of circumstances, tell the truth, the whole truth, and nothing but the truth"; or "never lie, under any circumstances." Imanuel Kant is the philosopher most often cited as a defender of absolutist moral principles prohibiting lying. But Kant's views on this matter lend themselves to varying interpretations, some of which construe his position as more flexible in matters of truth-telling than the standard interpretation allows. In any case, while there may be few defenders of an absolutist principle prescribing truth-telling, there are still two major areas where disagreement can arise. One concerns the circumstances or conditions that justify departures from truth-telling and how these are to be weighted in a specific case. The other lies in the type of justification offered by two different ethical theorists. Duty theorists, those who subscribe to a deontological ethical theory, claim that one of our *prima facie* duties as moral agents is to tell the truth. But, they would add, this duty can be overridden by other, more important duties, such as the duty to preserve life and health whenever possible. Utilitarians, or more generally, consequentialists, might agree both on the general principle that people ought to tell the truth and on just which particular circumstances justify departing from this moral principle. The justification offered by the utilitarian would be quite different from that of the deontologist, however. The utilitarian would say that truth-telling as a general moral practice, and perhaps in particular cases as well, is justified by the predominance of its good consequences over bad ones. (In this connection, see the Chapter 1 selection by Mill, pp. 35–51.) Departures from truth-telling are seen as justifiable, at least sometimes, if the good or benefit accomplished by lying outweighs whatever good accrues to adhering to the moral principle of telling the truth. Indeed, two persons, each of whom subscribes to a different moral theory, might agree on everything about a particular case except the moral justification for the action judged to be morally right or morally wrong. These sorts of disagreements are proper subjects of discussion for ethical theorists, but do not usually affect the sorts of problems faced by people who are involved in situations requiring moral decision-making.

It seems, not surprisingly, that few practitioners in the health sciences are concerned specifically with the application of abstract moral principles enjoining truth-telling—or anything else—to their daily practices. Instead, they view moral problems as arising directly out of situations they encounter where interests conflict or where people's rights are open to question. We observed earlier that there is much current concern about patients' rights; there is also a concern for the rights of other groups or classes of persons whose presumed rights have not been previously identified or claimed in medical situations, such as the rights of children, retarded persons, and prisoners used as experimental subjects. One specific right claimed on behalf of patients is their alleged "right to know." Just what it is that patients are supposed to have a right to know varies from case to case, and in some instances it is far from clear. Some obvious candidates for things a patient could be said to have the right to know are: the specific disease or ailment he has; what the prognosis is for him, in particular; general statistics about people who have this disease or condition, sometimes described in terms of the patient's "chances" for living or dying; and others that come readily to mind. There are many physicians who oppose telling a patient seriously bad news about his condition or his life chances. Of course, physicians do not usually couch their views in terms of the morality of lying to patients. Instead, they emphasize the importance of helping the patient maintain hope. Sometimes this is linked directly to the patient's medical condition; other times, it is seen as a separate yet significant aspect of the doctor's relationship with his patient.

We can readily see that the morality of telling the truth to a patient must be pitted against other values that are deemed important, in general, as well as in specific medical contexts: preservation of the health and well-being of fellow human beings. If it is, indeed, true that some patients are likely to be worse off—in any sense—as a result of knowing the severity of their condition or the prognosis, then perhaps these patients ought not be told. The difficulty lies in whether anyone can ascertain just which patients are likely to be harmed rather than benefited by knowing the truth.

Another set of reasons offered by those who advocate withholding information from terminally ill patients revolves around the notion of denial. Physicians frequently claim that the mechanism of denial with respect to our own death operates in most of us and that, furthermore, there are good psychological reasons why this defense exists and ought not be invaded by well-meaning doctors, family members, or others. Some writers on this subject add that the denial mechanism is so strong that even when a patient is told bluntly about his condition, he may not "process" the information correctly and thus may not really be aware of what he has been told. There is, however, another set of claims that urges the view that the dying know that they are dying, even without being told, and that terminally ill persons have guessed "the truth" even when everyone concerned has tried to hide the facts from them. This view is represented by a selection from Kübler-Ross' *On Death and Dying.*

So it appears that before we can directly confront the moral problem of what to tell seriously ill persons, we must address a number of factual questions: Might telling such patients the truth harm them more than it may benefit them? Is there a general answer to this question, or can the question only be asked appropriately for each particular patient? What criteria exist for determining whether or not a patient can "handle" the truth? If there are no easily identifiable criteria, then how do doctors themselves come to know these sorts of psychological facts about their patients? There are also some questions of a more or less factual sort regarding the issue of denial: does this mechanism operate in everyone? How can doctors tell whether or not the mechanism of denial is operative in a particular patient? If they cannot really know, should this inability affect their decision to tell or not to tell patients the truth?

Even apart from the philosophically problematic issues surrounding the notion of rights, the answer to the question of what doctors ought to tell patients is complicated by still other factors. These factors are related to some issues that are dealt with in the section concerning paternalism on the part of physicians. This sometimes takes the form of an appeal to the medical knowledge and therapeutic expertise of doctors; specifically, their medical knowledge and experience are cited as reasons why they know best when, what, and how much to tell patients. Occasionally other sorts of factors are mentioned—for example, the greater likelihood that the physician will be more rational and objective about the patient's condition than the patient himself; hence, whatever sorts of decisions might need to be made are more appropriately made by the doctor than by the patient, who may be highly emotional or under stress. But simply pointing these factors out does not provide a solution to the question of what to tell patients or whether or not to withhold information. An argument still needs to be offered to show that acts of paternalism are *justified* in such situations, in order to rebut the opposing view that patients have "the right to know" all the relevant facts about their own condition. If, as some people argue, the physician's obligation not to allow harm to befall his patients is the primary moral consideration, then the solution to this problem tends to favor the physician's discretionary judgments. If, on the other hand, insuring the rights of patients and maintaining the autonomy of adult persons are the major moral considerations, then the solution seems to be that physicians should tell patients all they want to know. But here again, there will always be debates about how to determine whether or not a patient "really" wants to know, so some judgments will inevitably have to be made by even the most frank and open physicians. As we shall see in some of the cases presented in this section, perhaps a measure of paternalism is justifiable; but this cannot simply be assumed, it must be demonstrated with cogent reasons.

Turning to the range of issues in the section entitled "Informed Consent and Coercion," we find that many of the same problems reappear. There are two closely related concerns to which the readings in this section are addressed: one of these is primarily ethical and the other is concerned with knowledge or belief. With respect to the latter, it is evident that the notion of "being informed" is none too clear. A great variation exists in both the amount and kind of information that one may possess, and as a result, there are different degrees of being informed. A question that demands some careful reflection is: *How much* information and *what specific sorts* of information ought a person have before his consent can properly be said to be "informed?" This question and a number of closely related ones are debated in the selections by Ingelfinger and Demy, while Preston Burnham responds to the problem satirically in his "consent form for hernia patients." Many physicians claim that patients, or lay persons in general, can never be fully informed in the requisite sense; in order to meet such a requirement, patients would have to know as much as the physician knows about diseases, risks, complications, statistics about similar cases, and perhaps a range of other facts. If being fully informed entails the possession of knowledge of this scope and depth, consent could rarely be given for most routine therapeutic procedures, much less for a variety of experimental procedures employing human subjects. We must, then, reasonably expect to adopt some standard other than "full and complete information" on which to base consent. A problem still remains in determining precisely what this standard should be. Focus should probably lie in the area of ascertaining what information is *relevant* to a patient's or experimental subject's granting consent, and even though judgments about relevance are also subject to dispute, the problem seems to be more manageable.

Aside from these issues concerning what it is to be informed and how we can tell in any specific case when a person really is informed, there are a number of closely related concerns that have moral implications. One is the question of the *ability or competence* of persons to give their consent; another issue is the *way* in which consent is obtained; and still another relates to the occasional *need to gain consent from someone other than the patient* himself. All these overlap and raise many of the same problems, but each has a somewhat different focus. In thinking about the topic of informed consent, we need to distinguish a variety of specific issues, conceptual as well as ethical. The conceptual ones include an inquiry into the concept of *competence,* in the sense required for a person to grant his consent for research or treatment. This, in turn, would probably lead to a discussion of the concept of *rationality:* Are the mentally ill, the emotionally disturbed, or children rational enough to be considered competent?

A somewhat different set of conceptual issues arises in connection with the notion of *voluntariness,* in the sense of "uncoerced" actions. In addition to being informed, consent must also be *voluntary,* or *uncoerced.* This is the area in which most of the moral problems concerning the use of prisoners as experimental subjects come up; some of these issues are also involved with other institutionalized populations such as the aged and the retarded. Several of our selections here are concerned with the ethics of experimenting on these special classes of persons, demonstrating the interrelationship of the various conceptual and ethical concerns just discussed. Two recent cases that achieved some prominence were: first, the case of the experiments at Willowbrook State School, in which hepatitis virus was injected into retarded youngsters in residence there; and second, the cancer research conducted on terminally ill, hospitalized old persons into whom living cancer cells were injected. In both cases, discussed below in the selection entitled "The Willowbrook Controversy" and in the article by Elinor Langer, the chief moral issue was the failure to obtain informed consent properly. However, it is worth noting that the circumstance of *dependency* on the part of these classes of persons is what rendered them much more accessible to medical researchers than normal persons in normal circumstances are likely to be.

We observed earlier how the patient role tends to confer a dependent status on those who occupy it. In addition, we may easily identify several special classes of "dependent persons" who suffer reduced autonomy. These categories include children, mentally retarded persons, the aged, prisoners, and the mentally ill—especially those emotionally disturbed persons who are institutionalized. Such people are generally considered less capable of autonomous decisions and actions than are normal adults; thus they are more susceptible to coercive measures and paternalistic acts undertaken on their behalf. But although some of these individuals are dependent because of less-than-normal capacity to think or reason or make judgments, others, such as prisoners, are rendered dependent in special ways by the actions of society. What is especially important about all these groups of persons is the way in which they have been used in medical research and scientific experimentation.

Our moral sentiments and beliefs in the field of medical ethics reflect the overall value scheme or ethical system that we hold, and such background assumptions need to be acknowledged explicitly. What are some of these background assumptions and how do they bear on moral problems in medicine, in particular? For one thing, our culture values highly the autonomy of persons—their independence and self-reliance, their ability to do things for themselves. Freedom from authoritarian rule and dislike of totalitarian practices serve to characterize not only our political democratic ideals but also, in large measure, our social institutions, including the family; one can readily observe the anti-authoritarian and anti-paternalistic bias that pervades American values.

In addition to the condition of being genuinely *informed,* a patient or experimental subject is supposed to give truly *voluntary* consent. But how can we tell when voluntariness is present or not? There are paradigm cases of coerced actions—such as yielding one's wallet to a gunman—which are performed under threat of violence or some other negative sanction. But we still have a problem in deciding what criteria to employ in judging when informed consent is truly voluntary and when it represents a decision under some form of coercion, however subtle.

If prisoners are told that they may be granted an early parole if they volunteer for some research, are they acting under a form of coercion if they volunteer? Suppose they are not even promised early parole, but rather, simply believe that volunteers will receive better treatment in general at the hands of prison officials. Can their consent to participate in experiments be viewed as truly voluntary? (These and other aspects of the ethical issues surrounding the use of prisoners in research are discussed in the selections by Jessica Mitford and Robert Marston.) Those who favor the continued use of prisoners in medical research argue that much basic medical research would not get done and medical science would not progress as rapidly, if at all, in some areas if prisoners were not used as subjects. Others object that it is never justifiable to use human beings in experimental situations that pose serious risks, even if one has taken all the steps possible to ensure that consent is truly voluntary and informed. As is often the case in these disputes, moral issues are inextricably intertwined with conceptual matters, and care is needed in sorting out the problems.

As we have observed, prisoners are not the only group of "dependent persons" about whom it is claimed that an element of coercion is always present in medical settings. The use of prisoners occurs chiefly in experimental and research activities, but questions of coercion arise also in treatment contexts. Here the most obvious class of dependent persons is that of children. Whether in therapeutic or in experimental settings, judgment about the proper handling of children remains a major problem in medical ethics. Conflicts concerning the treatment of children in therapeutic or experimental settings cannot be dismissed simply by pointing to the fact that parents or guardians are legally empowered to make decisions involving their minor children. The question is not what the law says in these issues, but rather, what is the morally best way to proceed in problematic cases. Do parents have the moral right to offer their minor children as experimental subjects in medical research where some risks to the child may be involved? Moreover, is there not a crucial difference between infants and young children and those who may still be legally minors but who in many other respects have attained full maturity? At what age is it appropriate to consider a child capable of making decisions for himself? And if, as is likely, no one specific chronological age can be deemed *the* correct age, what criteria are to be employed, and how, in practice, could these criteria be meaningfully applied? The fact that there is no clear and obviously correct answer to these and other problematic questions in medical ethics does not mean that we must despair of ever finding ethically sound solutions to such dilemmas. It does mean, however, that careful thought should continue to be given to these matters, in the hope of coming to a reasoned, reflective solution that is neither too dogmatic nor inclines too much toward a skeptical relativism.

One type of interference with the autonomous actions of other persons should be singled out for special attention. Such acts may involve coercive measures of various sorts, or they may be done in the absence of fully informed consent. What is special about this class of actions is its justification: acts of interference with other persons' autonomy are often justified by the claim that the acts are for the *benefit* or *welfare* of those who are being interfered with. The selections by Mill and Dworkin explore some general issues related to paternalism, and the essay by Anna Freud discusses a few of the less obvious aspects of paternalism in the doctor-patient relationship. Two specific examples of medical practices for which paternalistic justifications are offered are discussed in the remaining selections: sterilization of mentally retarded youth, and surgery on Jehovah's Witnesses who refuse blood transfusions on religious grounds.

In all classes of dependent persons, similar ethical issues arise. Both the aged and the retarded may suffer from impaired mental capacity, and both may also have physical disorders and deviant behavioral characteristics that make them significantly dependent on other people, whether family members or staff personnel in institutions. It is natural and, perhaps, even necessary in some instances to assume a paternalistic attitude toward such persons. And it is not uncommon to have the situation complicated when such an attitude is sensed by the dependent individuals; the situation may then be worsened rather than improved. This type of dependency makes the elderly and the retarded especially vulnerable to a variety of experimental treatments, only some of which might benefit them, and hence, could possibly be justified on paternalistic grounds.

The mentally ill and the mentally retarded are often treated in ways that primarily benefit society rather than themselves, although there may be arguable benefits, in many cases, for the treated persons themselves. Examples that come readily to mind are the enforced sterilization of retarded young adults, and involuntary confinement of persons believed to be mentally ill. It is clear why these activities pose moral problems, whichever position one adopts with respect to them. Confining persons deemed mentally ill to mental institutions without their consent—the practice known as civil commitment, or involuntary hospitalization—is a legally sanctioned practice in our society. But it is still an open question whether such a coercive measure is morally right or ethically permissible. Only if we believe that the "mentally ill" have lost their civil liberties by virtue of acting queerly —remember, not criminally—do we have an easy time justifying civil commitment. On the other side of the coin, of course, lie the legitimate interests of other family members and society at large, which must be weighed against the rights of a person who is to be involuntarily confined. The problem is complicated by the fact that individuals can be dependent in some respects and still be able to make some reflective judgments about their own capacities, as illustrated in "Who Will Tie My Shoe?."

Are mentally ill persons more like children or more like autonomous adults? If they are more like children, in relevant respects, then perhaps a measure of paternalism is justifiable. If, on the other hand, they are simply a bit more deviant in their ways than the rest of us, we need to question whether paternalistically motivated coercive measures are morally justifiable or whether they merely reflect our intolerance of certain forms of aberrant but noncriminal behavior.

Most people agree that consent for research or treatment must be voluntary, granted by mentally competent, rational agents, and properly informed. All of these concepts require clear analysis and explication so that we can develop useful and applicable criteria *in practice* when informed consent must be obtained. It is especially important to protect those individuals who are incapable of providing fully informed or fully voluntary consent on their own behalf, thus necessitating an inquiry into justifiable and unjustifiable modes of paternalism. In the absence of a careful analysis of these issues, we risk making our practical criteria too weak or too strong, too vague or too ambiguous, and therefore, inappropriate or hard to apply. Philosophical analysis can help us sharpen our thinking and reasoning, not only for abstract or theoretical purposes but also to aid in developing clear, practical criteria for *applying* the concept of informed consent, along with other central concepts in medical ethics.

R.M.

THE PHYSICIAN-PATIENT RELATIONSHIP

From "The Basic Models of the Doctor-Patient Relationship"

Thomas S. Szasz and Marc H. Hollender

The question naturally arises as to "What is a doctor-patient relationship?" It is our aim to discuss this question and to show that certain philosophical preconceptions associated with the notions of "disease," "treatment," and "cure" have a profound bearing on both the theory and the practice of medicine.

WHAT IS A HUMAN RELATIONSHIP?

The concept of a relationship is a novel one in medicine. Traditionally, physicians have been concerned with "things," for example, anatomical

Excerpted, with authors' and publisher's permission, from the *A.M.A. Archives of Internal Medicine* 97:585–92, 1956. Copyright 1956, American Medical Association.

structures, lesions, bacteria, and the like. In modern times the scope has been broadened to include the concept of "function." The phenomenon of a human relationship is often viewed as though it were a "thing" or a "function." It is, in fact, neither. Rather it is an abstraction, appropriate for the description and handling of certain observational facts. Moreover, it is an abstraction which presupposes concepts of both structure and function.

The foregoing comments may be clarified by concrete illustrations. Psychiatrists often suggest to their medical colleagues that the physician's relationship with his patient "per se" helps the latter. This creates the impression (whether so intended or not) that the relationship is a thing, which works not unlike the way that vitamins do in a case of vitamin deficiency. Another idea is that the doctor-patient relationship depends mainly on what the physician does (or thinks or feels). Then it is viewed not unlike a function.

When we consider a relationship in which there is joint participation of the two persons involved, "relationship" refers to neither a structure nor a function (such as the "personality" of the physician or patient). It is, rather, an abstraction embodying the activities of two interacting systems (persons).

THREE BASIC MODELS
OF THE DOCTOR-PATIENT RELATIONSHIP

The three basic models of the doctor-patient relationship . . . , which we will describe, embrace modes of interaction ubiquitous in human relationships and in no way specific for the contact between physician and patient. The specificity of the medical situation probably derives from a combination of these modes of interaction with certain technical procedures and social settings.

1. The Model of Activity-Passivity. Historically, this is the oldest conceptual model. Psychologically, it is not an interaction, because it is based on the effect of one person on another in such a way and under such circumstances that the person acted upon is unable to contribute actively, or is considered to be inanimate. This frame of reference (in which the physician does something to the patient) underlies the application of some of the outstanding advances of modern medicine (e.g., anesthesia and surgery, antibiotics, etc.). The physician is active; the patient, passive. This orientation has originated in—and is entirely appropriate for—the treatment of emergencies (e.g., for the patient who is severely injured, bleeding, delirious, or in coma). "Treatment" takes place irrespective of the patient's contribution and regardless of the outcome. There is a similarity here between the patient and a helpless infant, on the one hand, and between the physician and a parent, on the other. It may be recalled that psychoanalysis, too, evolved from a procedure (hypnosis) which was based on this model. Various physical measures to which psychotics are subjected today are another example of the activity-passivity frame of reference.

2. The Model of Guidance-Cooperation. This model underlies much of medical practice. It is employed in situations which are less desperate than those previously mentioned (e.g., acute infections). Although the patient is ill, he is conscious and has feelings and aspirations of his own. Since he suffers from pain, anxiety, and other distressing symptoms, he seeks help and is ready and willing to "cooperate." When he turns to a physician, he places the latter (even if only in some limited ways) in a position of power. This is due not only to a "transference reaction" (i.e., his regarding the physician as he did his father when he was a child) but also to the fact that the physician possesses knowledge of his bodily processes which he does not have. In some ways it may seem that this, like the first model, is an active-passive phenomenon. Actually, this is more apparent than real. Both persons are "active" in that they contribute to the relationship and what ensues from it. The main difference between the two participants pertains to power, and to its actual or potential use. The more powerful of the two (parent, physician, employer, etc.) will speak of guidance or leadership and will expect cooperation of the other member of the pair (child, patient, employee, etc.). The patient is expected to "look up to" and to "obey" his doctor. Moreover, he is neither to question nor to argue or disagree with the orders he receives. This model has its prototype in the relationship of the parent and his (adolescent) child. Often, threats and other undisguised weapons of force are employed, even though presumably these are for the patient's "own good." It should be added that the possibility of the exploitation of the situation—as in any relationship between persons of unequal power—for the sole benefit of the physician, albeit under the guise of altruism, is ever present.

   3. The Model of Mutual Participation.   Philosophically, this model is predicated on the postulate that equality among human beings is desirable. It is fundamental to the social structure of democracy and has played a crucial role in occidental civilization for more than two hundred years. Psychologically, mutuality rests on complex processes of identification—which facilitate conceiving of others in terms of oneself—together with maintaining and tolerating the discrete individuality of the observer and the observed. It is crucial to this type of interaction that the participants (1) have approximately equal power, (2) be mutually interdependent (i.e., need each other), and (3) engage in activity that will be in some ways satisfying to both.

   This model is favored by patients who, for various reasons, want to take care of themselves (at least in part). This may be an overcompensatory attempt at mastering anxieties associated with helplessness and passivity. It may also be "realistic" and necessary, as, for example, in the management of most chronic illnesses (e.g., diabetes mellitus, chronic heart disease, etc.). Here the patient's own experiences provide reliable and important clues for therapy. Moreover, the treatment program itself is principally carried out by the patient. Essentially, the physician helps the patient to help himself.

   In an evolutionary sense, the pattern of mutual participation is more highly developed than the other two models of the doctor-patient relationship. It requires a more complex psychological and social organization on the part of both participants. Accordingly, it is rarely appropriate for children or for those persons who are mentally deficient, very poorly educated, or profoundly immature. On the other hand, the greater the intellectual, educational, and general experiential similarity between physician and patient the more appropriate and necessary this model of therapy becomes.

THE BASIC MODELS AND
THE PSYCHOLOGY OF THE PHYSICIAN

Consideration of why physicians seek one or another type of relationship with patients (or seek patients who fit into a particular relationship) would carry us beyond the scope of this essay. Yet, it must be emphasized that as long as this subject is approached with the sentimental viewpoint that a physician is simply motivated by a wish to help others (not that we deny this wish), no scientific study of the subject can be undertaken. Scientific investigation is possible only if value judgment is subrogated, at least temporarily, to a candid scrutiny of the physician's actual behavior with his patients.

The activity-passivity model places the physician in absolute control of the situation. In this way it gratifies needs for mastery and contributes to feelings of superiority. At the same time it requires that the physician disidentify with the patient as a person.

Somewhat similar is the guidance-cooperation model. The disidentification with the patient, however, is less complete. The physician, like the parent of a growing child, could be said to see in the patient a human being potentially (but not yet) like himself (or like he wishes to be). In addition to the gratifications already mentioned, this relationship provides an opportunity to recreate and to gratify the "Pygmalion Complex." Thus, the physician can mold others into his own image, as God is said to have created man (or he may mold them into his own image of what they should be like, as in Shaw's "Pygmalion"). This type of relationship is of importance in education, as the transmission of more or less stable cultural values (and of language itself) shows. It requires that the physician be convinced he is "right" in his notion of what is "best" for the patient. He will then try to induce the patient to accept his aims as the patient's own.

The model of mutual participation, as suggested earlier, is essentially foreign to medicine. This relationship, characterized by a high degree of empathy, has elements often associated with the notions of friendship and partnership and the imparting of expert advice. The physician may be said to help the patient to help himself. The physician's gratification cannot stem from power or from the control over someone else. His satisfactions are derived from more abstract kinds of mastery, which are as yet poorly understood.

It is evident that in each of the categories mentioned the satisfactions of physician and patient complement each other. This makes for stability in a paired system. Such stability, however, must be temporary, since the physician strives to alter the patient's state. The comatose patient, for example, either will recover to a more healthy, conscious condition or he will die. If he improves, the doctor-patient relationship must change. It is at this point that the physician's inner (usually unacknowledged) needs are most likely to interfere with what is "best" for the patient. At this juncture, the physician either changes his "attitude" (not a consciously or deliberately assumed role) to complement the patient's emergent needs or he foists upon the patient the same role of helpless passivity from which he (allegedly) tried to rescue him in the first place. Here we touch on a subject rich in psychological and sociological complexities. The process of change the physician must undergo to have a mutually constructive experience with the patient is similar to a very familiar process: namely, the need for the parent to behave ever differently toward his growing child. . . .

The issue of agreement is of interest because it has direct bearing on the three models of the doctor-patient relationship. In the first two models "agreement" between physician and patient is taken for granted. The comatose patient obviously can not disagree. According to the second model, the patient does not possess the knowledge to dispute the physician's word. The third category differs in that the physician does not profess to know exactly what is best for the patient. The search for this becomes the essence of the therapeutic interaction. The patient's own experiences furnish indispensable information for eventual agreement, under otherwise favorable circumstances, as to what "health" might be for him. . . .

To illustrate this thesis let us consider some examples. A typical comparison, with which we can begin, is that of the various agents used in the treatment of lobar pneumonia: type-specific antisera, sulfonamides, and penicillin. Each superseded the other, as the increased efficacy of the newer preparations was demonstrated. This sort of comparison is meaningful because there is agreement as to what is being treated and as to what constitutes a "successful" result. There should be no need to belabor this point. What is important is that this conceptual model of therapeutic comparisons is constantly used in situations in which it does not apply; that is, in situations in which there is clear-cut disagreement as to what constitutes "cure." In this connection, the problem of peptic ulcer will exemplify a group of illnesses in which several therapeutic approaches are possible.

This question is often posed: Is surgical, medical or psychiatric treatment the "best" for peptic ulcer? Unless we specify conditions, goals, and the "price" we are willing to pay (in the largest sense of the word), the question is meaningless. In the case of peptic ulcer, it is immediately apparent that each therapeutic approach implies a different conception of "disease" and correspondingly divergent notions of "cure." At the risk of slight overstatement, it can be said that according to the surgical viewpoint the disease is the "lesion," treatment aims at its eradication (by surgical means), and cure consists of its persistent absence (nonrecurrence). If a patient undergoes a vagotomy and all evidence of the lesion disappears, he is considered cured even if he develops another (apparently unrelated) illness six months later. It should be emphasized that no criticism of this frame of reference is intended. The foregoing (surgical) approach is entirely appropriate, and accusations of "narrowness" are no more (nor less) justified than they would be against any other specialized branch of knowledge.

To continue our analysis of therapeutic comparisons, let us consider the same patient (with peptic ulcer) in the hands of an internist. This specialist might have a somewhat different idea of what is wrong with him than did the surgeon. He might regard peptic ulcer as an essentially chronic disease (perhaps due to heredity and other "predispositions"), with which the patient probably will have to live as comfortably as possible for years. This point is emphasized to demonstrate that the surgeon and the internist do not treat the "same disease." How then can the two methods of treatment and their results be compared? The most that can be hoped for is to be able to determine to what extent each method is appropriate and successful within its own frame of reference.

If we take our hypothetical patient to a psychoanalyst, the situation is even more radically different. This specialist will state that he is not treating the "ulcer" and might even go so far as to say that he is not treating the patient for his ulcer. The psychoanalyst (or psychiatrist) has his own ideas about what constitutes "disease," "treatment," and "cure."

From "The Doctor and Death"

August M. Kasper

The physician's training stresses "scientific objectivity," and physicians are often fond of mistaking themselves for scientists. There are some very useful similarities between science and medicine, but whereas a scientist is interested in death, a doctor is against it. It is indeed possible to be a physician and a scientist, but it is a rare combination in practice. The physician qua physician is committed to a credo which is far different from that of the scientist, even if we insist that such tenets as knowability, order, and inductive method are articles of faith. Medical practitioners have the wistful audacity, thank God, to blindly insist that pain is bad and life is to be preserved. This patent value judgment is the basis of medicine, and only coincidentally has it anything to do with knowledge of observable reality. Some doctors wish to be scientists in order to gain mastery over life by treating people as interesting things. It is this orientation which permits a doctor to speak of a "good" case of leukemia; that is, the case in question corresponds closely to the standard description of a certain disease entity, so that the adjective "good" is correctly, if disturbingly, used. This oddly inhuman perspective makes it possible for the doctor to observe, codify, diagnose, and treat, free from interfering preoccupations with horrors of disease and fear of death. The layman, hearing the doctor so speak and act, often gets the idea that the physician is cold and is treating the patient as a "thing," but the layman doesn't recognize that all such talk and activity is premised on the idea that life should be maintained and pain avoided. I cannot be sure whether it is a good thing or not, but the doctor will often conceal his own fear of pain and death behind his prerogative to be "objective" or "scientific." . . .

There is the frustration of the young doctor's orientation toward the hopelessly ill, toward those whom he knows can respond only with gratitude, and often not even that. These are the people in dreary wards and cheerless rooms. They lie quietly, dreaming perhaps, but looking for all the world like the doctor's "first patient." They need to have certain things done: indolent ulcers must be cleaned, draining wounds dressed, fetid mouths tended, fecal impactions removed, and very often, because no other way will do, they must be sustained by fluids dripped into failing, clogging veins. And this last tenderness gives a name to the whole tour of mercy: "watering the vegetables." The dying are thus not neglected, but they are very rarely approached with hope or even interest, because, I suppose, they simply will not feed the doctor's narcissism by responding and getting well. Their care is demanding, frustrating, and far from helpful to the medical magician's self-esteem.

Later, in the hospital years, one again sees clearly the formal, if unwritten, code: doctors should never become personally "involved" while working at their profession. This is sometimes carried to the extreme I witnessed while an intern. A very competent and kindly surgeon was performing an operation on a nine-year-old boy which could only extend the youngster's life a few weeks longer at the most. During surgery, the doctor remarked that it was a shame that this boy would not live to marry and have sons of his own. The interns, residents, and nurses who heard this remark later speculated about why it had been made. The consensus seemed to be that it was, at least, in bad taste and might even be explained by assuming that the surgeon had been drinking before surgery. They were wrong, I believe; but this very excellent doctor did often drink heavily *after* the day's work. He seemed to have reached the necessary truth, but like the fabled neurotic, he was unhappy about it.

. . . the doctor continues his maternal identification and vicarious dependency by caring for others. This ordinarily works very well because he helps people, and they are grateful and "like" him. But everyone knows how fickle is the affection of the "helped" person, how his dependency is felt as a weakness in which he has submitted to the helper, the physician; the doctor fears and the patient broods on the turning of the tables. The doctor works hard to keep the relationship from changing; traditionally, this omnipotent help is not even contaminated (made realistic) by talk of money for services rendered—as if both parties preferred the God-supplicant arrangement. Besides this, or as part of it, the doctor often is pretty unpleasant about people who don't understand how wonderful he is; on this point, one might consult nurses, curious patients, and Armed Forces personnel who had to command doctors. All this then to indicate that the doctor keeps his power, his patients' love, and his invulnerability by fending off death and illness. And when the magic doesn't work, the doctor who still believes the myth is in serious danger of disillusionment and disgrace. Such a doctor has often treated his patients so highhandedly that the latter will actually sense the situation and find some small comfort in the spiteful revenge of dying. We talk about positive and negative transference, but most doctors accept the first as their normal, just due, and any other reaction as recalcitrance or ingratitude. A convenient notion, an enviable viewpoint, but the doctor who subscribes to it simply cannot face the anger and rejection of the hurt and disappointed patient. Most doctors would rather not ever have to, but it is necessary at times—if only for the reason given by Hippocrates: "And by seeing and announcing beforehand those who will live and those who will die, he will thus escape censure." If we could, without censure, maintain our reputation for omnipotence, I wonder how often we would admit our inadequate skills.

If a doctor's death is dismayingly incredible to the dreamer in everyone, it is even more poignantly noted when a medical man hears of a psychiatrist's suicide, a surgeon's pancreatic cancer, or an internist's coronary occlusion. Here even the initiated are awed by the surrender of the specialist to his intimately familiar foe. Specialization would seem to offer some fascinating opportunities for more specific resolution of the search that leads men into the "noble art." I am not in a position to compare one specialty with another in this regard, but I would like to say a word about my own. Psychiatrists, often thought to be so far from organic disease, pain and death, hear a lot about how these things affect people. But if a surgeon hides behind his mask, a psychiatrist has an even more effective shield. I do not mean the couch, which is good in its way, but rather that wonderful step in intellectualization whereby we alter the quality of reality through nomenclature. This allows us to treat a man's fear of death as we would a fear of things in the dark. In practice, this is a good idea, i.e., it works because phobias are irrational fears. But where there isn't anything in the dark, there is death, and the man who doesn't recognize death is unlikely to preserve his life effectively. So it happens that the psychiatrist can deny death as he denies the apparent source of any other phobia, and some seem to take advantage of this possibility, although Freud wrote, "If you would endure life, be prepared for death." An even more elaborate formulation is often interpreted as meaning that we die because we "wish" it or are physically impelled toward it. Again this may be, but I imagine we would die whether or not it were so. It is the oversimplification and misunderstanding of such concepts that make the playwright and novelist depict us as unctious, smug possessors of secrets that would give man complete freedom from anxiety, guilt, and death. It seems to me however, that psychiatrists are less likely to give this impression now than previously, perhaps because we are understood better and understand more.

Almost all doctors are reluctant to make and reveal serious diagnoses. While touched by pain and saddened by each patient's death, they often contrive to show their feelings in devious and distorted ways. I recently saw a woman in consultation who gave a perceptive picture of the two types of doctors she had encountered during some twenty years of being treated for pulmonary tuberculosis. Doctors had assumed a God-like stature in her mind because her life literally depended on their judgment and treatment. Because of this she was unable to express any resentment directly to them. She said that at one extreme was the doctor who was solicitous, overly kind, protective, but afraid of her illness and its possible consequences. He seemed uncomfortable in touching her and took elaborate, sometimes extreme, precautions against becoming infected by her. He was so concerned and fearful that on many occasions he behaved too conservatively in his treatment and was reluctant to do anything that inconvenienced or hurt her. At the other pole, there was the doctor who was rough, brusque, and practically manhandled her. She liked being so treated to some extent because at least it made her feel respected as a person of some strength. However, this type of man told her very little about her progress, minimized her symptoms, and laughed at her complaints. Once when a chest X ray was made, he only told her that if anything was wrong, he would call her. He then let her worry for several weeks until she finally called him—only to be told that the chest plate was negative, and what the devil did she expect him to do: call every patient who had a negative X ray? The patient said she felt most doctors were probably inclined toward one or the other extreme, and that they were able to be pleasant, warm, and personable only as long as there was nothing seriously wrong with the patient, that is, so far as their own specialty was concerned. It is painfully evident to this woman that technical excellence cannot substitute for personal courage and warmth in the doctor's task to help his patient. She would be happy if she could deceive herself about her doctor, but her sensitivity to his feelings prevents it.

It is often unfortunately true that the seriously or hopelessly ill patient senses the doctor's emotions clearly. The doctor's disillusionment, depending on his maturity, will show as sympathy, anger, disgust, indifference, interest, disappointment, or embarrassment. Though not exhaustive, this list suggests the many ways a patient may perceive how his doom affects his physician. The hardest to bear is indifference because it is so defensive, so weak, that the patient cannot believe that which such a man tells him. I have sometimes seen attitudes closer to anger rouse a man from guilt and dread and keep him emotionally with his family until the real death. Those feelings at the opposite pole—true grief, sympathy—are most supportive for the dying one, not only because he feels loved, but because he then sees that the living need his help. He feels called upon to soothe the physician's hurt, to comfort those who will mourn, to assure men of their dignity. Such a man will live his life to the end, as well and as productively as he ever was able.

And the doctor will help to this end if he can know his own fear and weakness and hope. Realizing the human condition, he will not be too disturbed by his failure and disillusionment. He can function as comforter and, while not promising life, can offer hope.

From *Man, Mind, and Medicine*

Oliver Cope

Mutilation, particularly that involving sexual function, is another common problem encountered by physicians. Yet it has been considered almost not at all by those surgeons forced to practice it. Psychiatrists and an occasional physician are well aware of the emotional turmoil that many patients are thrown into by such mutilations as hysterectomy, mastectomy, orchidectomy, and radical prostatectomy. They understand something of the part the surgeon's personality may play in leading the patient to accept and subsequently manage the deficit, but rarely does the surgeon himself understand, and in his literature little of authoritative nature has been written.

The following account was written by a patient with cancer of the breast. This cancer is the commonest cancer afflicting women and the second commonest cancer known in the total population. Radical mastectomy has been the traditional approach to the management of this cancer for more than 50 years, yet I know of no article in the literature—by surgeon, physician or psychiatrist—dealing with the emotional consequences of the threat of losing the breast.

> My surgeon has asked me to write as directly as possible what I experienced when a lump was found in my right breast some months ago. I, like most other women, had been instructed to examine my breasts regularly to prevent just this emergency. This I had done from time to time, imagining that I did it regularly, so that when during a routine physical examination my medical doctor found a lump in my right breast, my reaction was one of disbelief rather than dismay. It could not be serious. It must just have started. Nothing to worry about, but what a nuisance.
>
> My doctor's suggestion that I should see a gynecologist did not increase my anxiety. His manner reassured me; he didn't seem worried. The gynecologist examined me carefully and he too identified the lump in my breast. His expression sobered. I should have a biopsy he said; the tumor was probably not malignant but should be checked immediately. This I knew was reasonable. I would have, I imagined, no more than the bother of a minor incision, a few days rest, and the incident would be behind me. He suggested that I see a younger man who, he said, did this operation, which he himself no longer performed.
>
> The younger doctor went over my breasts, my neck, my armpits. Then he stepped back. Yes, there was a lump there and I should have a biopsy to determine what it was. Probably it would be benign, but one could take no chances. And I should have it done as soon as possible.
>
> Well, there it was. I had better find out what was entailed. My husband and I were to leave in four days. How long would the biopsy take? If it were positive, how long would I be laid up? Would he please tell me exactly what to plan for?

Reprinted with permission of author and publisher from *Man, Mind, and Medicine* (Philadelphia: J. B. Lippincott Co., 1968), pp. 32–36.

Underneath the straightforwardness of my questions I was experiencing a mounting concern. Would it be cancer? Would I lose my breast? Inconceivable. But, then, the first operation, a biopsy, would be a minor one and should there be a malignancy, I would have time to prepare myself for the more serious operation and its consequences.

A biopsy? Well, this was done while the patient was under the anesthetic. A frozen section was made, and if this should show any malignancy he would proceed to remove the breast at once. Remove my breast, he said. I would go to sleep not knowing and wake up ineradicably altered. Forever. I pressed on, frightened now and angry, determined to know the worst at once in order to deal with it.

"You never do a biopsy first and then an operation?" No, they did not. "Why not?" Well, it was unnecessary to go under the anesthetic twice; easier to do it all at the same time. "Will you take more than the breast?" Well, sometimes, he explained standing there in front of me, it was necessary to remove the glands under the arm, and sometimes even the muscle underneath the arm. And then there would be radiation therapy afterwards to insure that there would be no spreading of the malignancy. "But my arm! It's my right arm! How much will I be able to use it afterwards?" He hesitated. Well, there would be almost normal use, he said, but perhaps the up and down forward movement would be slightly impaired. It would be almost normal.

Almost normal! What was he talking about? Take off your breast, cut out your muscles, and then assure you that you would be almost normal. I was furious. I looked at his young, calm face, and I thought You don't know, What conception have you of what this means? It's just the way it is always done. The way it has been done for years and years. Surgeons always want to tidy things up, anyway. I knew I was not being reasonable, that cancer was a fearsome disease, but at this moment of anguish the cool objectivity of his attitude struck me as being less than humane.

The next few days are a blank. When I told my husband, I made as light of the whole matter as I could; it would be only a minor operation and surely the tumor would be benign. Whether or not he believed me, he helped me by pretending that he did.

But my anxiety overwhelmed me. In the night, I awoke shaking. I would go back to my doctor and tell him that this was impossible, that there must be some other way. It was indecent to be caught like this with no alternatives. It was inhuman. I must be able to act in my own behalf, and make a reasonable choice. I understood now why women, when they found a lump in their breasts, refused to go to a doctor, refused to save their own lives. Rather dead than maimed. (It was never as conscious a choice as this, I suspected, but these were the roots of the delay.) Foolish, short-sighted, ignorant, perhaps, but deep down the intense desire to preserve one's own identity in physical form, to keep one's own life.

It still seemed incredible to me that there should be only one solution, with research going on all the time, impossible that the answer should still be no different from what it had been for fifty or more years. I would go to my doctor and see if he would help me.

Busy as he was, he showed me into his office and listened to my story blurted out rather incoherently. I was on the verge of tears. "If it could be more gradual," I told him, "first a biopsy and then the larger operation if it were necessary. That is how one does with plants. One acclimatizes them to changes in temperature and situation so that they will not die. Can't people be treated as sensitively? Or are there too many of us? Can't human beings be treated as other than bodies?" He looked at me sympathetically from where he sat on the other side of his desk. "Now, don't feel bad, dear. It will be all right." And that was it.

To add to my worry, I found out that my gynecologist did operate on patients with breast tumors but perhaps not on friends. I am his friend and neighbor. Is he avoiding me because my tumor is serious?

The following day the papers, which I was to fill out, came from the hospital. A night's sleep and resolve guided my hand on the page. My name, my address, my Blue Cross number. Did I want a television in the room? Slowly I filled in all the blanks. Plenty of women had this operation and survived very well. If they minded the loss of their breast or their arm muscles, they didn't say so. They stepped along as proudly as ever. Why was I making all this fuss? So what did it matter if you had only one breast? Probably your husband would not mind. Probably. Probably you would get used to it, even to the look of the scar. The scar, what did it look like? No, you would never get used to it. Never. You would just endure it. What lousy luck. I signed the paper.

That night, tossing in the darkness, an alternative came to me. I had a surgeon, a friend who had concern for me as a person. He had operated on my thyroid years ago, and when I had been threatened with a hysterectomy had given me good counsel and helped me to avoid it. He would perhaps help me this time.

My husband went with me to his office high in the new hospital building. Warmly he greeted us. My dossier lay on his desk. "Sit down," he said, "and tell me how you have been since you were last here." He listened quietly to what I had to say. "Suppose we see what is there," he said, "I should be very glad to take care of you."

Again the examining room, but what a difference. Already my confidence was rising, quite irrationally. With deft and skillful fingers he examined my breast. "Yes, you do have lumps, not one but several," and he showed me small, very small points under the surface of my breast. "How could I not have noticed?" I wondered.

When I had dressed, I went again into his office. He sat at his desk, hands folded. "Let me tell you what I do," he said. "I first operate, remove the tumor and do a frozen section. But I do nothing more surgically. I do not remove your breast. What I do is to treat the cancer with radiation therapy, first under your arm and the entire breast and then on the other side of the breast on the front of your chest. This prevents the spread of cancer without surgery. You will not have changed at all physically. You will be the same as ever. The radiation therapy will take about six weeks. You will have to be careful of being in the sun for some time afterwards, but that will be all. This, I believe, is just as effective a way of dealing with such a condition."

Later, I was to understand all the whys and wherefores, when he explained to me in detail the sound reasons why he found that this method of treatment was preferable to the other, and why ten years ago he had adopted it, and how statistically the results were the same, perhaps even a little better than when radical surgery was used. But at the moment, all I could feel was the intense flood of relief and gratitude that surged inside of me. I would not lose my breast. I would not be disfigured. I would have full use of my arm. I need not undergo a prolonged recovery, and never, never need face myself in the mirror with the right breast cut off. I was rescued.

From "Medical Ethics: Professional or Universal?"

Robert M. Veatch

There is an obvious tone of idealism in the claim that the individual layman's inputs into decision-making should be maximized. The professional would rightly claim that this, if carried to extremes, would complicate his task to the point of absurdity. He would have to spend hours explaining the technical details and policy options to each patient. For choices which are ethically trivial and technically complex this is just impossible. The more trivial the value alternatives involved, the less technically complex the choices have to be to make informed decision-making by the layman needlessly wasteful. Laymen are willing to spend more time and money paying professionals to clarify the options for them when the decision involves experimental heart surgery than when it involves which brand of antacid to use. This does not mean, however, that the layman should not be routinely consulted for decisions such as whether to use a generic name drug which should be cheaper but (under present FDA controls) perhaps more variable than the brand name drug.

Nevertheless, the professionals are right. It is logically and logistically impossible to defer every decision to the layman. This does not mean, however, that the decision reverts to the professional in his professional role because of his superior technical skills, his unique set of norms, or his superior ability in reaching ethical judgments. It may revert to him—it must in many cases—but it will revert to him as another human being with no necessarily superior decision-making skills. He may be using the layman's system of values. If he is dedicated, he will try to do so when it does not conflict with his own and will consciously withdraw from the case when it does; but he may be using a system which is quite at odds with the patient's. If the secondary factors of group identification and cultural system of meaning are significant in the decision-making process, the odds may be quite good that it is different from the patient's. When we are dealing in trivialities in medically serious situations such as the brand of compress to use to close a serious arterial wound, the value system conflict may be nearly irrelevant, but we should not overlook the fact that it is still there. A system of decision-making which is rooted in a universal, human ethic may still call on the professional to make many decisions; it certainly will insist that he practice his trade ethically; but the decisions he makes will be made within a universal frame of reference, one which is not unique to the profession he is practicing.

The conclusion to which one is led is that medical ethics must not be thought of as a special "professional ethic" at all, but as a specific application of the universal norms of ethical action. Those traditional and more modern codes of ethics and professional responsibility which are rooted in relativistic norms which cannot be universalized must be distinguished from those which have more universal foundations. The universally rooted principles of medical ethics are extremely important for curbing certain kinds of excesses and hastily-conceived actions. The professional codes of medical ethics, on the other hand, are not only irrelevant—if that were the case we could just ignore them. They are actually dangerous diversions which lead professionals to believe that there is a special type of ethics appropriate for their own professional discipline. Rather, we must first reject the fallacy of generalization of expertise—that expertise about the technical facts of a given area also gives one expertise in the evaluative factor required for decision-making in that area. ... Special norms or a special process of balancing norms cannot exist for a professional group without collapsing into ethical relativism and particularism. Expertise in ethical decision-making in questions relevant to a profession may reside in certain members of that profession, but other members of that profession may be particularly deficient in that skill, and on balance there is no evidence of a quantum difference in this regard between professionals and laymen. Finally, although professional review committees may be appropriate for certain limited functions, such as protecting the interests of the profession from the gross offenses of certain of its members, without the premises which have just been rejected, there is no theoretical reason for relying on these committees for adjudication of disputes within a professional area. There is some empirical evidence suggesting that they are not particularly effective and may actually be harmful by diverting the attention of other groups which may take up the cases. Let us hope that, if medical ethics is to emerge as an independent discipline, it is a special case of the universal norms of ethical behavior and not as a special professional ethic.

From "Philosophical Reflections on Experimenting with Human Subjects"

Hans Jonas

EXPERIMENTATION ON PATIENTS

So far we have been speaking on the tacit assumption that the subjects of experimentation are recruited from among the healthy. To the question "Who is conscriptable?" the spontaneous answer is: Least and last of all the

Reprinted with deletions from *Ethical Aspects of Experimentation with Human Subjects,* Spring 1969, by permission of author and *Daedalus,* Journal of the American Academy of Arts and Sciences, Boston, Massachusetts.

sick—the most available source as they are under treatment and observation anyway. That the afflicted should not be called upon to bear additional burden and risk, that they are society's special trust and the physician's particular trust—these are elementary responses of our moral sense. Yet the very destination of medical research, the conquest of disease, requires at the crucial stage trial and verification on precisely the sufferers from the disease, and their total exemption would defeat the purpose itself. In acknowledging this inescapable necessity, we enter the most sensitive area of the whole complex, the one most keenly felt and most searchingly discussed by the practitioners themselves. This issue touches the heart of the doctor-patient relation, putting its most solemn obligations to the test. Some of the oldest verities of this area should be recalled.

THE FUNDAMENTAL PRIVILEGE OF THE SICK

In the course of treatment, the physician is obligated to the patient and to no one else. He is not the agent of society, nor of the interests of medical science, the patient's family, the patient's co-sufferers, or future sufferers from the same disease. The patient alone counts when he is under the physician's care. By the simple law of bilateral contract (analogous, for example, to the relation of lawyer to client and its "conflict of interest" rule), he is bound not to let any other interest interfere with that of the patient in being cured. But manifestly more sublime norms than contractual ones are involved. We may speak of a sacred trust; strictly by its terms, the doctor is, as it were, alone with his patient and God.

There is one normal exception to this—that is, to the doctor's not being the agent of society vis-à-vis the patient, but the trustee of his interests alone—the quarantining of the contagious sick. This is plainly not for the patient's interest, but for that of others threatened by him. (In vaccination, we have a combination of both: protection of the individual and others.) But preventing the patient from causing harm to others is not the same as exploiting him for the advantage of others. And there is, of course, the abnormal exception of collective catastrophe, the analogue to a state of war. The physician who desperately battles a raging epidemic is under a unique dispensation that suspends in a nonspecifiable way some of the strictures of normal practice, including possibly those against experimental liberties with his patients. No rules can be devised for the waiving of rules in extremities. And as with the famous shipwreck examples of ethical theory, the less said about it the better. But what is allowable there and may later be passed over in forgiving silence cannot serve as a precedent. We are concerned with non-extreme, non-emergency conditions where the voice of principle can be heard and claims can be adjudicated free from duress. We have conceded that there are such claims, and that if there is to be medical advance at all, not even the superlative privilege of the suffering and the sick can be kept wholly intact from the intrusion of its needs. About this least palatable, most disquieting part of our subject, I have to offer only groping, inconclusive remarks.

THE PRINCIPLE OF "IDENTIFICATION" APPLIED TO PATIENTS

On the whole, the same principles* would seem to hold here as are found to hold with "normal subjects": motivation, identification, understanding on the part of the subject. But it is clear that these conditions are peculiarly difficult to satisfy with regard to a patient. His physical state, psychic preoccupation, dependent relation to the doctor, the submissive attitude induced by treatment—everything connected with his condition and situation makes the sick person inherently less of a sovereign person than the healthy one. Spontaneity of self-offering has almost to be ruled out; consent is marred by lower resistance or captive circumstance, and so on. In fact, all the factors that make the patient, as a category, particularly accessible and welcome for experimentation at the same time compromise the quality of the responding affirmation that must morally redeem the making use of them. This, in addition to the primacy of the physician's duty, puts a heightened onus on the physician-researcher to limit his undue power to the most important and defensible research objectives and, of course, to keep persuasion at a minimum.

Still, with all the disabilities noted, there is scope among patients for observing the rule of the "descending order of permissibility" that we have laid down for normal subjects, in vexing inversion of the utility order of quantitative abundance and qualitative "expendability." By the principle of this order, those patients who most identify with and are cognizant of the cause of research—members of the medical profession (who after all are sometimes patients themselves)—come first; the highly motivated and educated, also least dependent, among the lay patients come next; and so on down the line. An added consideration here is seriousness of condition, which again operates in inverse proportion. Here the profession must fight the tempting sophistry that the hopeless case is expendable (because in prospect already expended) and therefore especially usable; and generally the attitude that the poorer the chances of the patient the more justifiable his recruitment for experimentation (other than for his own benefit). The opposite is true.

NONDISCLOSURE AS A BORDERLINE CASE

Then there is the case where ignorance of the subject, sometimes even of the experimenter, is of the essence of the experiment (the "double blind"-control group-placebo syndrome). It is said to be a necessary element of the scientific process. Whatever may be said about its ethics in regard to normal subjects, especially volunteers, it is an outright betrayal of trust in regard to the patient who believes that he is receiving treatment. Only supreme importance of the objective can exonerate it, without making it less of a

*Early in this essay, Jonas argues that morally permissible use of human beings in medical experimentation requires that they be those persons with a maximum of identification, understanding, and spontaneity—the most highly motivated, the most highly educated, and the least "captive" members of the community. Ed.

transgression. The patient is definitely wronged even when not harmed. And ethics apart, the practice of such deception holds the danger of undermining the faith in the *bona fides* of treatment, the beneficial intent of the physician—the very basis of the doctor-patient relationship. In every respect, it follows that concealed experiment on patients—that is, experiment under the guise of treatment—should be the rarest exception, at best, if it cannot be wholly avoided.

This has still the merit of a borderline problem. This is not true of the other case of necessary ignorance of the subject—that of the unconscious patient. Drafting him for nontherapeutic experiments is simply and unqualifiedly impermissible; progress or not, he must never be used, on the inflexible principle that utter helplessness demands utter protection.

When preparing this paper, I filled pages with a casuistics of this harrowing field, but then scratched out most of it, realizing my dilettante status. The shadings are endless, and only the physician-researcher can discern them properly as the cases arise. Into his lap the decision is thrown. The philosophical rule, once it has admitted into itself the idea of a sliding scale, cannot really specify its own application. It can only impress on the practitioner a general maxim or attitude for the exercise of his judgment and conscience in the concrete occasions of his work. In our case, I am afraid, it means making life more difficult for him.

It will also be noted that, somewhat at variance with the emphasis in the literature, I have not dwelt on the element of "risk" and very little on that of "consent." Discussion of the first is beyond the layman's competence; the emphasis on the second has been lessened because of its equivocal character. It is a truism to say that one should strive to minimize the risk and to maximize the consent. The more demanding concept of "identification," which I have used, includes "consent" in its maximal or authentic form, and the assumption of risk is its privilege.

NO EXPERIMENTS ON PATIENTS UNRELATED TO THEIR OWN DISEASE

Although my ponderings have, on the whole, yielded points of view rather than definite prescriptions, premises rather than conclusions, they have led me to a few unequivocal yeses and noes. The first is the emphatic rule that patients should be experimented upon, if at all, *only* with reference to *their* disease. Never should there be added to the gratuitousness of the experiment as such the gratuitousness of service to an unrelated cause. This follows simply from what we have found to be the *only* excuse for infracting the special exemption of the sick at all—namely, that the scientific war on disease cannot accomplish its goal without drawing the sufferers from disease into the investigative process. If under this excuse they become subjects of experiment, they do so *because,* and only because, of *their* disease.

This is the fundamental and self-sufficient consideration. That the patient cannot possibly benefit from the unrelated experiment therapeutically, while he might from experiment related to his condition, is also true, but lies beyond the problem area of pure experiment. Anyway, I am discussing nontherapeutic experimentation only, where *ex hypothesi* the patient does not benefit. Experiment as part of therapy—that is, directed toward helping the subject himself—is a different matter altogether and raises its own problems, but hardly philosophical ones. As long as a doctor can say, even if only in his own thought: "There is no known cure for your condition (or: You have responded to none); but there is promise in a new treatment still under investigation, not quite tested yet as to effectiveness and safety; you will be taking a chance, but all things considered, I judge it in your best interest to let me try it on you"—as long as he can speak thus, he speaks as the patient's physician and may err, but does not transform the patient into a subject of experimentation. Introduction of an untried therapy into the treatment where the tried ones have failed is not "experimentation on the patient."

Generally, there is something "experimental" (because tentative) about every individual treatment, beginning with the diagnosis itself; and he would be a poor doctor who would not learn from every case for the benefit of future cases, and a poor member of the profession who would not make any new insights gained from his treatments available to the profession at large. Thus, knowledge may be advanced in the treatment of any patient, and the interest of the medical art and all sufferers from the same affliction as well as the patient may be served if something happens to be learned from his case. But this gain to knowledge and future therapy is incidental to the *bona fide* service to the present patient. He has the right to expect that the doctor does nothing to him just in order to learn.

In that case, the doctor's imaginary speech would run, for instance, like this: "There is nothing more I can do for you. But you can do something for me. Speaking no longer as your physician but on behalf of medical science, we could learn a great deal about future cases of this kind if you would permit me to perform certain experiments on you. It is understood that you yourself would not benefit from any knowledge we might gain; but future patients would." This statement would express the purely experimental situation, assumedly here with the subject's concurrence and with all cards on the table. In Alexander Bickel's words: "It is a different situation when the doctor is no longer trying to make [the patient] well, but is trying to find out how to make others well in the future."

But even in the second case of the nontherapeutic experiment where the patient does not benefit, the patient's own disease is enlisted in the cause of fighting that disease, even if only in others. It is yet another thing to say or think: "Since you are here—in the hospital with its facilities—under our care and observation, away from your job (or, perhaps, doomed), we wish to profit from your being available for some other research of great interest we are presently engaged in." From the standpoint of merely medical ethics, which has only to consider risk, consent, and the worth of the objective, there may be no cardinal difference between this case and the last one. I hope that my medical audience will not think I am making too fine a point when I say that from the standpoint of the subject and his dignity there is a cardinal difference that crosses the line between the permissible and the impermissible, and this by the same principle of "identification" I have been invoking all along. Whatever the rights and wrongs of any experimentation on any patient—in the one case, at least that residue of identification is left him that it is his own affliction by which he can contribute to the conquest of that affliction, his own kind of suffering which he helps to alleviate in others; and so in a sense it is his own cause. It is totally indefensible to rob the unfortunate of this intimacy with the purpose and make his misfortune a convenience for the furtherance of alien concerns. The observance of this rule is essential, I think, to attenuate at least the wrong that nontherapeutic experimenting on patients commits in any case.

CONFIDENTIALITY

From "Rights of Privacy in Medical Practice"

Leo J. Cass and William J. Curran

In discussing the relationship between physician and patient, we are brought back constantly to its basic foundations of mutual trust and confidentiality. In Anglo-American law, this is known as "a fiduciary relationship."[1]

In the United States there is a greater, perhaps excessive, interest in the subject of confidentiality: even so, perhaps more thought should be given to it in Britain.

The ethical and legal responsibilities of a confidential relationship for professional people have their narrowest application in what is called in America "a testimonial privilege." This privilege, which is statutory in about two-thirds of our States, allows a patient to prevent his physician from disclosing in court any information obtained as a result of the relationship.[2] In its broadest application, however, it is a part of the individual's *right of privacy.* This right is based on the idea that the details of a person's life are private and should be protected from intrusion; but that this right of privacy should be protected by law is a new concept. It is one of the few legal principles which the United States has *not* borrowed directly from English Common Law. It is a uniquely American doctrine. It had its origins in a paper by Warren and Brandeis.[3] (Louis D. Brandeis gained wide recognition

Reprinted, with deletions, from *The Lancet,* October 16, 1965.

[1]Prosser, W. L. The Law of Torts. St. Louis. 1958.

[2]Dewitt, C. Privileged Communications between Physician and Patient. Springfield. 1958.

[3]Warren, S. D., Brandeis, L. D. *Harvard Law Rev.* 1890, 4. 193.

through his service on the U.S. Supreme Court.) Despite the advocacy of these two lawyers, however, the American courts were slow to enforce the right. Even today, some of the American States still do not recognise its existence in a higher-court case.

A great surge forward in the enforcement of "privacy rights" may be expected soon, however, as a result of the recent decisions of the U.S. Supreme Court in a series of far-reaching civil-rights cases.

Most important of all is the case, decided in June, 1965, where the court struck down as unconstitutional the Connecticut statute barring the *use* of contraceptive devices or drugs even by married couples. The court held that no law could be used to punish acts of intimacy in marriage. In this case[4] the Supreme Court recognised the right of privacy as a fundamental human right guaranteed by the Bill of Rights in the Constitution.

In Britain this right of privacy has not yet received legal recognition.[5] There is, however, a great deal of interest in it. A Bill to establish the right was introduced in the House of Lords in 1961 by Lord Mancroft. It was supported by both Lord Denning and Lord Goddard and came very close to becoming law at that time. Support for this right is continuing to grow and it may soon join the long list of basic rights of man held in common by the United States, Great Britain, and the Commonwealth countries.

PHYSICIAN AND PATIENT

In this paper we concentrate on those aspects of the right of privacy contained in the confidential relationship of physician and patient. The basic ethics of the advisory professions support this concept of confidentiality. The trust of patients rests upon this expected silence. Physicians cannot otherwise demand the truth of patients.

Damage is done to a patient, client, friend, or colleague more often as the result of a careless or boastful revelation than from the evil design or the demands of others outside our professions.

Furthermore the patient's permission to reveal information does not release the physician entirely from his responsibility. The patient's privacy must sometimes be protected in his own interest in spite of appearances to the contrary. The patient must have full knowledge of what he is doing when giving permission and he must do so without coercion. For the physician, there should be an implied limitation on the scope of any release of confidential information—that what is revealed would not be harmful to him. Legally he may be protected in revealing information even though it proves harmful but he will have broken his code of ethics and abused his professional position by permitting a patient to do harm to himself.

One of us (L. J. C.) had a case which caused some concern. A patient, seen at a consultation three years ago, was an alcoholic with cirrhosis and

[4]Griswold *v.* The State of Connecticut. *U.S. Law Week,* 1965, 33, 4587.
[5]Britian, L. The Right of Privacy in England and the United States. *Tulane Law Review,* 1963.

a drug addict. A few months later he sent a health form from a life-insurance company enclosing permission to reveal the findings of the examination. When informed that a full disclosure of his condition would be obligatory and that he should either withdraw permission or recognise the results of a full disclosure the patient sent, by return, a letter of thanks and withdrew his permission. A request from the same insurance company, with permission granted by the widow, revealed that the company were contesting payment of a $200,000 policy. On this request no action was taken since it was felt that a man should not be called upon to give testimony against himself after death when he refused with full knowledge of the consequences during life.

The individual is entitled at all times and under all circumstances to the protection of his confidences when he reveals them to professional advisers. He has even some rights if he reveals confidences to anyone. If confidences are disclosed it may be in violation of the person's right of privacy. If no damage results, there may be no grounds for legal action, even though a breach of ethics has occurred. If the revelation were made by a physician it is a greater infringement and the physician can be held actionable for any damage his patient may suffer, be it to his reputation or to his physical or mental health.

WHEN INFORMATION SHOULD BE REVEALED

When do physicians have a duty to reveal information? The physician may have an obligation to reveal medical facts to other members of the clinical service or to another person in whom there is a legitimate interest in the medical problem, when, by doing so, the best interests of the patient are served. The policy underlying confidentiality is the promotion of the health and welfare of the patient and the reputation of the profession by engendering certainty in the mind of the patient and the public that intimate details or derogatory factors will never be disclosed to the embarrassment or disgrace of a patient.

There are instances, however, when a higher purpose or good outweighs this obligation to the patient. The most obvious example is the duty to inform public officials of a dangerous, contagious disease in a patient which is a threat to the general public. In the United States, such cases come under the statutes called "the reporting laws." These laws are binding upon physicians, who have no choice but to reveal this information to the public authorities responsible. . . .

Papers given at medical meetings concerning the legal aspects of a university health-service have in the past too frequently stressed only one area—protection from the legal risks of malpractice suits. This is an understandable concern for physicians. Like other human beings they are interested in protecting themselves. It is regrettable, however, that so much time and space has been given to this subject. The practice of medicine is the pursuit of a profession. By definition, this means physicians are bound by a code of ethics to act at all times in the best interests of those they serve.

The Law in America and in Britain enforces this responsibility in many aspects. One of the areas where the Law recognises and enforces this ethical imperative is that of keeping confidences by patients. Law and medicine therefore work together to assure what both desire to achieve—the maintenance of the highest standards of altruistic practice in the profession of medicine.

From "Confidentiality and Privileged Communication"

Neil L. Chayet

The murder of 8 student nurses in Chicago and the slaughter of 15 persons in Dallas share many common elements, not the least of which is the significant involvement of the medical profession. In the nurses' case it was a physician who was responsible for the apprehension of Richard Speck, calling the police after he noticed a resemblance to the composite sketch of the suspected killer and the tattoo, "Born to Raise Hell." In Dallas a psychiatrist became the subject of a national discussion when he let it be known that Charles Whitman had given expression to a fantasy of going up to the tower and shooting people.

Both incidents raise the subject of confidentiality, the disclosure of confidential information that a physician has learned from or about his patient during the course of the doctor-patient relation.

What is the responsibility of the physician to inform the police that a past crime has occurred or that a future crime is contemplated? There is no question that the physician who noticed the tattoo acted properly in informing the police, who were conducting a widespread manhunt for the killer, and it is equally evident that the Texas psychiatrist had no clear duty to inform the authorities of Charles Whitman's statement because of the circumstances under which it was made.

The reasons for imposing confidentiality upon the doctor-patient relation go to the very heart of that relation, which, without complete trust in one's physician, is seriously impaired. With Richard Speck, however, it could well be said that no doctor-patient relation had yet arisen, for Speck was treated by the doctor as an emergency case while he was incoherent, and under circumstances that negated any understanding of the relation that he bore to the physician. Even if it could be argued that the doctor-patient relation was established, the doctor would have been justified in going to the police because of the danger to the community that existed while the killer was at large and because of the huge manhunt in progress. It is always

Reprinted with permission of the author and *The New England Journal of Medicine* Vol. 275:18, 1009–10, November 3, 1966. Copyright Massachusetts Medical Society.

permissible to inform the police of the whereabouts of a wanted criminal. The principle of confidentiality may protect medical findings, but it does not serve to prevent the police from finding their suspect.

It is clear that in most jurisdictions the physician is not saddled with the legal responsibility of reporting all crimes which may come to his attention. A few states, such as New Jersey, require that any person who has knowledge of any crime must report such knowledge to the authorities, otherwise he becomes guilty of a crime himself. However, there are no reported cases arising under this statute and it is thus doubtful if it, or statutes similar to it, have ever been enforced. Most states adhere to the more realistic standard of requiring the reporting of certain criminal acts such as gunshot and stab wounds.

The question of confidentiality is a more difficult one for the psychiatrist, particularly when he is confronted by a patient who openly contemplates a future crime. Successful psychotherapy is usually predicated on complete trust by the patient that his statements will be held in strictest confidence. When a future crime is discussed, it often signifies that the therapy is succeeding, and it would be untenable to ask the psychiatrist to rush to the authorities each time a patient revealed thoughts that could be considered criminal in nature. The only exception to this rule is that if the psychiatrist is convinced that his patient is in fact going to commit a crime that will result in injury or harm to persons or property, he must then take appropriate action and must go to the authorities if he is not able to discourage the criminal intent to his satisfaction. No patient has the moral right to convince his psychiatrist that he is going to commit a crime and then expect him to do nothing because of the principle of confidentiality.

Closely related to confidentiality is the question of privileged communication. Confidentiality and privileged communication are often spoken of together and have similar roots, but they are distinctly different concepts. Privileged communication refers only to in-court testimony. It arises when a doctor is asked a question on the witness stand, the answer to which involves the releasing of confidential information that is in the possession of the doctor because of his professional relation with his patient. If his state is one that has a statute that grants "privilege" to the doctor-patient relation he has a privilege not to answer the question. Actually, the privilege belongs to the patient, who may waive it if he wishes. If the privilege is not waived, the doctor is not permitted to answer the question. Statutes making the psychiatrist-patient relation privileged are becoming more common although lawyers and judges often argue that valuable information may be lost to them.

An interesting question would have been posed if Charles Whitman had lived to be tried for his crime. Would his statements to the psychiatrist prior to the crime have been admissible against him to prove his intent to commit the crime? Hopefully not, since the basic right which the criminal defendant has is the right not to testify against himself. Calling to the stand a psychiatrist to whom an admission or confession is made would circumvent this right which is so basic to our legal system. The law should not penalize those who seek psychiatric help by later forcing their psychiatrist to testify.

"Role of Physician and Breach of Confidence"

Henry A. Davidson

The private practitioner is in the most delicate position of all. He is, after all, the patient's personally selected representative. Where the law requires disclosure (as in handling addicts, for instance), the physician's duty is clear: to obey the law. In the more typical case, the practitioner has to decide (1) the likelihood that the patient actually will carry out a threat that may be the product of fantasy only, (2) whether the doctor can persuade the patient to change his plans, (3) whether he can win the patient's agreement to notifying a responsible family member, or (4) whether concern for public safety requires an immediate disclosure. If the doctor keeps it confidential because he assumes that the patient is only playing a game in fantasy, he is taking a risk which he has to calculate himself. But then, medicine is full of risks, and the practitioner unwilling to take them had better move into another profession.

The industrial doctor is in an especially awkward position. He is an agent of both the patient and the employer. If he is to be effective, the patient must trust him. What does the industrial medical officer do when he learns that the executive vice-president is a homosexual or the sales manager is an alcoholic? If he doesn't do something about it, he may be violating a duty to the employer. If he does, he may be breaching a confidence and employees may never again trust him.

In its September, 1966, issue, the journal *Psychiatric Progress* interviewed several leading physicians on this matter and reported the following discussion:[1] "Under what circumstances, if any, is a breach of doctor-patient confidentiality justified? One doctor answered simply: whenever an innocent person might be harmed by keeping the confidence (spreading contagious disease, for example) or whenever the patient might do irreparable harm to himself if the secret were preserved."

Another doctor answered:

> The physician's fundamental purpose is to protect the patient. This includes protecting him from himself. It seems, therefore, that a breach is justified when it clearly benefits the patient. Thus it is incumbent upon us to protect him from becoming a murderer, because his act will not only *result in penalties and punishment to him,* but leads to our second obligation—to protect society when *it* is clearly in danger. When we have a firm feeling that something tragic *will* happen we must act and take whatever course is necessary. But cases differ and you can't make any hard and fast rules. Different physicians will interpret patient material differently.

Another practitioner replied:

Reprinted with permission from "Professional Secrecy" by Henry A. Davidson, in *Ethical Issues in Medicine,* ed. E. Fuller Torrey (Boston: Little, Brown and Co., 1968), pp. 190–94.

[1]Discussion. *Psychiatric Progress* 1:2, 1966.

If I were faced with the question, I would search my conscience and do what I thought was best under the circumstances. In the case of minors (such as some students) a breach of confidence is often permissible because the parents are legally responsible. I always explain to an adolescent that ordinarily I would never tell his parents anything he told me. But when a situation involves the parents I let the patient know that I am going to tell them, even though he may disapprove. I know that the law can demand information, but that doesn't really *justify* releasing it. Sometimes you have to do things for legal reasons that are not justified medically.

The medical director at a large university said:

There are some circumstances that call for a breach of confidence. At our university, we follow the policy of never violating a confidence except under subpoena: and then only after talking it over with the university's legal department. In other situations, one breaches confidentiality only in very unusual circumstances, as with homicide, suicide, or another action which, if not dealt with immediately, might damage the patient or others.

If possible, one tells the patient what is being done and why. If that isn't practical, he can tell the next of kin or another responsible person. If a confidence has to be violated, the doctor should consult with a well-versed person of integrity. It's better to share responsibility than to respond impulsively to being on the spot.

One of the country's leading forensic psychiatrists asserted that: A physician should report confidential information only if convinced of a real danger that the patient will carry out some dangerous act. Just being a nuisance is not enough. Another practitioner replied:

While circumstances vary, it is *never* justifiable to reveal contents of patients' fantasies or ideas when no valid purpose would be served.

But the doctor is justified in breaching a confidence when there is danger to the community or to the individual. The patient should be informed that the situation requires some other intervention and that information about his condition must be shared with a relative.

If the patient is incapable of making a rational decision about action to be taken, the physician is justified in going ahead, having first informed the patient of what is being done. At the same time one indicates to the authority, parent, or spouse, one's concern for the patient.

If a patient says he has committed a criminal act, the physician, after all, does not know whether the information is accurate—it might be delusional. False confessions often follow highly publicized murders. If a patient admits to a criminal act, the doctor has to decide if this is simply a fantasy-projection of guilt feelings, and if any good would be done by reporting it. If an innocent person is in prison when a patient confesses the crime, it would certainly be the duty of the doctor to tell the court. But if a patient says he assaulted someone 10 years ago and that no one has been convicted of the offense, there is scarcely any need to report it. Such decisions require a careful weighing of facts and possibilities, but that is the physician's job.

Another doctor said that it depends

> upon the nature of the crime. If a patient says he's going to forge a check, it wouldn't disturb me. If he says he is going to commit serious bodily injury, it *would* disturb me; my action would depend on whether I felt he was likely to do it.
>
> There are many women, for instance, who say they fear they might kill their children. Usually you know they won't. But if you give credence to such a statement, the first obligation is to inform the family that this is a serious problem and that they should be the motivating force in whatever is done. If they refuse and you still feel that a real danger is involved, you are obligated to report to the police.

An adult must be responsible for his own behavior, but if he cannot be, the physician has to share the responsibility, for the sake of both the individual and other persons.

In universities, the college or infirmary physician has a special problem. Release of intimate information by college authorities may well destroy the doctor's usefulness in the university. The college doctor generally has to decide to do one of three things: (1) absolutely refuse to release the information; (2) urge the student to see an outside (private) doctor and make only minimum notes in the college infirmary file; or (3) try to persuade the students that it would be best to permit the physician to discuss the matter with the dean, his parents, or a guidance counselor. When the chips are down, his college authorities can probably impound and read any record in their own infirmary.

With respect to private practitioners, the road may also be a rocky one. If we lived in a simple and tidy little world, it would be easy to say that the doctor's lips should be permanently sealed. But there are a dozen situations in which the question cannot be disposed of that readily. First, there is the legal requirement to report gunshot wounds and contagious disease. Furthermore, a doctor must not be an accomplice to a crime even in the negative sense of saying nothing. Then there is the problem of protecting public interest when it means revealing a confidence. If you know that the driver of a school bus is an alcoholic or epileptic, you should report it. Last year 30 people were killed when a bus driver had a heart attack and plunged his bus into the East River in New York City. The driver's physician had known about the bad heart, had cautioned him not to drive, but felt he could not report it to the company since the patient might lose his job. In New Jersey some years ago, six people were killed when a bus driver had a petit mal seizure. The treating doctor knew about the epilepsy, pleaded with the patient to stop driving, but didn't think he ought to report it to the motor vehicle department.

More and more patients' bills are being paid by third parties; for example, insurance companies. Medicare, welfare funds, Veterans Administration, relief administrations, Blue Shield, and many others. Most of these facilities will not pay the doctor unless they know the conditions which were treated. Furthermore, it is often no solution to get the patient's signature on an authorization or permission form, since this signature may be required if the patient is going to collect his benefits. In effect, the patient is told: either you waive the confidential nature of your doctor-patient relationship or you don't get the benefit, i.e., the award, the indemnity, the compensation, or whatever it is. Thus the patient may be blackmailed into waiving a precious right or may even be cajoled into signing a document, the import of which he simply does not understand. And once the seal of confidentiality is broken, the doctor-patient relationship is radically and irrevocably altered.

This is one problem that cannot be programmed into a computer. There is still no substitute for personal judgment, the facing of responsibility, and the path-pointing of the human conscience.

"What's an FBI Poster Doing in a Nice Journal Like That?"

Willard Gaylin

The pages of the *Archives of Dermatology*, with their full-color pictures of exotic skin diseases, are likely to strike the uninformed eye as bizarre and somewhat repellent. But even the best informed must have been startled by page 308 of the February 1972 issue. There, occupying almost the entire page, was an FBI wanted poster!

Appearing under the department heading, "News and Notes," the item looked identical to those appearing in police stations and post offices. But both of those are government agencies, and the *Archives* is an official publication of the American Medical Association. The graffiti that passes unnoticed in a subway station would outrage us if written on the wall of a church.

It seems ironic that the AMA, which has consistently opposed government intrusion into medical matters even where a legitimate public interest has been proved, should now have volunteered the services of organized medicine into a government function—and in an area so alien from the traditional medical mission as tracking down criminals.

Of course the thought occurs that it might not have been voluntary. The line between freedom and coercion is not so clearly drawn when the "petitioner" has the power of the Department of Justice. This thought, however, is only the first in the series of ethical and value questions inevitably raised by this eccentric utilization of a medical journal.

The notice, which also appeared in the *Archives of Internal Medicine,* described a 30-year-old woman indicted by a grand jury for "conspiring with another individual" in an act involving the interstate transportation of explosives. The alleged conspiracy violation occurred early in 1970. Along with the usual pictures in various poses, physical description, and biographical material, appeared the statement that she was known to be afflicted with an "acute and recurrent" skin condition. It further elaborates: "The recurrent aspect of this condition could necessitate treatment by a dermatologist." The reason for the FBI's wanting it in the *Archives of Dermatology* now becomes apparent. The reasons for the AMA's willingness to publish it are less immediately evident.

Before even the ethical questions, what is the legal responsibility of the physician reading this? Consultation with a professor of criminal law revealed that there were indeed open questions about liability and responsibility. If he had doubts—what of the average dermatologist?

The implications to the wanted person—who may or may not be a criminal—will also transcend ethical nicety. In this instance a fatal disease is not present—although it well might be in future cases, and it has been indicated that were the condition heart disease, diabetes, glaucoma, acute depression—the wanted notices would be referred to the appropriate journal. They would make it difficult, if not impossible, to get the necessary treatment.

The major question, however, seems to be whether medicine should be encouraged, or even allowed, to be an extension of the police functions of the society. There is no question that if this is seen as a legitimate function of medicine, it would represent a powerful and immense new ally for the police. In the files of physicians across the country are massive case records which would make an invaluable data bank (ready for computerization) of inestimable service in any police tracking function: the drugs one chronically uses, a tendency toward alcoholism, a hidden homosexual activity, proclivity for flirtations or other sexual idiosyncrasies, prescription glasses, specific allergies, dietary requirements, etc.

There is no question that all of this information would facilitate the police functions of the state. But is that the function of medicine? And in facilitating this other function *what would it do to the primary concern of medicine, which is relief of suffering, the treatment of illness, and the saving of life?* What happens to the tradition of confidentiality—so zealously protected over hundreds of years precisely because it has been seen as fundamental to the effective function of medicine? Such use of the profession by the police would represent the final destruction of the privacy, intimacy, and trust of a therapeutic relationship already seriously eroded.

It is conceivable that *in extremis* an institution must abandon its traditional role. The organized church has often supported the mass killing of war when it seemed essential for the survival of the state.

How are we to decide, however, *when* to violate our usual primary devotion and allegiance to the private person and his well-being, for the public purpose? How are we physicians to differentiate quantitatively

amongst the various crimes and conditions of criminality in which we have
no training? Are we prepared to assay indictment versus conviction, versus
material witness, versus "wanted for questioning"? What are the relevant
weights to be placed on conspiracy to blow up a heating system of the
Pentagon, versus armed robbery of a bank, versus possession of marijuana,
versus massive embezzlement? How do we weigh these public dangers
against the health or survival of a patient? Ought we be making these
decisions—or should they be left to public decision-making via the normal
legislative processes which, for example, now dictates that gunshot wounds
demand violation of confidentiality, but by implication of exclusion allows
a host of other material the protection of confidentiality?

Which raises the question of how such significant decisions should be
made. How, for example, are the power and responsibility which influence
the whole balance of medicine and government distributed by a major
organization such as the American Medical Association?

The Association is formed of elected delegates. These delegates, in
turn, as an organization, elect a board. There is an executive secretary who
administers the organization. There is a Judicial Council with its own legal
counsel that acts as an ethical watchdog. At what area of this complex
apparatus was the decision discussed, debated, considered, and finally decided? A call to the Editor of the *Archives of Dermatology* indicated that he had
authority and responsibility only over the scientific articles, and no responsibility for this particular poster. A call to the Director, Division of Scientific
Publications of the American Medical Association, confirmed that the editors
of the specialty journal controlled only that localized aspect. The Chairman
of the Judicial Council said the matter had never been brought to the
Council, and, indeed, he was unaware of the publication of the posters when
first consulted. He then suggested consulting the legal counsel of his committee who has had a long history of dealing with ethical issues and publication. *He* was unaware of the appearance of this FBI poster in the two
publications until he was advised of the fact and, further, he could not recall
its ever having been done before. He volunteered that when consulted in
the past by various state journals, he had cautioned great prudence in
publishing such material. Further calls to a variety of other sources in the
American Medical Association (who must remain anonymous) indicate that
it was "done somewhat experimentally" and spoke vaguely of "a great deal
of pressure," having been exerted.

It was finally established that a request had been made in writing by
the FBI to the Chief of the Division of Scientific Publication of the AMA, and
that he made the decision, seeing no need to consult the Judicial Council,
the representatives of the board of the American Medical Association, or the
Executive Secretary of the American Medical Association and his full-time
professional staff. He indicated that in his mind it was an "editorial decision" of no great moment and implied that it was a part of an ongoing
tradition that preceded his assumption of office three years ago. But Dr.
John Talbott, who formerly held the post, said that, to his memory, never
under his tenure was an FBI poster replicated in either the *Journal of the
American Medical Association* or any of its specialty journals. (This seems

indeed true, although investigation shows that three brief excerpts from "wanted" notices did appear in JAMA early in Dr. Talbott's editorship— 1961 and 1962. None, apparently, has appeared in the past ten years.)

Equally interesting was the gradual shift of the attitude of the staff of the Association when inquiries continued to indicate outside consternation. When they were first notified of the appearance of these pages, all seemed genuinely surprised, felt that the implications were of some moment, and suggested that, in a precedent-breaking move such as this, it seemed unlikely that one man, prudent though he be, would have initiated the action without extensive consultation.

But by the time this initial investigation was concluded, a new official profile was emerging, minimizing the innovation, suggesting it was a routine editorial-type decision, and denying even the presence of a problem. The man who made the decision stated that he would have no hesitation printing more such posters in the future, without advice or consultation, in whatever medical journals the AMA published, particularly when there was a specific medical potential for assisting the FBI, because *"no questions of medical ethics are involved."*

The assumption that there are "no ethical issues involved" seems at this time to be the collective stance of the AMA. A formal statement read over the phone by the Secretary of the AMA Judicial Council also starts with the statement that no issue of ethics is here involved. This may represent the most distressing aspect of this entire episode. Whether the publication of such material by an official medical journal is "ethical" or "unethical" may be debatable (and should be debated). That major ethical issues are raised, however, is indisputable. It involves such basic traditional questions as confidentiality and trust, private needs versus public rights, professional values versus personal ethics, the special role of the healer and saver of life, and the power of the state.

For an individual to want to avoid recognition of error is understandable. For a group to underestimate the implications of any ethical question is certainly no crime. If, however, an entire organization such as the AMA proves so insensitive to questions of ethics as to deny their existence here —it could be disastrous.

From "Ethical Duties Towards Others: Truthfulness"

Immanuel Kant

The exchange of our sentiments is the principal factor in social intercourse, and truth must be the guiding principle herein. Without truth social intercourse and conversation become valueless. We can only know what a man thinks if he tells us his thoughts, and when he undertakes to express them he must really do so, or else there can be no society of men. Fellowship is only the second condition of society, and a liar destroys fellowship. Lying makes it impossible to derive any benefit from conversation. Liars are, therefore, held in general contempt. Man is inclined to be reserved and to pretend. Reserve is *dissimulatio* and pretence *simulatio.* Man is reserved in order to conceal faults and shortcomings which he has; he pretends in order to make others attribute to him merits and virtues which he has not. Our proclivity to reserve and concealment is due to the will of Providence that the defects of which we are full should not be too obvious. Many of our propensities and peculiarities are objectionable to others, and if they became patent we should be foolish and hateful in their eyes. Moreover, the parading of these objectionable characteristics would so familiarize men with them that they would themselves acquire them. Therefore we arrange our conduct either to conceal our faults or to appear other than we are. We possess the art of simulation. In consequence, our inner weakness and error is revealed to the eyes of men only as an appearance of well-being, while we ourselves develop the habit of dispositions which are conducive to good conduct. No man in his true senses, therefore, is candid. Were man candid, were the request of Momus[1] to be complied with that Jupiter should place a mirror in each man's heart so that his disposition might be visible to all, man would have to be better constituted and to possess good principles. If all men were good there would be no need for any of us to be reserved; but since they are not, we have to keep the shutters closed. Every house keeps its dust-bin in a place of its own. We do not press our friends to come into our water-closet, although they know that we have one just like themselves. Familiarity in such things is the ruin of good taste. In the same way we make no exhibition of our defects, but try to conceal them. We try to conceal our mistrust by affecting a courteous demeanour and so accustom ourselves to courtesy that at last it becomes a reality and we set a good example by it. If that were not so, if there were none who were better than we, we should

Reprinted with permission of the publisher from Immanuel Kant, *Lectures on Ethics,* trans. Louis Infield (New York: Harper & Row, 1963), pp. 147–54.

[1]Momus, the god of mockery and censure, demanded that a little door be made in man's breast, that he might see his secret thoughts.

become neglectful. Accordingly, the endeavour to appear good ultimately makes us really good. If all men were good, they could be candid, but as things are they cannot be. To be reserved is to be restrained in expressing one's mind. We can, of course, keep absolute silence. This is the readiest and most absolute method of reserve, but it is unsociable, and a silent man is not only unwanted in social circles but is also suspected; every one thinks him deep and disparaging, for if when asked for his opinion he remains silent people think that he must be taking the worst view or he would not be averse from expressing it. Silence, in fact, is always a treacherous ally, and therefore it is not even prudent to be completely reserved. Yet there is such a thing as prudent reserve, which requires not silence but careful deliberation; a man who is wisely reserved weighs his words carefully and speaks his mind about everything excepting only those things in regard to which he deems it wise to be reserved.

We must distinguish between reserve and secretiveness, which is something entirely different. There are matters about which one has no desire to speak and in regard to which reserve is easy. We are, for instance, not naturally tempted to speak about and to betray our own misdemeanours. Every one finds it easy to keep a reserve about some of his private affairs, but there are things about which it requires an effort to be silent. Secrets have a way of coming out, and strength is required to prevent ourselves betraying them. Secrets are always matters deposited with us by other people and they ought not to be placed at the disposal of third parties. But man has a great liking for conversation, and the telling of secrets adds much to the interest of conversation; a secret told is like a present given; how then are we to keep secrets? Men who are not very talkative as a rule keep secrets well, but good conversationalists, who are at the same time clever, keep them better. The former might be induced to betray something, but the latter's gift of repartee invariably enables them to invent on the spur of the moment something non-committal. . . .

If I announce my intention to tell what is in my mind, ought I knowingly to tell everything, or can I keep anything back? If I indicate that I mean to speak my mind, and instead of doing so make a false declaration, what I say is an untruth, a *falsiloquium*. But there can be *falsiloquium* even when people have no right to assume that we are expressing our thoughts. It is possible to deceive without making any statement whatever. I can make believe, make a demonstration from which others will draw the conclusion I want, though they have no right to expect that my action will express my real mind. In that case I have not lied to them, because I had not undertaken to express my mind. I may, for instance, wish people to think that I am off on a journey, and so I pack my luggage; people draw the conclusion I want them to draw; but others have no right to demand a declaration of my will from me. Thus the famous Law[2] went on building so that people might not guess his intention to abscond. Again, I may make a false statement (*falsiloquium*) when my purpose is to hide from another what is in my mind and when the latter can assume that such is my purpose, his own purpose being

---

[2]The reference is to John Law (1671–1729) and his Mississippi venture.

to make a wrong use of the truth. Thus, for instance, if my enemy takes me by the throat and asks where I keep my money, I need not tell him the truth, because he will abuse it; and my untruth is not a lie (*mendacium*) because the thief knows full well that I will not, if I can help it, tell him the truth and that he has no right to demand it of me. But let us assume that I really say to the fellow, who is fully aware that he has no right to demand it, because he is a swindler, that I will tell him the truth, and I do not, am I then a liar? He has deceived me and I deceive him in return; to him, as an individual, I have done no injustice and he cannot complain; but I am none the less a liar in that my conduct is an infringement of the rights of humanity. It follows that a *falsiloquium* can be a *mendacium*—a lie—especially when it contravenes the right of an individual. Although I do a man no injustice by lying to him when he has lied to me, yet I act against the right of mankind, since I set myself in opposition to the condition and means through which any human society is possible. If one country breaks the peace this does not justify the other in doing likewise in revenge, for if it did no peace would ever be secure. Even though a statement does not contravene any particular human right it is nevertheless a lie if it is contrary to the general right of mankind. If a man spreads false news, though he does no wrong to anyone in particular, he offends against mankind, because if such a practice were universal man's desire for knowledge would be frustrated. For, apart from speculation, there are only two ways in which I can increase my fund of knowledge, by experience or by what others tell me. My own experience must necessarily be limited, and if what others told me was false, I could not satisfy my craving for knowledge. A lie is thus a *falsiloquium in praejudicium humanitatis*, even though it does not violate any specific *jus quaesitum* of another. In law a *mendacium* is a *falsiloquium in praejudicium alterius;* and so it must be in law; but morally it is a *falsiloquium in praejudicium humanitatis.* Not every untruth is a lie; it is a lie only if I have expressly given the other to understand that I am willing to acquaint him with my thought. Every lie is objectionable and contemptible in that we purposely let people think that we are telling them our thoughts and do not do so. We have broken our pact and violated the right of mankind. But if we were to be at all times punctiliously truthful we might often become victims of the wickedness of others who were ready to abuse our truthfulness. If all men were well-intentioned it would not only be a duty not to lie, but no one would do so because there would be no point in it. But as men are malicious, it cannot be denied that to be punctiliously truthful is often dangerous. This has given rise to the conception of a white lie, the lie enforced upon us by necessity—a difficult point for moral philosophers. For if necessity is urged as an excuse it might be urged to justify stealing, cheating and killing, and the whole basis of morality goes by the board. Then, again, what is a case of necessity? Everyone will interpret it in his own way, and, as there is then no definite standard to judge by, the application of moral rules becomes uncertain. Consider, for example, the following case. A man who knows that I have money asks me: "Have you any money on you?" If I fail to reply, he will conclude that I have; if I reply in the affirmative he will take it from me; if I reply in the negative, I tell a lie. What am I to do? If force is used to extort a confession from me, if my confession is improperly used against me, and if I cannot save myself by maintaining silence, then my lie is a weapon of defence. The misuse of a declaration extorted by force justifies me in defending myself. For whether it is my money or a confession that is extorted makes no difference. The forcing of a statement from me under conditions which convince me that improper use would be made of it is the only case in which I can be justified in telling a white lie. But if a lie does no harm to anyone and no one's interests are affected by it, is it a lie? Certainly. I undertake to express my mind, and if I do not really do so, though my statement may not be to the prejudice of the particular individual to whom it is made, it is none the less *in praejudicium humanitatis.* Then, again, there are lies which cheat. To cheat is to make a lying promise, while a breach of faith is a true promise which is not kept. A lying promise is an insult to the person to whom it is made, and even if this is not always so, yet there is always something mean about it. If, for instance, I promise to send some one a bottle of wine, and afterwards make a joke of it, I really swindle him. It is true that he has no right to demand the present of me, but in Idea it is already a part of his own property.

. . . But though we are entitled to form opinions about our fellows, we have no right to spy upon them. Everyone has a right to prevent others from watching and scrutinizing his actions. The spy arrogates to himself the right to watch the doings of strangers; no one ought to presume to do such a thing. If I see two people whispering to each other so as not to be heard, my inclination ought to be to get farther away so that no sound may reach my ears. Or if I am left alone in a room and I see a letter lying open on the table, it would be contemptible to try to read it; a right-thinking man would not do so; in fact, in order to avoid suspicion and distrust he will endeavour not to be left alone in a room where money is left lying about, and he will be averse from learning other people's secrets in order to avoid the risk of the suspicion that he has betrayed them; other people's secrets trouble him, for even between the most intimate of friends suspicion might arise. A man who will let his inclination or appetite drive him to deprive his friend of anything, of his fiancée, for instance, is contemptible beyond a doubt. If he can cherish a passion for my sweetheart, he can equally well cherish a passion for my purse. It is very mean to lie in wait and spy upon a friend, or on anyone else, and to elicit information about him from menials by lowering ourselves to the level of our inferiors, who will thereafter not forget to regard themselves as our equals. Whatever militates against frankness lowers the dignity of man.

From "Truthfulness and Uprightness"

Nicolai Hartmann

VALUATIONAL CONFLICTS BETWEEN TRUTHFULNESS
AND THE SO-CALLED "NECESSARY LIE"

Truthfulness as a value, with its specific moral claim, admits of no exception at all. What is called the necessary lie is always an anti-value—at least from the point of view of truthfulness as a value. No end can justify deliberate deception as a means—certainly not in the sense of causing it to cease to be a moral wrong.

Still we are confronted here with a very serious moral problem, which is by no means solved by the simple rejection of each and every lie. There are situations which place before a man the unescapable alternative either of sinning against truthfulness or against some other equally high, or even some higher, value. A physician violates his professional duty, if he tells a patient who is dangerously ill the critical state of his health; the imprisoned soldier who, when questioned by the enemy, allows the truth about his country's tactics to be extorted from him, is guilty of high treason; a friend, who does not try to conceal information given to him in strictest personal confidence, is guilty of breach of confidence. In all such cases the mere virtue of silence is not adequate. Where suspicions are aroused, mere silence may be extremely eloquent. If the physician, the prisoner, the possessor of confidential information will do their duty of warding off a calamity that threatens, they must resort to a lie. But if they do so, they make themselves guilty on the side of truthfulness.

It is a portentous error to believe that such questions may be solved theoretically. Every attempt of the kind leads either to a one-sided and inflexible rigorism concerning one value at the expense of the rest, or to a fruitless casuistry devoid of all significance—not to mention the danger of opportunism. Both rigorism and casuistry are offences against the intention of genuine moral feeling. The examples cited are so chosen that truthfulness always seems to be inferior to the other value which is placed in opposition to it. It is the morally mature and seriously minded person who is here inclined to decide in favour of the other value and to take upon himself the responsibility for the lie. But such situations do not permit of being universalized. They are extreme cases in which the conflict of conscience is heavy enough and in which a different solution is required according to the peculiar ethos of the man. For it is inherent in the essence of such moral conflicts that in them value stands against value and that it is not possible to escape from them without being guilty. Here it is not the values

From "Truthfulness and Uprightness" by Nicolai Hartmann, reprinted with permission from *Ethics*, vol. 2, trans. Stanton Coit (New York: Humanities Press; London: George Allen and Unwin Ltd., 1932), pp. 281–85.

as such in their pure ideality which are in conflict; between the claim of truthfulness as such and the duty of the soldier or friend there exists no antinomy at all. The conflict arises from the structure of the situation. This makes it impossible to satisfy both at the same time. But if from this one should think to make out a universal justification of the necessary lie, one would err, as much as if one were to attempt a universal justification for violating one's duty to one's country or the duty of keeping one's promise.

Nevertheless a man who is in such a situation cannot avoid making a decision. Every attempt to remain neutral only makes the difficulty worse, in that he thereby violates both values; the attempt not to commit oneself is at bottom moral cowardice, a lack of the sense of responsibility and of the willingness to assume it; and often enough is also due to moral immaturity, if not to the fear of others. What a man ought to do, when he is confronted with a serious conflict that is fraught with responsibility, is this: to decide according to his best conscience; that is, according to his own living sense of the relative height of the respective values, and to take upon himself the consequences, external as well as inward, ultimately the guilt involved in the violation of the one value. He ought to carry the guilt and in so doing become stronger, so that he can carry it with pride.

Real moral life is not such that one can stand guiltless in it. And that each person must step by step in life settle conflicts, insoluble theoretically, by his own free sense of values and his own creative energy, should be regarded as a feature of the highest spiritual significance in complete humanity and genuine freedom. Yet one must not make of this a comfortable theory, as the vulgar mind makes of the permissible lie, imagining that one brings upon oneself no guilt in offending against clearly discerned values. It is only unavoidable guilt which can preserve a man from moral decay.

"Truth, Honesty, and the Therapeutic Process"

Leon Salzman

A basic premise of a therapeutic relationship and an essential part of the contract the patient makes in establishing it is to be honest and truthful. Although the concepts of honesty and truth are rarely mentioned in the psychiatric or psychoanalytic literature, Freud referred to them constantly. He stated:

Reprinted with permission of author and publisher from the *American Journal of Psychiatry* 130: 11, 1281–82, November 1973. Copyright 1973, the American Psychiatric Association.

> The psychoanalytic treatment is founded on truthfulness. A great part of its educative effect and its ethical value lies in this very fact. . . . Since we demand strict truthfulness from our patients, we jeopardize our whole authority if we let ourselves be caught by them in a departure from the truth.[1]

In order for the therapeutic process to be useful to our patients, they must tell us what concerns them, with a minimum of distortion or withholding, to the extent that their emotional capacity and cognitive integrity permit. What is the therapist's part in this arrangement? How much should he tell or withhold from the patient? To communicate our feelings, attitudes, observations, or interpretations to our patients may be essential to the process of therapy, but at times such communication can be destructive. Is this countertransference or simply an essential part of the therapeutic arrangement?

THE DISTINCTION BETWEEN HONESTY AND TRUTH

First, we must clarify our concepts. Honesty is not the same as truth, although the two are related. Webster defines truth as "the state of being the case: fact," while honesty is defined as "fairness and straightforwardness of conduct or adherence to the facts." I would like to suggest that honesty is a dynamic concept that is based on an individual's sincere and objective attempt to appraise a total situation and that is limited by his inability to be totally unbiased. Truth, on the other hand, is a matter of definition and varies according to the framework in which it is established—whether scientifically, as in natural laws, or morally, as determined by man or God. As Oppenheimer has stated, "Truth is so largely defined by how you find it."[2] He meant simply that what is true depends upon how one sets out to determine the truth.

This distinction is crucial in a discussion of the place of truth, honesty, and trust in the therapeutic process. For example, we must recognize that honesty is not exclusively a moral issue, since it is determined by the degree of freedom the person has to explore, express, and determine the truths in his environment. A person's honesty is strongly influenced by the amount of neurotic defenses he has and the degree of distortion he unconsciously imposes on the environment by such behaviors as denial, projection, or dissociation. The degree of honesty a person expresses is determined by the amount of security and self-esteem he has, which allows him to be more or less honest in seeing a situation as it really is. Dishonesty, whether consciously elaborated or unconsciously demonstrated, is a defensive maneuver designed to support a neurotic system. We distinguish between the deliberate and the unconscious liar only because we still tend to assign moral judgments to those types of distortion.

Is the child lying when he tells you about the fire engine drawn by elephants and led by a maharajah, à la Dr. Seuss, or is he simply using his

---

[1]Freud S: Introductory lectures, in Complete Psychological Works, standard ed. Translated and edited by Strachey J. London, Hogarth Press, 1963.

[2]Oppenheimer JR: The Open Mind. New York, Simon and Schuster, 1955.

imagination? Are our patients being dishonest when they deny that they are irritated when we cut short their hours—because they are afraid we will get angry and terminate therapy? Is a patient being dishonest when he unconsciously falsifies a childhood experience by remembering it as having been bitten by a dog rather than as having kicked and hurt the dog?

These examples illustrate some of the vagaries of the concept of honesty and demonstrate why it cannot simply be appraised but must be understood in the context of the experience. Honesty is the potential to see a situation for what it is; it is achieved only when one has a minimal need to defend oneself against anxiety because one has sufficient self-regard. Whether we communicate this honest appraisal of a situation in a truthful statement or withhold it for reasons we believe are justified, our goal in the training of therapists should certainly be to encourage and develop basic honesty in our human contacts. Dishonesty is the inevitable consequence of the neurotic structure and occurs when a person's defenses demand some distortion of reality—by total reversal, slight distortion, exaggeration, minimizing, shading, etc. In therapy, this tendency is generally not categorized as dishonesty but rather is considered a problem of defense. The therapist should refrain from moralizing judgments and recognize that these distortions are a necessary activity in the neurotic state.

This link between neurosis and dishonesty has led many theorists, particularly Horney and Sullivan, to consider neuroses immoral and to classify them as "ethical diseases." Certainly the neurotic is dishonest but, since he is unable to make any choices, his dishonesty is imposed upon him by his neurosis. He does not wish it and would like to rid himself of it. The psychotic individual, whether his psychosis is of an organic or psychological origin, likewise describes events and experiences in a manner that deviates widely from fact. These reports are labeled delusions, hallucinations, faulty perceptions, confabulations, and the like. The issue of honesty or truth is not raised in regard to them, although we occasionally designate malingering as a deliberate attempt to deceive or defraud. In therapy we prefer to talk about defenses rather than honesty, since the problem of honesty is very loaded with ethical and theological judgments.

The matter of honesty leads us to an examination of the concept of truth. There are many interesting definitions of truth. All of them are true, yet none of them is entirely true. And this is precisely the limitation of the concept of truth, unless we believe in an absolute truth. To say that something is absolutely true is immediately to tell a lie, for truth is entirely dependent on our frame of reference, as Einstein plainly demonstrated in his experiments in relativity. Yet if we limit our definition of truth to some relativistic or indeterminate sense, we have chaos. Consequently, civilized societies have agreed on some basic truths as a foundation for morality.

HONESTY AND TRUTH IN THERAPY

In the therapeutic process honesty is an essential for patient and therapist. It is unthinkable that a rational, humanistic, nonauthoritarian healing process can take place without it. Yet it is too often demanded of the patient and not often enough required of the therapist. Many therapies, such as magic, proceed in an atmosphere that could be described as dishonest, but these are not subsumed under the strict category of psychotherapy by mutual exchange, as defined by Freud.

What needs to be clarified is not whether one should be honest, but how to use our honest evaluations in an effective way. This is exclusively a question of technique, or at least it should be. Although we should not knowingly deviate from honest appraisals in our therapeutic work, we must constantly decide how best to utilize these appraisals. The question is not when should we be honest but when should we communicate our honest observations so that they most effectively serve the therapeutic process. In the case of a patient with incipient schizophrenia, there is no question about *whether* we should interpret to him a dream caused by severe anxiety that presages emotional disorganization; it is only a matter of *when* to do it. Likewise, we must decide *when* to inform a patient that we dislike some behavior and find it obnoxious (not should we or should we not).

The therapist's honesty in appraising such situations must be assumed and required without question. *What* we communicate, however, is a different question from whether or not we honestly appraise the total situation. We must not confuse honesty with technique, for without a basic honesty the therapy itself is in jeopardy and the technical problem never arises.

Unfortunately, for many therapists this decision never occurs, for they automatically decide to withhold unpleasant or distressful observations from patients because of their own inability to handle the consequences. In such cases, however, we are not dealing with honesty or truth but with an incompetent or immature therapist who has greater concern for his own welfare than for that of his patient. At times, of course, it may be the overwhelming characterological problems of the patient that put the therapist on the defensive, and one must acknowledge that this can happen to any therapist, however skillful, experienced, or mature.

On the matter of truth I think we can be much clearer. I cannot visualize many situations in which an untruth can be justified in the healing profession. Certainly we can argue endlessly about the dilemma of the patient with incurable cancer, but, aside from this, I think we would all agree that in the psychotherapeutic process an untruth is never justified. This must be clearly distinguished from withholding the truth for definable reasons. Our rationalizations may be incorrect, our justifications fallacious, but withholding the truth is quite different from telling a patient a lie. Freud made this clear in his statement quoted above. Certainly it is easy to justify withholding the truth from patients for reasons ostensibly beneficial to them when we are really protecting ourselves. It is easy to blame failures in therapy on our patients when our own skills are at fault. But this is a matter of recognizing our own deficiencies. In my opinion our patients are better able to handle unpleasant material than we ever give them credit for.

Yet here again we must not confuse technique with truth. In the present state of development of psychological theory our interpretations and observations are a long way from being verifiable, and consequently we may not be withholding a *truth* if we refrain from making an interpretation, but only an *opinion*. We can establish some honesty in our appraisal only if we allow ourselves the freedom to examine human experience from a standpoint that is not biased or preconceived. The truthfulness of these observations will be determined somewhere far in the future.

At present we work only with skilled guesses, approximations, and rudimentary scientific observations and we must never fool ourselves about this fact. Frequently we present our educated guesses and approximations to our patients as though they were established truths. Such misrepresentations are as harmful as lying or withholding, and perhaps more so, since they occur so frequently. We must avoid the temptation to use our status to establish a set of "truths" that may be far removed from any acceptable definition of truth.

The purpose of distinguishing between honesty and truth in therapy is to stress the wisdom of using certain technical interventions in the therapeutic process. Although there is no virtue in a doctrine of absolute truthfulness in the therapeutic process, there seems never to be a justification for deception. But just as honesty is relative to the patient's sense of security, so must we recognize that the therapist is also human, and therefore subject to neurotic difficulties, defending himself with denials, and seeing less than the whole truth. We hope, however, that he has less need for such defenses than the patient does, and consequently we believe we have a right to expect less deception on his part.

"The Importance of Psychiatrists' Telling Patients the Truth"

William S. Appleton

A former professor of medicine at a leading university is said to have expelled a third-year student from the wards, the school, and medicine in front of 50 colleagues during grand rounds. The student's offense? He told a patient he had cancer.

As the student, frightened and near tears, was about to go, the professor called him back and said: "Now you have a small idea of what it is like to be told you have cancer."

I have always thought, as did many of the students who repeated it, that this story meant the professor did not believe in telling patients they were going to die. Looking back, it seems equally plausible that he wanted his students to understand the emotional impact of such a pronouncement on the patient.

To summarize current medical opinion on the matter: Tell the patient

Reprinted with permission of author and publisher from *American Journal of Psychiatry*, 129:6 742–45, December 1972.

the truth about whether or not he has a fatal illness if he really wants to know. (There is extensive discussion in the medical and psychiatric literature about how to tell which patients really do want to know, how the patient will react once informed, and how to identify those patients who should be protected from the truth about fatal illnesses.)

THE SPIRIT OF DIAGNOSIS

Psychiatrists have frequently criticized internists and surgeons for indulging in charades that not only do not fool the fatally ill patient but also confuse and disorient him. My colleagues often admonish physicians and surgeons to "communicate," to tell the patient the truth more often.

The irony of the psychiatrist's position in all this becomes overwhelmingly apparent as one examines the same problem in the field of mental illness. In the teaching hospital in which I work, in the many institutions I have visited, and in the hospitals where I have trained, too often psychiatric patients were told nothing about their illness.

The psychiatrist usually reasons that schizophrenia and depression are not predictable diseases with known causes. Therefore, to tell a patient he or she is so afflicted would have no therapeutic or prognostic meaning. He correctly believes the spirit of diagnosis to be not one of mere labeling but rather one of suggesting causation, therapeutic action, and outcome. Ironically, the internist or surgeon often employs similar reasoning to conceal the diagnosis of cancer: Why needlessly upset the patient when the disease may never recur or may be hopelessly malignant?

In most cases the patient, and perhaps his family, should be told what the psychiatrist concludes. If the diagnostic term is imperfect, it must be explained to the extent of the psychiatrist's knowledge; for example, "The schizophrenia is such that a relapse may occur within two years and the following symptoms should be watched for." The psychiatrist should do his best to warn the patient that "when you are stressed emotionally you have a tendency to confuse what is in your mind with what is real. Therefore, if a loved one were to die or if you were to move across country, you might be in danger of relapse." Perhaps out of an unwillingness to deemphasize the uniqueness of the individual and to view him statistically, psychiatrists collect little practical data of this kind. Surgeons know, for example, that if such and such a cancer has reached the lymph nodes or liver, the prognosis, on the average, is a certain number of months, which can be increased by a certain number of methods. Psychiatrists in American universities, however, do not tend to think that the schizophrenia of a 19-year-old with a good premorbid personality has "X" number of chances of recurring in five years, ten years, or never, and is subject to influence by "Y" number of means.

Psychiatrists have such strong feelings against supplying a diagnosis that they sometimes utter it out of despair. "You are borderline and will never be well," one analyst told his patient after three or four years of analysis. He thus avoided his medical obligation to cure her and at the same time released some of his frustration at being unable to do so.

THE PSYCHIATRIC MODEL

Another reason for withholding the diagnosis arises from the mistaken application of the psychiatric model, as opposed to the medical model. In the psychiatric model, the doctor allies himself with the healthy part of the patient's personality to observe and understand the causes of what both agree to be undesirable behavior or emotion. It is then up to the patient to change himself in the context of the psychiatric relationship. The medical patient submits his illness for diagnosis and is either told what to do or lets the doctor do something therapeutic to him.

Organically (biologically) oriented psychiatrists use the medical model. For example, they might say to a patient: "You have a depression with the following symptoms. Here is how to recognize it early and what to do about it." The analytic psychiatrist, predominant in the United States and especially in university centers, uses the psychiatric model and believes depression to be a "stance" to coerce help or love from a significant person. He does not regard his patient as having a depressive illness but regards him as not having abandoned the childlike expectation of being "given to" as opposed to the adult role of achieving for oneself. Even if this model is correct and if (as Thomas Szasz has stated) mental illness is a myth rather than a disease, schizophrenia does not exist, depression is a stance rather than a biochemical condition, and borderline means immaturity, I believe psychiatrists should nonetheless be sure to give the diagnosis, albeit in these "mythical" terms.

The word "diagnosis" means to distinguish or to know and refers in medicine to recognizing a disease from its symptoms. More than a mere label, it is the conclusion reached about causation from which therapeutic action is taken. The psychiatrist must tell the patient the result of his thinking. If he believes the patient's problems stem from misinterpretations of reality or from an unwillingness to put off the moment's pleasure for future reward, he ought to say so. If the physician believes that the patient is waiting in a depressed stance for others to take care of him, he should tell him. Being informed of his diagnosis helps the patient achieve the solution he desires; the doctor's thinking is also channeled more precisely. Once the diagnosis is stated, the patient may act immediately or, when he delays or forgets, his psychiatrist may remind him of it. In addition, a precise statement of the illness or problem helps the practitioner assess its outcome more accurately.

FEAR OF REINFORCEMENT

If full disclosure is such a good idea, then why do psychiatrists so often fail to give their patients the diagnosis? One reason is the psychiatrist's reluctance to repeat what angry families have been telling the patient for months or even years. "You want to be waited on. You won't take responsibility." Some psychiatrists are so troubled by members of their own families that they fear venting their anger and frustration on their patients and, as a result, go to the opposite extreme and say nothing at all. Others restrict themselves to obscure language for fear of producing the same reaction the patient has toward members of his family whom he either dislikes or mistrusts. If such reluctance represents true relationship-building attempts by the psychiatrist, it can be defended. For example, telling a paranoid that he is projecting (i.e., that his beliefs are unreal) is unwise if it alienates the therapist from the person he is trying to help. But if the psychiatrist's silence is due to fear of the patient's anger and results in avoiding transference reactions, it then defeats the whole purpose of the analytic therapist, which amounts to the analysis of the transference reaction itself. A fact frequently forgotten is that the patient will often listen to the trained and neutral physician when he will not listen to his wife or mother. Just because a patient's mother said something does not mean that it is necessarily wrong.

"But he won't listen," many of my colleagues would reply. Tell the patient what you think first, and if he does not listen, you can go on from there. Some psychiatrists believe that it is bad for the patient to know that he is schizophrenic because he may despair and stop trying. A diagnosis of schizophrenia is certainly depressing, and the patient may go through a stage of hopelessness. So does a newly diagnosed cancer patient. Psychiatrists and many medical doctors believe that most cancer patients know the nature of their illness without being told. Most schizophrenics do too, except for those too far out of contact. Telling a patient what he already knows has the added advantage of making him feel that the doctor is being honest.

The failure of psychiatrists to communicate with their patients has repeatedly come to my attention. In my clinic, psychiatric patients are given elaborate diagnostic exercises, including one-hour interviews but they are often denied a careful review of the physicians' clinical findings. A hospitalized patient recently called this to my attention when, after a conference lasting an hour and a half, she waited outside to ask me what was wrong and what she should do. This frequently happens and is usually followed by the conference chairman's hasty reply, "Ask your own doctor," as he rushes away. I decided that since this 60-year-old woman had patiently answered my questions in front of 35 colleagues, it was only fair to tell her what I thought. I did, and she was grateful and very much relieved.

A psychiatric resident whom I supervise presented the case of a 35-year-old virginal man who had been hospitalized with severe attacks of anxiety. The man repeatedly asked why he had palpitations and whether he was a homosexual. Doubt and fear prevented the doctor from answering these questions. He was uncertain whether the palpitations signaled suppressed aggression, he wanted the patient to develop his independence and a capacity for decision making, and he thought the patient, who liked to argue, would disagree.

Ironically, the resident shared the patient's concerns about himself. The resident believed that the patient's fear of becoming homosexual if he developed freedom of sexual expression was well founded. In spite of the therapist's silence, the patient thought he detected encouragement to ask a young woman for a date. "I didn't know you were interested in girls," the woman had said, refusing him, and the patient vowed never to invite another woman out. To this series of events, the resident showed no reaction. When the patient reported fantasizing a woman while masturbating for the first time in his life, he was greeted with more silence. As soon as the psychiatrist abandoned his uncertainty, took a stand, and openly encouraged his patient, the patient asked the young woman out again; this time she accepted.

A doctor ought not to allow himself to wait for complete certainty before giving his opinion, since this can become an excuse for silence. When a patient fears flying, the psychiatrist cannot guarantee that the plane will arrive safely but should, nonetheless, encourage him to try, especially if the physician has mastered his own fear. Some patients benefit by being told, "I worry in airplanes too. In fact 90 percent of all passengers are happier when the plane lands." Others require the assurance that the chances that one will die in a plane are less likely than in an automobile.

An important reason why psychiatrists withhold information, then, is doubt about really knowing the answers. The issue is one of epistemology: how do we know what we think we know, and when can we be sure we are right? Doctors are both intellectual and skeptical. They are aware of past medical certainties having turned into foolish relics, e.g., blood-letting, purgatives, and chaining the mentally ill. This leads them to shy away from being definite and risking an opinion that may later prove to be wrong.

But this cautious attitude can be harmful at times. This was manifested by an experiment in which psychiatrists were trained to give mood-elevating drugs to a group of depressed patients in two ways: (1) in a positive manner (this drug will help you and is very effective), and (2) in a scientific manner (this drug may or may not work, but try it and see). The cure rate for the first group was twice that of the second.

SUMMARY

Psychiatrists advocate honest and open communication by physicians with patients but too often do not practice what they preach. Their reasons for silence include uncertainty about the cause, treatment, and prognosis of psychiatric illnesses and unwillingness to depress, demoralize, anger, or alienate their patients.

If the psychiatrist can overcome his doubts and to the best of his ability honestly explain what is wrong with the patient and what is necessary to overcome the problem, then therapy will become more rapid and effective and its success or failure will be easier to evaluate. Giving the correct diagnosis and prescription may not make the psychiatrist popular with his listener, but this is not important as long as the patient can hear what is said and can learn to make use of it.

From *Man, Mind and Medicine*

Oliver M. Cope

DR. COPE: When I was a fourth-year student, William Sidney Thayer —the great professor of medicine at Hopkins, that wonderful understanding warm human being—came to Harvard and gave a *Care of the Patient* lecture. He described malignant disease and told how you handled it and how you always had to tell the patient the truth. This was a vivid experience for me. He described a patient who had come to him in Baltimore because he had been put off by physicians elsewhere. He knew he wasn't getting the answer, and so it was easy, I suppose, for Dr. Thayer to know that the thing to do was to tell him. The patient wanted it; that was why he came to Baltimore. So he told him. The fellow, of course, was upset; and his wife was angry with Dr. Thayer. He said she berated him: "What right did you have to tell him?" Then, two hours later, he got a telephone call. They had gone back to their hotel, and called Dr. Thayer to thank him for having told, because for the first time in several months, the two of them could sit down and talk.

That was a vivid model, and now I think of my mistakes. A woman had obvious cancer of the thyroid, and knew it. She knew it because of the way her physicians dodged telling her; everybody was alarmed. Any fool could see that her doctors were alarmed; so she made me promise the night before the operation, religiously promise, that I would tell her the truth. She suspected the truth; she outlined to me the number of reasons she needed to know. She was a widow; her children were not quite launched and so on; and I had to tell her for very practical reasons. So it was. It was a rapidly growing, undifferentiated carcinoma, the type with a wretched prognosis, perhaps nine months or a year, and it would have to be treated by radiation.

So I waited until she was over the anesthetic, and the next morning I came in, pulled up a chair next to her, sat down by her bedside, and said: "I will now do what you asked me to do. You have a serious condition: we are going to give you x-ray treatment. There is no doubt that these treatments will help you. It is possible we will manage to eliminate the trouble completely, but just the same you had better do what you said about rearranging your estate and taking care of your children and so on." She thanked me

Reprinted with permission of author and publisher from *Man, Mind, and Medicine* (Philadelphia: J. B. Lippincott Co., 1968), pp. 28–29.

very much, and I went out with great relief, thinking that I had carried it off. In the next two or three days, I was congratulating myself because she had taken it so well; I must have done a good job. On the fourth postoperative day, the nurse stopped me before I entered the room. "You know, Mrs. B is waiting. She wants to know when you are going to fulfill your promise and tell her what you found." I was younger then than I am now; I failed to take advantage of the broad hint offered me by the patient, namely, that she had shut out the bad news. So I went in and I said, "I hear from your nurse that I haven't told you. Don't you recall that the very day after operation I told you?" "Told me what?" So I went over it again. She, of course, went into a serious depression; and it was terrible. It ruined her life and, what is more, mistakes seem to be contagious. To make a long story short, the pathologist and I thought this was an undifferentiated carcinoma. It wasn't: it was one of those very peculiar tumors. The same type of tumor was found in the wall of her stomach four years later. She lived for 12 years after that to die of a coronary.

Most of us doctors don't have the understanding to manage these situations and we badly need to learn how.

DR. ZACHARIAS: Can you conceive of any kind of formal education that would have helped you with that?

DR. COPE: Yes, something, but certainly not what I had had. I acted on the single model given me, persuasively, by Dr. William Sidney Thayer.

DR. EISENBERG: Did you ever watch him do it instead of being told by him how to do it?

DR. COPE: No.

From "What to Tell Cancer Patients: A Study of Medical Attitudes"

Donald Oken

No problem is more vexing than the decision about what to tell the cancer patient. (Although the word cancer is neither a medical term nor a specific entity, common sense considerations provide a basis for use of this general

Reprinted with permission of author and publisher from the *Journal of the American Medical Association* 175, 86–94, April 1, 1961. Copyright 1961, American Medical Association.

term. As used in the present work, the term should be understood *to apply to all malignant neoplasms of characteristically grave prognosis.*) The situation is an ever recurring one and the questions involved are knotty. What should the patient be told? How and when should this be done? The manner in which such questions are handled is crucial for the patient and may determine his emotional status and capacity for function from that time on. It is easy enough to decide to follow a course which will "do least harm," but it is far from simple to determine just what course that is. The issues involved are complex factors which are difficult to assess, weigh, and place in proper perspective.

In his attempt to work out some solution, the doctor needs all the help he can get. The issues are a favorite and, often, heated topic of "corridor consultations." Often the opinion of a psychiatrist is sought: but psychiatric knowledge provides no clear and unequivocal answers. A considerable number of authors have attempted to provide assistance by describing their own views and approach. These writers, often wise and distinguished teachers drawing on long experience, offer solutions based on that experience. This too proves of insufficient help. Though many issues have become clarified, these experts differ widely about what to do. Opinions vary from one extreme to the other. A careful review of this literature discloses a further lack: the almost complete absence of systematic research. There is a plethora of opinion but a minimum of dependable fact. This is a curious situation in an area of so great importance. The present paper represents an initial attempt to provide some research data which bear on this situation and on the general issue of "telling." ...

"TELLING"

The initial undertaking in this research was the determination of whether or not physicians tell their patients they have cancer. It is evident, as seen in Table 1, that there is a strong and general tendency to *withhold* this information. Almost 90% of the group is within this half of the scale. Indeed, a majority tell only very rarely, if ever. No one reported a policy of informing every patient. ... No difference between specialities was uncovered; the small differences seen in Table 1, or involving the smaller groups of surgical subspecialties not detailed there, are far from significant statistically. (This lack of specialty differences was a consistent finding for all questionnaire items. Differences when present were small and off-set by wider divergencies within each specialty.) These findings also cut across the hospital staff rank and age. Younger and less experienced men did not have any greater inclination to tell than their seniors.

Use of a questionnaire, of course, forces answers into an artificially rigid mold. But, information derived from the interviews strengthens the finding. Answers indicating that patients are told often turned out to mean telling the patient that he had a "tumor," with strict avoidance of the terms cancer, malignancy, and the like. These more specific words were almost

TABLE 1   Physicians' Policies About "Telling" Cancer Patients

Usual Policy	Exceptions Made	Internists		Surgeons*		Generalists		Total Group	
		No.	%	No.	%	No.	%	No.	%
Do not tell	Never	7	8	7	8	4	15	18	9
	Very rarely	36	43	44	53	10	37	90	47
	Occasionally	28	34	21	25	7	26	56	29
	Often	4	5	1	1	0	0	5	3
Subtotal		75	90	73	87	21	73	169	88
Tell	Often	3	4	4	5	1	4	8	4
	Occasionally	4	5	4	5	2	7	10	5
	Very rarely	1	1	2	2	3	11	6	3
	Never	0	0	0	0	0	0	0	0
Subtotal		8	10	10	12	7	22	24	12
Total		83	100	83	100†	27	100	103	100

*Includes gynecologists and thoracic, genito-urinary, orthopedic, and neurosurgeons as well as general surgeons.

†Sum appears to equal 90% because of rounding to nearest %.

never used unless the patient's explicit and insistent questioning pushed the doctor's back to the wall.

Euphemisms are the general rule. These may extend from the vaguest of words ("lesion," "mass"); to terms giving a general indication that the process is neoplastic ("growth," "tumor," "hyperplastic tissue")—often tempered by a false explicit statement that the process is benign; to somewhat more suggestive expression (a "suspicious" or "degenerated" tumor). Where major surgical or radiation therapy is involved, especially if the patient is hesitant about proceeding, recourse may be had to such terms as "pre-cancerous," or a tumor "in the early curable stage." Some physicians avoid even the slightest suggestion of neoplasia and quite specifically substitute another diagnosis. Almost every one reported resorting to such falsification on at least a few occasions, most notably when the patient was in a far-advanced stage of illness at the time he was seen.

It is impossible to convey all the flavor of the diverse individual approaches. No two men use exactly the same technique. Each has his preferred plan, his select euphemisms, his favored tactics, and his own views about the optimal time for discussion and the degree of directness to be used. Some have a set pattern, while others vary their approach. But the general trend is consistent.

The modal policy is to tell as little as possible in the most general terms consistent with maintaining cooperation in treatment. Exceptions are made most commonly when the patient is in a position of financial responsibility which carries the necessity for planning. Questioning by the patient almost invariably is disregarded and considered a plea for reassurance unless persistent, and intuitively perceived as "a real wish to know." Even then it may be ignored. The vast majority of these doctors feel that almost all patients really do not want to know regardless of what people say. They approach the issue with the view that disclosure should be avoided unless there are positive indications, rather than the reverse. Intelligence and emotional stability are considered prerequisites for greater disclosure only if other "realistic" factors provide a basis for doing so. For the fewer physicians who tell with some frequency, these two factors assume more primary importance.

A few additional consistent themes emerge. Agreement was essentially unanimous that some family member must be informed if the patient is not made aware of the diagnosis. Legal and ethical considerations are by no means the only points of relevance here. Repeated instances were reported of patients who, dissatisfied with the progression of their disease in the face of treatment and desperate for help, were dissuaded from fruitless and unwise shifts to a new physician (or quack) only by the cooperation of an informed relative. Beyond this is the need to have someone to share the awful burden of knowledge. As one man put it, "I just can't carry the load alone." Few responsibilities are as heavy as knowing that someone is going to die; dividing it makes it easier to bear.

Variations in approach also converge to a single major goal: maintenance of hope. No inference was necessary to elicit this finding. Every single physician interviewed spontaneously emphasized this point and indicated his resolute and determined purpose is to sustain and bolster the patient's hope. Each in his own way communicates the possibility, even the likelihood, of recovery. Differences revolve about the range of belief about just how much information is compatible with the maintenance of hope. While some doctors believe "cancer means certain death and no normal person wants to die," others hold that "knowledge is power": power which can conquer fear. The crux of the divergence centers on two issues: whether cancer connotes certain death, and whether the expectation of death insurmountably deprives the patient of hope. The data indicate that an impressively large number of physicians would answer affirmatively to both. . . .

. . . It was the exception when a physician could report known examples of the unfavorable consequences of an approach which differed from his own. It was more common to get reports of instances in which different approaches had turned out satisfactorily. Most of the instances in which unhappy results were reported to follow a differing policy turned out to be vague accounts from which no reliable inference could be drawn.

Instead of logic and rational decision based on critical observation, what is found is opinion, belief, and conviction, heavily weighted with emotional justification. As one internist said: "I can't give a good reason except that I've always done it." Explanations are begun characteristically with such phrases as "I feel . . ." or "It is my opinion. . . ." Personal convictions were stated flatly and dogmatically as if they were facts. Thus, "Most people do not want to know," "It is my firm belief that they always know anyway," or "No one can be told without giving up and losing all hope." Highly charged emotional terms and vivid expressions were the rule, indicating the intensity and nature of feelings present. Knowledge of cancer is "a death sentence," "a Buchenwald," and "torture." Telling is "the cruelest thing in the world," "awful," and "hitting the patient with a baseball bat." It is not necessary even to read the words on the questionnaires. Heavy underlinings and a peppering of exclamation points tell the story. These are hardly cool scientific judgments. It would appear that personal conviction is the decisive factor. . . .

Another relevant finding is the doctor's wish to be told if he were the patient. As expected, those who tend to tell their patients wished to be told, themselves, more often than those who do not tell. But the total number of those who said they wished to be told (73 of 122) is far greater than those who tend to tell their patients. The explanation usually given was that, "I am one of those who can take it" or "I have responsibilities." That they did not feel this to be true for all physicians, however, is attested to by their treatment of other doctor-patients. Most of the group said they were neither more nor less likely to tell physicians than other patients. Of the group who did modify their policy, it was just as likely to find that they were *less* prone to tell doctors. It is impossible to draw any precise conclusion from this type of hypothetical question about one's self. But the inconsistency is characteristic of emotionally determined attitudes.

DEPRESSION AND SUICIDE

The pros and cons of telling have been discussed so often that there is little point in doing so again. Whatever the reasons for telling, the argument against doing so centers on the anticipation of profoundly disturbing psychological effects. There is no doubt that this disclosure has a profound and potentially dangerous impact. Questions do arise about the capacity of human beings to make a satisfactory adaptation to the expectation of death. Can anyone successfully handle such news without paying a price which mitigates whatever value this knowledge brings? If so, how widespread is the ability to call forth the necessary psychological defenses? What about time: does this readjustment take place within some reasonable span? Can the emotional cost of such a shattering experience, or of the effort required for mastering it, be weighed and predicted? The truth is that we know very little about these matters.

It has been repeatedly asserted that disclosure is followed by fear and despondency which may progress into overt depressive illness or culminate in suicide. This was the opinion of the physicians in the present study. Quite representative was the surgeon who stated, "I would be afraid to tell and have the patient in a room with a window." When it comes to actually documenting the prevalence of such untoward reactions, it becomes difficult to find reliable evidence. Instances of depression and profound upsets came quickly to mind when the subject was raised, but no one could report more than a case or two, or a handful at most. This may merely follow from the rarity with which patients are told. Such an explanation must be reconciled with the fact that these same doctors could remember many instances in which the patient was told and seemed to do well. It may also reflect the selection of those told. Or perhaps the knowledge produces covert psychological changes which are no less malignant for their sublety. But actually, the incidence and severity of depression and other psychological reactions in cancer patients, and their relation to being told, is not known.

The same situation holds with regard to suicide. Only 6 doctors could report definite known cases of suicide (2 of these reported two cases and 1 "several"), although about one-third of the group had "heard of" suicides after being told. Further investigation indicated that at least 2 of these patients had never been told. (And it is not altogether inconceivable that they would have felt better, not worse, had this been done.) Actually, the circumstances surrounding all but one or two of these cases are quite vague; it is impossible to feel any certainty about what lay behind the suicide. . . .

. . . The group who tell are equally vague in documenting that their patients do well. We simply do not have adequate data about the consequences of telling. As in any dreaded situation, emotion fills a vacuum with rumor, pseudofact, and projected fears. It is noteworthy that the question is posed: "can a patient stand being told," whereas "can the patient stand not being told" is almost never heard, although it is equally valid from the scientific viewpoint.

A physician who tells some of his patients uses certain rules of thumb to guide his decisions. It is striking how inconsistently these guides vary from one physician to another. Thus, some are more likely to tell the very aged while others especially avoid telling this group. Some are inclined to tell patients with a better prognosis and others only when the prognosis is poor. The disagreement about doctor-patients has already been noted. Such discrepancies may portray quite accurately chance differences in experience. More intriguing is the possibility that they reflect the doctor's personality. In any event they are typical of *a priori* judgments unsubstantiated by facts.

PESSIMISM

Cancer has many unconscious meanings and fantasies associated with it. Whatever the unconscious feelings which it stirs, typically it is feared consciously as a process equated with suffering and certain death. There was good general agreement among the physicians interviewed that these are what patients primarily fear. Other connotations (for example, that cancer is dirty or shameful) were far less prevalent. Many patients mouth statements about curability, and "know" neither suffering nor death are inevitable. But the physicians here report that this knowledge is only skin deep. People continue to think of cancer as "the killer."

What is impressive is that the doctors themselves feel very much the same way. It was not patients who described the diagnosis as a "death warrant" or "a date of execution." The internist who referred to cancer as an "incurable disease with an inevitable demise" expressed a view which was not atypical. The extent and intensity of this underlying pessimism stands out. The general feeling was that we can do very little to save lives and not a great deal to prevent suffering. Sighs and shrugging of the shoulders were the almost usual accompaniment of discussion in this area. Not that these men give up where the individual patient is concerned; on the contrary they fight ceaselessly and without compromise. But just below the surface is the feeling: "to me, it's like a stone wall—no prospects."

Early diagnosis is viewed with a not much more sanguine eye. Nearly all could remember a few cases, at least, where early diagnosis seemed of critical importance. (Breast and bowel lesions were singled out for special mention.) But a common feeling was that usually this makes no difference: "What's the use? You make an early diagnosis, the patient goes through a horrible operation and suffers, and two years later he's dead anyway." They are not convinced that it helps more than a handful.

"DEATH SHALL HAVE NO DOMINION"

Among the motivations for entering medicine, the wish to conquer suffering and death stands high on the list. Practicing physicians are not the kind of persons who can sit quietly by while nature pursues its course. One of the hardest things for a fledgling medical student to learn is watchful waiting. Few situations are as frustrating as sitting by impotently and "helplessly" in the face of illness. Fatal illness is felt as a major defeat. It is not uncommon to know at a glance that a colleague has recently lost a patient: it leaves its mark. . . .

The American Cancer Society has devoted vast effort and sums of money to public information campaigns. Publicity about the "danger signals" of cancer has led to howls of protest by some physicians who feel that such campaigns stimulate cancerophobia. Leaving aside any possible correctness of such contentions, why has the issue been so heated? Perhaps, we have here another manifestation of the wish to keep cancer out of sight and mind. For the most part, officials of the Society have responded to such complaints with defensive statements that the majority of the medical profession agrees that their approach has merit which exceeds the harm. The interviews here tend to support this view, although agreement was usually lukewarm. Reservations centered less on the problem of cancerophobia than on the positive value of public education. Part of this reflects the pessimism already described, but more is involved. The view expressed was that patients who respond to publicity are usually complaint (and cancer) free, while those with symptoms requiring attention are dominated by their irrational fears and are unaffected. The general conclusion was that education utilizing only a rational appeal is insufficient. New techniques must be developed which will modify emotional attitudes.

The same conclusion can be drawn about the education programs directed towards physicians. Cancer authorities cannot be lulled into complacency by the overt agreement of the profession with their goals or by their successes in providing technical information. Much more ingenuity and effort will be required to alter and surmount the formidable psychological barriers of physicians' covert attitudes. The medical profession plays a pivotal role in cancer control far beyond its direct functions in diagnosis and treatment. When doctors lose hope their patients know it. If doctors communicate the feeling that cancer is dreadful and irremediable, how can patients fail to despair? And frightened and despairing, how can they deal with the possibility that they have cancer? Their only recourse is to keep the possibility hidden—from themselves as well as their doctors. Thus, they court the very fate which they most fear. No physician, no matter how skillful, can treat the patient who stays away. Unwittingly, our own feelings reinforce the anxieties which keep them away, the very opposite of our intent. Perhaps the doctor, more than the patient, should be a target for emotional reeducation. . . .

"Playing Supergod"

Samuel Vaisrub

How should we tell a patient with a fatal disease the truth? And having told it, how do we prepare him for dying? These questions are discussed widely in current medical and lay publications as well as on televised panels in which physicians share concerns with attorneys, clergymen, and psychiatrists.

These concerns are not new. Until recently, however, the central question was not *how* to tell a patient the truth, but *whether* to tell it. Opinions were divided. Those who favored leveling with the patient marshalled persuasive arguments for so doing. After all, truth is considered to be a moral-religious imperative. To withhold it is sinful, as well as harmful and impractical. Why deprive the patient of a compelling incentive for setting his business affairs in order and making his peace with God?

Less self-righteous, those who oppose informing the patient were often too self-conscious to present their views with convincing forcefulness. Yet, they have a strong case. The truth about imminent death is not a philosophical abstraction to be discussed with cool detachment. It is a statement which may be as lethal to the spirit as its message is to the body. To many patients—even to those who insist on being told the truth—certitude of impending death may prove to be an unbearable burden. The emotional state provoked by the revelation may dim rather than brighten judgment for setting one's house in order or for preparing to face one's Creator.

It may even be argued that foreknowledge of death is contrary to Nature's plan or God's will. No mortal to-date has received a Divine estimate of his remaining days on earth. Nor has Nature provided this kind of information. Unlike fear or pain which often serve a protective purpose, intimation of mortality, apparently, has no survival value in the evolutionary process of natural selection.

Must, then, the physician set himself above Nature and play Supergod?

"The Dying As Teachers"

Elisabeth Kübler-Ross

To tell or not to tell, that is the question.

In talking to physicians, hospital chaplains, and nursing staff, we are often impressed about their concern for a patient's tolerance of "the truth." "Which truth?" is usually our question. The confronting of patients after the diagnosis of a malignancy is made is always difficult. Some physicians favor telling the relatives but keeping the facts from the patient in order to avoid an emotional outburst. Some doctors are sensitive to their patient's needs and can quite successfully present the patient with the awareness of a serious illness without taking all hope away from him.

I personally feel that this question should never come up as a real conflict. The question should not be "Should we tell . . . ?" but rather "How do I share this with my patient?" I will try to explain this attitude in the following pages. I will therefore have to categorize crudely the many experiences that patients have when they are faced with the sudden awareness of their own finality. As we have outlined previously, man is not freely willing to look at his own end of life on earth and will only occasionally and half-heartedly take a glimpse at the possibility of his own death. One such occasion, obviously, is the awareness of a life-threatening illness. The mere fact that a patient is told that he has cancer brings his possible death to his conscious awareness.

It is often said that people equate a malignancy with terminal illness and regard the two as synonymous. This is basically true and can be a blessing or a curse, depending on the manner in which the patient and family are managed in this crucial situation. Cancer is still for most people a terminal illness, in spite of increasing numbers of real cures as well as meaningful remissions. I believe that we should make it a habit to think about death and dying occasionally, I hope before we encounter it in our own life. If we have not done so, the diagnosis of cancer in our family will brutally remind us of our own finality. It may be a blessing, therefore, to use the time of illness to think about death and dying in terms of ourselves, regardless of whether the patient will have to meet death or get an extension of life.

If a doctor can speak freely with his patients about the diagnosis of malignancy without equating it necessarily with impending death, he will do the patient a great service. He should at the same time leave the door open for hope, namely, new drugs, treatments, chances of new techniques and new research. The main thing is that he communicates to the patient that all is not lost; that he is not giving him up because of a certain diagnosis; that it is a battle they are going to fight together—patient, family, and doctor —no matter the end result. Such a patient will not fear isolation, deceit, rejection, but will continue to have confidence in the honesty of his physi-

Reprinted, with permission of the author and publisher, from *On Death and Dying* by Elisabeth Kübler-Ross (N.Y.: The Macmillan Co., 1970). Copyright © 1969 by Elisabeth Kübler-Ross.

cian and know that if there is anything that can be done, they will do it together. Such an approach is equally reassuring to the family who often feel terribly impotent in such moments. They greatly depend on verbal or non-verbal reassurance from the doctor. They are encouraged to know that everything possible will be done, if not to prolong life at least to diminish suffering.

If a patient comes in with a lump in the breast, a considerate doctor will prepare her with the possibility of a malignancy and tell her that a biopsy, for example, will reveal the true nature of the tumor. He will also tell her ahead of time that a more extensive surgery will be required if a malignancy is found. Such a patient has more time to prepare herself for the possibility of a cancer and will be better prepared to accept more extensive surgery should it be necessary. When the patient awakens from the surgical procedure the doctor can say, "I am sorry, we had to do the more extensive surgery." If the patient responds, "Thank God, it was benign," he can simply say, "I wish that were true," and then silently sit with her for a while and not run off. Such a patient may pretend not to know for several days. It would be cruel for a physician to force her to accept the fact when she clearly communicates that she is not yet ready to hear it. The fact that he has told her once will be sufficient to maintain confidence in the doctor. Such a patient will seek him out later when she is able and strong enough to face the possible fatal outcome of her illness.

Another patient's response may be, "Oh, doctor, how terrible, how long do I have to live?" The physician may then tell her how much has been achieved in recent years in terms of extending the life span of such patients, and about the possibility of additional surgery which has shown good results; he may tell her frankly that nobody knows how long she can live. I think it is the worst possible management of any patient, no matter how strong, to give him a concrete number of months or years. Since such information is wrong in any case, and exceptions in both directions are the rule, I see no reason why we even consider such information. There may be a need in some rare instances where a head of a household should be informed of the shortness of his expected life in order to bring his affairs in order. I think even in such cases a tactful, understanding physician can communicate to his patient that he may be better off putting his affairs in order while he has the leisure and strength to do so, rather than to wait too long. Such a patient will most likely get the implicit message while still able to maintain the hope which each and every patient has to keep, including the ones who say that they are ready to die. Our interviews have shown that all patients have kept a door open to the possibility of continued existence, and not one of them has at all times maintained that there is no wish to live at all.

When we asked our patients how they had been told, we learned that all the patients knew about their terminal illness anyway, whether they were explicitly told or not, but depended greatly on the physician to present the news in an acceptable manner.

What, then, is an acceptable manner? How does a physician know which patient wants to hear it briefly, which one with a long scientific explanation, and which one wants to avoid the issue all together? How do we know when we do not have the advantage of knowing the patient well enough before being confronted with such decisions?

The answer depends on two things. The most important one is our own attitude and ability to face terminal illness and death. If this is a big problem in our own life, and death is viewed as a frightening, horrible, taboo topic, we will never be able to face it calmly and helpfully with a patient. And I say "death" on purpose, even if we only have to answer the question of malignancy or no malignancy. The former is always associated with impending death, a destructive nature of death, and it is the former that evokes all the emotions. If we cannot face death with equanimity, how can we be of assistance to our patients? We, then, hope that our patients will not ask us this horrible question. We make rounds and talk about many trivialities or the wonderful weather outside and the sensitive patient will play the game and talk about next spring, even if he is quite aware that there will be no next spring for him. These doctors then, when asked, will tell us that their patients do not want to know the truth, that they never ask for it, and that they believe all is well. The doctors are, in fact, greatly relieved that they are not confronted and are often quite unaware that they provoked this response in their patients.

Doctors who are still uneasy about such discussions but not so defensive may call a chaplain or priest and ask him to talk to the patient. They may feel more at ease having passed on the difficult responsibility to someone else, which may be better than avoiding it altogether. They may, on the other hand, be so anxious about it that they leave explicit orders to the staff and chaplain not to tell the patient. The degree of explicitness in such orders will reveal more about the doctors' anxiety than they wish to recognize.

There are others who have less difficulty with this issue and who find a much smaller number of patients unwilling to talk about their serious illness. I am convinced, from the many patients with whom I have spoken about this matter, that those doctors who need denial themselves will find it in their patients and that those who can talk about the terminal illness will find their patients better able to face and acknowledge it. The need of denial is in direct proportion with the doctor's need for denial. But this is only half of the problem.

We have found that different patients react differently to such news depending on their personality makeup and the style and manner they used in their past life. People who use denial as a main defense will use denial much more extensively than others. Patients who faced past stressful situations with open confrontation will do similarly in the present situation. It is, therefore, very helpful to get acquainted with a new patient, in order to elicit his strengths and weaknesses. I will give an example of this:

Mrs. A., a thirty-year-old white woman, asked us to see her during her hospitalization. She presented herself as a short, obese, pseudo-gay woman who smilingly told us of her "benign lymphoma" for which she had received a variety of treatments including cobalt and nitrogen mustard, known by most people in the hospital to be given for malignancies. She was very familiar with her illness and readily acknowledged having read the literature about it. She suddenly became quite weepy and told a rather pathetic story of how her doctor at home told her of her "benign lymphoma" after receiving the biopsy results. "A benign lymphoma?" I repeated, expressing some doubt in my voice and then sitting quietly for an answer. "Please, doctor, tell me whether it's malignant or benign?" she asked but without waiting for my answer, she began a story of a fruitless attempt to get pregnant. For nine years she had hoped for a baby, she went through all possible tests, finally through agencies in the hope of adopting a child. She was turned down for many reasons, first because she had been married only two and a half years, later because of emotional instability perhaps. She had not been able to accept the fact that she could not even have an adopted child. Now she was in the hospital and was forced to sign a paper for radiation treatment with the explicit statement that this would result in sterility, thus rendering her finally and irrevocably unable to bear a child. It was unacceptable to her in spite of the fact that she had signed the paper and had undergone the preliminary work-up for the radiation. Her abdomen was marked and she was to have her first treatment the following morning.

This communication revealed to me that she was not able to accept the fact yet. She asked the question of the malignancy but did not wait for an answer. She also told me of her inability to accept the fact of her childlessness in spite of her acceptance of the radiation treatment. She went on at great length to tell about all the details of her unfulfilled wish and kept on looking at me with big question marks in her eyes. I told her that she might be talking about her inability to face her illness rather than her inability to face being barren. I told her that I could understand this. I also said that both situations were difficult but not hopeless and left her with the promise to return the next day after the treatment.

It was on the way to the first radiation treatment that she confirmed her knowledge of her malignancy, but she hoped that this treatment might cure it. During the following informal, almost social visits, she fluctuated between talking about babies and her malignancy. She became increasingly tearful and dropped her pseudo-gay appearance during these sessions. She asked for a "magic button" which would enable her to get rid of all her fears and free her from the heavy burden in her chest. She was deeply concerned about the expected new roommate, "worrying to death" as she called it that she would get a terminally sick woman. Since the nursing staff on her ward was very understanding, we related her fears to them, and she became the companion of a cheerful young woman who was a great relief to her. The nursing staff also encouraged her to cry when she felt like it, rather than expecting her to smile all the time, which the patient appreciated. She had a great capacity to determine with whom she could talk about her malignancy and chose the less willing ones for her conversations about babies. The staff was quite surprised to hear of her awareness and ability to discuss her future realistically.

It was after a few very fruitful visits that the patient suddenly asked me if I had children and when I acknowledged this, she asked to terminate the visit because she was tired. The following visits were filled with angry, nasty remarks at the nursing staff, psychiatrists, and others until she was able to admit her feelings of envy for the healthy and the young, but especially towards me since I seemed to have everything. When she realized that she was not rejected in spite of becoming at times a rather difficult patient, she became increasingly aware of the origin of her anger and expressed it quite directly as anger at God for allowing her to die so young and so unfulfilled. The hospital chaplain fortunately was not a punitive but a very understanding man and talked with her about this anger in much the same terms as I did until her anger subsided to make room for more depression and, it is hoped, final acceptance of her fate.

Until the present time, this patient still maintains this dichotomy in regard to her chief problem. To one group of people she only relates as a conflicted woman in terms of her childlessness; to the chaplain and me, she talks about the meaning of her short life and the hopes she still maintains (rightfully so) for prolonging it. Her greatest fear at the time of this writing is the possibility of her husband marrying another woman who might bear children, but then she laughingly admits, "He is not the shah of Persia, though a really great man." She still has not completely coped with her envy for the living. The fact that she does not need to maintain denial or displace it onto another tragic but more acceptable problem allows her to deal with her illness more successfully.

Another example of a problem of "to tell or not to tell" is Mr. D., of whom nobody was sure whether he knew the nature of his illness. The staff was convinced that the patient did not know the great seriousness of his condition, since he never allowed anybody to get close to him. He never asked a question about it, and seemed in general rather feared by the staff. The nurses were ready to bet that he would never accept an invitation to discuss the matter with me. Anticipating difficulties, I approached him hesitantly and asked him simply, "How sick are you?" "I am full of cancer . . ." was his answer. The problem with him was that nobody ever asked a simple straightforward question. They mistook his grim look as a closed door; in fact, their own anxiety prevented them from finding out what he wanted to share so badly with another human being.

If malignancy is presented as a hopeless disease which results in a sense of "what's the use, there is nothing we can do anyway," it will be the beginning of a difficult time for the patient and for those around him. The patient will feel the increasing isolation, the loss of interest on the part of his doctor, the isolation and increasing hopelessness. He may rapidly deteriorate or fall into a deep depression from which he may not emerge unless someone is able to give him a sense of hope.

The family of such patients may share their feelings of sorrow and uselessness, hopelessness and despair, and add little to the patient's well-being. They may spend the short remaining time in a morbid depression instead of an enriching experience which is often encountered when the physician responds as outlined earlier.

I have to emphasize, though, that the patient's reaction does not depend solely on how the doctor tells him. The way in which the bad news is communicated is, however, an important factor which is often underestimated and which should be given more emphasis in the teaching of medical students and supervision of young physicians.

In summary, then, I believe the question should not be stated, "Do I tell my patient?" but should be rephrased as, "How do I share this knowledge with my patient?" The physician should first examine his own attitude toward malignancy and death so that he is able to talk about such grave matters without undue anxiety. He should listen for cues from the patient which enable him to elicit the patient's willingness to face the reality. The more people in the patient's environment who know the diagnosis of a malignancy, the sooner the patient himself will realize the true state of affairs anyway, since few people are actors enough to maintain a believable mask of cheerfulness over a long period of time. Most if not all of the patients know anyway. They sense it by the changed attention, by the new and different approach that people take to them, by the lowering of voices or avoidance of rounds, by a tearful face of a relative or an ominous, smiling member of the family who cannot hide their true feelings. They will pretend not to know when the doctor or relative is unable to talk about their true condition, and they will welcome someone who is willing to talk about it but allows them to keep their defenses as long as they have the need for them.

Whether the patient is told explicitly or not, he will nevertheless come to this awareness and may lose confidence in a doctor who either told him a lie or who did not help him face the seriousness of his illness while there might have been time to get his affairs in order.

It is an art to share this painful news with any patient. The simpler it is done, the easier it is usually for a patient who recollects it at a later date, if he can't "hear it" at the moment. Our patients appreciated it when they were told in the privacy of a little room rather than being told in the hallway of a crowded clinic.

What all of our patients stressed was the sense of empathy which counted more than the immediate tragedy of the news. It was the reassurance that everything possible will be done, that they will not be "dropped," that there were treatments available, that there was a glimpse of hope—even in the most advanced cases. If the news can be conveyed in such a manner, the patient will continue to have confidence in the doctor, and he will have time to work through the different reactions which will enable him to cope with this new and stressful life situation.

INFORMED CONSENT AND COERCION

From *Schloendorff v. New York Hospital*

Benjamin N. Cardozo

. . . Every human being of adult years and sound mind has a right to determine what shall be done with his own body; and a surgeon who performs an operation without his patient's consent commits an assault, for which he is liable in damages. (*Pratt* v. *Davis*, 224 Ill. 300; *Mohr* v. *Williams*, 95 Minn. 261.) This is true except in cases of emergency where the patient is unconscious and where it is necessary to operate before consent can be obtained. . . .

From "Viral Hepatitis: New Light on an Old Disease"

Saul Krugman and Joan P. Giles

Our studies on the natural history and prevention of viral hepatitis have been in progress since 1956. During the past 14 years we have collected and stored more than 25,000 serum specimens from more than 700 patients who were exposed to hepatitis in an institution where the disease has been highly endemic. Serial samples of serum were obtained before exposure, during the incubation period, and for many months and years after infection. This hepatitis serum bank has been a valuable source of materials for the study of the natural history of infectious hepatitis and serum hepatitis.

The discovery of Australia antigen by Blumberg and associates has opened a new chapter in hepatitis research. The association of this serum antigen with viral hepatitis has been confirmed by many investigators. The specific association with serum hepatitis has been demonstrated by Prince and by Giles and associates. The availability of a simple agar-gel precipitin test and a quantitative complement fixation test for the detection of Australia or hepatitis-associated antigen (HAA) and antibody (anti-HAA) represents an important technological advance. The use of these procedures for the reevaluation of the specimens in our hepatitis serum bank has enabled us to shed new light on an old disease.

From B. N. Cardozo, *Schloendorff* v. *N.Y. Hospital* 211 N.Y. 127, 129, 105 N.E. 92, 93 (1914) as it appears in Jay Katz, *Experimentation with Human Beings* (New York: Russell Sage Foundation, 1972), p. 526.
Reprinted from *Journal of the American Medical Association* 212:6, 1019–21, May 11, 1970. © 1970, American Medical Association.

Background for Willowbrook Hepatitis Studies. The Willowbrook State School is an institution for mentally retarded children located in Staten Island, N.Y. The nature of endemic hepatitis, first recognized in Willowbrook in 1949, has been described in detail in previous reports. Subsequently, the constant admission of many susceptible children in a population which increased to more than 5,000 patients by 1960 provided fertile soil for a continuing endemic situation. In the absence of an effective, specific prophylactic agent, it has been impossible to prevent the spread of this infection. As indicated in a previous report,* "under the chronic circumstance of multiple and repeated natural exposure, it has been shown that most newly admitted children become infected within the first 6 to 12 months of residence in the institution." Studies reported in 1967 revealed evidence of two distinctive immunological types of viral hepatitis, MS-1 which resembled infectious hepatitis (IH) and MS-2 which resembled serum hepatitis (SH).

The most important source of serum specimens was children whose hepatitis infection followed artificial exposure to the Willowbrook strains of virus which have been prevalent in the institution. The decision to conduct these studies was reached after consideration of many factors.

It was inevitable that susceptible children would become infected in the institution. Hepatitis was especially mild in the 3- to 10-year age group at Willowbrook. These studies would be carried out in a special unit with optimum isolation facilities to protect the children from other infectious diseases such as shigellosis, and parasitic and respiratory infections which

TABLE 2   Incidence of Hepatitis-Associated Antigen (HAA) in Patients at the Willowbrook State School From 1965 to 1970

Group	Description	Age Yr.	Time in Institution	No. Tested	HAA-Positive No.	HAA-Positive %
1.	Retarded adult men, all types, 1965*	19–36	> 6 yr	150	23	15.3
2.	Retarded adult male mongoloids, 1970	19–36	> 6 yr	86	16	18.6
3.	Retarded children, all types, 1968–1969	< 5	0–7 mo	130	13	10.0
4.	Retarded children, all types, 1968–1969†	< 10	0–5 yr	210	58	32.8
5.	Retarded children, congenital rubella, 1970	< 10	0–7 yr	45	11	24.4

* Of 150 adults in group 1, 17 had Down's syndrome and 133 had other causes of mental retardation. The HAA was detected in 3 of 17 (18%) of those with Down's syndrome and in 20 of 133 (15%) of other retarded adults. Sixteen HAA-positive patients were retested in 1969; 14 were still abnormal.

† Of 210 children in group 4, 44 had Down's syndrome; 43% were HAA-positive. Of the remaining 166 mentally retarded children, 24.4% were HAA-positive.

*Krugman S, Giles JP, Hammond J: Infectious hepatitis: Evidence for two distinctive clinical, epidemiological, and immunological types of infection. *JAMA* 200:365–73, 1967.

are prevalent in the institution. It should be emphasized that the artificial induction of hepatitis implies a "therapeutic" effect because of the immunity which is conferred.

The study groups have included only children whose parents gave written consent. Our method of obtaining informed consent has changed progressively since 1956. At that time the information was conveyed to individual parents by letter or personal interview. More recently, we have used the group technique of obtaining consent. The following procedure has been employed: First, a psychiatric social worker discusses the project with parents during a preliminary interview. Those who are interested are invited to attend a group session at the institution to discuss the project in greater detail. These sessions are conducted by the staff responsible for the program, including the physician, supervising nurse, staff attendants, and psychiatric social workers. Meetings have been frequently attended by outside physicians who have expressed interest. Parents in groups of six to eight are given a tour of the facilities. The purposes, potential benefits, and potential hazards of the program are discussed with them, and they are encouraged to ask questions. Thus, all parents can hear the response to questions posed by the more articulate members of the group. After leaving this briefing session parents have an opportunity to talk with their private physicians who may call the unit for more information. Approximately two weeks after the visit, the psychiatric social worker contacts the parents for their decision. If the decision is in the affirmative, the consent is signed but parents are informed that signed consent may be withdrawn any time before the beginning of the program. It has been clear that the group method has enabled us to obtain more thorough informed consent. Children who are wards of the state or children without parents have never been included in our studies.

Since 1956 the hepatitis studies have been reviewed and sanctioned by various local, state, and federal agencies. These studies have been reviewed and approved by the New York University and Willowbrook State School committees on human experimentation since their formation in February 1967. Prior to this date the functions of the present University Committee on Human Experimentation were performed by the Executive Faculty of the School of Medicine for studies of this type. The initial proposal in 1956 was reviewed and approved by the following groups: Executive Faculty, New York University School of Medicine, New York State Department of Mental Hygiene, New York State Department of Health, and Armed Forces Epidemiological Board. It is of interest that the guidelines which were adopted for the hepatitis studies at its inception in 1956 conformed to the World Medical Association's Draft Code of Ethics on Human Experimentation which was presented to its general assembly in September 1961, five years later.

Letters: Experiments at the Willowbrook State School

SIR,—You have referred to the work of Krugman and his colleagues at the Willowbrook State School in three editorials. In the first article the work was cited as a notable study of hepatitis and a model for this type of investigation. No comment was made on the rightness of attempting to infect mentally retarded children with hepatitis for experimental purposes, in an institution where the disease was already endemic.

The second editorial again did not remark on the ethics of the study, but the third sounded a note of doubt as to the justification for extending these experiments. The reason given was that some children might have been made more susceptible to serious hepatitis as the result of the administration of previously heated icterogenic material.

I believe that not only this last experiment, but the whole of Krugman's study, is quite unjustifiable, whatever the aims, and however academically or therapeutically important are the results. I am amazed that the work was published and that it has been actively supported editorially by the *Journal of the American Medical Association* and by Ingelfinger in the 1967–68 *Year Book of Medicine.* To my knowledge only the *British Journal of Hospital Medicine* has clearly stated the ethical position on these experiments and shown that it was indefensible to give potentially dangerous infected material to children, particularly those who were mentally retarded, with or without parental consent, when no benefit to the child could conceivably result.

Krugman and Giles have continued to publish the results of their study, and in a recent paper go to some length to describe their method of obtaining parental consent and list a number of influential medical boards and committees that have approved the study. They point out again that, in their opinion, their work conforms to the World Medical Association Draft Code of Ethics on Human Experimentation. They also say that hepatitis is still highly endemic in the school.

This attempted defence is irrelevant to the central issue. Is it right to perform an experiment on a normal or mentally retarded child when no benefit can result to that individual? I think that the answer is no, and that the question of parental consent is irrelevant. In my view the studies of Krugman serve only to show that there is a serious loophole in the Draft Code, which under General Principles and Definitions puts the onus of consent for experimentation on children on the parent or guardian. It is this section that is quoted by Krugman. I would class his work as "experiments conducted solely for the acquisition of knowledge," under which heading the code states that "Persons retained in mental hospital or hospitals for mental defectives should not be used for human experiment." Krugman may believe that his experiments were for the benefit of his patients, meaning the individual patients used in the study. If this is his belief he has a difficult case to defend. The duty of a pediatrician in a situation such as exists at Willowbrook State School is to attempt to improve that situation,

Letters reprinted from *The Lancet,* April 10, May 8, and July 10, 1971.

not to turn it to his advantage for experimental purposes, however lofty the aims.

Every new reference to the work of Krugman and Giles adds to its apparent ethical respectability, and in my view such references should stop, or at least be heavily qualified. The editorial attitude of *The Lancet* to the work should be reviewed and openly stated. The issue is too important to be ignored.

If Krugman and Giles are keen to continue their experiments I suggest that they invite the parents of the children involved to participate. I wonder what the response would be.

Stephen Goldby

SIR,—Dr. Stephen Goldby's critical comments (April 10, p. 749) about our Willowbrook studies and our motives for conducting them were published without extending us the courtesy of replying in the same issue of *The Lancet*. Your acceptance of his criticisms without benefit of our response implies a blackout of all comment related to our studies. This decision is unfortunate because our recent studies on active and passive immunisation for the prevention of viral hepatitis, type B, have clearly demonstrated a "therapeutic effect" for the children involved. These studies have provided us with the first indication and hope that it may be possible to control hepatitis in this institution. If this aim can be achieved, it will benefit not only the children, but also their families and the employees who care for them in the school. It is unnecessary to point out the additional benefit to the world-wide populations which have been plagued by an insoluble hepatitis problem for many generations.

Dr. Joan Giles and I have been actively engaged in studies aimed to solve two infectious-disease problems in the Willowbrook State School—measles and viral hepatitis. These studies were investigated in this institution because they represented major health problems for the 5000 or more mentally retarded children who were residents. Uninformed critics have assumed or implied that we came to Willowbrook to "conduct experiments on mentally retarded children."

The results of our Willowbrook studies with the experimental live attenuated measles vaccine developed by Enders and his colleagues are well documented in the medical literature. As early as 1960 we demonstrated the protective effect of this vaccine during the course of an epidemic. Prior to licensure of the vaccine in 1963 epidemics occurred at two-year intervals in this institution. During the 1960 epidemic there were more than 600 cases of measles and 60 deaths. In the wake of our ongoing measles vaccine programme, measles has been eradicated as a disease in the Willowbrook State School. We have not had a single case of measles since 1963. In this regard the children at the Willowbrook State School have been more fortunate than unimmunised children in Oxford, England, other areas in Great

Britain, as well as certain groups of children in the United States and other parts of the world.

The background of our hepatitis studies at Willowbrook has been described in detail in various publications. Viral hepatitis is so prevalent that newly admitted susceptible children become infected within 6 to 12 months after entry in the institution. These children are a source of infection for the personnel who care for them and for their families if they visit with them. We were convinced that the solution of the hepatitis problem in this institution was dependent on the acquisition of new knowledge leading to the development of an effective immunising agent. The achievements with smallpox, diphtheria, poliomyelitis, and more recently measles represent dramatic illustrations of this approach.

It is well known that viral hepatitis in children is milder and more benign than the same disease in adults. Experience has revealed that hepatitis in institutionalised, mentally retarded children is also mild, in contrast with measles, which is a more severe disease when it occurs in institutional epidemics involving the mentally retarded. Our proposal to expose a small number of newly admitted children to the Willowbrook strains of hepatitis virus was justified in our opinion for the following reasons: (1) they were bound to be exposed to the same strains under the natural conditions existing in the institution; (2) they would be admitted to a special, well-equipped, and well-staffed unit where they would be isolated from exposure to other infectious diseases which were prevalent in the institution—namely, shigellosis, parasitic infections, and respiratory infections—thus, their exposure in the hepatitis unit would be associated with less risk than the type of institutional exposure where multiple infections could occur; (3) they were likely to have a subclinical infection followed by immunity to the particular hepatitis virus; and (4) only children with parents who gave informed consent would be included.

The statement by Dr. Goldby accusing us of conducting experiments exclusively for the acquisition of knowledge with no benefit for the children cannot be supported by the true facts.

Saul Krugman

SIR.—I am astonished at the unquestioning way in which *The Lancet* has accepted the intemperate position taken by Dr. Stephen Goldby (April 10, p. 749) concerning the experimental studies of Krugman and Giles on hepatitis at the Willowbrook State School. These investigators have repeatedly explained—for over a decade—that natural hepatitis infection occurs sooner or later in virtually 100% of the patients admitted to Willowbrook, and that it is better for the patient to have a known, timed, controlled infection than an untimed, uncontrolled one. Moreover, the wisdom and human justification of these studies have been repeatedly and carefully examined and verified by a number of very distinguished, able individuals who are respected leaders in the making of such decisions.

The real issue is: Is it not proper and ethical to carry out experiments in children, which would apparently incur no greater risk than the children were likely to run by nature, in which the children generally receive better medical care when artificially infected than if they had been naturally infected, and in which the parents as well as the physician feel that a significant contribution to the future well-being of similar children is likely to result from the studies? It is true, to be sure, that the W.M.A. code says, "Children in institutions and not under the care of relatives should not be the subjects of human experiments." But this unqualified *obiter dictum* may represent merely the well-known inability of committees to think a problem through. However, it has been thought through by Sir Austin Bradford Hill, who has pointed out the unfortunate effects for these very children that would have resulted, were such a code to have been applied over the years.

Geoffrey Edsall

"Children in Institutions"

Paul Ramsey

Even if one granted the right of parents to consent for their children to be used in medical investigations having unknown present and future risks to them and promising future possible benefits only for others, it would still be possible to argue that children in institutions and not directly and continuously under the care of parents or relatives should *never* be so used. If we are not persuaded that *because they are children* children cannot consent (nor should anyone else consent in their behalf) to experiments primarily for the accumulation of knowledge, we at least should be convinced that such experiments ought not to be performed upon children in orphanages, reformatories, or homes for the retarded *because they are a captive population.*

In discussions of the consent-requirement more attention has been paid to the question of whether and under what possible circumstances adult prisoners can validly consent to research trials than to the question of whether and under what possible circumstances there can be valid consent for children who cannot consent at all. Some authors seem to find it easier to include children by proxy, reducing consent to a merely formal requirement which can be met by someone else other than the real subject, than to include prisoners who may be under undue duress (but who, to suppose

Reprinted with permission of author and publisher from Paul Ramsey, *The Patient as a Person* (New Haven: Yale University Press, 1970), pp. 40–58.

the worst, do themselves conditionally consent). In an otherwise excellent article, Professor John Fletcher of Virginia Theological Seminary, for example, comes closest to ever saying "never" in ethics when he is discussing the use of prisoners, while accepting as standard the substitution of the consent of an incompetent's legal representative.[1] This anomaly or contrast in the literature of medical ethics is worth pondering.

The usual reasons offered for not accepting prisoner volunteers are only cautionary, even if very severe, warnings. It is not impossible in local situations to overcome them so as to secure from prisoners a reasonably free as well as an adequately informed consent. It is duress that has to be avoided —the duress to give a particular consent because of too great hope of parole. This should not be an automatic "payment." Even a pattern of always weighing heavily the consent of prisoners in considering them for parole has to be avoided. Still it is not impossible to arrange things so that a man in prison may freely volunteer to become a joint adventurer in an experiment for the sake of the knowledge and good to come, and not for the sake of the reward. It is not impossible to protect his will from duress to cooperate in such medical undertakings. To do this, some would require in the case of prisoners the complete exclusion of any possibility of reward, or of earlier parole. This seems unfairly severe on prisoners. No one who has read the noble words of Nathan Leopold concerning the purposefulness of his own and other prisoners' participation in the malaria experiments in the Illinois State Prison during World War II can deny that prisoners *may* be as free in volunteering as persons in normal life.

If the consent of prisoners to medical experimentation is not inherently or always necessarily invalid, there may still be decisive objection to the general practice of using them. This was the most persuasive argument made by Professor David Daube in the Ciba Symposium in morally forbidding the use of prisoners as donors of organs for transplantation. Daube allowed that the pressure upon familial donors may be greater than that placed upon prisoners, but "the pressure in one's family or circle belongs to the normal burden and dignity of social existence"; this is "a pressure consonant with the dignity and responsibility of free life." This we deny to prisoners. Lord Kilbrandon made something of the same point (appealing to what philosophers call *fairness*-considerations) when he said that "when

---

[1]Fletcher, "Human Experimentation," pp. 620–49. The author "agrees with those who would put the sharpest restrictions upon the use of prisoner populations in medical research, since by virtue of their imprisonment they cannot be truly said to possess an active capacity to consent. . . . [Those who have suffered] the loss of public liberty through imprisonment, should not then be made to go through the charade of seeming to possess what has been temporarily removed" ibid., p. 636. I suggest that a child, by virtue of his childhood, cannot be truly said to possess all active capacity to consent; and that it is a dangerous charade for anyone to go through the motions of consenting for him when this is not truly done *in his behalf medically.* Particularly in regard to children in institutions, to say "never" to the consents of their legal representatives when these are not even ostensibly in the children's behalf medically would not be "to remove oneself from historical possibility" (*ibid.*, p. 636, n. 46). It would rather be to place upon ourselves the moral requirement that other historical possibilities for the accumulation of knowledge be looked for or designed.

we put a man in prison we deprive him of a large number of his consents, therefore it is perhaps distasteful to confer upon him a consent which is not for his benefit but for our own." In any case, from these considerations, Professor Daube drew a strict conclusion: "No person under any restraint whatsoever should be allowed to give consent"; "a person under restraint cannot be presumed to consent."[2] These statements—as we shall see in a moment—are applicable as well to children in institutions.

But the reasons so far cited that lend support to this sweeping conclusion are not adequate, unless imprisonment means that a man has been altogether drummed out of the human community. Since it does not, one might argue for quite the opposite conclusion. It can be contended that since we have deprived a prisoner of a large number of his consents, we should yield to his consent to do good if it is an understanding, voluntary consent. It can be contended that there are dignity and responsibilities consonant with prison life, and that under proper precautions participation in medical experimentation may be among them.

Interwoven with these considerations, however, was another that was more convincing. As Professor Daube put it: "Not all prison authorities throughout the world deserve the fullest trust"; ". . . it would be fatal to lower standards in an indirect manner, however laudable the purposes"; "I have no doubt that 99 out of 100 prisoners would have done this freely, but I wouldn't take the chance on the 100th."[3]

Dr. T. E. Starzl, and the other transplant surgeons at the University of Colorado, had used prisoner donors. He remained convinced of the *voluntariness* of their action. The program was announced in a low key, by a simple notice on the bulletin board of the prison. No pay or pardon or reduction of length of servitude was offered, and none was given. The incidence of enlistment was low. Many of those who volunteered had only a few weeks or months left to serve. These facts support the view that the prisoners' actions were volitional. They also lead us to question again whether the opportunity to make this consent should be withheld from prisoners if it is an opportunity to be presented to anyone. Still, Dr. Starzl was persuaded by Professor Daube for the reason stated above, and the practice was discontinued. Dr. Starzl summarized the argument very well indeed: "The use of penal volunteers, however equitably handled in a local situation, would inevitably lead to abuse if accepted as a reasonable precedent and applied broadly."[4]

This asks and gives one answer to the question: Which rule of medical practice or institutional practice, if widely adopted, can be foreseen to lead on the whole to the violation of men and to their self-violation, even if this need not be the case in each instance? Where, for example, the payment of money for blood tissue is practiced, and prisoners are not excluded from this payment, one does not have to travel far even in this enlightened land

[2]Wolstenholme and O'Connor, *Ethics in Medical Progress*, pp. 198, 204, 205, 197, 204.
[3]Ibid., pp. 198, 204.
[4]Ibid., pp. 75–77.

to hear rumors that local or state politicians have a concession or a kickback on the prisoner blood supply! That is wrong and was predictable, even if payment, and payment to prisoners, is not wrong in each instance.

To return to the question of investigations involving children in institutions as subjects in trials having no relation to their care, we can now say that even if this would not be (as I have argued) inherently or always necessarily wrong, still the use of captive populations in children, however equitably and safely handled in a local situation, would inevitably lead to abuse if accepted as a reasonable precedent and applied broadly. A rule of practice prohibiting the use of children in institutions simply as experimental subjects in the accumulation of knowledge for the benefit of others should govern the institutions set up to care for them. Some philosophers would call this a rule-utilitarian-rule. It is rather a rule of fidelity, expressing in a specific practice mankind's minimum loyalty to children.

The Kefauver-Harris amendments to the Federal Food, Drug, and Cosmetic Act passed in 1962 do not so rule; and the use of captive populations of children in pharmacological investigations is a practice that is not only widespread but predictably abused in this country. The bill that went before Congress for vote contained no provision for patient or subject consent. Senator Jacob Javits proposed to amend the bill to require that in investigations of a new drug the patients or subjects be "appropriately advised that such drug had not been determined to be safe in use for human beings." The outcome of debate in the House and Senate was to make subject consent mandatory while lodging the certification of this in the investigators, not in the Food and Drug Administration. The provision finally enacted introduced proxy consent and two exceptions to the procuring of consent. As finally adopted the provision requires:

> . . . that experts using such drugs for investigational purposes certify to such manufacturer or sponsor that they will inform any human beings to whom such drugs, or any controls used in connection therewith, are being administered, or their representatives, that such drugs are being used for investigational purposes and will obtain the consent of such human beings or their representatives, except [1] where they deem it not feasible or, [2] in their professional judgment, contrary to the best interests of such human beings.[5]

The first interpretative ruling by the FDA concerning this consent requirement was not issued until August 30, 1966. Meantime, a number of investigators had thought that "not feasible" allowed them to dispense with consent if this inconvenienced the research design. In short, the provision was thought to have enacted the supremacy of *another* duty of medical experimenters, namely, to ensure that the quality of the research design is such as to secure the scientific results being sought.

The 1966 interpretative ruling, however, limited the intention of this stipulation to care for the patients or subjects consenting to drug investiga-

[5]Federal Food, Drug, and Cosmetic Act, Section 505 (i).

tions. It adopted the distinction in the Helsinki Declaration between research primarily for the accumulation of knowledge and research in therapeutic situations. No exception to the requirement of consent of the subject or his representative was allowed in the first instance. The two exceptions applied only to research having patient care primarily in view. Finally, the meaning of these exceptions was determined largely by reference to the debates in the House and Senate in 1962. "Not feasible" meant patients in coma or patients otherwise incapable of consenting whose legal representative was unavailable in an emergency. "Contrary to the best interests of such human beings" was meant to permit beneficial investigations on, for example, cancer patients without upsetting such a patient's well-being when in a physician's discretion the patient does not know he has cancer.

This interpretative ruling concerning the meaning of these exceptions is dangerous if it is taken to sanction unrelated experimentation on the seriously ill or the dying without the patient's prior participatory consent. But the main thing to be said is that these stipulations are largely irrelevant to drug research. The interpretation of the "exceptions" followed the debate in Congress; but that debate about seriously ill and dying patients was also largely irrelevant to the majority of drug research. Therefore, even after these interpretations were issued, it could fairly be said of the FDA "exceptions": "Better loopholes may be invented, but this seems a good start."[6] However, seriously ill or dying patients may need an insufficiently tested drug. Then medical ethics would require that the efficacy of the new drug be predictable with some confidence; it must be more likely to work than an established remedy. But we may allow that in the course of new-drug investigations there may be cases in which, all other therapies having failed or estimated to be likely to prove less beneficial than the new drug, a patient's consent can be constructively implied as the basis of Good Samaritan emergency treatment.

Ordinarily, however, drug research is more deliberate and preplanned. What is needed are human beings willing to consent to take the drugs or to serve as anonymous controls. What is needed is an easily controlled population. The legal representative of children in institutions would ordinarily be available, if he is to be vested with the power of consent for them but not in their medical behalf. The children themselves are ordinarily under no necessity to have the drug used without delay. Reference to the use of drugs in emergencies among the specifications of a law governing investigations in drugs is exceedingly likely to come to mean that anything that delays the solution of medical problems is unethical. The research consequences are likely to become overriding. This may happen if investigators are tempted to transfer the exceptions to the consent requirement in cases of beneficial (emergency) research to the bulk of drug research, which is nonbeneficial, and which should proceed only with the understanding of

[6]Oscar D. Ratnoff and Marian F. Ratnoff, "Ethical Responsibility in Clinical Investigation," *Perspectives in Biology and Medicine*, Autumn 1967, p. 89.

the subject. The crux, therefore, is the admission that a subject's consent can be satisfied by *his representative*.[7] This opens the door to the use of children in institutions for experimental purposes and not for drug testing that is incidental to the course of their medical care.

In 1958 and 1959 the *New England Journal of Medicine* reported a series of experiments performed upon patients and new admittees to the Willowbrook State School, a home for retarded children in Staten Island, New York.[8] These experiments were described as "an attempt to control the high prevalence of infectious hepatitis in an institution for mentally defective patients." The experiments were said to be justified because, under conditions of an existing controlled outbreak of hepatitis in the institution, "knowledge obtained from a series of suitable studies could well lead to its control." In actuality, the experiments were designed to duplicate and confirm the efficacy of gamma globulin in immunization against hepatitis, to develop and improve or improve upon that inoculum, and to learn more about infectious hepatitis in general.

The experiments were justified—doubtless, after a great deal of soul searching—for the following reasons: there was a smoldering epidemic throughout the institution and "it was apparent that most of the patients at Willowbrook were naturally exposed to hepatitis virus"; infectious hepatitis is a much milder disease in children; the strain at Willowbrook was especially mild; only the strain or strains of the virus already disseminated at Willowbrook were used: and only those small and incompetent patients whose parents gave consent were used.

The patient population at Willowbrook was 4478, growing at a rate of one patient a day over a three-year span, or from 10 to 15 new admissions per week. In the first trial the existing population was divided into two groups: one group served as uninoculated controls, and the other group was inoculated with 0.01 ml. of gamma globulin per pound of body weight. Then for a second trial new admittees and those left uninoculated before were again divided: one group served as uninoculated controls and the other was inoculated with 0.06 ml. of gamma globulin per pound of body weight. This

[7]By contrast, the statement on "Clinical Investigations Using Human Beings as Subject" issued by the U.S. Public Health Service severely limits the consent of such human beings' legal representatives. "No subject may participate in an investigative procedure," it says, "unless: (a) He is mentally competent and has sufficient mental and communicative capacity to understand his choice to participate; and (b) He is 21 years of age or more, except that if the individual be less than 21, he may participate in a procedure intended and designed to protect or improve his personal health or otherwise for his personal benefit or advantage if the informed written consent of his parents or legal guardian be obtained as well as the written consent of the subject himself if he be mature enough to appreciate the nature of the procedure and the risks involved" (Department of Health, Education and Welfare, Bureau of Medical Services Circular No. 38, June 23, 1966).

[8]Robert Ward, Saul Krugman, Joan P. Giles, A. Milton Jacobs, and Oscar Bodansky, "Infectious Hepatitis: Studies of Its Natural History and Prevention," *New England Journal of Medicine* 258, no. 9 (February 27, 1958): 407–16; Saul Krugman, Robert Ward, Joan P. Giles, Oscar Bodansky, and A. Milton Jacobs, "Infectious Hepatitis: Detection of the Virus during the Incubation Period and in Clinically Inapparent Infection," *New England Journal of Medicine* 261, no. 15 (October 8, 1959): 729–34. The following account and unannotated quotations are taken from these articles.

proved that Stokes et al. had correctly demonstrated that the larger amount would give significant immunity for up to seven or eight months.[9]

Serious ethical questions may be raised about the trials so far described. No mention is made of any attempt to enlist the adult personnel of the institution, numbering nearly 1,000 including nearly 600 attendants on ward duty, and new additions to the staff, in these studies whose excusing reason was that almost everyone was "naturally" exposed to the Willowbrook virus. Nothing requires that major research into the natural history of hepatitis be first undertaken in children. Experiments have been carried out in the military and with prisoners as subjects. There have been fatalities from the experiments; but surely in all these cases the consent of the volunteers was as valid or better than the proxy consent of these children's "representatives." There would have been no question of the understanding consent that might have been given by the adult personnel at Willowbrook, if significant benefits were expected from studying that virus.

Second, nothing is said that would warrant withholding an inoculation of some degree of known efficacy from part of the population, or for withholding in the first trial less than the full amount of gamma globulin that had served to immunize in previous tests, except the need to test, confirm, and improve the inoculum. That, of course, was a desirable goal; but it does not seem possible to warrant withholding gamma globulin for the reason that is often said to justify controlled trials, namely, that one procedure is *as likely* to succeed as the other.

Third, nothing is said about attempts to control or defeat the low-grade epidemic at Willowbrook by more ordinary, if more costly and less experimental, procedures. Nor is anything said about admitting no more patients until this goal had been accomplished. This was not a massive urban hospital whose teeming population would have to be turned out into the streets, with resulting dangers to themselves and to public health, in order to sanitize the place. Instead, between 200 and 250 patients were housed in each of 18 buildings over approximately 400 acres in a semirural setting of fields, woods, and well-kept, spacious lawns. Clearly it would have been possible to secure other accommodation for new admissions away from the infection, while eradicating the infection at Willowbrook building by building. This might have cost money, and it would certainly have required astute detective work to discover the source of the infection. The doctors determined that the new patients likely were not carrying the infection upon admission, and that it did not arise from the procedures and routine inoculations given them at the time of admission. Why not go further in the search for the source of the epidemic? If this had been an orphanage for normal

[9]J. Stokes, Jr., et al., "Infectious Hepatitis: Length of Protection by Immune Serum Globulin (Gamma Globulin) during Epidemics," *Journal of the American Medical Association* 147 (1951): 714–19. Since the half-life of gamma globulin is three weeks, no one knows exactly why it immunizes for so long a period. The "highly significant protection against hepatitis obtained by the use of gamma globulin," however, had been confirmed as early as 1945 (see Edward B. Grossman, Sloan G. Stewart, and Joseph Stokes, "Post-Transfusion Hepatitis in Battle Casualties," *Journal of the American Medical Association* 129. no. 15 [December 8, 1945]: 991–94). The inoculation *withheld* in the Willowbrook experiments had, therefore, proved vaulable.

children or a floor of private patients, instead of a school for mentally defective children, one wonders whether the doctors would so readily have accepted the hepatitis as a "natural" occurrence and even as an opportunity for study.

The next step was to attempt to induce "passive-active immunity" by feeding the virus to patients already protected by gamma globulin. In this attempt to improve the inoculum, permission was obtained from the parents of children from 5 to 10 years of age newly admitted to Willowbrook, who were then isolated from contact with the rest of the institution. All were inoculated with gamma globulin and then divided into two groups: one served as controls while the other group of new patients were fed the Willowbrook virus, obtained from feces, in doses having 50 percent infectivity, i.e., in concentrations estimated to produce hepatitis with jaundice in half the subjects tested. Then twice the 50 percent infectivity was tried. This proved, among other things, that hepatitis has an "alimentary-tract phase" in which it can be transmitted from one person to another while still "inapparent" in the first person. This, doubtless, is exceedingly important information in learning how to control epidemics of infectious hepatitis. The second of the two articles mentioned above describes studies of the incubation period of the virus and of whether pooled serum remained infectious when aged and frozen. Still the small, mentally defective patients who were deliberately fed infectious hepatitis are described as having suffered mildly in most cases: "The liver became enlarged in the majority, occasionally a week or two before the onset of jaundice. Vomiting and anorexia usually lasted only a few days. Most of the children gained weight during the course of hepatitis."

That mild description of what happened to the children who were fed hepatitis (and who continued to be introduced into the unaltered environment of Willowbrook) is itself alarming, since it is now definitely known that cirrhosis of the liver results from infectious hepatitis more frequently than from excessive consumption of alcohol! Now, or in 1958 and 1959, no one knows what may be other serious consequences of contracting infectious hepatitis. Understanding human volunteers were then and are now needed in the study of this disease, although a South American monkey has now successfully been given a form of hepatitis, and can henceforth serve as our ally in its conquest. But not children who cannot consent knowingly. If Peace Corps workers are regularly given gamma globulin before going abroad as a guard against their contracting hepatitis, and are inoculated at intervals thereafter, it seems that this is the least we should do for mentally defective children before they "go abroad" to Willowbrook or other institutions set up for their care.

Discussions pro and con of the Willowbrook experiments that have come to my attention serve only to reinforce the ethical objections that can be raised against what was done simply from a careful analysis of the original articles reporting the research design and findings. In an address at the 1968 Ross Conference on Pediatric Research, Dr. Saul Krugman raised the question, Should vaccine trials be carried out in adult volunteers before subjecting children to similar tests?[10] He answered this question in the negative. The reason adduced was simply that "a vaccine virus trial may be a more hazardous procedure for adults than for children." Medical researchers, of course, are required to minimize the hazards, but not by moving from consenting to unconsenting subjects. This apology clearly shows that adults and children have become interchangeable in face of the overriding importance of obtaining the research goal. This means that the special moral claims of children for care and protection are forgotten, and especially the claims of children who are most weak and vulnerable. (Krugman's reference to the measles vaccine trials is not to the point.)

The *Medical Tribune* explains that the 16-bed isolation unit set up at Willowbrook served "to protect the study subjects from Willowbrook's other endemic diseases—such as shigellosis, measles, rubella and respiratory and parasitic infections—while exposing them to hepatitis."[11] This presumably compensated for the infection they were given. It is not convincingly shown that the children could by no means, however costly, have been protected from the epidemic of hepatitis. The statement that Willowbrook "had endemic infectious hepatitis and a sufficiently open population so that the disease could never be quieted by exhausting the supply of susceptibles" is at best enigmatic.

Oddly, physicians defending the propriety of the Willowbrook hepatitis project soon begin talking like poorly instructed "natural lawyers"! Dr. Louis Lasagna and Dr. Geoffrey Edsall, for example, find these experiments unobjectionable—both, for the reason stated by Edsall: "the children would apparently incur no greater risk than they were likely to run by nature." In any case, Edsall's examples of parents consenting with a son 17 years of age for him to go to war, and society's agreement with minors that they can drive cars and hurt themselves were entirely beside the point. Dr. David D. Rutstein adheres to a stricter standard in regard to research on infectious hepatitis: "It is not ethical to use human subjects for the growth of a virus for any purpose."[12]

[10]Saul Krugman, "Reflections on Pediatric Clinical Investigations," in *Problems of Drug Evaluation in Infants and Children,* Report of the Fifty-eighth Ross Conference on Pediatric Research, Dorado Beach, Puerto Rico, May 5–7, 1968 (Columbus: Ross Laboratories), pp. 41–42.

[11]"Studies with Children Backed on Medical, Ethical Grounds," *Medical Tribune and Medical News* 8, no. 19 (February 20, 1967): 1, 23.

[12]*Daedalus,* Spring 1969, pp. 471–72, 529. See also pp. 458, 470–72. Since it is the proper business of an ethicist to uphold the proposition that only retrogression in civility can result from bad moral reasoning and the use of inept examples, however innocent, it is fair to point out the startling comparison between Edsall's "argument" and the statement of Dr. Karl Brandt, plenipotentiary in charge of all medical activities in the Nazi Reich: "Do you think that one can obtain any worth-while, fundamental results without a definite toll of lives? The same goes for technological development. You cannot build a great bridge, a gigantic building—you cannot establish a speed record without deaths!" (quoted by Leo Alexander, "War Crimes: Their Social-Psychological Aspects," *American Journal of Psychiatry* 105, no. 3 [September 1948]: 172). Casualties to progress, or injuries accepted in setting speed limits, are morally quite different from death or maiming or even only risks, or unknown risks, directly and deliberately imposed upon an unconsenting human being.

The latter sweeping verdict may depend on knowledge of the effects of viruses on chromasomal difficulties, mongolism, etc., that was not available to the Willowbrook group when their researches were begun thirteen years ago. If so, this is a telling point against appeal to "no discernible risks" as the sole standard applicable to the use of children in medical experimentation. That would lend support to the proposition that we always know that there are unknown and undiscerned risks in the case of an invasion of the fortress of the body—which then can be consented to by an adult in behalf of a child only if it is in the child's behalf medically.

When asked what she told the parents of the subject-children at Willowbrook, Dr. Joan Giles replied, "I explain that there is no vaccine against infectious hepatitis. . . . I also tell them that we can modify the disease with gamma globulin but we can't provide lasting immunity without letting them get the disease."[13] Obviously vaccines giving "lasting immunity" are not the only kinds of vaccine to be used in caring for patients.

Doubtless the studies at Willowbrook resulted in improvement in the vaccine, to the benefit of present and future patients. In September 1966, "a routine program of GG [gamma globulin] administration to every new patient at Willowbrook" was begun. This cut the incidence of icteric hepatitis 80 to 85 percent. Then follows a significant statement in the *Medical Tribune* article: "A similar reduction in the icteric form of the disease has been accomplished among the employees, who began getting routine GG earlier in the study."[14] Not only did the research team (so far as these reports show) fail to consider and adopt the alternative that new admittees to the staff be asked to become volunteers for an investigation that might improve the vaccine against the strand of infectious hepatitis to which they as well as the children were exposed. Instead, the staff was routinely protected earlier than the inmates were! And, as we have seen, there was evidence from the beginning that gamma globulin provided at least some protection. A "modification" of the disease was still an inoculum, even if this provided no lasting immunization and had to be repeated. It is axiomatic to medical ethics that a known remedy or protection—even if not perfect or even if the best exact administration of it has not been proved—should not be withheld from individual patients. It seems to a layman that from the beginning various trials at immunization of all new admittees might have been made, and controlled observation made of their different degrees of effectiveness against "nature" at Willowbrook. This would doubtless have been a longer way round, namely, the "anecdotal" method of investigative treatment that comes off second best in comparison with controlled trials. Yet this seems to be the alternative dictated by our received medical ethics, and the only one expressive of minimal care of the primary patients themselves.

Finally, except for one episode the obtaining of parental consent (on the premise that this is ethically valid) seems to have been very well handled. Wards of the state were not used, though by law the administrator at Willow-

---

[13] *Medical Tribune*, February 20, 1967, p. 23.
[14] *Medical Tribune*, February 20, 1967, p. 23.

brook could have signed consent for them. Only new admittees whose parents were available were entered by proxy consent into the project. Explanation was made to groups of these parents, and they were given time to think about it and consult with their own family physicians. Then late in 1964 Willowbrook was closed to all new admissions because of overcrowding. What then happened can most impartially be described in the words of an article defending the Willowbrook project on medical and ethical grounds:

> Parents who applied for their children to get in were sent a form letter over Dr. Hammond's signature saying that there was no space for new admissions and that their name was being put on a waiting list.
>
> But the hepatitis program, occupying its own space in the institution, continued to admit new patients as each new study group began. "Where do you find new admissions except by canvassing the people who have applied for admission?" Dr. Hammond asked.
>
> So a new batch of form letters went out, saying that there were a few vacancies in the hepatitis research unit if the parents cared to consider volunteering their child for that.
>
> In some instances the second form letter apparently was received as closely as a week after the first letter arrived.[15]

Granting—as I do not—the validity of parental consent to research upon children not in their behalf medically, what sort of consent was that? Surely, the duress upon these parents with children so defective as to require institutionalization was far greater than the duress on prisoners given tobacco or paid or promised parole for their cooperation! I grant that the timing of these events was inadvertent. Since, however, ethics is a matter of criticizing institutions and not only of exculpating or making culprits of individual men, the inadvertence does not matter. This is the strongest possible argument for saying that even if parents have the right to consent to submit the children who are directly and continuously in their care to nonbeneficial medical experimentation, this should not be the rule of practice governing institutions set up for their care.

Such use of captive populations of children for purely experimental purposes ought to be made legally impossible. My view is that this should be stopped by legal acknowledgement of the moral invalidity of parental or legal proxy consent for the child to procedures having no relation to a child's own diagnosis or treatment. If this is not done, canons of loyalty require that the rule of practice (by law, or otherwise) be that children in institutions and not directly under the care of parents or relatives should *never* be used in medical investigations having present pain or discomfort and unknown present and future risks to them, and promising future possible benefits only for others.

In 1967, after a study of twenty-one New York City municipal hospitals, State Senator Seymour R. Thaler proposed an amendment to the New

[15]*Medical Tribune,* February 20, 1967, p. 23.

York State Civil Rights bill that would apply sweepingly to all medical research and to all research involving children as subjects. Some of the provisions of his amendment could be applied more narrowly to captive populations of children. Senator Thaler would require the "voluntary informed written consent of adult patients used in medical experiment and would prohibit research on children unless authorized by a 'court of competent jurisdiction.' " His bill stipulated that the court may authorize a medical experiment or other medical research upon a minor when such experiment or research is related to the minor's physical or mental ailment and upon a finding by the court that the best interests of the minor would thereby be served. It was the provision placing all research upon children under courts of competent jurisdiction that caused the furor. Dr. Saul Krugman, chairman of pediatrics at New York University, called the bill "a disaster—a real disaster," if passed.[16]

The version of this bill introduced by Senators Thaler and Lent in 1969 does not entirely invalidate parental consent. This, however, is set within the context of the creation of a state board on human research charged with responsibility to formulate rules and regulations and to require the establishment of institutional and regional screening committees. The bill provides that "no person shall be used in human research without his or his parent's, guardian's or legal representative's prior written informed consent, but the board may make such exceptions as it may prescribe where the proposed subject is incompetent to give such consent . . ."[17]

The objection to this legislation can be only the resistance of researchers to the development of public policy in this regard, by law and through regulatory agencies. There are more regulations governing animal experimentation than govern human experimentation; more laws regulating the interstate transportation of bodies than regulate the interstate transportation of dying patients (who may be eligible organ donors when they are pronounced dead); a great mass of case law having to do with medical negligence in cases of treatment but little that deals with investigations primarily for the accumulation of knowledge. This situation is not likely long to endure.

For this reason, let us look briefly at another attempt to draft appropriate legislation—this time not by a state senator but by Frank P. Grad, Adjunct Professor of Legislation and Associate Director of the Legislative Drafting Research Fund at Columbia University Law School. In a paper before a conference sponsored by the New York Academy of Sciences, Professor Grad stated the principle that runs throughout our legal and moral tradition. "The rationale," he wrote, "which allows parents or guardians to consent on behalf of their children or wards in the therapeutic situation are not clearly applicable to the non-therapeutic one. . . . There is

[16]*New York Times,* January 20, 1967. Krugman was one of the physicians who conducted the Willowbrook experiments.

[17]An Act To Amend the Education Law, in Relation to the Regulation of Research on Human Subjects, In Senate, 1969–70 Regular Session, Cal. No. 1865, 4652–A. February 14, 1969.

no clear reason why a parent should be given the power to consent to expose his child to a risk, where taking the risk is not clearly in the child's interest or for his benefit. Nor is there any reason why a lawyer-guardian sitting in his downtown office ought to be free to expose his incompetent ward in a state hospital to hazards which he has neither chosen, nor which he has the competency to choose, for himself. Consent on behalf of minors and incompetents has, therefore, been rather closely circumscribed."[18]

But in the model legislation accompanying his paper, Professor Grad suggested the unqualified enactment of this principle only in the case of incompetents other than children as such. "Valid consent for an incompetent to become a subject may be given by his legal guardian," the draft legislation reads, "only if the human experimentation or research bears directly upon such incompetent's disability." That statement might have been repeated with regard to subjects judged incompetent for reasons of age. Instead, the draft reads: "Valid consent for a person under the age of eighteen years may be given by his parent or legal guardian only if there is no reason to believe that the human experimentation or research will result in physical or psychological injury or harm."

In other words, these legislative proposals would bring under public scrutiny both the parental consents obtained and the physiologically describable acts to be used in medical research. Neither would actually rule out the power of the consent of parents to enter their children into nontherapeutic medical trials. I suggest that—short of prohibiting the latter—our legislation would still need to go further than these proposals. Parental responsibility is necessarily weakened when children are institutionalized, when they are no longer directly, daily, and continuously under our care.

If we are going to count on parental and familial consent as sufficient protection of child-life, this should be only when parents are constantly placed on their mettle in the daily life of the home. If we then fail our children, this may be, as Professor Daube said, among the normal burdens, hazards, and dignity of a child's daily life. But surely we have the wisdom to know that even ordinary parental care must slacken when children are away in institutions; this is even more true when parents grievously need to place a child in an institution in order to provide at all for his care.

If, then, we are not going to invalidate the consents of parents and relatives except in the case of investigations proximately or remotely related

[18]Frank P. Grad, "Regulation of Clinical Research by the State," Conference on New Dimensions in Legal and Ethical Concepts for Human Research, New York Academy of Sciences, New York City, May 19–21, 1969. Professor Grad resolved the alleged problem of drawing the line between therapeutic and nontherapeutic research by imagining a patient to ask: " '*Doctor, are you doing this for me, or am I doing this for you?*' If the physician can truthfully answer that he is doing it for the patient, then it is clearly therapeutic research. If, on the contrary, the subject is undergoing a particular procedure not for his own benefit but for that of the researcher in the pursuit of a scientific goal, then the procedure is non-therapeutic." The thesis of this chapter is that since the child patient cannot ask that question, what he is doing for the researcher is simply being done to him, while what is done to him by way of treatment or investigational treatment, with legitimate parental or guardian consent or by his implied consent, has the patient as an end in view.

to a child's own treatment, there can be no valid argument against doing exactly this in the limited case of children in orphanages, reformatories, or homes for the retarded. The legal representatives of such children—even if parents—should be able to make decisions only in the stated medical interests of the children themselves if they are part of a captive population. To require a showing that this in fact is what is being done would be a proper additional arrangement guaranteeing that institutions for the care of children exist in fact only to care for them according to the canons of the highest loyalty, and not for the accumulation of knowledge having no stated benefit to these children themselves. Then parents and medical experimentation in general in the case of children might be moved to come up to the standards of our institutions.

"Human Experimentation: New York Verdict Affirms Patient's Rights"

Elinor Langer

New York, N.Y. Two years ago this month, New York City's yellow and not-so-yellow journalists had a feast with the disclosure that, as part of a research project, live cancer cells were being injected into hospitalized patients under circumstances in which the nature of their consent to the proceedings was exceedingly ambiguous (*Science,* 7 February 1964). A number of circumstances made the case particularly newsworthy. The patients in question were 22 seriously ailing and debilitated inhabitants of a relatively obscure Brooklyn institution, the Jewish Chronic Disease Hospital (JCDH). The research in question, studies in cancer immunology, was generally rated within the scientific community as among the most significant of all lines of research on malignant diseases. And both the researcher in question, Chester Southam, and his institution, Sloan-Kettering, held unassailable positions in the forefront of American medical science.

After considerable time the sensational charges and accusations of "Nazi tactics" disappeared from the headlines, although an article on the case, entitled "How doctors use patients as guinea pigs," appeared in a national women's magazine as recently as last fall. But in the labyrinths of New York State's administrative machinery, under the direction of a unit of the department of education known as the Division of Professional Conduct, the case was being subjected to intensive review. Last month the Regents of the University of the State of New York, acting under this responsibility

Reprinted with permission from *Science* 151:11, 663–66, February 1966. Copyright 1966 by the American Association for the Advancement of Science.

for licensing the medical profession, issued their verdict.* Southam and Emanuel Mandel, medical director of the Chronic Disease Hospital, were found guilty of "unprofessional conduct" and of "fraud and deceit in the practice of medicine." Their licenses were suspended for 1 year, although execution of the sentences has been stayed. The men will be on probation, but allowed to practice.

In the course of their review, the Regents and the medical grievance committee which advised them explored many questions of serious importance to the entire medical research community. On two key questions— when is consent "informed," and how far may the physician exercise his physician's authority when he is acting in the role of experimenter—the Regents have developed definitions which, while not legal precedents (except perhaps in New York), represent a major attempt to put some precision into the vague ethical concepts now governing experimentation with human subjects.

Some of the arguments raised by the defense lawyers are also important, for they suggest that Southam and Mandel were stumbling through a signless desert and that, if they lost their way, they did no more than other researchers have done before them or than, in the absence of clearer standards, researchers will continue to do after them.

Finally, the fact of the proceedings is in itself significant, confirming what the large-scale publicity itself hinted—that the question of medical experimentation is already outside the house of science. The Regents' decision is an affirmation that there is a public interest to be protected in the field of medical research; it is an omen that the public may begin to set the rules. (The body of the Regents' decision is given on pages 148–50.)

The nondisputed facts in the case are these: Southam's work involved the injection of tissue-cultured cancer cells into human subjects and measurement of the speed with which the injected substance was rejected by the body. Earlier phases of the work had established that healthy persons would reject the tissue culture in 4 to 6 weeks, and that individuals already ill with advanced cancer would reject them in a longer period, ranging from 6 weeks to several months. To test the hypothesis that the slower rate of rejection in the cancer patients was in fact attributable to their cancer and not to the general debility that accompanies any chronic illness, it was necessary to perform the experiment on patients severely ill with nonmalignant diseases. A chronic-disease hospital was a logical place to look for patients with the required characteristics. Southam approached Mandel, who agreed to the collaboration, and, in July 1963, 22 patients (including three cancer patients

*The Board of Regents consists of 15 individuals elected by joint resolution of the two houses of New York's legislature for terms of 15 years. The Regents have jurisdiction over all education in the state, public and private, and over all licensed professions excluding the law. The three Regents most intimately involved in this decision were the three members of a special committee on discipline: Joseph W. McGovern, a lawyer; Joseph T. King, a lawyer; and Carl H. Pforzheimer, Jr., an investment banker. The remaining Regents, who concurred in the decision, are drawn from a variety of business and professional interests, including law, banking, education and philanthropy.

used as controls) were subjected to the experiment. The patients were asked by Mandel, Southam, and their assistants if they would consent to an injection which was described as a test to discover their resistance or immunity to disease. They were told that a lump would form, and that in a few weeks it would go away. They were not told in plain language that the procedure was a research project unrelated to medical treatment of their own condition. And they were not told that the substance to be injected consisted of live cancer cells. The record indicates that all the patients approached agreed to the injection and, further, that none suffered any ill effects other than the transient discomfort of the injection and the nodule it produced.

MOTIVATIONS

Both men had reasons for acting as they did. Their thinking is extensively set out in the records of the administrative hearings, and their views were restated in interviews with *Science* last week.

Southam's practices, developed in the earlier experimentation on cancer patients at Memorial and James Ewing hospitals in New York, rested on the conviction that the procedure involved no risk of transplanting cancer to the experimental subjects. "I saw no reason why we should use [the word *cancer*] because it is not pertinent to the phenomenon which is going to follow," he told the hearing board. "We are not doing something which is going to induce cancer. We are not going to do something which is going to cause them any harm. . . . We are going to observe the growth and rejection of these transplanted cancer cells. The fact then that they are cancer cells does not mean that there is any risk of cancer to this patient." In addition, Southam believes that the word *cancer* "has a tremendous emotive value, disvalue, to everybody. . . . What the ordinary patient, what the nonmedical person, and even many doctors . . . whose knowledge of the basic science behind transplantation is not great—to them the use of a cancer cell might imply a risk that it will grow and produce cancer, and the fear that this word strikes in people is very great." The suggestion was raised in the hearing that, having recognized the emotional impact of the word *cancer*, the doctors avoided it through fear that its use would discourage consent and thus hinder the research. But Southam sees his action as an act of professional judgment and solicitude, based on an unwillingness to scare or arouse the patients when such fright was not in fact relevant to the objective situation. And he believes that his formula gave the patients all the information they needed to make an intelligent decision about participation.

On the basic question of the type of explanation to be given to the patients, Mandel followed, and endorsed, the practice described to him by Southam. But many factors influenced Mandel's agreement to the project. A relative newcomer to the Chronic Disease Hospital, he was alarmed by what seemed to him disastrously insufficient medical attention to the long-term, chronically ill patients. "I could tell you stories which would curdle your blood," he told *Science* last week, and he did. The experiment involved a number of visits to the patients by the JCDH resident working with

Southam to check on the development and regression of the nodules, and Mandel believed that the added attention would improve their care. He saw some hope of using the injections as a diagnostic device, to discover undetected cancer in patients hospitalized for other illnesses. And he looked forward to the possibility of a more prolonged collaboration with the Sloan-Kettering, which would contribute to upgrading his own institution.

Within the hospital, Mandel's decision to permit the experiment to proceed became the focus of an intense disagreement which led to a battle with one of the hospital's directors over the confidentiality of patients' records and to the resignation of several staff physicians. The bad feeling between Mandel and the physicians, whether it preceded the Sloan-Kettering issue, as Mandel contends, or was the result of it, as the physicians imply, seriously impeded the efforts of the examining committees to evaluate one of the ugliest charges in the case—that the patients used were in such a debilitated physical and mental state that they were incapable of giving informed consent. Almost every patient became the subject of conflicting testimony from the opposing sides. In his report to the Regents, a physician member of the medical grievance committee which conducted the bulk of the hearings summarized descriptions of patients that had been supplied by the physicians who resigned. Patient No. 26 is fairly typical: "Suffering from advanced Paget's disease, with overgrowth of bone, pressing on the brain. This patient was suffering from severe deafness, blindness, mental condition." Another patient was described as suffering from "Parkinson's disease, lung abscess, was running and falling, speech was unintelligible." A chart stated that the patient "was misunderstood by the orderly, drools, and tries to avoid speech." Another patient, a 75-year-old man described as senile, was diagnosed as "impaired mentally, with easy crying and laughing, tendency to repeat the same sentence several times. Also it is difficult to obtain the patient's attention." In all these cases, Mandel and the resident, supported by Southam, testified basically that, if you knew the patients (as the resident did), it was possible to communicate adequately with them and that they had an alert appreciation of what was going on.

Although the Regents were unable to come to a definitive conclusion about the alertness of all the patients, they did find that at least "some . . . were incapable of understanding the nature of this experiment or of giving informed consent thereto." While agreeing with Southam's contention that he was not responsible for the internal practices of the Chronic Disease Hospital, the Regents argued that he had a clear responsibility nonetheless: "As a physician in charge of the experiment, it was his duty to pay enough attention to what was going on to make sure that he was dealing with persons capable of being volunteers and sufficiently informed to consent to the use of their bodies for the experiment and not merely with people who were too confused or too sick or too resigned to object to the injection." Southam believes, the Regents continued, that "it is important to make it clear to the patients that what is being done is an experiment and is not for the treatment or diagnosis of their own condition, yet he was present, this was not adequately done, and he did not complain. A physician may not shirk his ethical responsibility or violate basic human rights so easily." As

for Mandel, the Regents concluded that although he had, legitimately, delegated responsibility for the actual conduct of the experiment to a resident,
he was nonetheless "directly responsible for the determination of the procedure followed" in the selection of patients and the explanations he permitted them to be offered. In addition to the substantive arguments, lawyers
for Mandel and Southam raised two technical points of some interest. First,
they claimed that, because "no clear-cut medical or professional standards
were in force or were violated" by the two physicians, the attempt to find
them guilty had an ex post facto quality. They also argued that the charges
did not accurately fit the case. Testimony was introduced from well-known
cancer and other professional researchers, including I. S. Ravdin, vice president for medical affairs of the University of Pennsylvania, and George E.
Moore, director of Roswell Park Memorial Institute, to the effect that Southam's practices did not differ dramatically from those of other researchers.
"If the whole profession is doing it," one of the lawyers remarked in an
interview, "how can you call it 'unprofessional conduct' "? The lawyers also
argued that the "fraud and deceit" charge was more appropriate to low-
brow scoundrels, such as physicians who cheat on insurance, supply illegal
narcotics, or practice medicine without a license, than to their respectable
and well-intentioned clients.

VOICE OF THE PUBLIC

To all arguments of humane motivations, extenuating circumstance, conflicting testimony, or legal ambiguities, the final answer of the Regents was
very simple: It is no excuse. There was never any disagreement on the
principle that patients should not be used in experiments unrelated to
treatment unless they have given informed consent. But in the Regents'
decision, two refinements of that principle are heavily stressed. The first is
that it is the patient, and not the physician, who has the right to decide what
factors are or are not relevant to his consent, regardless of the rationality
of his assessment. "Any fact which might influence the giving or withholding
of consent is material," the Regents said. "A patient has the right to know
he is being asked to volunteer and to refuse to participate in an experiment
for any reason, intelligent or otherwise, well-informed or prejudiced. A
physician has no right to withhold from a prospective volunteer any fact
which he knows may influence the decision. It is the volunteer's decision to
make, and the physician may not take it away from him by the manner in
which he asks the question or explains or fails to explain the circumstances.
There is evidenced in the record . . . an attitude on the part of some physicians that they can go ahead and do anything which they conclude is good
for the patient, or which is of benefit experimentally or educationally and
is not harmful to the patient, and that the patient's consent is an empty
formality. With this we cannot agree."

The second principle stressed by the Regents is that the physician,
when he is acting as experimenter, has no claim to the doctor-patient relationship that, in a therapeutic situation, would give him the generally ac-

knowledged right to withhold information if he judged it in the best interest of the patient. In the absence of a doctor-patient relationship, the Regents said, "there is no basis for the exercise of their usual professional judgment applicable to patient care." Southam, in an interview, disagreed. "An experimental relation has some elements of a therapeutic relationship," he said last week. "The patients still think of you as a doctor, and I react to them as a doctor, and want to avoid frightening them unnecessarily." Mandel takes a similar position. In a letter to the editor of a medical affairs newspaper he stated: "In accordance with the age-old motto—primum non nocere —it would seem that consideration of the patient's well-being may, at times, supersede the requirement for disclosure of facts if such facts lack pertinence and may cause psychologic harm." But on this point, the Regents are clear: "No person can be said to have volunteered for an experiment unless he had first understood what he was volunteering for. Any matter which might influence him in giving or withholding his consent is material. Deliberate nondisclosure of the material fact is no different from deliberate misrepresentation of such a fact."

In closing their case, and acknowledging that the penalties imposed were severe—they might have just authorized a censure and reprimand— the Regents were pointed and succinct: "We trust that this measure of discipline will serve as a stern warning that zeal for research must not be carried to the point where it violates the basic rights and immunities of a human person."

What the impact of the case will be is by no means clear. The Regents' decision outlines clear rules for a very narrow situation and attempts to set out some broad principles as well. But it is by no means binding, and it by no means covers the variety of situations with which researchers seeking to use human subjects are faced. The question is, What will cover these situations? Codes and declarations, of which there are already several, are too general to offer specific guidance. Researchers and patients alike are too vulnerable to await a slow case-by-case accretion of specific rulings. One alternative is the development within each hospital or research institution of "ethical review committees" that could define the consent-and-disclosure requirements for each proposed experiment and see that they were adhered to. In theory, this is already taking place. During the Southam-Mandel hearings, the state attempted to prove that Southam, a recipient of an NIH grant, had violated regulations of the Public Health Service. In fact, the regulations in question govern only the normal volunteer program of the NIH Clinical Center in Bethesda. The PHS response to an inquiry from New York's Attorney General made clear that the rules were not generally applicable and stated that, "in supporting extramural clinical investigations, it is the position of the Public Health Service that proper ethical and moral standards are more effectively safeguarded by the processes of review and criticism by an investigator's peers than by regulation."

That is the theory, but the trouble is, it is not yet being done. And, given the tremendous growth and variety of medical research involving human beings, if it is not done by the scientific community, someone else will start to do it. The New York Regents may be only the beginning.

THE REGENT'S DECISION

We are of the opinion that there are certain basic ethical standards concerning consent to human experimentation which were involved in this experiment and which were violated by the respondents. When a patient engages a physician or enters a hospital he may reasonably be deemed to have consented to such treatment as his physician or the hospital staff, in the exercise of their professional judgment, deem proper. Consent to normal diagnostic tests might similarly be presumed. Even so, doctors and hospitals as a matter of routine obtain formal written consents before surgery, and in a number of other instances, and whether or not a specific consent is required for a specific act must be decided on the facts of the particular case.

No one contends that these 22 patients, by merely being in the hospital, had volunteered their bodies for any purpose other than treatment of their condition. These injections were made as a part of a cancer research project. The incidental and remote possibility, urged by Dr. Mandel, that the research might have been beneficial to a patient is clearly insufficient to bring these injections within the area of procedures for which a consent could be implied. Actual consent was required.

What form such an actual consent must take is a matter of applying common sense to the particular facts of the case. No consent is valid unless it is made by a person with legal and mental capacity to make it, and is based on a disclosure of all material facts. Any fact which might influence the giving or withholding of consent is material. A patient has the right to know he is being asked to volunteer and to refuse to participate in an experiment for any reason, intelligent or otherwise, well-informed or prejudiced. A physician has no right to withhold from a prospective volunteer any fact which he knows may influence the decision. It is the volunteer's decision to make, and the physician may not take it away from him by the manner in which he asks the question or explains or fails to explain the circumstances. There is evidenced in the record in this proceeding an attitude on the part of some physicians that they can go ahead and do anything which they conclude is good for the patient, or which is of benefit experimentally or educationally and is not harmful to the patient, and that the patient's consent is an empty formality. With this we cannot agree.

In his testimony . . . Dr. Mandel took the position that he regards these experiments as beneficial to the patients both because the experiment might result in a diagnosis of an advanced cancer which had not been discovered by the hospital, and also because the participation in the experiment would result in extra medical attention to the patients involved and possibly other patients in the hospital.

The record indicates that the only additional medical care any of these patients received as a result of this experiment was that the injections were made and they were occasionally checked thereafter as to the progress of the growth and disappearance of the nodule. The inference that participation in the experiment benefited the patients because of such additional medical care is without foundation in the record. Since the purpose of the experiment was to obtain verification of Dr. Southam's hypothesis that diseased patients would reject the implant in the same manner as healthy patients and that their rejection would not be delayed as was that of patients suffering from an advanced cancer, it is somewhat inconsistent for Dr. Mandel to say before the experiment was completed that he authorized it as a diagnostic measure. In any event, it was clearly not treatment, not experimental therapy, and not a diagnostic test which would reasonably be given to these particular patients. Nevertheless, from the manner in which they were asked for their consent and from the statement made to them that this was a test to determine their immunity or resistance to disease, the patients could naturally assume that it was being given to help in the diagnosis or treatment of their condition. They were not clearly and unequivocally asked if they wanted to volunteer to participate in an extraneous research project.

There is one point which is undisputed, namely, that the patients were not told that the cells to be injected were live cancer cells. From the respondents' standpoint this was not considered to be an important fact. They regarded the experiment as medically harmless. There was not appreciable danger of any harmful effects to the patients as a result of the injection of these cancer cells. It is not uncommon for a doctor to refrain from telling his patient that he had cancer where the physician in his professional judgment concludes that such a disclosure would be harmful to the patient. The respondents testified that they felt that telling these patients that the material did consist of live cancer cells would upset them and was immaterial to their consent. They overlooked the key fact that so far as this particular experiment was concerned, there was not the usual doctor-patient relationship and, therefore, no basis for the exercise of their usual professional judgment applicable to patient care. No person can be said to have volunteered for an experiment unless he has first understood what he was volunteering for. Any matter which might influence him in giving or withholding his consent is material. Deliberate nondisclosure of the material fact is no different from deliberate misrepresentation of such a fact. The respondents maintain that they did not withhold the fact that these were cancer cells because they thought that some of the patients might have refused to consent to the injection of live cancer cells into their bodies. This was, however, a possibility and a decision that had to be made by the patients and not for them. Accordingly, the alleged oral consents that they obtained after deliberately witholding this information were not informed consents and were, for this reason, fraudulently obtained.

Although there is conflicting testimony and evidence in this point, it is our opinion that some of these patients were in such a physical and mental condition that they were incapable of understanding the nature of this experiment or of giving an informed consent thereto. . . . We note that in no case were any relatives of any of these patients told about the experiment nor were any of these patients asked if they wished to think the matter over or discuss it with their relatives. It is noteworthy that one of these same patients was operated on two days after the injections and that prior to making the operation, which was a part of the patient's treatment, the hospital obtained two separate written consents each signed by both the patient and a relative. If there was any doubt at all concerning a patient's ability to fully comprehend and consent to this experiment, it was the duty of the physicians involved to resolve that doubt before proceeding further. . . . We do not say that it is necessary in all cases of human experimentation to obtain consents from relatives or to obtain written consents, but certainly upon the fact of this case and in view of the fact that the patients were debilitated, the performance of this experiment on the basis of alleged oral consents from these particular patients falls short of the ethical standards of the medical profession.

From "Medical Experimentation on Humans"

Preston J. Burnham

Having read the News and Comment headed "Human experimentation: New York verdict affirms patient's rights," I believe I understand the situation well enough to attempt to help lay committees develop a series of forms for obtaining patients' informed consent. I am working now on forms . . . for our standard operations. . . .

CONSENT FORM FOR HERNIA PATIENTS:

I, _____, being about to be subjected to a surgical operation said to be for repair of what my doctor thinks is a hernia (rupture or loss of belly stuff—intestines—out of the belly through a hole in the muscles), do hereby give said doctor permission to cut into me and do duly swear that I am giving my informed consent, based upon the following information:

Operative procedure is as follows: The doctor first cuts through the skin by a four-inch gash in the lower abdomen. He then slashes through the other things—fascia (a tough layer over the muscles) and layers of muscle —until he sees the cord (tube that brings the sperm from testicle to outside) with all its arteries and veins. The doctor then tears the hernia (thin sac of bowels and things) from the cord and ties off the sac with a string. He then pushes the testicle back into the scrotum and sews everything together, trying not to sew up the big arteries and veins that nourish the leg.

Possible complications are as follows:
1. Large artery may be cut and I may bleed to death.

Reprinted with permission from *Science* 152:22, 448–50, April 1966. Copyright 1966 by the American Association for the Advancement of Science.

2. Large vein may be cut and I may bleed to death.

3. Tube from testicle may be cut. I will then be sterile on that side.

4. Artery or veins to testicles may be cut—same result.

5. Opening around cord in muscles may be made too tight.

6. Clot may develop in these veins which will loosen when I get out of bed and hit my lungs, killing me.

7. Clot may develop in one or both legs which may cripple me, lead to loss of one or both legs, go to my lungs, or make my veins no good for life.

8. I may develop a horrible infection that may kill me.

9. The hernia may come back again after it has been operated on.

10. I may die from general anesthesia.

11. I may be paralyzed if spinal anesthesia is used.

12. If ether is used, it could explode inside me.

13. I may slip in hospital bathroom.

14. I may be run over going to the hospital.

15. The hospital may burn down.

I understand: the anatomy of the body, the pathology of the development of hernia, the surgical technique that will be used to repair the hernia, the physiology of wound healing, the dietetic chemistry of the foods that I must eat to cause healing, the chemistry of body repair, and the course which my physician will take in treating any of the complications that can occur as a sequel of repairing an otherwise simple hernia.

_____

Patient

_____

Lawyer for Patient

_____

Lawyer for Doctor

_____

Lawyer for Hospital

_____

Lawyer for Anesthesiologist

_____

Mother-in-Law

_____

Notary Public

From "Informed (But Uneducated) Consent"

Franz J. Ingelfinger

The trouble with informed consent is that it is not educated consent. Let us assume that the experimental subject, whether a patient, a volunteer, or otherwise enlisted, is exposed to a completely honest array of factual detail. He is told of the medical uncertainty that exists and that must be resolved by research endeavors, of the time and discomfort involved, and of the tiny percentage risk of some serious consequences of the test procedure. He is also reassured of his rights and given a formal, quasi-legal statement to read. No exculpatory language is used. With his written signature, the subject then caps the transaction, and whether he sees himself as a heroic martyr for the sake of mankind, or as a reluctant guinea pig dragooned for the benefit of science, or whether, perhaps, he is merely bewildered, he obviously has given his "informed consent." Because established routines have been scrupulously observed, the doctor, the lawyer, and the ethicist are content.

But the chances are remote that the subject really understands what he has consented to—in the sense that the responsible medical investigator understands the goals, nature, and hazards of his study. How can the layman comprehend the importance of his perhaps not receiving, as determined by the luck of the draw, the highly touted new treatment that his roommate will get? How can he appreciate the sensation of living for days with a multi-lumen intestinal tube passing through his mouth and pharynx? How can he interpret the information that an intravascular catheter and radiopaque dye injection have an 0.01 per cent probability of leading to a dangerous thrombosis or cardiac arrhythmia? It is moreover quite unlikely that any patient-subject can see himself accurately within the broad context of the situation, to weigh the inconveniences and hazards that he will have to undergo against the improvements that the research project may bring to the management of his disease in general and to his own case in particular. . . .

Nor can the information given to the experimental subject be in any sense totally complete. It would be impractical and probably unethical for the investigator to present the nearly endless list of all possible contingencies; in fact, he may not himself be aware of every untoward thing that might happen. Extensive detail, moreover, usually enhances the subject's confusion. Epstein and Lasagna showed that comprehension of medical information given to untutored subjects is inversely correlated with the elaborateness of the material presented.[1] The inconsiderate investigator, indeed, conceivably could exploit his authority and knowledge and extract

Reprinted with permission from *The New England Journal of Medicine* 287, 465–66, August 31, 1972. Copyright 1972, Massachusetts Medical Society.

[1]Epstein LC, Lasagna L: Obtaining informed consent: form or substance. Arch Intern Med 123:682–688, 1969

"informed consent" by overwhelming the candidate-subject with information.

Ideally, the subject should give his consent freely, under no duress whatsoever. The facts are that some element of coercion is instrumental in any investigator-subject transaction. Volunteers for experiments will usually be influenced by hopes of obtaining better grades, earlier parole, more substantial egos, or just mundane cash. These pressures, however, are but fractional shadows of those enclosing the patient-subject. Incapacitated and hospitalized because of illness, frightened by strange and impersonal routines, and fearful for his health and perhaps life, he is far from exercising a free power of choice when the person to whom he anchors all his hopes asks, "Say, you wouldn't mind, would you, if you joined some of the other patients on this floor and helped us to carry out some very important research we are doing?" When "informed consent" is obtained, it is not the student, the destitute bum, or the prisoner to whom, by virtue of his condition, the thumb screws of coercion are most relentlessly applied; it is the most used and useful of all experimental subjects, the patient with disease.

When a man or woman agrees to act as an experimental subject, therefore, his or her consent is marked by neither adequate understanding nor total freedom of choice. The conditions of the agreement are a far cry from those visualized as ideal. Jonas would have the subject identify with the investigative endeavor so that he and the researcher would be seeking a common cause: "Ultimately, the appeal for volunteers should seek . . . free and generous endorsement, the appropriation of the research purpose into the person's [i.e., the subject's] own scheme of ends."[2] For Ramsey, "informed consent" should represent a "covenantal bond between consenting man and consenting man [that] makes them . . . joint adventurers in medical care and progress."[3] Clearly, to achieve motivations and attitudes of this lofty type, an educated and understanding, rather than merely informed, consent is necessary.

Although it is unlikely that the goals of Jonas and of Ramsey will ever be achieved, and that human research subjects will spontaneously vounteer rather than be "conscripted,"[4] efforts to promote educated consent are in order. In view of the current emphasis on involving "the community" in such activities as regional planning, operation of clinics, and assignment of priorities, the general public and its political leaders are showing an increased awareness and understanding of medical affairs. But the orientation of this public interest in medicine is chiefly socioeconomic. Little has been done to give the public a basic understanding of medical research and its requirements not only for the people's money but also for their participation. The public, to be sure, is being subjected to a bombardment of sensation-mongering news stories and books that feature "breakthroughs," or

[2]Jonas H: Philosophical reflections on experimenting with human subjects. Daedalus 98:219–247, Spring, 1969

[3]Ramsey P: The ethics of a cottage industry in an age of community and research medicine. N Engl J Med 284:700–706, 1971

[4]Jonas, Philosophical reflections.

that reveal real or alleged exploitations—horror stories of Nazi-type experimentation on abused human minds and bodies. Muckraking is essential to
expose malpractices, but unless accompanied by efforts to promote a
broader appreciation of medical research and its methods, it merely compounds the difficulties for both the investigator and the subject when "informed consent" is solicited.

The procedure currently approved in the United States for enlisting
human experimental subjects has one great virtue: patient-subjects are put
on notice that their management is in part at least an experiment. The
deceptions of the past are no longer tolerated. Beyond this accomplishment,
however, the process of obtaining "informed consent," with all its regulations and conditions, is no more than an elaborate ritual, a device that, when
the subject is uneducated and uncomprehending, confers no more than the
semblance of propriety on human experimentation. The subject's only real
protection, the public as well as the medical profession must recognize,
depends on the conscience and compassion of the investigator and his
peers.

From "Informed Opinion on Informed Consent"

Nicholas J. Demy

To the Editor.—As a radiologist who has been sued, I have reflected earnestly
on advice to obtain Informed Consent but have decided to "take the risks
without informing the patient" and trust to "God, judge, and jury" rather
than evade responsibility through a legal gimmick. . . .

President Truman had a sign on his desk to remind him that "the buck
stops here." So with the physician. He may not be God, judge, and jury, but
he is their surrogate and must speak alone with the patient as Moses did with
God on Mt. Sinai. Think what the Ten Commandments would be if a
committee or a TEAM had gone up there to discuss the terms.

Alfidi's form and arguments are appropriate for the patient with a
serious problem who is referred to the Cleveland Clinic or to some other
medical Mecca for a special examination. Such patients have already been
primed and know the score, but in a general radiologic practice many of our
patients are uninformable and we would never get through the day if we had
to obtain their consent to every potentially harmful study. We do not have
the resident and nursing staff to act as our angels and interpreters. The
practice of medicine is a matter of individual communication and good
rapport with the patient. . . .

Reprinted with permission of author and publisher from *Journal of the American Medical Association*
217:5, 696–97, August 2, 1971. Copyright 1971, the American Medical Association.

We still have patients with language problems, the uneducated and the unintelligent, the stolid and the stunned who cannot form an Informed Opinion to give an Informed Consent; we have the belligerent and the panicky who do not listen or comprehend. And then there are the Medicare patients who comprise 35% of general hospital admissions. The bright ones wearily plead to be left alone; protoplasm grows old and awfully tired, and longs for immortality elsewhere; they do not even want the Routine Profile of gall bladder, intravenous pyelogram, barium enema, and gastrointestinal tract, much less the Rule Out angiogram. As for the apathetic rest, many of them were kindly described by Richard Bright as not being able to comprehend because "their brains are so poorly oxygenated." Try talking cold turkey to them. Asking a patient with the Sword of Damocles hanging over his head to sign an Informed Consent may be smart protection but it sounds as gruesome as an Executioner getting a pardon from his victim before the axe descends.

Why instill fear and then argue to allay it? Patients—like lovers— change their minds or their vows.

> "Yes," I answered you last night;
>   "No," this morning, sir, I say.
> Colors seen by candle-light
>   Will not look the same by day.

If a complication arises after the procedure, patients can deny, and have denied, that they understood what they were signing or that the Informed Consent included the complication they suffered despite the adjuvant paragraph to cover the unexpected: "It would be impractical and probably misleading . . . to describe in detail all the complications . . ." The law says you cannot sign away your rights in advance of a procedure and the courts have upheld awards in the face of signed Informed Consents. You may still be sued.

A lawyer will see to that.

From "Ethical Issues
in Psychiatric Follow-Up Studies"

Scott H. Nelson and Henry Grunebaum

An inevitable conflict exists in behavioral research between the value of preserving patients' human and medical rights and the desire to increase knowledge and thereby improve treatment. This paper attempts to make an empirical rather than theoretical contribution to this subject by reporting

Reprinted with permission of author and publisher from the *American Journal of Psychiatry*, 128:11, 1358–62, May 1972. Copyright 1972, the American Psychiatric Association.

the actual ethical problems we encountered in a follow-up study of former psychiatric patients.

We had been concerned about several ethical issues before beginning our study. How would patients who were no longer in treatment react to being reminded of their past symptoms? Would, or should, professionals who were still seeing these patients be willing to give information about them without the patients' permission? Could patient consent given in a single telephone conversation be regarded as truly informed consent? What happened in the course of our study suggests certain answers to these and other similar questions.

METHOD

We conducted a five- to six-year follow-up study of wrist slashers[1] from January to June 1969 at the Massachusetts Mental Health Center (MMHC), a community mental health center in Boston. Our sample consisted of 23 patients: 17 patients who were treated at MMHC, three who were treated elsewhere, and three who received no psychiatric attention. (One of us [H.G.] had studied these patients' charts from January 1, 1963, to December 31, 1964.[2]) All patients were originally seen in the emergency room of a nearby general hospital, where they had come for treatment of self-inflicted lacerations.

Records from the general hospital and MMHC (both of which are teaching hospitals of Harvard Medical School) were reviewed for past and current clinical and social data. All possible avenues for locating patients were noted, including contact with psychiatrists, social workers, other physicians, and various social and welfare agencies. The last professional to see the patient was then contacted. If he had an ongoing relationship with the patient and was willing to give pertinent information, the patient was not contacted directly.

One of us (S.H.N.) wrote to the 15 patients for whom there was no evidence of a current professional relationship; there was no return address or other identification on the envelope. The letter described the objectives of the study and the reasons for which the patient had been selected. The patient was asked to contact the interviewer for a single appointment if he was willing to participate. Confidentiality was assured, and the patient was offered reimbursement for travel expenses.

Six persons responded directly to the letter; four came for interviews. One man said that he wanted to "help the hospital, since it helped me." The three other former patients seemed to have come with the underlying wish for obtaining psychiatric help. At the time of the interview all four patients were offered referral to the clinic for further evaluation; however, none actually used the clinic facility. A fifth patient agreed to speak to the inter-

[1]Nelson SH, Grunebaum HU: A follow-up study of wrist slashers. Amer J Psychiat 127:1345–1349, 1971

[2]Goldwyn RM, Cahill JL, Grunebaum HU: Self-inflicted injury to the wrist. Plast Reconstr Surg 39:583–589, 1967

viewer by telephone since he lived out of the state. A sixth patient who lived overseas asked if she could write us about her experiences. We sent her a questionnaire, which she completed and returned.

Three subjects responded to the letter indirectly. One, a chronic schizophrenic, asked her private psychiatrist to telephone us and supply information we had requested. The other two patients reacted in negative ways. The psychiatrist of a paranoid schizophrenic man reported that his patient had become incensed that the chart describing his emergency-room treatment had been studied without his consent. The psychiatrist refused to give any information without his patient's consent. An acquaintance of the other patient, who was in prison at the time she received the letter, threatened one of us with personal harm. This angry response was perhaps due to the fact that the letter was read by the prison superintendent, who was required to censor all incoming mail.

Attempts were made to locate the six patients who did not answer the letter. The mothers of two women were contacted by telephone. They were told only that the caller was a physician trying to reach the patient for purposes of follow-up of previous outpatient general hospital treatment. Both relayed this information to their daughters, but neither mother would give information as to where the daughter herself could be contacted. An uncle readily gave us another former patient's address and telephone number without knowing the identity of the caller.

A letter was written to the father of a fourth patient; he contacted his daughter, who called the interviewer long-distance. The study was explained to her at that time, and she hesitantly agreed to participate by telephone conversation. Another patient, located through her college alumni office, was contacted by telephone in a distant state. One patient was lost to follow-up altogether, despite various attempts to locate him.

Ethical Issues

From the outset it was clear that although the study could increase our knowledge about wrist slashing, it could also disrupt the personal lives of former patients. In the follow-up we were concerned about respect for three basic rights of patients: the right to adequately informed consent, the right to confidentiality, and the right to privacy.

The Right to Informed Consent

One of our major ethical considerations was whether or not certain subjects could, in fact, give truly informed consent. We were especially sensitive about patients with whom we expected to establish contact only once—to explain the study, obtain consent, and conduct the interview forthwith over the telephone. Although such patients voluntarily agreed to participate, several were hesitant about doing so.

Conflict arose in these situations because of our feelings that patients contacted by telephone may not and often cannot have sufficient time to reflect upon or discuss with others the psychological implications of talking about their previous symptoms, despite the fact that when asked to participate they have agreed to do so. In some instances our subjects were plunged immediately into an emotionally stressful experience. One woman became progressively psychotic as she reviewed her feelings over the telephone.

It is a matter of judgment, therefore, as to what constitutes "informed" consent. Physicians are advised generally by legal authorities to inform their patients about the possible hazards of a procedure insofar as possible.[3] Our procedure was to try to anticipate reactions to our questions from a patient's history of response to similar emotional stresses. We also tried to avoid arousing difficult feelings by emphasizing to the subjects that questions which might cause emotional upset did not have to be answered. Adverse reactions were unusual however and, in general, we were direct and matter-of-fact about our questions. In addition, it must be recognized that for purposes of a follow-up study, an overly cautious approach may lead to inadequate or incomplete data, as well as to the loss of a subject altogether.

The Right to Confidentiality

The conduct of the study posed several questions of patient confidentiality: Do professionals in a hospital (especially in a teaching institution) have the special right to examine the charts of patients other than those they themselves treated? Do professionals have the right to divulge information to a research investigator without the patient's consent? Does an investigator have the right to contact anyone other than the patient in attempts to locate him?

Teaching hospitals frequently allow their records, not to mention their patients, to be used in a variety of ways because of the potential benefits to training and education. Research activities frequently are included under this philosophy. It is argued that patients who are treated at teaching hospitals receive the benefit of care by several physicians, rather than only one. Theoretically, and perhaps practically, this leads to better medical care. In return, these patients by tradition give implicit permission for their case records to be used in teaching and research, in ways to be determined by the institution.

As mentioned earlier, the specific concern of one of the patients in our study was that his emergency-room chart had been read without his permission. This caused us to observe that teaching hospitals have few specific rules as to who may review patient records. In addition, there are few safeguards with regard to the identification and credentials of the reviewer, much less the purposes of the review. In our study one of us (S.H.N.) told the secretary of the general hospital record room only that he was a psychiatrist from another institution. Without hesitation, she made available all patient records that he requested.

Another issue about patient confidentiality arose from our contacting several professionals (without the patients' consent) and asking them to give information. We were concerned not only about the ethical aspects of such contacts, but also about the implications for the conduct of the study, should

[3]Bellamy WA: Psychiatric malpractice, in American Handbook of Psychiatry, vol 3. Edited by Arieti S. New York, Basic Books, 1966, pp. 615–628

our request for such information be refused. However, 14 of the 15 professionals agreed to give information, taking the interviewer's word that he was a psychiatrist pursuing a research study.

Legally, except in special circumstances, medical privilege remains with the patient rather than with the physician or professional. According to law, professionals are enjoined from giving out information without the patient's formal consent. Our rationale for contacting professionals rather than the patients themselves was to avoid undue emotional distress for the patients. This was explained in detail to each professional before inquiring about specific information. The patient whose psychiatrist refused to give information had already received our letter directly, so that protection could not be offered in that case.

It was our considered opinion that it was more ethical to avoid patient distress by contacting a professional than to ask first for the consent of each individual patient, particularly those who had not received treatment recently. Some may disagree with this value choice and argue that each patient should have the right to decide whether or not information about him may be used. The optimal way of dealing with this ethical issue is clearly open to debate.

We were also concerned about maintaining confidentiality in our attempts to locate former patients. Frequently, we had to contact relatives or friends to learn where a patient could be reached. Doing this without mentioning the subject's former status as a psychiatric patient was often a thorny matter. We gave only a general explanation for our call. If further questions were asked, the person was told that any other information regarding the nature of our mission would have to be discussed directly with the patient.

Although it was likely that most of the friends and/or relatives contacted knew about the patient's psychiatric history, we could not assume this to be true in every case. A person often does not admit a history of psychiatric care to new friends, employers, or even spouses because of feelings of embarrassment or fear of rejection. Follow-up studies in which such new acquaintances are often inadvertently contacted increase the possibility that the patient's secret will become known.

Therefore, even though we risked losing significant follow-up data, we adopted the policy of discussing psychiatric matters only with the patient himself. We had been doubtful of the necessity for this until one recently married woman, who was finally reached by telephone after her husband had been contacted twice, commented that she had appreciated our attention to confidentiality, since her husband knew nothing about her previous psychiatric treatment.

The Right to Privacy

Our concern about genuinely informed consent and maintenance of confidentiality in gaining patient information led us to consider an even more fundamental question: Do current or former patients have the right not to be contacted in *any* way by any professionals?.

It is understandable that former patients often do not wish to be reminded of past emotional symptoms. In many cases, defenses have been erected to deal with previously troublesome thoughts and feelings. There may be relative contentment with the degree of adjustment achieved. Should research investigators be allowed to contact former patients at will and risk disturbing their intrapsychic and interpersonal equilibrium? We believe that the ethical aspects of this question, which involves a fundamental human right, have not been sufficiently considered.

A related question may arise in psychiatric follow-up studies when a patient who is later discovered to be under psychiatric treatment is contacted directly. Since it is often impossible to ascertain from a patient's hospital record whether or not he is currently in psychotherapy, one cannot always follow the procedure of contacting a professional in order to avoid emotional distress for a patient. Serious repercussions to the patient-doctor relationship may result.

For example, the negative reactions of the aforementioned schizophrenic man, according to his psychiatrist, placed considerable strain on the patient-physician relationship. Our letter had at first led the patient to believe that his doctor had released information to us without his consent. In addition, the physician was obviously annoyed that we had contacted his patient without *his* prior knowledge.

DISCUSSION

Several authors have implied that research studies should be concerned with more than the traditional criteria of informed consent and preservation of confidentiality. Rutstein has aptly termed this the patient's "right to be subjected to minimal risk."[4] Although he was referring to medical problems, his discussion is relevant to psychiatric studies as well. The Group for the Advancement of Psychiatry has stated that "the physician has the responsibility that no harm come to anyone within the range of his professional activity even though there may be no direct treatment obligation."[5]

The Judicial Council of the American Medical Association has suggested that confidences entrusted to a physician should not be revealed "unless required . . . by law or unless it becomes necessary in order to protect the welfare of the individual or the community."[6] The Panel on Privacy and Behavioral Research (appointed by the President's Office of Science and Technology in 1966) stated that few investigators have given sufficient thought to the serious ethical questions of propriety in relation to the privacy and dignity of their subjects.[7]

[4]Rutstein DD: The ethical design of human experiments. Daedalus 98:523–541. Spring 1969

[5]Group for the Advancement of Psychiatry: Confidentiality and Privileged Communication in the Practice of Psychiatry. Report 45. New York, GAP, 1960

[6]American Medical Association: Opinions and Reports of the Judicial Council, Section 9. Chicago, AMA, 1969, pp. 55–57.

[7]Panel on Privacy and Behavioral Research: Privacy and behavioral research. Int J Psychiat 5:496–502, 1968.

This seeming lack of concern appears to be true as well for follow-up studies. Such a situation is unfortunate both for the subjects and for the field of psychiatric research. If attention is not given to patients' rights, it will not be long before such studies will not be feasible at all, either because of increased legal sanctions or because patients may become aware of the discomfort that may result from participation.

Another area of concern is the preservation of the ongoing doctor-patient relationship. In psychiatry, a relationship based on mutual respect and trust is itself a prerequisite for successful treatment. Unsolicited probing by research investigators into therapeutic situations may be disruptive.

The ethical problems described in this paper do not yield easy solutions. However, concrete changes in the current administration of programs in teaching hospitals and other research facilities could prevent some of the difficulties we encountered.

Hospital Record-Room Guidelines

All hospitals should have specific criteria as to who may and may not view patients' records. Specific identification may be required. Viewers could be asked to specify in writing the intended use of the records and to sign a form that releases the hospital from liability for improper use of information obtained.

Patient-Teaching Hospital Agreements

Obtaining patients' consent for follow-up upon hospital admission or discharge would obviate many difficulties later encountered. Permission could be included in the routine procedures for medical as well as psychiatric patients. In the clinic or emergency room, consent for follow-up could be obtained in the signed form that gives consent for treatment. It also should be explained clearly to the patient that to accept and authorize treatment at a teaching hospital carries with it the specific provision for later follow-up. This obviously can be a problem when there are no readily available alternative facilities.

Adequate Planning of Investigations

Many ethical pitfalls can be avoided by anticipating ethical problems before starting an experimental procedure. In addition, as Rutstein has pointed out, the experimental design of a study usually reflects the degree to which ethical problems have been considered (4). A well-planned study usually has taken into account legitimate ways in which data may be obtained. A poorly designed project, on the other hand, is unethical in itself since information obtained will be of little use.

Research studies should maintain truly informed consent insofar as possible. Confidentiality also should be maximized, particularly for patients currently in treatment. One might ask professionals directly whether or not patient consent should be obtained before information is divulged. Certainly it seems clear that after treatment is concluded, psychiatric issues should only be discussed with patients directly.

It would seem, however, that an investigator should go even farther. He should engage in the more fundamental practice of weighing the risks of disturbing patients' privacy and well-being against the potential benefits of his study. When should patients' feelings and sense of well-being be subjected to the scrutiny of behavioral scientists' constant quest for data? The answers to such fundamental questions remain far from resolved.

It is not our intent to make the regulation of medical or psychiatric research more restrictive. However, it *is* our purpose to call professional attention to our experiences before the American public begins to demand redress. Through such considerations as those we have presented, patients' rights and dignity can be increasingly safeguarded, while at the same time behavioral knowledge and treatment can continue to be promoted. It seems to us that both are valid concerns for psychiatric research.

From "Experiments Behind Bars: Doctors, Drug Companies, and Prisoners"

Jessica Mitford

Before a new drug can be marketed in the United States, it must, according to Food and Drug Administration rules, be tested on human beings. In recent years, most of the early testing of our increasingly exotic drugs has been done in prisons. And prisoners have been the subjects of other medical experiments as well.

For some time, international medical societies have attempted to prohibit the use of prisoners as subjects, but these efforts have been effectively frustrated by American medical experimenters. The World Medical Association proposed in 1961 that prisoners "being captive groups should not be used as the subject of experiments." The recommendation was never formally adopted, largely because of the opposition of American doctors. "Pertinax" writes in the *British Medical Journal* for January, 1963: "I am disturbed that the World Medical Association is now hedging on its clause about using criminals as experimental material. The American influence has been at work on its suspension." He adds wistfully, "One of the nicest American scientists I know was heard to say, 'Criminals in our penitentiaries are fine experimental material—and much cheaper than chimpanzees.' I hope the chimpanzees don't come to hear of this."[1]

Although few involved in prison experiments like to talk openly about them, alarming stories crop up in the press with sufficient regularity to give

    [1]See M. H. Pappworth, M.D., *Human Guinea Pigs*, Beacon Press, 1967.

some indication of the scope and nature of the experiments. In 1963, *Time* magazine reported that the federal government was using prisoner "volunteers" for large-scale research, dispensing rewards ranging from a package of cigarettes to $25 in cash plus reduction of sentence; that prisoners in Ohio and Illinois were injected with live cancer cells and with blood from leukemia patients to determine whether these diseases could be transmitted; that doctors in Oklahoma were grossing an estimated $300,000 a year from deals with pharmaceutical companies to test out new drugs on prisoners; that the same doctors were paying prisoners $5 a quart for blood which they retailed at $15.

In July, 1969, Walter Rugaber of the *New York Times* reported that "the Federal Government has watched without interference while many people sickened and some died in an extended series of drug tests and blood plasma operations . . . the immediate damage has been done in the penitentiary systems of three states. Hundreds of inmates in voluntary programs have been stricken with serious disease. An undetermined number of the victims have died."

The stakes in prison research are high. The drug companies, usually operating through private physicians with access to the prisons, can obtain healthy human subjects living in controlled conditions that are difficult, if not impossible, to duplicate elsewhere. In addition, the companies can buy these for a fraction—less than one-tenth, according to many medical authorities—of what they would have to pay medical students or other "free-world" volunteers. They can conduct experiments on prisoners that would not be sanctioned for student-subjects at any price because of the degree of risk and pain involved. Guidelines for human experimentation established by HEW and other agencies are easily disregarded behind prison walls.

When the studies are carried out in the privacy of prison, if a volunteer becomes seriously ill, or dies, as a result of the procedures to which he is subjected, the repercussions will likely be smaller than they would be on the outside. As Rugaber discovered when trying to trace deaths resulting from the "voluntary programs," prison medical records that might prove embarrassing to the authorities have a habit of conveniently disappearing. There is minimal risk that subjects disabled by the experiments will bring lawsuits against the drug companies. Prisoners are often required to sign a waiver releasing those responsible from damage claims that may result. Such waivers have been held legally invalid as contrary to public policy and are specifically prohibitied by FDA regulations, but the prisoner is unlikely to know this. The psychological effect of signing the waiver, along with the general helplessness of prisoners, make lawsuits a rarity.

For the prisoner, the pittance he gets from the drug company—generally around $1 a day for the more onerous experiments—represents riches when viewed in terms of prison pay scales: $30 a month compared with the $2 to $10 a month he might make in an ordinary prison job.

Dr. Robert Batterman, a clinical pharmacologist, told me, "The prisoner-subject gets virtually nil." He cited an estimate given him for experimenting on prisoners in Vacaville, California: $15 a month for three months to be *lowered* to $12.50 a month should the experiment run for six months. "We would normally do it the other way around with free-world volunteers. We'd give them more money if the experiment ran longer." Dr. Batterman makes considerable use of student-subjects from a nearby Baptist divinity school. For a comparatively undemanding experiment—one requiring a weekly withdrawal of blood—he would pay a student at least $100 a month, he said.

However, the problem as seen by some leaders of the American medical profession is not that the prisoner-subjects are paid too little, but rather that they may be paid too much. That a dollar-a-day stipend to a healthy adult can be so overwhelmingly attractive as to invalidate the results of medical research is a possibility only in the topsy-turvy world of prisons. Yet the fear that this will happen is precisely what is expressed by some spokesmen for the profession. Thus Dr. Herbert L. Ley, Jr., then commissioner of the Food and Drug Administration, testified in 1969 before the Senate Select Committee on Small Business:

> The basic problem here, Mr. Chairman, is that the remuneration to the prisoner was too much. This meant that the prisoner had a very strong pressure not to report and not to withdraw from the study. Therefore he would decline to say that he felt any adverse reactions. This is bad for the prisoner in that it exposes him to unnecessary risk, it is bad for our records in that it does not provide us full information.

Prisoners do indeed view the small sums paid as largesse. In a series of interviews conducted in 1969 at Vacaville prison, California, by Martin Miller, a graduate student at the University of California Department of Criminology, some of the prisoners commented: "Yeah, I was on research but I couldn't keep my chow down. Like I lost about thirty-five pounds my first year in the joint, so I started getting scared. I hated to give it up because it was a good pay test." . . . "Hey, man, I'm making $30 a month on the DMSO thing [Chronic Topical Application of Dimethylsulfoxide]. I know a couple of guys had to go to the hospital who were on it—and the burns were so bad they had to take *everyone* off it for a while. But who gives a shit about that, man? Thirty is a full canteen draw and I wish the thing would go on for years—I'd be lost without it." . . . "I was on DMSO last year. It paid real good and it was better than that plague thing [Bubonic Plague Vaccine Immunization Study] that fucked with guys last year. There was a lot of bad reactions to DMSO but I guess that's why it paid so good." Of DMSO Morton Mintz, staff writer for the Washington *Post,* had written three years earlier: "Human testing has now been severely curbed by FDA because of reports of serious adverse effects" (*Washington Post,* July 24, 1966).

The participating physician cashes in on the programs in various ways. He may make a direct deal with the drug company for financial backing, out of which he pays the expenses of research and pockets the rest as his fee. An individual research grant might run from $5000 to more than $50,000, enabling a doctor with good prison contacts to double or triple his regular income. Or if he is, as many are, a faculty member in a medical school, he can route the grant through his university, to the acclaim of his colleagues. His prestige will be enhanced when the results of his research appear in a professional journal. . . .

Dr. Hodges becomes almost lyrical in his discussion of the moral and ethical aspects of such experimentation. The prisoner-volunteers, he says, are "our companions in medical science and adventure"; the subject "in whatever degree derelict or forlorn has sacred rights which the physician must always put ahead of his burning curiosity." Dr. Hodges, without elaborating on these sacred rights, concludes: "A system of voluntary participation firmly based on legal and ethical standards has provided a rich opportunity for clinical investigators who wish to study metabolic, physiologic, pharmacologic, and medical problems. This has been a rewarding experience both for the physicians and for the subjects."

One such experience is described by Dr. Hodges in one of his papers: "Clinical Manifestations of Ascorbic Acid Deficiency in Man," in the *American Journal of Clinical Nutrition* of April, 1971. The object: "to define the metabolism of this vitamin in the face of severe dietary deficiency." For the study, which consisted of experimentally induced scurvy, five companions in medical science and adventure were recruited from the Iowa State Penitentiary "and their informed consent was obtained." For periods ranging from 84 to 97 days they were fed by stomach tube a liquid formula free of ascorbic acid: "Because of the unpalatability of this formula, the men took it thrice daily via polyethylene gastric tube." They were exposed in a cold-climate "control room" to a temperature of fifty degrees for four hours each day. The volume of blood drawn "for laboratory purposes" was large enough to "cause mild anemia in all the men." In a throwaway line, Dr. Hodges observes that "the mineral supplement [recommended by the National Research Council] was inadvertently omitted from the diets during the first 34 days of the depletion period."

The experiment was a great success. It was the second of its kind, Dr. Hodges having tried it once before with far less favorable results: "Despite a somewhat shorter period of deprivation in the second scurvy study, the subjects in the second study developed a more severe degree of scurvy . . . although none of the subjects in the first scurvy study developed arthralgia, this was a complaint in four out of five men who participated in the second scurvy study. Joint swelling and pain made themselves evident in Scurvy II, but had not been observed in the subjects participating in Scurvy I."

The gradual onset of scurvy in the five prisoners is traced by Dr. Hodges with some enthusiasm. "The first sign of scurvy to appear in both studies was petechial hemorrhage [hemorrhages in the skin]. Coiled hairs were observed in two of the men and first appeared on the 42nd and 74th days, respectively. The first definite abnormalities of the gums appeared between the 43rd and 84th days of depletion and progressed after the plasma ascorbic acid levels fell. . . . The onset of joint pains began between the 67th and 96th days. . . . Beginning on the 88th day of deprivation there was a rapid increase in weight followed by swelling of the legs in the third man, who had the most severe degree of scurvy."

By the time it was all over, Dr. Hodges was able to chalk up these significant accomplishments: all five subjects suffered joint pains, swelling of the legs, dental cavities, recurrent loss of new dental fillings, excessive loss of hair, hemorrhages in the skin and whites of the eyes, excess fluid in the joint spaces, shortness of breath, scaly skin, mental depression, and abnormalities in emotional responses. The youngest, a twenty-six-year-old, "became almost unable to walk as a result of the rapid onset of arthropathy [painful joints] superimposed on bilateral femoral neuropathy [disease in both large nerves to the thighs and legs plus hemorrhage into nerve sheaths]. The onset of scurvy signaled a period of potentially rapid deterioration." Dr. Hodges' anticlimactic conclusion: "Once again our observations are in accord with those of the British Medical Research Council."

To other doctors, the "Ascorbic Acid Deficiency" study appears as a senseless piece of cruelty visited on the five volunteers. "This study was totally pointless," Dr. Ephraim Kahn of the California Department of Public Health said of Dr. Hodges' publication. "The cause and cure of scurvy have been well known in the medical profession for generations. Some of the side effects he lists may well be irreversible—the young man who had the most severe case of scurvy may never have recovered. There's a clue here to the degree of competence of these so-called 'researchers'—they 'inadvertently' omitted a mineral supplement from the diets. This no doubt weakened the men and exacerbated the other side effects. It might cause them to go into shock, and to suffer severe cardiac abnormalities." Among effects of the experiment recorded in the publication that could be permanent, Dr. Kahn cited heart damage, loss of hair, damage to teeth, hemorrhage into femoral nerve sheaths—the latter is "terribly painful and could lead to permanent nerve damage."

I asked Dr. Hodges, now a professor of internal medicine at the University of California medical school at Davis, how much he had paid the scurvy test volunteers. "I think it was one dollar or maybe two dollars a day," he replied. "Over the years, when I was in Iowa, as the cost of cigarettes and razor blades went up, we increased prisoners' pay somewhat. It's unethical to pay an amount of money that is too attractive. Oh, we had the money, we could have paid much more, of course—but we weren't just being cheap, we were considering the ethics of the situation. The prisoners got a bit extra for really unpleasant things—if we had to put a tube down their throats for several hours, or take a biopsy of the skin the size of a pencil eraser, we'd give them a few dollars more." . . .

In 1947 fifteen German doctors, all distinguished leaders of their profession, were tried and convicted at Nuremberg for their cruel and frequently murderous "medical experiments" performed on concentration camp inmates. The barbarity of these crimes is of course unparalleled, but the Nuremberg tribunal established standards for medical experimentation on humans, which, if observed, would end altogether the practice of using prisoners as subjects: "The voluntary consent of the human subject is absolutely essential. This means the person involved should have legal capacity to give consent; should be so situated as to be able to exercise free power of choice . . . and should have sufficient knowledge and comprehension of the elements of the subject matter involved as to enable him to make an understanding, enlightened decision." Are prisoners, stripped of their civil rights when they enter the gates, subjected to years or decades of confinement, free agents capable of exercising freedom of choice? Can we trust that they are furnished by the experimenters with "knowledge and comprehension" to enable them to make "understanding and enlightened" decisions? To ask these questions is, I believe, to answer them.

From "Research on Minors, Prisoners and the Mentally III"

Robert Q. Marston

In the chain of events stretching from the first biomedical research concept to ultimate delivery of improved medical services, the most critical link is the human research subject. If through lack of care or an excess of investigative zeal, we allow abuse of the human subject, we endanger the beneficial forward march of research and fall short as professionals. However, we must make it clear that there is immorality in not carrying out research involving human subjects. It follows that we must ensure that all those involved as subjects in medical research be as fully protected as humanly possible. . . .

Medical-research trials frequently require that a convenient stable subject population be followed over a period of weeks or months rather than days or hours. The medical scientist naturally turns to groups whose availability can be controlled—hospitalized patients, institutionalized patients, medical students, and prisoners. Much research, particularly that involving appreciable risks and requiring frequent monitoring, is concentrated in such groups. I have therefore proposed additional regulations to cover these situations.

If a grant proposal from a medical school or other research institution entails work involving human subjects in prisons or in hospitals for the mentally ill and retarded, an award of a National Institutes of Health grant or contract would be contingent on assurances from these institutions as well as from the grantee or contractor. The institution where the research actually is done would also be required to establish broadly based institutional committees with the responsibility and expertise for reviewing research proposals and for assuring compliance with Department's policy.

Any financial compensation to subjects in such institutions would be reasonably related to the amounts paid for other services and not so high as to constitute undue inducement. We would require a clear statement that neither participation in the proposed research project nor withdrawal from it will materially affect the conditions or terms of any subject's confinement.

In hospitals for the mentally ill and retarded, the research supported would be restricted to the following: research that is directly concerned with the issues of mental illness, mental health or mental retardation, or that will potentially benefit a class of persons commonly confined to a hospital for the mentally ill or retarded, or will lead to such knowledge that may reasonably be expected to reduce the need for hospitalization for mental illness or retardation. . . .

If, in a specific case, I were forced to make a choice between the individual and the general welfare of society, I would choose to protect the individual. But in the real world we must have both individual and social welfare. And in the real world the day-by-day decisions are not made in Washington but by the individual investigator, the individual physician, the individual institution. The responsibility ultimately rests with them. They need to appreciate, gather, and apply new knowledge. But the new knowledge, designed to benefit all society, must not be gained at the expense of any individual or any segment of society.

"On the Justifications for Civil Commitment"

Joseph M. Livermore, Carl P. Malmquist, and Paul E. Meehl

Involuntary confinement is the most serious deprivation of individual liberty that a society may impose. The philosophical justifications for such a deprivation by means of the criminal process have been thoroughly explored. No such intellectual effort has been directed at providing justifications for societal use of civil commitment procedures.

When certain acts are forbidden by the criminal law, we are relatively comfortable in imprisoning those who have engaged in such acts. We say that the imprisonment of the offender will serve as an example to others and thus deter them from violating the law. If we even stop to consider the morality of depriving one man of his liberty in order to serve other social ends, we usually are able to allay anxiety by referring to the need to incarcerate to protect society from further criminal acts or the need to reform the criminal. When driven to it, at last, we admit that our willingness to permit such confinement rests on the notion that the criminal has justified it by his crime. Eligibility for social tinkering based on guilt, retributive though it may be, has so far satisfied our moral sensibilities.

It is, we believe, reasonably clear that the system could not be justified were the concept of guilt not part of our moral equipment. Would we be comfortable with a system in which any man could go to jail if by so doing

Reprinted with permission from *University of Pennsylvania Law Review* 117, 75–96, November 1968. Copyright 1968 by U. Pa.

he would serve an overriding social purpose? The normal aversion to punishment by example, with its affront to the principle of equality, suggests that we would not. Conversely, could we abide a rule that only those men would be punished whose imprisonment would further important social ends? Again, the thought of vastly different treatment for those equally culpable would make us uneasy.

Similarly, if we chose to justify incarceration as a means of isolating a group quite likely to engage in acts dangerous to others, we would, without the justification of guilt, have difficulty explaining why other groups, equally or more dangerous in terms of actuarial data, are left free. By combining background environmental data, we can identify categories of persons in which we can say that fifty to eighty per cent will engage in criminal activity within a short period of time. If social protection is a sufficient justification for incarceration, this group should be confined as are those criminals who are likely to sin again.

The same argument applies when rehabilitative considerations are taken into account. Most, if not all, of us could probably benefit from some understanding psychological rewiring. Even on the assumption that confinement should be required only in those cases where antisocial acts may thereby be averted, it is not at all clear that criminals are the most eligible for such treatment. In addition, most people would bridle at the proposition that the state could tamper with their minds whenever it seemed actuarially sound to do so.

Fortunately, we can by reason of his guilt distinguish the criminal from others whom we are loathe to confine. He voluntarily flouted society's commands with an awareness of the consequences. Consequently, he may serve utilitarian purposes without causing his imprisoners any moral twinge.

This same sort of analysis is not available once we move beyond the arena of the criminal law. When people are confined by civil process, we cannot point to their guilt as a basis for differentiating them from others. What can we point to?

The common distinguishing factor in civil commitment is aberrance. Before we commit a person we demand either that he act or think differently than we believe he should. Whether our label be inebriate, addict, psychopath, delinquent, or mentally diseased, the core concept is deviation from norms.* Our frequently expressed value of individual autonomy, how-

*The concept "abnormal" or "aberrant" is sorely in need of more thorough logical analysis than it has, to our knowledge, as yet received. It seems fairly clear that several components—perhaps even utterly distinct kinds of meaning—can be discerned in the current usage of medicine and social science. The most objective meaning is the purely statistical one, in which "abnormal" designates deviation from the (statistical) "norm" of a specified biological or social population of organisms. Whether an individual specimen, or bit of behavior, is abnormal in this sense is readily ascertained by adequate sampling methods plus a more or less arbitrary choice of cutting score (*e.g.*, found in less than 1 in 100 cases). But for legal purposes this purely statistical criterion does not suffice, because the *kind* and *direction* of statistical deviation from population norms, as well as the *amount* of deviation which threatens a protected social interest sufficiently to justify legal coercion, are questions not answerable by statistics alone. Thus, anyone who has an IQ of 180, or possesses absolute pitch, or is color-blind, is statistically abnormal but hardly rendered thereby a candidate for incarceration, mandatory

ever, renders us unable to express those norms, however deeply they may be felt, in criminal proscriptions. We could not bring ourselves to outlaw senility, or manic behavior, or strange desires. Not only would this violate the common feeling that one is not a criminal if he is powerless to avoid the crime, but it might also reach conduct that most of us feel we have a right to engage in. When a man squanders his savings in a hypomanic episode, we may say, because of our own beliefs, that he is "crazy," but we will not say that only reasonable purchases are allowed on pain of criminal punishment. We are not yet willing to legislate directly the Calvinist ideal.

What we are not willing to legislate, however, we have been willing to practice through the commitment process. That process has been used to reach two classes of persons, those who are mentally ill and dangerous to themselves or others and those who are mentally ill and in need of care, custody or treatment. While those terms seem reasonably clear, on analysis that clarity evaporates.

---

treatment, or deprivation of the usual rights and powers of a "normal" individual. A second component in the concept of normality relies upon our (usually inchoate or implicit) notions of biological health, of a kind of proper functioning of the organism conceived as a teleological system of organs and capacities. From a biological viewpoint, it is not inconsistent to assert that a sizable proportion—conceivably a majority—of persons in a given population are abnormal or aberrant. Thus, if an epidemiologist found that 60% of the persons in a society were afflicted with plague or avitaminosis, he would (quite correctly) reject an argument that "Since most of them have it, they are okay, *i.e.*, not pathological and not in need of treatment." It is admittedly easier to defend this non-statistical, biological-fitness approach in the domain of physical disease, but its application in the domain of behavior is fraught with difficulties. *See* W. Schofield, *Psychotherapy: The Purchase of Friendship* 12 (1964). Yet even here there is surely something to be said for it in extreme cases, as, for example, the statistically "normal" frigidity of middle-class Victorian women, which any modern sexologist would confidently consider a biological maladaptation in need of repair, induced by "unhealthy" social learnings. A third component invokes some sort of subjective norm, such as an aesthetic, religious, ethical, or political ideal or rule. Finally, whether an a priori concept of "optimal psychological adjustment" should be considered as yet a fourth meaning of normality, or instead subsumed under one or more of the preceding, is a difficult question. In any event, it is important to keep alert to hidden fallacies in legal and policy arguments that rely upon the notion of abnormality or aberration, such as subtle transitions from one of these criteria to another. It is especially tempting to the psychiatrist or clinical psychologist, given his usual clinical orientation, to slip unconsciously from the idea of "sickness," where treatment of a so-called "patient" is the model, to an application that justifies at most a statistical or ideological or psychological-adjustment usage of the word "norm." Probably the most pernicious error is committed by those who classify as "sick" behavior that is aberrant in *neither* a statistical sense *nor* in terms of any defensible biological or medical criterion, but solely on the basis of the clinician's personal ideology of mental health and interpersonal relationships. Examples might be the current psychiatric stereotype of what a good mother or a healthy family must be like, or the rejection as "perverse" of forms of sexual behavior that are not biologically harmful, are found in many infra-human mammals and in diverse human cultures, and have a high statistical frequency in our own society. *See generally* F. Beach, *Sexual Behavior in Animals and Men* (1950); H. Ellis, *Studies in the Psychology of Sex* (1936); C. Ford & F. Beach, *Patterns of Sexual Behavior* (1951); A. Kinsey, W. Pomeroy & C. Martin, *Sexual Behavior in the Human Male* (1948); A. Kinsey, W. Pomeroy, C. Martin & P. Gebhard, *Sexual Behavior in the Human Female* (1953); W. Masters & V. Johnson, *Human Sexual Response* (1966); Ellis, "What is 'Normal' Sexual Behavior," 28 *Sexology* 364 (1962); S. Freud, "Three Essays on the Theory of Sexuality," in 7 *Complete Psychological Works* 123 (J. Strachey ed. 1962).

MENTAL ILLNESS

One need only glance at the diagnostic manual of the American Psychiatric Association to learn what an elastic concept mental illness is. It ranges from the massive functional inhibition characteristic of one form of catatonic schizophrenia to those seemingly slight aberrancies associated with an emotionally unstable personality, but which are so close to conduct in which we all engage as to define the entire continuum involved. Obviously, the definition of mental illness is left largely to the user and is dependent upon the norms of adjustment that he employs. Usually the use of the phrase "mental illness" effectively masks the actual norms being applied. And, because of the unavoidably ambiguous generalities in which the American Psychiatric Association describes its diagnostic categories, the diagnostician has the ability to shoehorn into the mentally diseased class almost any person he wishes, for whatever reason, to put there.

    All this suggests that the concept of mental illness must be limited in the field of civil commitment to a necessary rather than a sufficient condition for commitment. While the term has its uses, it is devoid of that purposive content that a touchstone in the law ought to have. Its breadth of meaning makes for such difficulty of analysis that it answers no question that the law might wish to ask.

DANGEROUSNESS TO OTHERS

The element of dangerousness to others has, at least in practice, been similarly illusive. As Professors Goldstein and Katz have observed, such a test, at a minimum, calls for a determination both of what acts are dangerous and how probable it is that such acts will occur. The first question suggests to a criminal lawyer the answer: crimes involving a serious risk of physical or psychical harm to another. Murder, arson and rape are the obvious examples. Even in criminal law, however, the notion of dangerousness can be much broader. If one believes that acts that have adverse effects on social interests are dangerous, and if one accepts as a generality that the criminal law is devoted to such acts, any crime can be considered dangerous. For example, speeding in a motor vehicle, although traditionally regarded as a minor crime, bears great risk to life and property, and thus may be viewed as a dangerous act. Dangerousness can bear an even more extensive definition as well. An act may be considered dangerous if it is offensive or disquieting to others. Thus, the man who walks the street repeating, in a loud monotone, "fuck, fuck, fuck," is going to wound many sensibilities even if he does not violate the criminal law. Other examples would be the man, found in most cities, striding about town lecturing at the top of his lungs, or the similar character in San Francisco who spends his time shadow boxing in public. If such people are dangerous, it is not because they threaten physical harm but because we are made uncomfortable when we see aberrancies. And, of course, if dangerousness is so defined, it is at least as broad a concept as mental illness. The cases are unfortunately silent about what meaning the concept of danger bears in the commitment process.

Assuming that dangerousness can be defined, the problem of predictability still remains. For the man who can find sexual release only in setting fires, one may confidently predict that dangerous acts will occur. For the typical mentally aberrant individual, though, the matter of prediction is not susceptible of answer. However nervous a full-blown paranoiac may make us, there are no actuarial data indicating that he is more likley to commit a crime than any normal person. Should he engage in criminal activity, his paranoia would almost certainly be part of the etiology. But on a predictive basis we have, as yet, nothing substantial to rely on.

Even if such information were available, it is improbable that it would indicate that the likelihood of crime within a group of individuals with any particular psychosis would be any greater than that to be expected in a normal community cross-section. Surely the degree of probability would not be as high as that in certain classes of convicted criminals after their release from prison or that in certain classes of persons having particular sociological or psychological characteristics.

DANGEROUSNESS TO SELF

The concept of "dangerousness to self" raises similar problems. The initial thought suggested by the phrase is the risk of suicide. But again it can be broadened to include physical or mental harm from an inability to take care of one's self, loss of assets from foolish expenditures, or even loss of social standing or reputation from behaving peculiarly in the presence of others. Again, if read very broadly this concept becomes synonymous with that of mental illness. And, of course, reliable prediction is equally impossible.

IN NEED OF CARE, CUSTODY, OR TREATMENT

The notion of necessity of care or treatment provides no additional limitation beyond those imposed by the concepts already discussed. One who is diagnosably mentally ill is, almost by definition, in need of care or treatment. Surely the diagnostician reaching the first conclusion would reach the second as well. And, if a man is dangerous, then presumably he is in need of custody. The problem, of course, lies with the word "need." If it is defined strictly as, for example, "cannot live without," then a real limitation on involuntary commitment is created. In normal usage, however, it is usually equated with "desirable," and the only boundary on loss of freedom is the value structure of the expert witness.

It is difficult to identify the reasons that lie behind incarceration of the mentally ill. Three seem to be paramount:

1. It is thought desirable to restrain those people who may be dangerous;
2. It is thought desirable to banish those who are a nuisance to others;

3. It is thought humanitarian to attempt to restore to normality and productivity those who are not now normal and productive.

Each of these goals has social appeal, but each also creates analytic difficulty.

As already mentioned, in order to understand the concept of danger one must determine what acts are dangerous and how likely is it that they will occur. There is a ready inclination to believe that experts in the behavioral sciences will be able to identify those members of society who will kill, rape, or burn. The fact is, however, that such identification cannot presently be accomplished. First, our growing insistence on privacy will, in all but a few cases, deny the expert access to the data necessary to the task of finding potential killers. Second, and of much greater importance, even if the data were available it is unlikely that a test could be devised that would be precise enough to identify only those individuals who are dangerous. Since serious criminal conduct has a low incidence in society, and since any test must be applied to a very large group of people, the necessary result is that in order to isolate those who will kill it is also necessary to incarcerate many who will not. Assume that one person out of a thousand will kill. Assume also that an exceptionally accurate test is created which differentiates with ninety-five per cent effectiveness those who will kill from those who will not. If 100,000 people were tested, out of the 100 who would kill 95 would be isolated. Unfortunately, out of the 99,900 who would not kill, 4,995 people would also be isolated as potential killers.* In these circumstances, it is clear that we could not justify incarcerating all 5,090 people. If, in the criminal law, it is better that ten guilty men go free than that one innocent man suffer, how can we say in the civil commitment area that it is better that fifty-four harmless people be incarcerated lest one dangerous man be free?

The fact is that without any attempt at justification we have been willing to do just this to one disadvantaged class, the mentally ill. This practice must rest on the common supposition that mental illness makes a man more likely to commit a crime. While there may be some truth in this, there is much more error. Any phrase that encompasses as many diverse concepts as does the term "mental illness" is necessarily imprecise. While the fact of paranoid personality might be of significance in determining a heightened probability of killing, the fact of hebephrenic schizophrenia probably would not. Yet both fit under the umbrella of mental illness.

Even worse, we have been making assessments of potential danger on the basis of nothing as precise as the psychometric test hypothesized. Were we to ignore the fact that no definition of dangerous acts has been agreed upon, our standards of prediction have still been horribly imprecise. On the armchair assumption that paranoids are dangerous, we have tended to play safe and incarcerate them all. Assume that the incidence of killing among

---

*See Meehl & Rosen, "Antecedent Probability and the Efficiency of Psychometric Signs, Patterns, or Cutting Scores," 52 *Psychological Bull.* 194 (1955): Rosen, "Detection of Suicidal Patients: An Example of Some Limitations in the Prediction of Infrequent Events," 18 *J. Consulting Psychology* 397 (1954).

paranoids is five times as great as among the normal population. If we use paranoia as a basis for incarceration we would commit 199 non-killers in order to protect ourselves from one killer. It is simply impossible to justify any commitment scheme so premised. And the fact that assessments of dangerousness are often made clinically by a psychiatrist, rather than psychometrically and statistically, adds little if anything to their accuracy.

We do not mean to suggest that dangerousness is not a proper matter of legal concern. We do suggest, however, that limiting its application to the mentally ill is both factually and philosophically unjustifiable. As we have tried to demonstrate, the presence of mental illness is of limited use in determining potentially dangerous individuals. Even when it is of evidentiary value, it serves to isolate too many harmless people. What is of greatest concern, however, is that the tools of prediction are used with only an isolated class of people. We have alluded before to the fact that it is possible to identify, on the basis of sociological data, groups of people wherein it is possible to predict that fifty to eighty per cent will engage in criminal or delinquent conduct. And, it is probable that more such classes could be identified if we were willing to subject the whole population to the various tests and clinical examinations that we now impose only on those asserted to be mentally ill. Since it is perfectly obvious that society would not consent to a wholesale invasion of privacy of this sort and would not act on the data if they were available, we can conceive of no satisfactory justification for this treatment of the mentally ill.

One possible argument for different treatment can be made in terms of the concept of responsibility. We demonstrate our belief in individual responsibility by refusing to incarcerate save for failure to make a responsible decision. Thus, we do not incarcerate a group, eighty per cent of whom will engage in criminal conduct, until those eighty per cent have demonstrated their lack of responsibility—and even then, the rest of the group remains free. The mentally diseased, so the argument would run, may be viewed prospectively rather than retrospectively because for them responsibility is an illusory concept. We do not promote responsibility by allowing the dangerous act to occur since, when it does, we will not treat the actor as responsible. One way of responding to this is to observe that criminal responsibility and mental illness are not synonymous, and that if incarceration is to be justified on the basis of irresponsibility, only those mentally ill who will probably, as a matter of prediction, commit a crime for which they will not be held responsible should be committed. A more fundamental response is to inquire whether susceptibility to criminal punishment is reasonably related to any social purpose. Granted that there is a gain in social awareness of individual responsibility by not incarcerating the responsible in advance of their crime, it does not necessarily follow that it is sufficiently great to warrant the markedly different treatment of the responsible and the irresponsible.

The other possible justification for the existing differential is that the mentally diseased are amenable to treatment. We shall explore the ramifications of this at a later point. It is sufficient now to observe that there is no reason to believe that the mentally well, but statistically dangerous, individ-

ual is any less amenable to treatment, though that treatment would undoubtedly take a different form.

Another basis probably underlying our commitment laws is the notion
that it is necessary to segregate the unduly burdensome and the social
nuisance. Two cases typify this situation. The first is the senile patient whose
family asserts inability to provide suitable care. At this juncture, assuming
that the family could put the person on the street where he would be unable
to fend for himself, society must act to avoid the unpleasantness associated
with public disregard of helplessness. This caretaking function cannot be
avoided. Its performance, however, is a demonstration of the psychological
truth that we can bear that which is kept from our attention. Most of us
profess to believe that there is an individual moral duty to take care of a
senile parent, a paranoid wife, or a disturbed child. Most of us also resent
the bother such care creates. By allowing society to perform this duty,
masked in medical terminology, but frequently amounting in fact to what
one court has described as "warehousing," we can avoid facing painful
issues.

The second case is the one in which the mentally ill individual is simply
a nuisance, as when he insists on sharing his paranoid delusions or hallucinations with us. For reasons that are unclear, most of us are extremely
uncomfortable in the presense of an aberrant individual, whether or not we
owe him any duty, and whether or not he is in fact a danger to us in any
defensible use of that concept. Our comfort, in short, depends on his banishment, and yet that comfort is equally dependent on a repression of any
consciousness of the reason for his banishment. It is possible, of course, to
put this in utilitarian terms. Given our disquietude, is not the utility of
confinement greater than the utility of liberty? Perhaps so, but the assertions
either that we will act most reasonably if we repress thinking about why we
are acting or, worse yet, that our legislators will bear this knowledge for us
in order to preserve our psychic ease make us even more uncomfortable
than the thought that we may have to look mental aberrance in the eye.

Again, we do not wish to suggest that either burden or bother is an
inappropriate consideration in the commitment process. What we do want
to make clear is that when it is a consideration it ought to be advertently so.
Only in that way can intelligent decisions about care, custody, and treatment
be made.

The final probable basis for civil commitment has both humanitarian
and utilitarian overtones. When faced with an obviously aberrant person, we
know, or we think we know, that he would be "happier" if he were as we
are. We believe that no one would want to be a misfit in society. From the
very best of motives, then, we wish to fix him. It is difficult to deal with this
feeling since it rests on the unverifiable assumption that the aberrant person, if he saw himself as we see him, would choose to be different than he
is. But since he cannot be as we, and we cannot be as he, there is simply no
way to judge the predicate for the assertion.

Our libertarian views usually lead us to assert that treatment cannot
be forced on anyone unless the alternative is very great social harm. Thus
while we will require smallpox vaccinations and the segregation of conta-

gious tuberculars, we will not ordinarily require bed rest for the common cold, or a coronary, or even require a pregnant woman to eat in accordance with a medically approved diet. Requiring treatment whenever it seemed medically sound to do so would have utilitarian virtues. Presumably, if death or serious incapacitation could thereby be avoided society would have less worry about unsupported families, motherless children, or individuals no longer able to support themselves. Similarly, if the reasoning were pursued, we could insure that the exceptionally able, such as concert violinists, distinguished scholars, and inspiring leaders would continue to benefit society. Nonetheless, only rarely does society require such treatment. Not only does it offend common notions of bodily integrity and individual autonomy, but it also raises those issues of value judgment which, if not insoluble, are at least discomforting. For example, is the treatment and cure of the mentally ill individual of more benefit to society than the liberty of which he is deprived and the principle (lost, or tarnished) that no one should assert the right to control another's beliefs and responses absent compelling social danger?

The reason traditionally assigned for forcing treatment on the mentally ill while making it voluntary for other afflicted persons is that the mentally ill are incapable of making a rational judgment whether they need or desire such help. As with every similar statement, this depends on what kind of mental illness is present. It is likely that a pederast understands that society views him as sick, that certain kinds of psychiatric treatment may "cure" him, and that such treatment is available in certain mental institutions. It is also not unlikely that he will, in these circumstances, decide to forego treatment, at least if such treatment requires incarceration. To say that the pederast lacks insight into his condition and therefore is unable to intelligently decide whether or not to seek treatment is to hide our real judgment that he ought to be fixed, like it or not. It is true that some mentally ill people may be unable to comprehend a diagnosis and, in these instances, forced treatment may be more appropriate. But this group is a small proportion of the total committable population. Most understand what the clinician is saying though they often disagree with his view.

We have tried to show that the common justifications for the commitment process rest on premises that are either false or too broad to support present practices. This obviously raises the question of alternatives. Professor Ehrenzweig has suggested in another context that the definition of mental illness ought to be tailored to the specific social purpose to be furthered in the context in question. That is what we propose here.

Returning to the first of our considerations supporting commitment, we suggest that before a man can be committed as dangerous it must be shown that the probabilities are very great that he will commit a dangerous act. Just how great the probabilities need be will depend on two things: how serious the probable dangerous act is and how likely it is that the mental condition can be changed by treatment. A series of hypotheticals will indicate how we believe this calculus ought to be applied.

Case 1: A man with classic paranoia exhibits in clinical interview a fixed belief that his wife is attempting to poison him. He calmly states that on release he will be forced to kill her in self-defense. The experts agree that his condition is untreatable. Assume that statistical data indicate an eighty per cent probability that homicide will occur. If society will accept as a general rule of commitment, whether or not mental illness is present, that an eighty per cent probability of homicide is sufficient to incarcerate, then this man may be incarcerated. In order to do this, of course, we must be willing to lock up twenty people out of 100 who will not commit homicide.

Case 2: Assume the same condition with only a forty per cent probability of homicide. We do not know whether, if the condition is untreatable, commitment is justified in these circumstances. If lifetime commitment is required because the probabilities are constant, we doubt that the justification would exist. Our own value structure would not allow us to permanently incarcerate sixty harmless individuals in order to prevent forty homicides. On the other hand, if incarceration for a year would reduce the probability to ten per cent, then perhaps it is justified. Similarly, if treatment over the course of two or three years would substantially reduce the probability, then commitment might be thought proper.

Case 3: A man who compulsively engages in acts of indecent exposure has been diagnosed as having a sociopathic personality disturbance. The probability is eighty per cent that he will again expose himself. Even if this condition is untreatable, we would be disinclined to commit. In our view, this conduct is not sufficiently serious to warrant extended confinement. For that reason, we would allow confinement only if "cure" were relatively quick and certain.

The last case probably is more properly one of nuisance than of danger. The effects of such conduct are offensive and irritating but it is unlikely that they include long-term physical or psychical harm. That does not mean, however, that society has no interest in protecting its members from such upset. Again, the question is one of alternatives. Much nuisance behavior is subject to the control of the criminal law or of less formal social restraints. In mental institutions patients learn that certain behavior or the recounting of delusions or hallucinations will be met with disapproval. Accordingly, they refrain from such behavior or conversation. There is no reason to believe that societal disapproval in the form of criminal proscriptions or of less formal sanctions will be less effective as a deterrent. And, from our standpoint, the liberty of many mentally ill individuals is worth far more than the avoidance of minor nuisances in society.

Case 4: A person afflicted with schizophrenia walks about town making wild gestures and talking incessantly. Those who view him are uncomfortable but not endangered. We doubt that commitment is appropriate even though it would promote the psychic ease of many people. Arguably we would all be happier if our favorite bogey man, whether James Hoffa, Rap Brown, Mario Savio, or some other, were incarcerated. Most of us would be outraged if any of these men were committed on such a theory. If we cannot justify such a commitment in these cases, we doubt that it is any more justifiable when social anxiety is a consequence of seeing mentally ill individuals. While it might be proper to commit if speedy cure were possible, such cures are, as a matter of fact, unavailable. Moreover, we have some difficulty distinguishing the prevention of psychic upset based on cure of the mentally ill and prevention based on neutralizing other upsetting behavior.

The next justification of commitment is more solid, though it too presents the question of the necessity of utilizing less burdensome alternatives. This is the rationale of care for the person who is unable to care for himself and who has no one else to provide care for him. As we suggested earlier, such care must be provided if we are unwilling to allow people to die in the streets.

Case 5: An elderly woman with cerebro-vascular disease and accompanying cerebral impairment has the tendency to leave her home, to become lost, and then to wander helplessly about until someone aids her. At other times she is perfectly able to go shopping or visit friends. She has no relatives who will care for her in the sense that they will prevent her from wandering or will find her when she has become lost. In some ways, this is another case of a public nuisance and it may well be that it is impossible to find a justification for incarcerating this woman. On the other hand, to allow this woman to die from exposure on one of her forays is as disquieting as the loss of her freedom. Since her condition is untreatable, provision of treatment offers no justification for confinement. It might be justifiable to exercise some supervision over her, but surely that justification will not support total incarceration. In these circumstances, we believe that if the state wishes to intervene it must do so in some way that does not result in a total loss of freedom. The desire to help ought not to take the form of simple jailing.

Case 6: A schizophrenic woman is causing such an upset in her family that her husband petitions for commitment. It is clear that the presence of this woman in the family is having an adverse effect on the children. Her husband is simply unwilling to allow the situation to continue. The alternatives here are all unpleasant to contemplate. If the husband gets a divorce and custody, he may accomplish his end. But the social opprobrium attaching to that solution makes it unlikely. The question, then, is whether the state should provide a socially acceptable alternative. If that alternative is her loss of freedom, we find it hard to justify. Assuming that the condition is untreatable, that the woman is not dangerous, and that her real sin is her capacity to disrupt, it is almost incomprehensible that she should be subject to a substantial period of incarceration. Yet that is what it has meant. Presumably, in order to isolate the woman from her family, it is necessary to transport her to a location where she will no longer bother her family. Then, if she is able to support herself she could have complete freedom. If she is not able, the state will have to provide care. That care, of course, need not involve a total deprivation of freedom.

The final justification for commitment—the need to treat—is in many ways the most difficult to deal with. As we have said before, society has not traditionally required treatment of treatable diseases even though most people would agree that it was "crazy" for the diseased person not to seek treatment. The problem has been complicated by the fact that religious beliefs against certain forms of treatment often are present and by the fact that most cases of stubborn refusal to accept treatment never come into public view. There is, however, a competing analogy that suggests that mandatory treatment may sometimes be appropriate.

Without going into unnecessary detail, we think it can be said that one of the reasons society requires compulsory education is that it believes a certain minimum amount of socialization is necessary for everyone lest they be an economic burden or a personal nuisance. That principle can also be used to support mandatory psychiatric rewiring if the individual to be refurbished is in fact a burden or nuisance and can be fixed. The difficulty, of course, lies in the extent to which the principle can be carried. To take a mild example outside the field of mental disease, assume an unemployable individual who is unable to support his large and growing family. Could society incarcerate him until he had satisfactorily acquired an employable skill? In the context of mental disease, then, can society demand that an individual obtain an employable psyche?

Case 7: An individual has been suffering from paranoid schizophrenia for several years without remission and has lost his job because of his behavior. He is divorced, but he is able to support himself from prior savings. He is not dangerous, and if he is committed it is unlikely that he will be cured since the recovery rates from such long-term schizophrenia are very low. In addition, the availability of treatment in a state mental institution is problematic. We doubt that he can justifiably be committed. If treatment is an adequate basis for confinement, it surely ceases to be so either when the illness is untreatable or when treatment is in fact not given or given in grossly insufficient amounts. No other basis for commitment being present, it is unjustifiable.

Case 8: A distinguished law school professor, known for a series of brilliant articles, is suffering from an involutional depression. His scholarship has dried up, and, while he is still able to teach, the spark is gone and his classes have become extremely depressing. There is a chance, though probably not more than twenty-five per cent, that he will commit suicide. He has been told that he would recover his old élan if he were subjected to a series of electro-shock treatments but this he has refused to do. In fact, in years past when he was teaching a course in law and psychology, he stated that if he ever became depressed he wanted it known that before the onset of depression he explicitly rejected such treatment. Should he be compelled to undergo treatment? The arguments of social utility would suggest that he should. Yet we are unable to dislodge the notion that potential added productivity is not a license for tampering.

Case 9: A woman suffers from a severe psychotic depression resulting in an ability to do little more than weep. Again shock treatment is recommended with a reasonable prospect of a rapid recovery. The woman rejects the suggestion saying that nothing can make her a worthy member of society. She is, she claims, beyond help or salvation. It is possible to distinguish this from the preceding case on the ground that her delusional thought processes prevent her from recognizing the desirability of treatment. But any distinction based on a proposed patient's insight into her condition will probably be administered on the assumption that any time desirable treatment is refused, insight is necessarily lacking. And that, of course, would destroy the distinction.

These cases suggest that the power to compel treatment is one that rarely ought to be exercised. We are unable to construct a rationale that will not as well justify remolding too many people to match predominant ideas of the shape of the ideal psyche. We recognize, of course, that we are exhibiting a parade of horrors. In this instance, however, we believe such reference justified. The ease with which one can be classified as less than mentally healthy, and the difficulty in distinguishing degrees of sickness, make us doubt the ability of anyone to judge when the line between minimum socialization and aesthetically pleasing acculturation has been passed. Regardless of our views, however, it seems clear that if society chooses to continue to exercise the power to compel treatment, it ought to do so with constant awareness of the threat to autonomy thus posed.

Different considerations are present when commitment is not based on the need to treat. If one is committed as dangerous, or as a nuisance, or as unable to care for oneself, and treatment can cure this condition, then it is easier to strike the balance between deprivation of liberty and the right to refuse treatment in favor of compulsory treatment. If told that this is the price of freedom, the patient may accede; if he prefers confinement to treatment, perhaps the state ought not to override his wishes. But at least in this situation the question is ethically a close one.

The difficulty with present commitment procedures is that they tend to justify all commitments in terms that are appropriate only to some, and to prescribe forms of treatment that are necessary in only some cases. Thus, while danger stemming from mental illness may be a proper basis for commitment, it does not follow that all mentally ill are dangerous, or that the standards of danger should be markedly less rigid in cases of mental illness. Similarly, because mentally ill people may be a nuisance and some means of preventing such nuisance must be found, it does not follow that nuisance commitments ought to involve the same restraints as commitments based upon potential danger. Finally, because treatment is humanitarian when applied to those confined for danger, nuisance, or care, does not in itself suggest that treatment can be applied whenever administrators believe it proper or humane to do so.

We recognize that many people will not agree with the manner in which we have drawn the balance in individual cases. We hope that few will disagree that the balance must be drawn. We suggest, therefore, that in each case of proposed commitment, the following questions be asked:

I.   What social purpose will be served by commitment?

A.   If protection from potential danger, what dangerous acts are threatened? How likely are they to occur? How long will the individual have to be confined before time or treatment will eliminate or reduce the danger so that he may be released?

B.   If protection from nuisance, how onerous is the nuisance in fact? Ought that to justify loss of freedom? If it should, how long will confinement last before time or treatment will eliminate or reduce the risk of nuisance so that release may occur?

C.   If the need for care, is care in fact necessary? If so, how long will confinement last before time or treatment will eliminate the need for care so that release may occur?

II.   Can the social interest be served by means less restrictive than total confinement?

III.   Whatever standard is applied, is it one that can comfortably be applied to all members of society, mentally ill or healthy?

IV.   If confinement is justified only because it is believed that it will be of short term for treatment, is the illness in fact treatable? If it is, will appropriate treatment in fact be given?

If these questions are asked—and we view it as the duty of the attorney for the potential patient to insure that they are—then more intelligent commitment practices may follow.

From the Position Statement on Involuntary Hospitalization of the Mentally Ill (Revised)

American Psychiatric Association

The American Psychiatric Association is convinced that most persons who need hospitalization for mental illness can be and should be informally and voluntarily admitted to hospitals in the same manner that hospitalization is afforded for any other illness.

Moreover, modern concepts of psychiatric treatment emphasize the use of community-based outpatient facilities for the treatment and care of the mentally ill who voluntarily seek these services. Psychiatrists attempt to avoid hospitalization to every possible extent, although for some patients a period of hospitalization, usually brief, continues to be the indicated treatment.

Unfortunately, a small percentage of patients who need hospitalization are unable, because of their mental illness, to make a free and informed decision to hospitalize themselves. Their need for and right to treatment in a hospital cannot be ignored. In addition, public policy demands that some form of involuntary hospitalization be available for those mentally ill patients who constitute a danger either to themselves or to others.

PATERNALISM

From *Buck* v. *Bell*

Oliver Wendell Holmes

We have seen more than once that the public welfare may call upon its best citizens for their lives. It would be strange if it could not call upon those who already sap the strength of the State for these lesser sacrifices, often not felt to be such by those concerned, in order to prevent our being swamped with incompetence. It is better for all the world, if instead of waiting to execute degenerate offspring for crime, or to let them starve for their imbecility, society can prevent those who are manifestly unfit from continuing their kind. The principle that sustains compulsory vaccination is broad enough to cover cutting the Fallopian tubes. (*Jacobson* v. *Massachusetts,* 197 U.S. 11, 25 S.Ct. 358, 49 L.Ed. 643, 3 Ann.Cas. 765). Three generations of imbeciles are enough.

From *On Liberty*

John Stuart Mill

The object of this essay is to assert one very simple principle, as entitled to govern absolutely the dealings of society with the individual in the way of compulsion and control, whether the means used be physical force in the form of legal penalties or the moral coercion of public opinion. That principle is that the sole end for which mankind are warranted, individually or collectively, in interfering with the liberty of action of any of their number is self-protection. That the only purpose for which power can be rightfully exercised over any member of a civilized community, against his will, is to prevent harm to others. His own good, either physical or moral, is not a sufficient warrant. He cannot rightfully be compelled to do or forbear because it will be better for him to do so, because it will make him happier, because, in the opinions of others, to do so would be wise or even right. These are good reasons for remonstrating with him, or reasoning with him, or persuading him, or entreating him, but not for compelling him or visiting him with any evil in case he do otherwise. To justify that, the conduct from which it is desired to deter him must be calculated to produce evil to someone else. The only part of the conduct of anyone for which he is amenable to society is that which concerns others. In the part which merely concerns himself, his independence is, of right, absolute. Over himself, over his own body and mind, the individual is sovereign.

From O. W. Holmes, *Buck v. Bell* 274 U.S. 200; 47 S.Ct. 584, 71 L.Ed. 1000 (1927).
From John Stuart Mill, *On Liberty,* edited by Currin V. Shields. Copyright © 1956, by The Liberal Arts Press, Inc. Reprinted by permission of The Bobbs-Merrill Company, Inc.

It is, perhaps, hardly necessary to say that this doctrine is meant to apply only to human beings in the maturity of their faculties. We are not speaking of children or of young persons below the age which the law may fix as that of manhood or womanhood. Those who are still in a state to require being taken care of by others must be protected against their own actions as well as against external injury. For the same reason we may leave out of consideration those backward states of society in which the race itself may be considered as in its nonage. The early difficulties in the way of spontaneous progress are so great that there is seldom any choice of means for overcoming them; and a ruler full of the spirit of improvement is warranted in the use of any expedients that will attain an end perhaps otherwise unattainable. Despotism is a legitimate mode of government in dealing with barbarians, provided the end be their improvement and the means justified by actually effecting that end. Liberty, as a principle, has no application to any state of things anterior to the time when mankind have become capable of being improved by free and equal discussion. Until then, there is nothing for them but implicit obedience to an Akbar or a Charlemagne, if they are so fortunate as to find one. But as soon as mankind have attained the capacity of being guided to their own improvement by conviction or persuasion (a period long since reached in all nations with whom we need here concern ourselves), compulsion, either in the direct form or in that of pains and penalties for noncompliance, is no longer admissible as a means to their own good, and justifiable only for the security of others.

It is proper to state that I forego any advantage which could be derived to my argument from the idea of abstract right as a thing independent of utility. I regard utility as the ultimate appeal on all ethical questions; but it must be utility in the largest sense, grounded on the permanent interests of man as a progressive being. Those interests, I contend, authorize the subjection of individual spontaneity to external control only in respect to those actions of each which concern the interest of other people. If anyone does an act hurtful to others, there is a *prima facie* case for punishing him by law or, where legal penalties are not safely applicable, by general disapprobation. There are also many positive acts for the benefit of others which he may rightfully be compelled to perform, such as to give evidence in a court of justice, to bear his fair share in the common defense or in any other joint work necessary to the interest of the society of which he enjoys the protection, and to perform certain acts of individual beneficence, such as saving a fellow creature's life or interposing to protect the defenseless against ill usage—things which whenever it is obviously a man's duty to do he may rightfully be made responsible to society for not doing. A person may cause evil to others not only by his actions but by his inaction, and in either case he is justly accountable to them for the injury. The latter case, it is true, requires a much more cautious exercise of compulsion than the former. To make anyone answerable for doing evil to others is the rule; to make him answerable for not preventing evil is, comparatively speaking, the exception. Yet there are many cases clear enough and grave enough to justify that exception. In all things which regard the external relations of the individual, he is *de jure* amenable to those whose interests are concerned, and, if need be, to society as their protector. There are often good reasons for not holding him to the responsibility; but these reasons must arise from the special expediencies of the case: either because it is a kind of case in which he is on the whole likely to act better when left to his own discretion than when controlled in any way in which society have it in their power to control him; or because the attempt to exercise control would produce other evils, greater than those which it would prevent. When such reasons as these preclude the enforcement of responsibility, the conscience of the agent himself should step into the vacant judgment seat and protect those interests of others which have no external protection; judging himself all the more rigidly, because the case does not admit of his being made accountable to the judgment of his fellow creatures.

But there is a sphere of action in which society, as distinguished from the individual, has, if any, only an indirect interest: comprehending all that portion of a person's life and conduct which affects only himself or, if it also affects others, only with their free, voluntary, and undeceived consent and participation. When I say only himself, I mean directly and in the first instance; for whatever affects himself may affect others through himself; and the objection which may be grounded on this contingency will receive consideration in the sequel. This, then, is the appropriate region of human liberty. It comprises, first, the inward domain of consciousness, demanding liberty of conscience in the most comprehensive sense, liberty of thought and feeling, absolute freedom of opinion and sentiment on all subjects, practical or speculative, scientific, moral, or theological. The liberty of expressing and publishing opinions may seem to fall under a different principle, since it belongs to that part of the conduct of an individual which concerns other people, but, being almost of as much importance as the liberty of thought itself and resting in great part on the same reasons, is practically inseparable from it. Secondly, the principle requires liberty of tastes and pursuits, of framing the plan of our life to suit our own character, of doing as we like, subject to such consequences as may follow, without impediment from our fellow creatures, so long as what we do does not harm them, even though they should think our conduct foolish, perverse, or wrong. Thirdly, from this liberty of each individual follows the liberty, within the same limits, of combination among individuals; freedom to unite for any purpose not involving harm to others: the persons combining being supposed to be of full age and not forced or deceived.

No society in which these liberties are not, on the whole, respected is free, whatever may be its form of government; and none is completely free in which they do not exist absolute and unqualified. The only freedom which deserves the name is that of pursuing our own good in our own way, so long as we do not attempt to deprive others of theirs or impede their efforts to obtain it. Each is the proper guardian of his own health, whether bodily *or* mental and spiritual. Mankind are greater gainers by suffering each other to live as seems good to themselves than by compelling each to live as seems good to the rest.

"Paternalism"

Gerald Dworkin

> Neither one person, nor any number of persons, is warranted in saying to another human creature of ripe years, that he shall not do with his life for his own benefit what he chooses to do with it. *Mill*

> I do not want to go along with a volunteer basis. I think a fellow should be compelled to become better and not let him use his discretion whether he wants to get smarter, more healthy or more honest. *General Hershey*

I take as my starting point the "one very simple principle" proclaimed by Mill in *On Liberty* ... "That principle is, that the sole end for which mankind are warranted, individually or collectively, in interfering with the liberty of action of any of their number, is self-protection. That the only purpose for which power can be rightfully exercised over any member of a civilized community, against his will, is to prevent harm to others. ... He cannot rightfully be compelled to do or forbear because it will be better for him to do so, because it will make him happier, because, in the opinion of others, to do so would be wise, or even right."[1]

This principle is neither "one" nor "very simple." It is at least two principles; one asserting that self-protection or the prevention of harm to others is sometimes a sufficient warrant and the other claiming that the individual's own good is *never* a sufficient warrant for the exercise of compulsion either by the society as a whole or by its individual members. I assume that no one with the possible exception of extreme pacifists or anarchists questions the correctness of the first half of the principle. This essay is an examination of the negative claim embodied in Mill's principle —the objection to paternalistic interferences with a man's liberty.

I

By paternalism I shall understand roughly the interference with a person's liberty of action justified by reasons referring exclusively to the welfare, good, happiness, needs, interests or values of the person being coerced. One is always well-advised to illustrate one's definitions by examples but it is not easy to find "pure" examples of paternalistic interferences. For almost any piece of legislation is justified by several different kinds of reasons and even if historically a piece of legislation can be shown to have been introduced for purely paternalistic motives, it may be that advocates of the legislation with an anti-paternalistic outlook can find sufficient reasons justifying the legislation without appealing to the reasons which were originally

Reprinted with permission of author and publisher from the *Monist* 56:1, 64–84, June 1972.

[1] J. S. Mill, *Utilitarianism* and *On Liberty* (Fontana Library Edition, ed. by Mary Warnock, London, 1962), p. 135. All further quotes from Mill are from this edition unless otherwise noted.

adduced to support it. Thus, for example, it may be that the original legisla-tion requiring motorcyclists to wear safety helmets was introduced for purely paternalistic reasons. But the Rhode Island Supreme court recently upheld such legislation on the grounds that it was "not persuaded that the legislature is powerless to prohibit individuals from pursuing a course of conduct which could conceivably result in their becoming public charges," thus clearly introducing reasons of a quite different kind. Now I regard this decision as being based on reasoning of a very dubious nature, but it illus-trates the kind of problem one has in finding examples. The following is a list of the kinds of interferences I have in mind as being paternalistic.

II

1. Laws requiring motorcyclists to wear safety helmets when operating their machines.

2. Laws forbidding persons from swimming at a public beach when life-guards are not on duty.

3. Laws making suicide a criminal offense.

4. Laws making it illegal for women and children to work at certain types of jobs.

5. Laws regulating certain kinds of sexual conduct, e.g. homosexuality among consenting adults in private.

6. Laws regulating the use of certain drugs which may have harmful conse-quences to the user but do not lead to anti-social conduct.

7. Laws requiring a license to engage in certain professions, with those not receiving a license subject to fine or jail sentence if they do engage in the practice.

8. Laws compelling people to spend a specified fraction of their income on the purchase of retirement annuities. (Social Security).

9. Laws forbidding various forms of gambling (often justified on the grounds that the poor are more likely to throw away their money on such activities than the rich who can afford to).

10. Laws regulating the maximum rates of interest for loans.

11. Laws against duelling.

In addition to laws which attach criminal or civil penalties to certain kinds of action, there are laws, rules, regulations, and decrees which make it either difficult or impossible for people to carry out their plans and which also are justified on paternalistic grounds. Examples of this are:

1. Laws regulating the types of contracts which will be upheld as valid by the courts, e.g. (an example of Mill's to which I shall return) no man may make a valid contract for perpetual involuntary servitude.

2. Not allowing as a defense to a charge of murder or assault the consent of the victim.

3. Requiring members of certain religious sects to have compulsory blood transfusions. This is made possible by not allowing the patient to have re-course to civil suits for assault and battery, and by means of injunctions.

4. Civil commitment procedures, when these are specifically justified on the basis of preventing the person being committed from harming himself. (The D.C. Hospitalization of the Mentally Ill Act provides for involuntary hospitalization of a person who "is mentally ill, and because of that illness, is likely to injure *himself* or others if allowed to remain at liberty." The term injure in this context applies to unintentional as well as intentional injuries.)

5. Putting fluorides in the community water supply.

All of my examples are of existing restrictions on the liberty of individuals. Obviously one can think of interferences which have not yet been imposed. Thus one might ban the sale of cigarettes, or require that people wear safety-belts in automobiles (as opposed to merely having them installed), enforcing this by not allowing motorists to sue for injuries, even when caused by other drivers, if the motorist was not wearing a seat-belt at the time of the accident.

I shall not be concerned with activities which, though defended on paternalistic grounds, are not interferences with the liberty of persons; *e.g.* the giving of subsidies in kind rather than in cash, on the grounds that the recipients would not spend the money on the goods which they really need; or not including a $1000 deductible provision in a basic protection automobile insurance plan, on the ground that the people who would elect it could least afford it. Nor shall I be concerned with measures such as "truth-in-advertising" acts and the Pure Food and Drug legislation, which are often attacked as paternalistic but which should not be considered so. In these cases all that is provided—it is true by the use of compulsion—is information which it is presumed that rational persons are interested in having in order to make wise decisions. There is no interference with the liberty of the consumer, unless one wants to stretch a point beyond good sense and say that his liberty to apply for a loan without knowing the true rate of interest is diminished. It is true that sometimes there is sentiment for going further than providing information, for example, when laws against usurious interest are passed, preventing those who might wish to contract loans at high rates of interest from doing so; and these measures may correctly be considered paternalistic.

III

Bearing these examples in mind, let me return to a characterization of paternalism. I said earlier that I meant by the term, roughly, interference with a person's liberty for his own good. But as some of the examples show, the class of persons whose good is involved is not always identical with the class of persons whose freedom is restricted. Thus in the case of professional licensing, it is the practitioner who is directly interfered with and it is the would-be patient whose interests are presumably being served. Not allowing the consent of the victim to be a defense to certain types of crime primarily affects the would-be aggressor, but it is the interests of the willing victim that we are trying to protect. Sometimes a person may fall into both classes, as would be the case if we banned the manufacture and sale of cigarettes and a given manufacturer happened to be a smoker as well.

Thus we may first divide paternalistic interferences into "pure" and "impure" cases. In "pure" paternalism, the class of persons whose freedom is restricted is identical with the class of persons whose benefit is intended to be promoted by such restrictions. Examples: the making of suicide a crime, requiring passengers in automobiles to wear seat-belts, requiring a Jehovah's Witness to receive a blood transfusion. In the case of "impure" paternalism, in trying to protect the welfare of a class of persons we find that the only way to do so will involve restricting the freedom of other persons besides those who are benefitted. Now it might be thought that there are no cases of "impure" paternalism since any such case could always be justified on non-paternalistic grounds, i.e., in terms of preventing harm to others. Thus we might ban cigarette manufacturers from continuing to manufacture their product, on the grounds that we are preventing them from causing illness to others in the same way that we prevent other manufacturers from releasing pollutants into the atmosphere, thereby causing danger to members of the community. The difference is, however, that in the former, but not the latter case the harm is of such a nature that it could be avoided by those individuals affected, if they so chose. The incurring of the harm requires, so to speak, the active co-operation of the victim. It would be mistaken theoretically, and hypocritical in practice, to assert that our interference in such cases is just like our interference in standard cases of protecting others from harm. At the very least someone interfered with in this way can reply that no one is complaining about his activities. It may be that impure paternalism requires arguments or reasons of a stronger kind in order to be justified, since there are persons who are losing a portion of their liberty and they do not even have the solace of having it be done "in their own interest." Of course in some sense, if paternalistic justifications are ever correct, then we are protecting others, we are preventing some from injuring others, but it is important to see the differences between this and the standard case.

Paternalism then will always involve limitations on the liberty of some individuals in their own interest, but it may also extend to interferences with the liberty of parties whose interests are not in question.

IV

Finally, by way of some more preliminary analysis, I want to distinguish paternalistic interferences with liberty from a related type with which it is often confused. Consider, for example, legislation which forbids employees to work more than, say, 40 hours per week. It is sometimes argued that such legislation is paternalistic for, if employees desired such a restriction on their hours of work, they could agree among themselves to impose it voluntarily. But because they do not, the society imposes its own conception of their best interests upon them by the use of coercion. Hence this is paternalism.

Now it may be that some legislation of this nature is, in fact, paternalistically motivated. I am not denying that. All I want to point out is that there is another possible way of justifying such measures, which is not paternalistic in nature. It is not paternalistic because, as Mill puts it in a similar context, such measures are "required not to overrule the judgment of individuals respecting their own interest, but to give effect to that judgment: they being unable to give effect to it except by concert, which concert again cannot be effectual unless it receives validity and sanction from the law."[2]

The line of reasoning here is a familiar one, first found in Hobbes and developed with great sophistication by contemporary economists in the last decade or so. There are restrictions which are in the interests of a class of persons taken collectively, but are such that the immediate interest of each individual is furthered by his violating the rule when others adhere to it. In such cases the individuals involved may need the use of compulsion, to give effect to their collective judgment of their own interest by guaranteeing each individual compliance by the others. In these cases compulsion is not used to achieve some benefit which is not recognized to be a benefit by those concerned, but rather because it is the only feasible means of achieving some benefit which *is* recognized as such by all concerned. This way of viewing matters provides us with another characterization of paternalism in general. Paternalism might be thought of as the use of coercion to achieve a good which is not recognized as such by those persons for whom the good is intended. Again, while this formulation captures the heart of the matter —it is surely what Mill is objecting to in *On Liberty*—the matter is not always quite like that. For example, when we force motorcyclists to wear helmets we are trying to promote a good—the protection of the person from injury —which is surely recognized by most of the individuals concerned. It is not that a cyclist doesn't value his bodily integrity; rather, as a supporter of such legislation would put it, he either places, perhaps irrationally, another value or good (freedom from wearing a helmet) above that of physical well-being or, perhaps, while recognizing the danger in the abstract, he either does not fully appreciate it or he underestimates the likelihood of its occurring. But now we are approaching the question of possible justifications of paternalistic measures, and the rest of this essay will be devoted to that question.

V

I shall begin for dialectical purposes by discussing Mill's objections to paternalism and then go on to discuss more positive proposals.

An initial feature that strikes one is the absolute nature of Mill's prohibitions against paternalism. It is so unlike the carefully qualified admonitions of Mill and his fellow Utilitarians on other moral issues. He speaks of self-protection as the *sole* end warranting coercion, of the individuals own goals as *never* being a sufficient warrant. Contrast this with his discussion of the prohibition against lying in *Utilitarianism.*

[2]J. S. Mill, *Principles of Political Economy* (New York: P. F. Collier and Sons, 1900), p. 442.

Yet that even this rule, sacred as it is, admits of possible exception, is acknowledged by all moralists, the chief of which is where the with-holding of some
fact . . . would save an individual . . . from great and unmerited evil.[3]

The same tentativeness is present when he deals with justice.

It is confessedly unjust to break faith with any one: to violate an engagement,
either express or implied, or disappoint expectations raised by our own conduct, at least if we have raised these expectations knowingly and voluntarily.
Like all the other obligations of justice already spoken of, this one is not
regarded as absolute, but as capable of being overruled by a stronger obligation of justice on the other side.[4]

This anomaly calls for some explanation. The structure of Mill's argument
is as follows:

1.   Since restraint is an evil the burden of proof is on those who propose
such restraint.

2.   Since the conduct which is being considered is purely self-regarding, the
normal appeal to the protection of the interests of others is not available.

3.   Therefore we have to consider whether reasons involving reference to
the individual's own good, happiness, welfare, or interests are sufficient to
overcome the burden of justification.

4.   We either cannot advance the interests of the individual by compulsion,
or the attempt to do so involves evil which outweighs the good done.

5.   Hence the promotion of the individual's own interests does not provide
a sufficient warrant for the use of compulsion.

Clearly the operative premise here is (4) and it is bolstered by claims
about the status of the individual as judge and appraiser of his welfare,
interests, needs, etc.

With respect to his own feelings and circumstances, the most ordinary man or
woman has means of knowledge immeasurably surpassing those that can be
possessed by any one else.[5]

He is the man most interested in his own well-being: the interest which any
other person, except in cases of strong personal attachment, can have in it, is
trifling, compared to that which he himself has.[6]

These claims are used to support the following generalizations concerning
the utility of compulsion for paternalistic purposes.

The interferences of society to overrule his judgment and purposes in what
only regards himself must be grounded on general presumptions; which may

[3]Mill, *Utilitarianism* and *On Liberty*, p. 174.

[4]*Ibid.*, p. 299.

[5]*Ibid.*, p. 207

[6]*Ibid.*, p. 206.

be altogether wrong, and even if right, are as likely as not to be misapplied to individual cases.[7]

But the strongest of all the arguments against the interference of the public with purely personal conduct is that when it does interfere, the odds are that it interferes wrongly and in the wrong place.[8]

All errors which the individual is likely to commit against advice and warning are far outweighed by the evil of allowing others to constrain him to what they deem his good.[9]

Performing the utilitarian calculation by balancing the advantages and disadvantages we find that:

Mankind are greater gainers by suffering each other to live as seems good to themselves, than by compelling each other to live as seems good to the rest.[10]

From which follows the operative premise (4).

This classical case of a utilitarian argument with all the premises spelled out is not the only line of reasoning present in Mill's discussion. There are asides, and more than asides, which look quite different and I shall deal with them later. But this is clearly the main channel of Mill's thought, and it is one which has been subjected to vigorous attack from the moment it appeared—most often by fellow Utilitarians. The link that they have usually seized on is, as Fitzjames Stephen put it, the absence of proof that the "mass of adults are so well acquainted with their own interests and so much disposed to pursue them that no compulsion or restraint put upon them by any others for the purpose of promoting their interest can really promote them."[11] Even so sympathetic a critic as Hart is forced to the conclusion that:

In Chapter 5 of his essay Mill carried his protests against paternalism to lengths that may now appear to us as fantastic. . . . No doubt if we no longer sympathise with this criticism this is due, in part, to a general decline in the belief that individuals know their own interest best.[12]

Mill endows the average individual with "too much of the psychology of a middle-aged man whose desires are relatively fixed, not able to be artificially stimulated by external influences; who knows what he wants and what gives him satisfaction of happiness; and who pursues these things when he can."[13]

Now it is interesting to note that Mill himself was aware of some of the limitations on the doctrine that the individual is the best judge of his own

---

[7] *Ibid.*, p. 207.

[8] *Ibid.*, p. 214.

[9] *Ibid.*, p. 207

[10] *Ibid.*, p. 138.

[11] J. F. Stephens, *Liberty, Equality, Fraternity* (New York: Henry Holt & Co., n.d.), p. 24

[12] H. L. A. Hart, *Law, Liberty and Morality* (Stanford: Stanford University Press, 1963), p. 32.

[13] *Ibid.*, p. 33.

interests. In his discussion of government intervention in general (even where the intervention does not interfere with liberty but provides alternative institutions to those of the market), after making claims which are parallel to those just discussed, e.g.:

> People understand their own business and their own interests better, and care for them more, than the government does, or can be expected to do,[14]

he goes on to an intelligent discussion of the "very large and conspicuous exceptions" to the maxim that:

> Most persons take a juster and more intelligent view of their own interest, and of the means of promoting it, than can either be prescribed to them by a general enactment of the legislature, or pointed out in the particular case by a public functionary.[15]

Thus there are things

> of which the utility does not consist in ministering to inclinations, nor in serving the daily uses of life, and the want of which is least felt where the need is greatest. This is peculiarly true of those things which are chiefly useful as tending to raise the character of human beings. The uncultivated cannot be competent judges of cultivation. Those who most need to be made wiser and better, usually desire it least, and, if they desired it, would be incapable of finding the way to it by their own lights.
>
> . . . A second exception to the doctrine that individuals are the best judges of their own interest, is when an individual attempts to decide irrevocably now what will be best for his interest at some future and distant time. The presumption in favor of individual judgment is only legitimate, where the judgment is grounded on actual, and especially on present, personal experience; not where it is formed antecedently to experience, and not suffered to be reversed even after experience has condemned it.[16]

The upshot of these exceptions is that Mill does not declare that there should never be government interference with the economy but rather that

> . . .in every instance, the burden of making out a strong case should be thrown not on those who resist but on those who recommend government interference. Letting alone, in short, should be the general practice: every departure from it, unless required by some great good, is a certain evil.[17]

In short, we get a presumption, not an absolute prohibition. The question is why doesn't the argument against paternalism go the same way?

I suggest that the answer lies in seeing that in addition to a purely utilitarian argument Mill uses another as well. As a Utilitarian Mill has to show, in Fitzjames Stephen's words, that:

[14]Mill, *Principles,* II, 448.
[15]*Ibid.,* II, 458.
[16]*Ibid.,* II, 459.
[17]*Ibid.,* II, 451.

> Self-protection apart, no good object can be attained by any compulsion which is not in itself a greater evil than the absence of the object which the compulsion obtains.[18]

To show this is impossible; one reason being that it isn't true. Preventing a man from selling himself into slavery (a paternalistic measure which Mill himself accepts as legitimate), or from taking heroin, or from driving a car without wearing seat-belts may constitute a lesser evil than allowing him to do any of these things. A consistent Utilitarian can only argue against paternalism on the grounds that it (as a matter of fact) does not maximize the good. It is always a contingent question that may be refuted by the evidence. But there is also a non-contingent argument which runs through *On Liberty*. When Mill states that "there is a part of the life of every person who has come to years of discretion, within which the individuality of that person ought to reign uncontrolled either by any other person or by the public collectively" he is saying something about what it means to be a person, an autonomous agent. It is because coercing a person for his own good denies this status as an independent entity, that Mill objects to it so strongly and in such absolute terms. To be able to choose is a good that is independent of the wisdom of what is chosen. A man's "mode of laying out his existence is the best, not because it is the best in itself, but because it is his own mode."[19]

> It is the privilege and proper condition of a human being, arrived at the maturity of his faculties, to use and interpret experience in his own way.[20]

As further evidence of this line of reasoning in Mill consider the one exception to his prohibition against paternalism.

> In this and most civilised countries, for example, an engagement by which a person should sell himself, or allow himself to be sold, as a slave, would be null and void; neither enforced by law nor by opinion. The ground for thus limiting his power of voluntarily disposing of his own lot in life, is apparent, and is very clearly seen in this extreme case. The reason for not interfering, unless for the sake of others, with a person's voluntary acts, is consideration for his liberty. His voluntary choice is evidence that what he so chooses is desirable, or at least endurable, to him, and his good is on the whole best provided for by allowing him to take his own means of pursuing it. But by selling himself for a slave, he abdicates his liberty; he foregoes any future use of it beyond that single act.
>
> He therefore defeats, in his own case, the very purpose which is the justification of allowing him to dispose of himself. He is no longer free; but is thenceforth in a position which has no longer the presumption in its favour, that would be afforded by his voluntarily remaining in it. The principle of freedom

[18]Stephen, p. 49.
[19]Mill, *Utilitarianism* and *On Liberty*, p. 197.
[20]*Ibid.*, p. 186.

cannot require that he should be free not to be free. It is not freedom to be allowed to alienate his freedom.[21]

Now leaving aside the fudging on the meaning of freedom in the last line, it is clear that part of this argument is incorrect. While it is true that *future* choices of the slave are not reasons for thinking that what he chooses then is desirable for him, what is at issue is limiting his immediate choice; and since this choice is made freely, the individual may be correct in thinking that his interests are best provided for by entering such a contract. But the main consideration for not allowing such a contract is the need to preserve the liberty of the person to make future choices. This gives us a principle —a very narrow one—by which to justify some paternalistic interferences. Paternalism is justified only to preserve a wider range of freedom for the individual in question. How far this principle could be extended, whether it can justify all the cases in which we are inclined upon reflection to think paternalistic measures justified, remains to be discussed. What I have tried to show so far is that there are two strains of argument in Mill—one a straight-forward Utilitarian mode of reasoning and one which relies not on the goods which free choice leads to, but on the absolute value of the choice itself. The first cannot establish any absolute prohibition but at most a presumption, and indeed a fairly weak one, given some fairly plausible assumptions about human psychology; the second, while a stronger line of argument, seems to me to allow on its own grounds a wider range of paternalism than might be suspected. I turn now to a consideration of these matters.

VI

We might begin looking for principles governing the acceptable use of paternalistic power in cases where it is generally agreed that it is legitimate. Even Mill intends his principles to be applicable only to mature individuals, not those in what he calls "non-age." What is it that justifies us in interfering with children? The fact that they lack some of the emotional and cognitive capacities required in order to make fully rational decisions. It is an empirical question to just what extent children have an adequate conception of their own present and future interests, but there is not much doubt that there are many deficiencies. For example it is very difficult for a child to defer gratification for any considerable period of time. Given these deficiencies and given the very real and permanent dangers that may befall the child, it becomes not only permissible but even a duty of the parent to restrict the child's freedom in various ways. There is however an important moral limitation on the exercise of such parental power, which is provided by the notion of the child eventually coming to see the correctness of his parent's interventions. Parental paternalism may be thought of as a wager by the parent on the child's subsequent recognition of the wisdom of the restric-

[21] *Ibid.*, pp. 235–236.

tions. There is an emphasis on what could be called future-oriented consent —on what the child will come to welcome, rather than on what he does welcome.

The essence of this idea has been incorporated by idealist philosophers into various types of "real-will" theory as applied to fully adult persons. Extensions of paternalism are argued for by claiming that in various respects, chronologically mature individuals share the same deficiencies in knowledge, capacity to think rationally, and the ability to carry out decisions that children possess. Hence in interfering with such people we are in effect doing what they would do if they were fully rational. Hence we are not really opposing their will, hence we are not really interfering with their freedom. The dangers of this move have been sufficiently exposed by Berlin in his Two Concepts of Liberty. I see no gain in theoretical clarity nor in practical advantage in trying to pass over the real nature of the interferences with liberty that we impose on others. Still the basic notion of consent is important and seems to me the only acceptable way of trying to delimit an area of justified paternalism.

Let me start by considering a case where the consent is not hypothetical in nature. Under certain conditions it is rational for an individual to agree that others should force him to act in ways in which, at the time of action, the individual may not see as desirable. If, for example, a man knows that he is subject to breaking his resolves when temptation is present, he may ask a friend to refuse to entertain his requests at some later stage.

A classical example is given in the Odyssey when Odysseus commands his men to tie him to the mast and refuse all future orders to be set free, because he knows the power of the Sirens to enchant men with their songs. Here we are on relatively sound ground in later refusing Odysseus' request to be set free. He may even claim to have changed his mind, but since it is just such changes that he wished to guard against we are entitled to ignore them.

A process analogous to this may take place on a social rather than individual basis. An electorate may mandate its representatives to pass legislation which when it comes time to "pay the price" may be unpalatable. I may believe that a tax increase is necessary to halt inflation, though I may resent the lower pay check each month. However in both this case and that of Odysseus the measure to be enforced is specifically requested by the party involved and at some point in time there is genuine consent and agreement on the part of those persons whose liberty is infringed. Such is not the case for the paternalistic measures we have been speaking about. What must be involved here is not consent to specific measures but rather consent to a system of government, run by elected representatives, with an understanding that they may act to safeguard our interests in certain limited ways.

I suggest that since we are all aware of our irrational propensities, deficiencies in cognitive and emotional capacities, and avoidable and unavoidable ignorance it is rational and prudent for us to in effect take out "social insurance policies." We may argue for and against proposed paternalistic measures in terms of what fully rational individuals would accept as forms of protection. Now clearly, since the initial agreement is not about specific measures, we are dealing with a more-or-less blank check, and therefore there have to be carefully defined limits. What I am looking for are certain kinds of conditions which make it plausible to suppose that rational men could reach agreement to limit their liberty even when other men's interests are not affected.

Of course as in any kind of agreement schema there are great difficulties in deciding what rational individuals would or would not accept. Particularly in sensitive areas of personal liberty, there is always a danger of the dispute over agreement and rationality being a disguised version of evaluative and normative disagreement.

Let me suggest types of situations in which it seems plausible to suppose that fully rational individuals would agree to having paternalistic restrictions imposed upon them. It is reasonable to suppose that there are "goods" such as health which any person would want to have in order to pursue his own good—no matter how that good is conceived. This is an argument that is used in connection with compulsory education for children but it seems to me that it can be extended to other goods which have this character. Then one could agree that the attainment of such goods should be promoted even when not recognized to be such, at the moment, by the individuals concerned.

An immediate difficulty that arises stems from the fact that men are always faced with competing goods and that there may be reasons why even a value such as health—or indeed life—may be overridden by competing values. Thus the problem with the Jehovah's Witness and blood transfusions. It may be more important for him to reject "impure substances" than to go on living. The difficult problem that must be faced is whether one can give sense to the notion of a person irrationally attaching weights to competing values.

Consider a person who knows the statistical data on the probability of being injured when not wearing seat belts in an automobile and knows the types and gravity of the various injuries. He also insists that the inconvenience attached to fastening the belt every time he gets in and out of the car outweighs for him the possible risks to himself. I am inclined in this case to think that such a weighing is irrational. Given his life-plans which we are assuming are those of the average person, his interests and commitments already undertaken, I think it is safe to predict that we can find inconsistencies in his calculations at some point. I am assuming that this is not a man who for some conscious or unconscious reasons is trying to injure himself nor is he a man who just likes to "live dangerously." I am assuming that he is like us in all the relevant respects but just puts an enormously high negative value on inconvenience—one which does not seem comprehensible or reasonable.

It is always possible, of course, to assimilate this person to creatures like myself. I, also, neglect to fasten my seat belt and I concede such behavior is not rational, but not because I weigh the inconvenience differently from those who fasten the belts. It is just that having made (roughly) the same calculation as everybody else I ignore it in my actions. (Note: a much better case of weakness of the will than those usually given in ethics texts.) A plausible explanation for this deplorable habit is that, although I know in some intellectual sense what the probabilities and risks are, I do not fully appreciate them in an emotionally genuine manner.

We have two distinct types of situation in which a man acts in a non-rational fashion. In one case he attaches incorrect weights to some of his values; in the other he neglects to act in accordance with his actual preferences and desires. Clearly there is a stronger and more persuasive argument for paternalism in the latter situation. Here we are really not—by assumption—imposing a good on another person. But why may we not extend our interference to what we might call evaluative delusions? After all in the case of cognitive delusions we are prepared, often, to act against the expressed will of the person involved. If a man believes that when he jumps out the window he will float upwards—Robert Nozick's example—would not we detain him, forcibly if necessary? The reply will be that this man doesn't wish to be injured and if we could convince him that he is mistaken as to the consequences of his action he would not wish to perform the action. But part of what is involved in claiming that a man who doesn't fasten his seat-belts is attaching an irrational weight to the inconvenience of fastening them is that if he were to be involved in an accident and severely injured, he would look back and admit that the inconvenience wasn't as bad as all that. So there is a sense in which if I could convince him of the consequences of his action, he also would not wish to continue his present course of action. Now the notion of consequences being used here is covering a lot of ground. In one case it's being used to indicate what will or can happen as a result of a course of action, and in the other it's making a prediction about the future evaluation of the consequences—in the first sense—of a course of action. And whatever the difference between facts and values—whether it be hard and fast or soft and slow—we are genuinely more reluctant to consent to interferences where evaluative differences are the issue. Let me now consider another factor which comes into play in some of these situations, which may make an important difference in our willingness to consent to paternalistic restrictions.

Some of the decisions we make are of such a character that they produce changes which are in one or another way irreversible. Situations are created in which it is difficult or impossible to return to anything like the initial stage at which the decision was made. In particular, some of these changes will make it impossible to continue to make reasoned choices in the future. I am thinking specifically of decisions which involve taking drugs that are physically or psychologically addictive and those which are destructive of one's mental and physical capacities.

I suggest we think of the imposition of paternalistic interferences in situations of this kind as being a kind of insurance policy which we take out against making decisions which are far-reaching, potentially dangerous, and irreversible. Each of these factors is important. Clearly there are many decisions we make that are relatively irreversible. In deciding to learn to play chess I could predict, in view of my general interest in games, that some portion of my free-time was going to be pre-empted and that it would not be easy to give up the game once I acquired a certain competence. But my whole life-style was not going to be jeopardized in an extreme manner. Further it might be argued that even with addictive drugs such as heroin one's normal life plans would not be seriously interfered with if an inexpensive and adequate supply were readily available. So this type of argument might have a much narrower scope than appears to be the case at first.

A second class of cases concerns decisions which are made under extreme psychological and sociological pressures. I am not thinking here of the making of the decision as being something one is pressured into—e.g., a good reason for making duelling illegal is that unless this is done many people might have to manifest their courage and integrity in ways in which they would rather not do so—but rather of decisions such as that to commit suicide, which are usually made at a point where the individual is not thinking clearly and calmly about the nature of his decision. In addition, of course, this comes under the previous heading of all-too-irrevocable decision. Now there are practical steps which a society could take if it wanted to decrease the possibility of suicide—for example, not paying social security benefits to the survivors or, as religious institutions do, not allowing such persons to be buried with the same status as natural deaths. I think we may count these as interferences with the liberty of persons to attempt suicide, and the question is whether they are justifiable.

Using my argument schema the question is whether rational individuals would consent to such limitations. I see no reason for them to consent to an absolute prohibition but I do think it is reasonable for them to agree to some kind of enforced waiting period. Since we are all aware of the possibility of temporary states, such as great fear or depression, that are inimical to the making of well-informed and rational decisions, it would be prudent for all of us if there were some kind of institutional arrangement whereby we were restrained from making a decision which is (all too) irreversible. What this would be like in practice is difficult to envisage, and it may be that if no practical arrangements were feasible then we would have to conclude that there should be no restriction at all on this kind of action. But we might have a "cooling off" period, in much the same way that we now require couples who file for divorce to go through a waiting period. Or, more far-fetched, we might imagine a Suicide Board composed of a psychologist and another member picked by the applicant. The Board would be required to meet and talk with the person proposing to take his life, though its approval would not be required.

A third class of decisions—these classes are not supposed to be disjoint —involves dangers which are either not sufficiently understood or appreciated correctly by the persons involved. Let me illustrate, using the example of cigarette smoking, a number of possible cases.

1.   A man may not know the facts—e.g., smoking between 1 and 2 packs a day shortens life expectancy 6.2 years, the costs and pain of the illness caused by smoking, etc.

2.   A man may know the facts, wish to stop smoking, but not have the requisite will-power.

3.   A man may know the facts but not have them play the correct role in his calculation because, say, he discounts the danger psychologically, because it is remote in time, and/or inflates the attractiveness of other consequences of his decision which he regards as beneficial.

In case 1 what is called for is education, the posting of warnings, etc. In case 2 there is no theoretical problem. We are not imposing a good on someone who rejects it. We are simply using coercion to enable people to carry out their own goals. (Note: There obviously is a difficulty in that only a subclass of the individuals affected wish to be prevented from doing what they are doing.) In case 3 there is a sense in which we are imposing a good on someone since, given his current appraisal of the facts, he doesn't wish to be restricted. But in another sense we are not imposing a good, since what is being claimed—and what must be shown or at least argued for—is that an accurate accounting on his part would lead him to reject his current course of action. Now we all know that such cases exist, that we are prone to disregard dangers that are only possibilities, that immediate pleasures are often magnified and distorted.

If in addition the dangers are severe and far-reaching, we could agree to allowing the state a certain degree of power to intervene in such situations. The difficulty is in specifying in advance, even vaguely, the class of cases in which intervention will be legitimate.

A related difficulty is that of drawing a line so that it is not the case that all ultra-hazardous activities are ruled out, e.g., mountain-climbing, bull-fighting, sports-car racing, etc. There are some risks—even very great ones—which a person is entitled to take with his life.

A good deal depends on the nature of the deprivation—e.g., does it prevent the person from engaging in the activity completely or merely limit his participation—and how important to the nature of the activity is the absence of restriction, when this is weighed against the role that the activity plays in the life of the person. In the case of automobile seat belts, for example, the restriction is trivial in nature, interferes not at all with the use or enjoyment of the activity, and does, I am assuming, considerably reduce a high risk of serious injury. Whereas, for example, making mountain climbing illegal prevents completely a person engaging in an activity which may play an important role in his life and his conception of the person he is.

In general the easiest cases to handle are those which can be argued about in the terms which Mill thought to be so important—a concern not just for the happiness or welfare, in some broad sense, of the individual, but rather a concern for the autonomy and freedom of the person. I suggest that we would be most likely to consent to paternalism in those instances in which it preserves and enhances for the individual his ability rationally to consider and carry out his own decisions.

I have suggested in this essay a number of types of situations in which it seems plausible that rational men would agree to granting the legislative powers of a society the right to impose restrictions on what Mill calls "self-regarding" conduct. However, rational men knowing something about the resources of ignorance, ill-will, and stupidity available to the law-makers of a society—a good case in point is the history of drug legislation in the United States—will be concerned to limit such intervention to a minimum. I suggest in closing two principles designed to achieve this end.

In all cases of paternalistic legislation there must be a heavy and clear burden of proof placed on the authorities to demonstrate the exact nature of the harmful effects (or beneficial consequences) to be avoided (or achieved) and the probability of their occurrence. The burden of proof here is twofold—what lawyers distinguish as the burden of going forward and the burden of persuasion. That the authorities have the burden of going forward means that it is up to them to raise the question and bring forward evidence of the evils to be avoided. Unlike the case of new drugs where the manufacturer must produce some evidence that the drug has been tested and found not harmful, no citizen has to show with respect to self-regarding conduct that it is not harmful or promotes his best interests. In addition the nature and cogency of the evidence for the harmfulness of the course of action must be set at a high level. To paraphrase a formulation of the burden of proof for criminal proceedings—better 10 men ruin themselves than one man be unjustly deprived of liberty.

Finally I suggest a principle of the least restrictive alternative. If there is an alternative way of accomplishing the desired end without restricting liberty then, although it may involve great expense, inconvenience, etc., the society must adopt it.

From "The Doctor-Patient Relationship"

Anna Freud

... Even if the doctor contributes a good deal to [the doctor-patient relationship] I think it is only fair to say that the patient contributes more. ... Your patients will be ill and therefore they need a doctor. They will have bodily pains; they expect you to cure them. ... One would expect that this is a straight-forward relationship, that the doctor ... enters the patient's life as a new person with new qualities, that the patient reacts to him as such, that the patient values his knowledge, appreciates his attitude, and chooses him like one chooses other professional people in life. ... But curiously enough the relationship between ... patient and doctor does not remain the same. Elements enter it which cannot be explained by the present reality at all. We are surprised by it, we have to search for the origin. For example ... many patients over-evaluate their doctors. ... Their doctor is the best in the world. Their dentist is the best. Enormous expectations are raised— he will help, he will cure, he will fulfill all expectations. This gives you a

Reprinted with permission of the author, as it appears in Jay Katz, *Experimentation with Human Beings* (N.Y.: Russell Sage Foundation, 1972), pp. 635–37. Copyright by A. Freud, 1964.

warm glow of satisfaction. It's nice to be thought such a remarkable person until, a week later, the scene changes. You are no good at all—such an ignorant person has never existed. You don't fulfill the expectations. You have promised something and you can't carry it out. The patient is deeply disappointed in you, and you become dejected. Am I really as bad as that? . . . Until, when this same sequence has repeated itself a number of times, you become alerted to it and you realize this is not you at all. You are neither as good, nor as bad, neither as efficient nor as inefficient as the patient sees you. He evidently has turned you into somebody else. And this belief is strengthened by further discoveries, namely that the patient doesn't only expect you to fulfill the contract to be cured by you, but that he expects you to like him or, if it is in analysis, even to love him, to be interested in him, to prefer him to other patients. He comes to you with details of his life, which have really nothing to do with the doctor-patient relationship on a reality basis, and you realize that now you have ceased to be what you set out to be—the person to cure this particular individual; you have become an important person in his life, somebody who is loved, hated, on whom demands are made, from whom the patient wants interest, intimacy, preference, and suddenly you feel this must be somebody quite definite from the patient's past. He treats you as if you were his parent. He obeys you as if you had authority over him, or he fights against you as if he were a rebellious child. And suddenly you find that instead of having a sensible patient before you, you have become what we call an object of his transference, namely the whole load of feeling left over from earlier years—unfulfilled, disappointed —has been unloaded onto you. You are in the center of his interest, and he expects you to play the role that you are given.

What can you do with this most disturbing doctor-patient relationship? . . .

I think that all doctors use the transferred positive relationships from the patients for their own advantage. The patient is in a state of submission, admiration, obedient to the doctor. All the better. So long as this whole trend is positive, you can use it for your own ends; you will find that your prescriptions work better, your commands are obeyed, and at least the psychological side of the patient's illness—and we know there is mostly a psychological side—will be influenced favorably. Doctors have done that always. They have done it without knowing it. It's only when this attitude becomes negative that you are in trouble. . . .

To understand what is going on can be of enormous help in your profession. It will save you a lot of annoyance. It will make you very careful how to act or how to make use of the patient's personal relationship. It will do something to your self-esteem when you know that this changing picture of yourself is not your fault. It will help you to stand firm and, as in so many other walks of life, understanding the difficulties of the situation will ease them. It will ease it especially with regard to one particular point. The patient uses the doctor . . . not only to replace people of a lost past, he also uses him to represent in the outside world parts of his own person. For instance, a patient may be quite aware of the fact that either his eating habits or his drinking habits, or any other habits are injurious to his health, but he doesn't feel that he has the strength inside to combat the injurious habits. Then he will give you the role, to represent that part of himself which should control the eating and drinking. Many women who want to lose weight look for a doctor who gives them a diet, where they could diet themselves by eating less. But that is very difficult. It is easier to have the figure of the forbidding agency outside, and then either to obey or to revolt. The same is true about drinking. The same is true about people with heart trouble who cannot bring themselves to be really careful of their bodies. It's easier to have the forbidding agency outside, which in itself does not yet guarantee obedience. . . .

But even that isn't the whole story yet. I have another point to make for you. [You will discover] how badly adult and sensible people take care of their own bodies. After all, our body, our health is one of our most valuable possessions, if not the most valuable one altogether. Wouldn't you expect all your patients to take the greatest care of their bodies, never to do anything that is injurious to their health, carefully to avoid infections, damage, dangers and, if they are ill, to take the right measures immediately. Wouldn't that be eminently sensible behavior? But there are very few adults, reasonable as they may be otherwise, who show such sensible behavior. This lack of good sense in health matters will make your future work extremely difficult. It will make it all the more difficult because you will feel, "I just can't understand it. After all it's his body. Why doesn't he take better care of it? Why does he expect me to do it instead of doing it himself?" You wouldn't be at all astonished about that point, if you had the opportunity to watch the human being's relationship to his body from the very beginning. . . .

If you have the chance to observe children in their second year of life, you will make the surprising discovery that they treat their bodies as if they were not their own. Their bodies belong to their mothers which is only natural since it is not so very long ago—in the intrauterine stage—that the infant's body was actually part of the mother's. Neither in his first nor in his second year can the infant do anything for the care of his body. There is, in the beginning, even no barrier to self-injury and the baby would draw blood from his face if the mother did not see to the cutting of his nails. What we call the pain barrier is established gradually during the first year and the child's aggression deflected with it from his own body to the world outside.

We even think that the infant begins to love and respect his own body to the degree it is loved and respected by the mother, i.e., for the mother's sake. As regards the toddler, we certainly feel that he needs more than our guardian angel to keep alive in spite of the attractions of heights, stairs, water, fire, scissors, knives, and whatever other dangerous objects he may meet. He has, at this time of life, no appreciation of danger and he will inevitably injure himself unless he is protected. Pediatricians, child analysts and other workers in the field have learned to judge the quality of mothering available to a young child by the numbers of accidents in which he has been involved.

The child's intelligence has to mature before he learns to appreciate that fire burns and water drowns, that not everything is edible, etc. What he learns last of all is submission to the rules of hygiene and obedience in medical matters. At school age even, and right up to adolescence, many children act as if it were their privilege to do the most harmful and danger-ous things to their bodies, while it is the parents' duty and privilege to protect them. [You] know how difficult it is to keep a child in bed with a fever, with an infection, that the dietary rules are felt by the child as a deep offense, a deprivation, a sign of not being liked. Even the ill child would eat what is bad for him, or the child would, for its own reasons, not eat even if he were starving himself. . . .

But what about you and the doctor-patient relationship? I only tell you these stories so that you can understand where all the irrational attitudes of your adult patients towards their health and towards their bodies come from. It is true you deal with adults, but every adult who is ill, who has fever, who is in pain, or who expects an operation, returns to childhood in some way. He feels small and helpless, and due to the ease with which he transfers feelings of the past onto you, you become the parent, you own his body. It is now your duty to look after him, and it is his privilege to be naughty about it: he feels well protected by you because he feels that somehow you will see to it that he doesn't do the wrong thing. You may get angry about it, but you will not be angry, if you remember that this adult before you is in reality a child, once more the child who has entrusted his body for safe-keeping to an adult.

This brings us to the end point and perhaps to one of the most difficult tasks of the doctor in the doctor-patient relationship. The patient, as you see from the various points I made, will do his best to push you into the place of parental authority, and he will make use of you as parental authority to the utmost. You must understand that. On the other hand, you must not be tempted to treat him as a child. You must be tolerant towards him as you would be towards a child and as respectful as you would be towards a fellow adult, because he has only gone back to childhood so far as he's ill. He also has another part of his personality which has remained intact, and that part of him will resent it deeply, if you make too much use of your authority.

From "Compulsory Sterilization"*

Angela R. Holder

Many states enacted statutes several decades ago which provided for the compulsory sterilization of mental defectives. While these statutes are not as widely invoked as in former years and the number of decisions in which they are involved has diminished, they remain on the books in many areas and are far from a dead issue in some courts.

THE POLICE POWER OF THE STATE

In 1927 the US Supreme Court upheld as constitutional state statutes providing for compulsory sterilization of retarded persons. The decision included the famous sentence "Three generations of imbeciles are enough" (*Buck* v. *Bell*, 247 US 200).

Numerous state court decisions of the same vintage approved the statutes as necessary in the public interest (e.g., *State ex rel Smith* v. *Shaffer*, 270 P 604, Kan 1928). There was, apparently, a consensus that the police power of the state could be used in requiring sterilization for the good of the community as a whole (e.g., *State* v. *Troutman*, 229 Pac 668, Idaho 1931; *In re Clayton*, 234 NW 630, Neb 1931). There was, either expressly or impliedly, an understanding in these opinions that there was no right to bear children which was transgressed by these statutes (e.g., *In re Main*, 19 P 2d 152, Okla 1933).

As the court stated in *Smith* v. *Command* (204 NW 140, Mich 1925), "No citizen has any right superior to the common welfare." In that case the mother of a retarded 16-year-old girl had petitioned the court to have her daughter sterilized, and the court allowed the procedure.

The number of decisions involving compulsory sterilization has declined sharply in recent years, but two fairly modern ones have upheld these statutes. *In re Simpson* (180 NE 2d 206, Ohio 1962) also involved a petition by a mother to have her daughter sterilized. The court concluded that the procedure would serve both the welfare of the woman and of sociey and allowed it to take place.

In re Cavitt (157 NW 2d 171, Neb 1968) involved a retarded woman who had already had eight children and who was confined to a state institution for the mentally deficient. Her sterilization was made a prerequisite of her release. The constitutional attack on the statute failed when the state supreme court upheld it as a valid exercise of the state's police power. It

Reprinted with permission of the author and publisher from the *Journal of the American Medical Association* 221:2, 229–30, July 10, 1972. Copyright 1972, the American Medical Association.

*[Since this article first appeared, many significant decisions on the subject have been handed down. Ms. Holder calls attention particularly to Doug Comer's "Sterilization of Mental Defectives: Compulsion and Consent," 27 *Baylor Law Review* No. 1, Winter 1975, pp. 174–98, as a valuable discussion. Ed.]

further pointed out that while there is a natural right to have children, which in and of itself was a departure from older decisions, no individual's right to do so is superior to the common good. The court also held that the state did not have to demonstrate that the children the woman might have if she were not sterilized would inherit her retardation.

Where no statute exists, however, the state has no power to order sterilization. In fact, since the would-be patient is legally incompetent to consent even if she wants it, the procedure may not be permissible at all (e.g., *Holmes* v. *Powers*, 439 SW 2d 579, Ky 1969). In *Frazier* v. *Levi* (440 SW 2d 393, Tex 1969), the mother of a retarded daughter petitioned for her sterilization. The daughter already had two children. The court denied the request, holding that in the absence of a statute, an incompetent ward did not have the legal capacity to give a valid consent and her guardian had no authority. In some states, however, on a petition from the natural guardian of an incompetent, the courts might deem the consent of the guardian sufficient, as would be the case if the incompetent required an appendectomy, tonsillectomy, or any other form of surgery.

In a recent Ohio trial court decision, the judge who ordered a compulsory sterilization in the absence of any enabling statute was found personally liable for damages. The woman had been sterilized pursuant to the court's order and over her objections. The judge argued that he was immune from suit. The court found that if he had merely exceeded his jurisdiction, his point would have been well taken, but if, as in this case, he had no jurisdiction at all to begin with, ordinary judicial immunity did not apply (*Wade* v. *Bethesda Hospital*, Civil Action #70-225, DC Ohio 1971, *The Citation*, 24:50). . . .

DUE PROCESS OF LAW

Before compulsory sterilization can be performed, constitutional guarantees of due process of law mandate that the would-be patient be given notice, a guardian be appointed, and a hearing be held (e.g., *State ex rel Smith* v. *Shaffer; In re Opinion of the Justices*, 162 So 123, Ala 1935; *In re Hendrickson*, 123 P 2d 322, Wash 1942; *Brewer* v. *Walk*, 167 SE 638, NC 1933). No decisions can be located which dealt with the right to counsel at these hearings but presumably such a right would exist if the patient could afford one. The right to appointed counsel for indigents has been restricted to criminal prosecutions until the present time, but a good case could be made for appointment of counsel in these cases since the persons involved are almost inevitably indigent and of necessity incompetent.

NEW DEVELOPMENTS IN THE LAW

An interesting analogy can be drawn between new concepts apparent in decisions involving abortion laws and laws requiring compulsory sterilization. Several decisions within the past few years have indicated that a woman who wants an abortion may have a constitutional right to have one. She may, in short, have a constitutional right not to bear an unwanted child (e.g., *Babbitz* v. *McCann*, 310 F Supp 293, DC Wisc, 320 F Supp 219, 1970; *People* v. *Belous*, 458 P 2d 194, Cal 1969). The same reasoning, applied conversely, might make it quite likely that laws providing for compulsory sterilization for economic or genetic reasons would be declared unconstitutional. If a woman who wants an abortion has the right not to bear a child, then the woman who might be compulsorily sterilized might well be held to have an equal right to have as many children as she wants. No decisions can be found in which the point has been argued, since there are no compulsory sterilization cases on the appellate level, at least in those states where this right has been declared, which do not predate the abortion decisions by many years. This type of challenge may be expected, however, in any state in which the issue of compulsory sterilization is brought before the courts.

CONCLUSION

The decline in the number of cases involving compulsory sterilization since the 1920s and 1930s is probably attributable to three factors. In the first place, modern medical research in genetics and new knowledge on environmental and hereditary factors in retardation has served to provide new answers to the problems. Second, modern methods of contraception which are effective for those who are mentally deficient have provided an alternative to sterilization. Third, and most important, however, World War II brought the American people into contact with an enemy who systematically enforced compulsory sterilization against groups the government wished to eliminate. . . . Since that time a great many people in this country might well feel that any system of compulsory sterilization is too near Naziism to be acceptable in a democratic society.

Where these statutes exist, however, the state still has the power to employ sterilization against the mentally deficient, at least until new constitutional challenges are made. The entire question is not simply a medical issue. It has always been and will remain a moral, religious, legal, and sociological issue, as much if not more than a medical one. Changing concepts of social justice, due process of law, and individual freedom inevitably change the court's outlooks on these issues of fundamental freedoms. Greater respect for the rights of the mentally retarded also has been demonstrated in this country in the last few years. This, too, will have an inevitable effect on future developments on the law of compulsory sterilization.

A Considered Approach to Sterilization of Mentally Retarded Youth

Jane C. S. Perrin, Carolyn R. Sands, Dorris E. Tinker,
Bernadette C. Dominguez, Janet T. Dingle, and
Mariamma J. Thomas

Recent publicity of tubal ligation of two mentally retarded minors has posed anew the problem of sterilization to the public. It is pertinent at this time to communicate our experience in developing criteria and a protocol for sterilization of the retarded juvenile. Ohio has neither obligatory, enabling, nor prohibitive statutes for surgical sterilization, so we have proceeded cautiously with 20 patients from May 1970 to February 1973, with a 38- to 5-month follow-up. No operations have been performed since the moratorium announced by the Department of Health, Education and Welfare in July 1973.

A premise for permanent birth control is that certain young women have the right to be protected from pregnancy with which they cannot cope, resulting in children which they cannot rear.

SETTING

All patients lived at home and were active in, or referred to, the Comprehensive Care Program,[1] a multidisciplinary pediatric program for the handicapped child based in a county hospital that is also a medical school teaching hospital. Program personnel include those in medical, nursing, psychology, social service, speech pathology, and sex education counseling disciplines.

Along with the clinical services offered by the Program, sex education and family planning services have been developed in recent years. Objectives of this project are to increase the juvenile's understanding of and control over his/her own body, to prevent and treat venereal disease, to prevent unwanted pregnancy and assist in long-term reproductive planning and birth control.

CRITERIA FOR STERILIZATION

The first indication for considering a retarded minor for sterilization is when: (1) parents *request* the procedure because of deep concern over possible unwanted pregnancy in their offspring who are unable to make use of

Reprinted with permission of the authors. Unpublished paper from the Departments of Pediatrics (Comprehensive Care Program) and Reproductive Biology, Case Western Reserve School of Medicine at Cleveland Metropolitan General Hospital. A shorter version of this paper will appear in *The American Journal of Diseases of Children.*

[1]Perrin et al.: Evaluation of a ten-year experience in a comprehensive care program for handicapped children, *Pediatrics,* 50:793–800, 1972.

birth control techniques, unable to nurture children, and often unable to manage menstrual hygiene. We then proceed to evaluate the following: (2) protection offered against sexual exploitation in home environment; (3) parental estimate of degree of dependency, provocative behavior, and risk of pregnancy; (4) intelligence of patient; (5) social maturity; (6) presence of high risk hereditary condition; (7) degree of physical handicap. Criteria 3 to 7 are considered in combination after initial determination that a retarded girl is in an environment offering the best possible protection from sexual assault or molestation by members of the family or outsiders.

In general our female patients have been those who are lifetime dependents and very passive or provocative of sexual overtures, making them high risk for pregnancy. Most have intelligence quotients under 50, but the psychological assessment is coupled with results of social maturity assessment in deciding function.

Social maturity determination was based on history from parents and teachers. For our last six cases we have added data from the patient's score on the Cain-Levine Social Competency Scale,[2] and parent and patient responses on the Personal Inventory. The Cain-Levine Scale ranks skills in personal care, mealtime, general tasks, interpersonal relations, and communication in comparison to those of previously tested mentally retarded groups. The Personal Inventory is a questionnaire on knowledge of body and sex function, menstrual hygiene, and social skills developed by two of us (CRS and DET).

Genetic disease that results in severe handicap is determined by family pedigree, physical examination, and appropriate laboratory tests for definitive diagnosis. A hereditary disease was considered high risk if there is $\geq$ 50% risk of transmission, such as an autosomal dominant condition (50% risk to offspring), chromosomal trisomy (50% risk to offspring), or the homozygote whose condition damages the fetus (phenylketonuric mother with 88% risk of retarded offspring).

Physical handicap of the individual is considered severe if there is major interference with sensory and/or motor function that impedes self-care.

CASE REPORTS

Case # 1

B., a 13-year-old girl, the youngest of 10 children, was a premature baby with Trisomy 21 Down's syndrome complicated by pneumococcal meningitis at five months, and severe myopia. She has been known to the Comprehensive Care Program for 10 years, and serial psychological testing has shown an IQ of 30 with minimal speech development.

At age 7½ goiter was noted without hyperthyroidism, age 10 thelarche and 10-½ menarche with heavy flow. During menses B. became frightened and with-

[2]L. F. Cain, S. Levine, F. F. Elzey: Cain-Levine Social Competency Scale. Palo Alto, Consulting Psychologists Press, 1963.

drawn, refusing to eat and going to bed or crawling under the bed. She did not understand repeated explanation of menses by mother, could not cope with menstrual hygiene, and had to be kept home from school during menstrual periods.

The mother's request for a hysterectomy for B. was deemed appropriate by the pediatric team, director of Family Planning Clinic, and director of the Department of Obstetrics and Gynecology. B. had total abdominal hysterectomy under general anesthesia without difficulty at age 11. Postoperatively she had a urinary tract infection which cleared rapidly with treatment. In the two years since surgery B. is reported to have a happier personality at home with no episodes of withdrawal, and she has not missed school. There is no history of sexual activity or molestation.

Case # 2

R. is an 18½-year-old girl who survived tuberculous meningitis at age 3 with residual bilateral optic atrophy and 20/200 vision, right spastic hemiplegia, and trainable level of mental retardation; known to the Program 11 years.

In March 1972 the mother expressed concern about the presence in the home of R's two half-brothers in their twenties, but she did not think birth control for R. was necessary. R. presented in June 1972 with a 10-week pregnancy, and both parents requested abortion and tubal ligation.

R. was able to describe several experiences of sexual intercourse with a brother, but did not relate these to pregnancy. On psychological testing she scored an IQ of 48 on the Wechsler Adult Intelligence Scale and a social maturity age equivalent of 3 years 10 months. She was described by the psychiatrist as being unaware of the meaning of pregnancy (she said her stomach hurt), by the psychologist as relating to individuals by excess body contact, and by the pediatrician as an immature dependent girl with severe visual impairment and poor function of one arm so that caring for her own needs such as dressing was difficult. The family and professionals concluded that R. was totally incapable of mothering a child; the fetus was at some risk for genetic abnormality as the product of an incestuous mating.

Intrauterine suction curettage followed by laparoscopic tubal cautery and transection was performed without complication under general anesthesia at age 17½ years. Postoperatively she returned to her job in workshop training without any problems and has been considered well-adjusted at home the ensuing year; the two half-brothers have been moved from the home.

Case # 3

E., a 20-year-old retarded female with seizure disorder, was presented by both parents for birth control at age 15½ following an incident of sexual activity with a boy in her class. E. was described by parents and teacher as very affectionate and seductive (she pursued boys relentlessly) and parents feared pregnancy. On the Stanford-Binet LM E. achieved a mental age of 8 and IQ of 55.

Case counseling of the entire family was initiated when assessment revealed disturbed relationships. E. was placed on Norinyl 1+80 for contraception plus attempt at control of irregular menses, menorrhagia, and dysmenorrhea. At 17 the parents discontinued the pill because of side effects and enrolled E. in a private residential school out of state; she was lost to follow-up to age 19 when she returned with "possible pregnancy following a pick-up," continued menstrual irregularity with heavy flow, and inability to manage menstrual hygiene. She was not pregnant, but parents requested hysterectomy because of the combination of her high risk for pregnancy and her menstrual symptoms.

On psychosocial assessment at this time, she was able to read with second grade level comprehension, had poor memory for self-care routines, good verbal language but little content, and abstract reasoning and judgment on the 5–6 year level. She could not describe differences between males and females in spite of previous sex education. During extensive preoperative preparation for hysterectomy, E. expressed great relief that she would stop having periods. At operation (age 19½ years) there was a didelphic uterus with two cervical openings, a bipartate right fallopian tube with separate fimbria, a right hemorrhagic corpus luteum cyst and multiple follicular cysts: hysterectomy and right oophoretomy were performed.

Postoperatively she developed a urinary tract infection which responded to treatment. During the six-month follow-up period, she has shown great pleasure in her increased independence in self-care since being free of menses, and there has been no history of sexual exploitation.

DISCUSSION

At issue are civil liberties and legal rights of an individual who undergoes a procedure which falls somewhere between compulsory sterilization (many states retain eugenic sterilization statutes) and voluntary sterilization (the volunteering is done by the parent or guardian for the defective minor or incompetent young adult).

A sense of justice and morality dictates great caution in subjecting a mentally handicapped individual to any different legal or medical standards from those for the normal individual. A bill enacted in Ohio in 1974 (SB336, effective as law on July 1, 1975) specifically guarantees rights of the retarded person, including the right to informed consent and to refuse consent for surgery.

But if the retarded female has the right to child-bearing, does she not also have the right to reliable uncomplicated control over reproduction? If sterilization is withheld because a person is mentally incapable of making his/her own decisions, the individual will be protected against surgical violation but will be denied protection against reproduction.

One of the conclusions of the 1963 White House Conference on Mental Retardation was that retarded persons may function in society if not burdened by children. Bass,[3] in advocating sterilization, points out that in marriages of mentally retarded persons home conditions and child care improved as the number of children decreased; and that such marriages permitted normal interpersonal relationships and were stable when not overtaxed by the responsibility of parenthood.

Current approved alternate forms of contraception are untenable for

[3]M. S. Bass: Marriage for the mentally deficient. *Ment Retard* 1–2:198–202, 1963–64.

constant and reliable use over a 30-year reproductive span in a retarded female. The retarded girl does not remember to take the pill; users run the risk of thromboembolism. Failure rate of the intrauterine device is up to 20%[4] and is less effective in nulliparous patients and not well-tolerated. The diaphragm and the condom (for the retarded male) are not used regularly or correctly.

Considerations in addition to the reproductive rights of the retarded individual are pertinent. One is the risk of producing retarded offspring.

Reid[5] describes a several-generation family study in Minnesota in which 42 probands produced 1450 retarded descendants at a rate of 14.3%, with the risk of retarded offspring 40% for a union of two retardates, 10% for a union of retarded male with normal female, and 18% for a union of a retarded female with normal male. In comparison, the risk of retarded offspring to normal parents with normal siblings was 0.5%.

Other considerations are of the unborn child and the guardian. Pilpel[6] places contraception, abortion, and sterilization all under the family planning category and sets forth the family planning concept as including the interest of the patient, spouse, living siblings, unborn child, and community. A parent so handicapped that he/she cannot maintain self-care will be unable to nurture children. The unborn child then faces the sure prospect of rearing by persons other than his natural parents, often to the detriment of quality of his life and hardship to relatives. If the guardian of the retarded person will have to assume all responsibilities for offspring of that person, then should he not have a voice in controlling the reproductive life of that person?

CONCLUSIONS AND SPECULATION

Serious adverse effects are absent in the follow-up of 20 sterilized patients in our study, and parent satisfaction is high. Sterilization of the mentally handicapped should neither be obligatory nor prohibited.

In the absence of statutes we have performed sterilization of retarded individuals on a carefully individualized basis involving a multidisciplinary approach and agreement between the family of the retarded patient and medical personnel. After developing our own guidelines, we have come to recognize that legal clarification is necessary. Existing statutes for compulsory sterilization, whatever the question of their basic scientific and social validity, constitutionality, and morality, do not apply to those patients whose parents petition for permanent birth control.

A competent individual has a right to undergo voluntary sterilization,

[4]H. J. Davis: Performance of loop and shield intrauterine contraceptive devices. Proc. Family Planning Research Conf., Amsterdam, Excerpta Medica: 44–46, 1972.

[5]E. W. Reed: Mental retardation and fertility. *Soc Biol* 18 suppl: S42–S49, 1971.

[6]H. Pilpel: Family planning and the law. *Soc Biol* 18 suppl: S127–S133, 1971.

but how is the incompetent person to be both assured the right and protected against coercion? We agree with the recommendation of Brakel and Rock[7] that statutes for voluntary sterilization for the mentally disabled should afford every reasonably substantive and procedural protection to assure that sterilization is truly voluntary. When the person is incapable of valid consent and the volunteering is substituted by the responsible parent, protection should apply but accessible pathways be left open for consideration of the request.

Our experience dictates the following guidelines: that

1. Patients considered for sterilization by substituted consent be severely handicapped by dint of an IQ below 50, or retardation caused by a high risk genetic condition, or retardation complicated by emotional disturbance or physical disability so that he/she would be unable to nurture children beyond any reasonable doubt.

2. Interests of the parent requesting and consenting for the sterilization coincide with those of the retardate.

3. If medical evaluation supports the request for sterilization, a court hearing be held promptly with legal counsel freely available to both retardate and parent.

To be tested is the recently proposed HEW sterilization guideline[8] requiring a five-person review committee whose members are not associated with the medical project to deal with the medical, legal, social, and ethical issues of sterilization cases. It is uncertain that such a committee inserted between the medical institution and the court will add to the protection of rights of both retarded individual and parent.

In states where no sterilization laws exist, medical personnel who consider sterilization of the retardate by either direct or substituted consent, even with sanction of the court, have now been shown to be vulnerable to litigation (*Wade* v. *Bethesda Hospital,* 40 U. S. Law Week 2165 D.C. D. S. Ohio September 8, 1971).[9] This dilemma will not be solved by federal regulations or even by lower court hearings, but requires action by state legislatures. Perhaps the best guidelines would result from joint efforts by mental retardation experts in the medical and behavioral sciences, legal experts, and parents of the retarded to advise legislative committees.

[7]Eugenic sterilization: The mentally disabled and the law, ed. by S. J. Brakel and R. S. Rock. Chicago, University of Chicago Press, 1971, pp. 207–225.

[8]C. C. Edwards: Sterilization guidelines. Federal Register 38:20930–20931, 3 Aug. 1973.

[9]A. H. Bernstein: The law and sterilization. *Hospitals* 46:160–164 and 180, 1972.

From "Who Will Tie My Shoe?"

Training Center and Workshop of the New York City Association for the Help of Retarded Children

Sometime in November 1965, six retarded young people and a social worker got together in a television studio of station WABC in New York City and held a two hour discussion. This is an abridged script of that discussion.

The discussion was conducted in the form of a panel rather than a counseling session. The group leader was much more directive than she would have been in a counseling session, actively canvassed the group for opinions and attitudes and refrained from actively encouraging the members to explore significant thought and feeling in depth.

About twenty minutes of this discussion were telecast the following month as part of an hour long program on mental retardation which a year later won an Emmy Award of the New York City Chapter of the National Academy of Television Arts and Sciences. The program, which was largely concerned with the projects of the New York City Association for the Help of Retarded Children, was called "Who Will Tie My Shoe?" The title originated in a line spoken by one of the discussants.

The program dealt mainly with the Shop* and with the habilitation program of Dr. Jack Gootzeit. The Shop was primarily represented by this panel discussion. The discussants—all young adults—were either trainees at the Shop at the time or had once been trainees and were still very much involved with it as members of the Alumni Club which is operated by the Shop Friday evenings. The leader of the discussion, Mrs. Gerda Corvin, the chief of social service at the Shop, had been the social worker for four of the discussants and knew the other two very well through Alumni Club contacts. We are giving the six discussants pseudonyms in this paper and they will be known as Beth, George, Jack, Jim, Joan and Rose.

Perhaps the main point of the entire discussion is that many mentally retarded people, with prolonged periods of intensive help and encouragement and opportunity, can come to express important thoughts and feelings about themselves and the world around them. This expression is part of a process which enables them to modify their behavior and attitudes so that they can become more mature and socially competent and happier people. I doubt that these six persons are particularly atypical. They all show strong signs of organicity, have IQs in the sixties, and had failed to make vocational, educational and other social adjustments before coming to the Shop. These are not "pseudoretarded" people.

From "Who Will Tie My Shoe?" Training Center and Workshop, New York City Association for the Help of Retarded Children (New York, 1967), pp. 1–10. By permission of the Association.

*The Shop is what we call the Training Center and Workshop of the New York City Association for the Help of Retarded Children. This is an agency which provides remunerative work as the core of a training and treatment program for some 250 mentally retarded young adults who are helped to achieve outside employment or adapt to sheltered employment, and in any case, who are helped to improve their social competence and emotional stability. The Shop has three centers, two smaller ones in Brooklyn and Queens, and the central setting—which has between 160 and 200 trainees—in Manhattan.

Of the six, four are single. Two, the only Negroes in the group, were already married when the discussion took place but have no children. All come from working class families with low to low middle incomes and one comes from a family receiving public assistance.

The discussion was spontaneous although the group had met together one afternoon a few days earlier to consider the issues they would explore. Actually much of the material in the televised discussion had not been anticipated. Of course all of the discussants had had intensive individual and group counseling so that it was not new for them to talk about significant experiences, thoughts and feelings. Had it been their first exposure to such a discussion—particularly for television—they probably would have frozen.

The Shop brought to bear upon them a certain climate and a constellation of programs and services. All of the trainees had intensive individual and group counseling, as did some of their parents. The trainees were exposed to treatment-oriented individualized relationships with their non-professional work supervisors. They participated in a number of group activity programs. Work assignments were often made for psychological rather than directly vocational reasons, especially in the early phase of their training. They experienced a range of monetary, status and recognition rewards on the one hand and another range of deprivations, limitations and restrictions on the other. Some were examined by our neuropsychiatrist and given medication. All were tested by our psychologist. Some received instruction in traveling in the streets and subways and some were tutored in work-related reading, writing and arithmetic. They attended job orientation classes and went through a bimonthly treatment-oriented evaluation process. When designated employable, they received selective placement services which included in some cases intervention with the employer to salvage jobs which seemed headed for disaster.

All were actively encouraged to understand themselves and express themselves and to be creative in ways useful to themselves as persons and to the Shop. They were all paid. They were given opportunities for leadership and helping roles. While encouraged to verbalize problems, they were also expected to participate in their solution. And of course staff tried to relate to them with real patience, a genuine acceptance of their retardation and their trying personalities, a sensitive recognition of their worthwhileness simply by virtue of their being people, and with a warmth and humor which hopefully imparted to their whole experience in the Shop a pervasive quality of humaneness and optimism.

Almost all of these young people in varying degrees came to the Shop immature, tight, angry, suspicious and pessimistic. Judging from the outcomes and from the discussion which follows, something worthwhile did happen inside them. What happened to them is happening to other retarded persons receiving similar treatment and training, and would happen to many more if they could be provided with adequate resources for similar habilitation processes.

January 27, 1967

Jerome Nitzberg, MSW
Assistant Director

CORVIN Well, look, if you remember, when we talked last time on Tuesday, we discussed the question, "Suppose you had to have a handicap, which handicap would you pick?" Would you want to be retarded rather than anything else?

JOAN Of course. I can use my hands and I can see and I can do plenty of things, help around the house, and you know, when I'm married, to help out. I can do more things. That's why I'd pick retarded.

CORVIN How about George?

GEORGE You can use your hands. You can work. That's about it. About everything else that you would do.

CORVIN You think that retarded people can work and use their hands and do many things which other people mightn't be able to do—other handicapped people mightn't be able to do?

GEORGE Yes.

CORVIN How about you, Jim?

JIM I agree with George. I think it's the same thing. Because when you're crippled in a wheelchair, you can't walk. At least I'm retarded. I can walk and move my hands and work with my hands.

CORVIN How about Beth?

BETH I agree with all of them. Retarded, I can do a lot of things —hold a job, do all different kinds of work, take care of housework, shop and do everything.

CORVIN Make a budget. (Laughter)

JACK I feel the same way as everybody else. Because you can use your hands. You can move around and do a lot of things. Where, if you were the other way you wouldn't be able to do it.

CORVIN And Rose?

ROSE I agree with all of them because people that are in wheelchairs and some of them can't see, they can't do nothing for themselves. They need somebody to work for them. And us, we could work for ourselves. We can help around the house with the cooking and cleaning, and go to the store sometimes, and sometimes go out with friends. Like them that can't see and can't walk, they can't go out by themselves.

CORVIN You think they need someone to take care of them all the time?

ROSE   Yes, yes.

CORVIN   Now all of you have been saying that retarded people can work, they can use their hands, they can do many kinds of different things. In what way would you say then are retarded people different from normal people?

ROSE   Well, some retarded people like myself are slow in work. Some—I can't say which ones—but I know myself, like when I went to school, I was slow, so they put me in a special class.

CORVIN   Uh-huh. How did you feel about being put in a special class?

ROSE   Oh, I didn't feel so bad because there was others like myself in the class. And I didn't feel so bad. But when the kids in the street used to tease me I felt real bad, and sometimes started to cry.

CORVIN   Beth is nodding her head and George is nodding. Did you have a similar experience?

BETH   Yes.

CORVIN   You mean the kids teased you?

BETH   Yes.

CORVIN   And what else happened?

BETH   Well, I—when I went to school my high school years, the teacher always told me not to feel sorry for myself, to go out and try, because you can do if you want to.

CORVIN   Well, how would you say, Beth—in what way would you say a retarded person is different from a normal person?

BETH   Well, some retarded people—they can use their hands and walk around but they can't concentrate. A lot of them have slow concentration.

CORVIN   Why do you think they have slow concentration?

BETH   Well, some of them feel sorry for themselves and that makes a conflict on them, makes them feel that they can't do, but they can.

CORVIN   Jim, you're nodding as if you agreed.

JIM   I do.

CORVIN   That's unusual for Jim to agree with us.

JIM   Especially with women.

CORVIN   Especially with women.

JIM   I used to feel sorry for myself all the time. It's no good.

CORVIN   Well, do you remember when you stopped feeling sorry for yourself?

JIM   I guess when I came to the Shop and started learning things that I didn't know before, got away from the house. When you're sitting around the house watching television and don't know what to do with yourself, you start feeling sorry you got nothing else to do.

CORVIN   Before you came to this Shop, you were just sitting around, doing nothing, watching TV? I hope it was Channel 7. (Laughter)

What about you, Joan? In what way would you say retarded people are different from normal people?

JOAN   Well, they're slow with their hands.

CORVIN   Well, think of the people in the Shop or of yourself, for that matter. In what way would you say that you are different from a normal person?

JOAN   I'm slow.

CORVIN   What are you slow in?

JOAN   Slow in my work, using my hands.

CORVIN   You're pretty fast in many ways, aren't you?

JOAN   Yes, in clerical work.

CORVIN   How about Jack? In what way do you think retarded people are different from normals?

JACK   Just that they're slow, I think.

CORVIN   When you say they're slow, really what do you mean?

JACK   Like they're not as fast as other people. Like if you put a not retarded person next to a retarded person and you gave them something to write or something they feel, probably they could do it faster than the other one, the other person.

CORVIN   You mean the normal person could write it down faster?

JACK   Yes, yes, that's right.

CORVIN   And suppose the retarded person were given enough time? Do you think he might be able to write things down or read things just as fast as everybody else?

ROSE   Yes.

CORVIN   You think—

JACK   Learning is actually what it means. I mean slow in learning things.

CORVIN   Rose, I think you wanted to say something.

ROSE   I found out when I went out to make an application one time that some bright people can't write, neither, because one man came over to the man at the desk and said, "Would you make this out for me?" He said, "Can't you try and write your name?" He says, "I don't know how." And I said to myself there, "I try." I make out the form. If I don't know, I just leave it and they help you.

CORVIN   Who helps you?

ROSE   The person that interviews you. I had it already.

CORVIN   So you had a very nice interviewer and he helped you fill out the application?

ROSE   Yes.

CORVIN   I think some of you have had different experiences when you were asked to fill out forms. Jim?

JIM   I was looking for a job and I tried and filled out a form and I said I couldn't fill it out because I couldn't read, so they said they couldn't use me, and that was that.

CORVIN   Did anybody try to help you fill out the form?

JIM   No.

CORVIN   They just said nothing doing.

JIM   "If you can't read, we can't use you. Tell him we can't use him," the boss said to his secretary.

CORVIN   Were you angry at them?

JIM   Well, if they can't use me, they can't use me, that's all. What can I do about it?

CORVIN   How about Jack there? Were you ever asked to fill out anything that you couldn't fill out or you didn't know how to read—didn't understand the paper?

JACK   A couple of times. But they helped me.

CORVIN   Did you feel badly about having to ask them to help you fill out the forms? Yes, Rose?

ROSE   Well, I didn't because I know I told them I couldn't understand, and some words I couldn't read. Like my birthday I put down, and the year I was born, and my social security number. And he said if I had a phone. I couldn't read that because I didn't understand that. So he helped me.

CORVIN   You mean it's a long word—telephone number?

ROSE   Yes. So I said—I went over to him. He gave me a number and he said as soon as he called me he'll help me make it out. He said do I feel bad about asking somebody this? I said, "Well, they always tell us if we need help we should always come and ask somebody."

CORVIN   Who tells you this?

ROSE   This is what we were taught in the orientation group in the Shop. If we need to go to somebody, they help us with a form. And I learned it.

CORVIN   Well, what about this—you know, having trouble reading things and understanding things? Do you feel that this is something that makes retarded people different from normals?

JIM   Yes, very much. Most normal people know how to read and write, I think.

CORVIN   Well, how do you feel about not being able to read so well, Jim?

JIM   Lousy, miserable.

CORVIN   Miserable?

JIM   Like a stupid little kid.

CORVIN   Have you been able to learn anything in class at the Shop within the last year or so?

JIM   Learned a little bit of reading, and how to write my name. The Shop aide taught me.

CORVIN   Do you think she helped you feel any better about reading than you felt before, or do you still feel so miserable?

JIM   Well, I feel a little bit better because I know how to read a little bit but not enough, as much as I should or want to know.

CORVIN   Do you feel that not being able to read might make it difficult for you to find a job?

JIM   Yes.

CORVIN Have you ever looked for work?

JIM Especially in the thing I've been trained for—as a messenger. It's very hard. I found that out for myself. It's very hard to get a job as a messenger on the outside if you can't read because most messenger jobs call for reading.

CORVIN Are you actually saying that it's not a good idea to train you as a messenger because you can't read?

JIM Well, yes, in a way, because when I first came to the Shop I didn't think I could do it because I couldn't read. But the supervisor said I could. There were other boys there that could, but it's a little hard. It's much better if you know how to read better. It might be much easier to be a messenger.

CORVIN But we also know that some of our very best messengers are people unable to read and somehow they get around.

JIM Yes.

CORVIN And you get around beautifully.

JIM Yes, because they tell me how to travel.

CORVIN How can you travel if you don't know how to read?

JIM You travel—know how to take the trains to different places.

CORVIN How do you know where to get off?

JIM Well, if somebody prints the name of the station, prints it the way it is on the sign, I can read it, but if they write it in regular writing, I can't make head or tail of it. But if they print it, I can find it.

CORVIN Tell me, when did you first find out—any of you—first find out that you were retarded? In school?

JOAN In school.

CORVIN Do you remember how old you were?

JOAN I was around ten years old. And I was up—I was in a regular class in the fifth grade and then I couldn't catch up with the other class. I was slow. The teacher told me that I had to go down to a special class. And the following month I was in a special class ever since.

CORVIN But you didn't like it?

JOAN I didn't like it.

CORVIN Did you like it in the regular classes and not being able to keep up with them?

JOAN   Yes, because I wanted to catch up with them, but I couldn't. I was too slow.

CORVIN   Well, you couldn't keep up with the other kids in the regular classes?

JOAN   In the reading and arithmetic.

CORVIN   What about the special classes? Were you able to do as well as the others there?

JOAN   In the special classes?

CORVIN   Yes.

JOAN   I did very good in the special classes. It was easy work but I didn't like the idea of being sent to one, because I felt I could do the work. But I was there in special classes ever since.

CORVIN   You stayed in special classes until you left school?

JOAN   Until I left high school.

CORVIN   How about you, Rose? When did you first find out?

ROSE   When I was nine, when I was nine years old. My mother—no, my father—took me to a doctor to see why I used to cry. Every time I come from school I always complained that one of the little boys or girls used to hit me in school. And I would never want to hit them back. I was one of those that never wanted to defend themselves. So my father one day kept me from school and took me to the doctor and the doctor took all sorts of tests. He even took a how-do-you-call-it?

CORVIN   Electroencephalogram?

ROSE   No, brain wave. And he told my father that I had some kind of a seizure and they told my mother. My father had to bring my mother and they told my father and mother that you should be put in some institution until I grow out of it. But I was away from nine, from nine and a half until about seventeen.

CORVIN   That's when you were sent to Willowbrook?

ROSE   Yes, I was there for six years straight. I didn't learn no reading, no writing, but I learned how to sew and cook and how to keep a house.

CORVIN   So you think that in a way maybe it was good that they sent you away?

ROSE   No, no.

CORVIN No?

ROSE It was a waste of time.

CORVIN You think it was?

ROSE I feel that it was just a waste of time and waste of money.

CORVIN Did you get along with the kids in Willowbrook?

ROSE I never got into trouble. I got along with everybody. I still have friends that write to me from the school.

CORVIN They're still there?

ROSE Yes. That they don't have nobody—no parents, no brothers, no sisters. They're all by themselves. They work. I feel that people like us should be proud of ourselves what we can do for ourselves, and what the state or what anybody can do, the social workers and everybody.

CORVIN You're really saying you're sorry for the people who still are at Willowbrook?

ROSE Yes.

CORVIN And who have no families to go back to?

ROSE That's right.

CORVIN We'll get back to this a little bit later. But let's get to Jack. When did you first find out about being retarded?

JACK When I was in grammar school. See, I stayed in the same class and the kids were, you know, they were going ahead of me and I couldn't understand it. And my mother told me and she took me to doctors and they said that I was, but it wasn't, you know, a real bad case. But I was. And then that's when I was in about the fourth grade, not even that.

CORVIN Do you remember how you felt when—

JACK Well, I felt a little bad because the other kids were going to other grades and I was just sitting there, and at the beginning I didn't, you know, care. But then later on as the time went by I felt down, you know. Like they were better than me. And why was this happening? And I never used to want to go to school.

CORVIN You know, this must be a question I think all of you must ask yourselves again and again—why is this happening? Why did it have to happen to me of all people? Yes, Rose?

ROSE You know, a lot of my friends—they're braver than me and they say to me that I don't act like I'm retarded because I have a mind, that I talk to people clear as day, they tell me. Like my friend yesterday, I told her I was going on a show. I told her I don't know when they were going to show it on television. She said to me I don't act like I was retarded or anything, because I talk like a normal person should, like a normal adult should.

CORVIN Wait again. We'll come back to this, Rose, O.K.? But let's get to George. When did you first find out about being retarded?

GEORGE Well, I think when I was about nine.

CORVIN Also in public school?

GEORGE In public school, yes.

CORVIN Well, how did you find out about it?

GEORGE Well, when I went to this special class there, and all the other kids were there. I felt pretty bad then.

CORVIN Did they tell you why they were sending you to special classes?

GEORGE No, they didn't tell me that. I was sent there. I knew why, though.

CORVIN You knew why, but you didn't ask them? You didn't want to be told?

GEORGE No.

CORVIN How about you, Beth?

BETH Well, I came all the way through elementary, all the way through high school, and I graduated. But I was a little slow. But all the tests that the doctors had given me say that I am mostly handicapped more than retarded.

CORVIN You mean with your arm?

BETH Yes, because they say you are very, very, you're slow, but you're very, very smart in some ways.

CORVIN I think this is true of everybody here. How about Jim? When did you first find out about being retarded?

JIM I think I found out when I was about fifteen.

CORVIN Fifteen?

JIM   Although I was going to grammar school and I kept getting left back in classes, but I didn't know why. Nobody ever told me. They just thought I was playing stupid, that's all.

CORVIN   They thought that you were playing stupid?

JIM   That's what the kids used to call me, too. I just thought they were right. But I went into a special school for one hour a week when I was fifteen. That's how I found out I had to go to special school to learn how to read, but it didn't do too good.

CORVIN   Well, did you go to any doctor or psychologist?

JIM   There was one in the special school. He told my mother, and I was standing there, he told my mother that I would never work in the school. Like a psychologist I think he was.

CORVIN   He told your mother in your presence that you would never be able to work?

JIM   Yes.

CORVIN   Well, you fooled him, didn't you?

JIM   (Depressed) I fooled him. I'm working in the Shop, though. I had one or two jobs on the outside but never really kept them.

CORVIN   You don't feel that the psychologist was wrong?

JIM   Well, I do in a way. I proved that I can work but so far I haven't been able to keep a job yet.

CORVIN   What happened when you were in school, Jim? Or any of you, when you were in school as long as you were in regular classes, and all of you were in regular classes to begin with at least.

ROSE   For two weeks.

CORVIN   For two weeks?

ROSE   I went from the sixth to the fifth.

CORVIN   Well, you said something before, Rose, that the kids would tease you.

ROSE   Uh-huh.

CORVIN   What did they say? Just what did they do to you?

ROSE   "You're stupid. You can't read and can't write, ha-ha." So I used to say, "If I can't read . . ."

CORVIN   Sounds familiar.

ROSE I used to say to them like this—tears used to come out. I used to say, "If I can't read, do you think you could do better?" Then they used to gang up on me and then I'd run home. Of course, I don't like to fight with nobody. Now I go to school now, night classes, three nights a week, and well, my mother said I am improving in my reading and writing now.

CORVIN Do you feel that you are improving?

ROSE Yes. Now this year I am in a class that I am going to graduate and I am proud of myself. I've been going for three years. Like this year to study. But after I make . . .

CORVIN That's a big project.

ROSE If I pass the test this year, I go into Junior High School in nights.

CORVIN Uh-huh.

ROSE So I said to my mother, "If I pass, it will be a miracle."

CORVIN You don't think you'll be able to pass?

ROSE Well, last year I passed all the tests that he gave me—the teacher—except one, except one.

CORVIN Which one was that?

ROSE Spelling.

CORVIN Spelling?

ROSE Four, four. I passed my arithmetic, my reading and my social studies, but my spelling was poor. He said I got a 53.

CORVIN Oh.

ROSE But I didn't feel so bad. I didn't feel so bad as long as I knew I passed my writing.

CORVIN I think George is sympathetic. How's your spelling? I really don't know. No good?

GEORGE No good.

CORVIN Is it keeping you from working now? When you were in school, George, do you remember when you were in regular classes the first two or three years? Did the kids tease you? Did they get after you?

GEORGE No, they didn't bother me.

CORVIN They didn't bother you. How about later on? Were you ever teased by anybody?

GEORGE No.

CORVIN He was lucky huh? IIow about Beth? Did you ever get teased by people?

BETH No. I wasn't because I always felt to myself that if I can learn how to be faster and do things then I wouldn't be teased. But the teachers always said, "No matter what anyone says, you are just as good as anyone else is, and you can learn to do and you can take care of your own self. Don't never let no one tell you that you can't, because you can."

CORVIN And you believed them?

BETH Yes.

CORVIN And you proved that you can.

BETH That's right.

CORVIN How about Jim? You had a rough time?

JIM Yes, a very rough time.

CORVIN Well, do you want to talk about it a little bit?

JIM Well, they used to always tease me, call me stupid, can't read and all that stuff. Big guys used to beat me up and all because I couldn't fight too good either. They never wanted to let me play ball. They said, "You can't catch. You can't play." I went through a lot of stuff when I was a kid.

CORVIN Did they tease you any other way at all?

JIM What do you mean? What other way?

CORVIN I don't know. I can think of many other ways in which people can tease others.

JIM I don't know.

CORVIN Did they make fun of the way you talk?

JIM Sometimes. Some say I got buck teeth and everything else.

CORVIN Buck teeth?

ROSE I don't think that was nice. Not nice at all.

CORVIN Well, what did you do?

ROSE Ignore them.

CORVIN You can ignore them?

JIM I wasn't much for ignoring. I had a bad temper when I was a kid. I used to throw things at them.

CORVIN You threw things at them?

JIM I once threw a lunch chair at one guy once. Missed him.

CORVIN Did you ever hurt anybody?

JIM Sometimes. Not real bad, but I hurt them. I think I got beat up more times than I fought back. I used to be—I'd more or less run away. I was a coward, as the saying goes.

CORVIN What about you, Jack, when you got teased, or did you get teased at all?

JACK Oh, I didn't get teased. Not much. Once in a while the kids in the neighborhood like if they were running for something, like, you know, running around and I couldn't go so fast, they'd say, "What's the matter?" And I'd say, "Well, I can't help it. What do you want me to do?" Then they won't say nothing to you. Like I more or less ignored them, you know, and they'd say, they ask me something to which I had no answer. And they'd say, "Well, how come?" Well, I could try the best I can, that's all I used to say to them. But I didn't get teased.

CORVIN Do you feel, any of you, later on, after you left school and you went to special classes and then later on when you came to the Shop, that people made fun of you? Yes, Jack?

JACK Well, if they made fun of you at the Shop, they were talking about themselves, too, because if they did that they were there for the same reason we were, or some other reason. Because everybody that comes here has a reason, that's true.

CORVIN What kind of reason?

JACK Maybe they're a little slow, maybe, you know. It's all different cases, I guess.

CORVIN You don't agree Jim?

JIM I agree some of them are different. They say you're stupid or something. You say, "Well, what are *you* doing here? You must be the same thing." And they shut up.

CORVIN Three hands at the same time. All right, Joan.

JOAN That's why we're all at the Shop, because we're all slow—no one special. So if they make fun of us, they're only talking about themselves, like Jack said. They call us retarded. They're retarded, themselves.

CORVIN Do people use the word "retarded"—do you think—as a kind of cuss word?

JOAN   When they get mad—as an expression. But they only talk about themselves when they call other people that.

CORVIN   How about Rose?

ROSE   This is one of the things you was talking about when I came for my interview.

You said if somebody would ever call you names, they'd be calling themselves names because, like yesterday, a boy was calling another boy stupid. And I interrupted. I says, "That's not right. If he's stupid, so are you stupid." I said, "Because if you call another person stupid, you're calling it to yourself," I said. So the boss told us that if you call another person stupid, that's not nice anyway. You're making fun of another person. They act like children there.

CORVIN   Who acts like children?

ROSE   A lot of them.

CORVIN   Anybody at the Shop acts like children?

SEVERAL   Yes.

CORVIN   When they tease you, they're like children?

JIM   They're just acting like children, growing up.

JOAN   They like to make others get mad. They tease. Others can't take it and some can take it. And they tease you.

CORVIN   Do you think they like to see people get mad?

JIM   Sort of.

JOAN   Sort of, yes. (Laughter.)

CORVIN   What's so funny?

JIM   Temperamental.

CORVIN   Temperamental, huh. That rings a bell.

JOAN   Of course, it makes you feel very bad about being in the Shop.

CORVIN   Jack?

JACK   I think the reason why they say that is because they're not thinking and they're not realizing—well, they're calling it to somebody else, but if they stop to think, it's themselves, too. I mean the ones that are saying it to you at the Shop, it's themselves, too, and they're not thinking about themselves being that way and they wouldn't want no one else to say it to them.

CORVIN Well, Beth, you have your hand up.

BETH Well, I feel this way. If you hear them say that in order to avoid a fight or argument, walk away. Because it's better to walk away than to fight. Because you have always told us in the Shop if we feel that it's going to be an argument or they say something against us, our social workers are there, and that's what they're there for, to get us both together and discuss our problems and to see what it's all about. Because if you get mad at each other and fight all the time, then you'll never be able to be friends. You'll always constantly remember that same fight every time you get together.

CORVIN So you are really saying they ought to have it out with the social worker?

BETH Yes.

CORVIN You did?

BETH Isn't this the truth, Mrs. Corvin, that that's what the social workers are there for, to help the trainees with problems like this here? And that's what the supervisors are around for, to watch your work, what you do, and to prevent fights? Whoever gets into a fight, you're supposed to stop it and bring them to their social worker.

CORVIN That's right. And then what does the social worker do?

BETH Well, the social worker talks to you, and if she can't talk to you, they suspend you. That's what I guess. I don't know. I was never suspended.

CORVIN I think Joan disagrees.

JOAN The social workers don't suspend you. The social workers will talk to you, you know, and try to help you see what's wrong. But if it continues, if they keep getting into the same fight and you have to keep talking to them and it doesn't do any good, then it's either to the director of the Shop to suspend the trainee if he should continue fighting. You know, like I say, he gets into a fight every day and loses his temper, or there's something wrong.

CORVIN Would you say that retarded people have more fights or get into hot water more easily than other people?

JOAN No. Other people—normal people—get into just as many fights as we do. Millions fight all over the city.

JIM Even social workers.

CORVIN Even social workers.

JIM   Guys who want to work, fight. Who's going to talk to social workers when they fight?

CORVIN   That's a good question, Jim. The social workers' social worker?

ROSE   This isn't true. I've seen a picture one time on TV. I don't remember, I remember it was about a social worker. He went to a psychiatrist and the psychiatrist told him that he was going to have a breakdown. I don't want to say anything else, no more.

CORVIN   Do what you are saying is that social workers have problems just like trainees or other people.

ROSE   There's another thing. That normal people I've read in the papers, that·people that are, you know, okay and all of that stuff—normal—they rob things, they take dope, they take, I don't know, all sorts of things. They get in trouble with the law and all that.

CORVIN   You think retarded people get into this kind of trouble, too? It could happen.

JIM   I never said it. I never seen anybody or heard anybody, but it could happen.

ROSE   At least we have a Shop to come to.

From "Application of President and Directors of Georgetown College"

J. Skelly Wright

Mrs. Jones was brought to the hospital by her husband for emergency care, having lost two thirds of her body's blood supply from a ruptured ulcer. She had no personal physician, and relied solely on the hospital staff. She was a total hospital responsibility. It appeared that the patient, age 25, mother of a seven-month-old child, and her husband were both Jehovah's Witnesses, the teachings of which sect, according to their interpretation, prohibited the injection of blood into the body. When death without blood became imminent, the hospital sought the advice of counsel, who applied to the District Court in the name of the hospital for permission to administer

Excerpted from the decision 331 F.2d 1000. (D.C. Cir.), certiorari denied, 377 U.S. 978 (1964). Reprinted as it appeared in *Experimentation with Human Beings,* ed. J. Katz (N.Y.: Russell Sage Foundation, 1972), pp. 551–52.

blood. Judge Tamm of the District Court denied the application, and counsel immediately applied to me, as a member of the Court of Appeals, for an appropriate writ.

I called the hospital by telephone and spoke with Dr. Westura, Chief Medical Resident, who confirmed the representations made by counsel. I thereupon proceeded with counsel to the hospital, where I spoke to Mr. Jones, the husband of the patient. He advised me that, on religious grounds, he would not approve a blood transfusion for his wife. He said, however, that if the court ordered the transfusion, the responsibility was not his. I advised Mr. Jones to obtain counsel immediately. He thereupon went to the telephone and returned in 10 or 15 minutes to advise that he had taken the matter up with his church and that he had decided that he did not want counsel.

I asked permission of Mr. Jones to see his wife. This he readily granted. Prior to going into the patient's room, I again conferred with Dr. Westura and several other doctors assigned to the case. All confirmed that the patient would die without blood and that there was a better than 50 per cent chance of saving her life with it. Unanimously they strongly recommended it. I then went inside the patient's room. Her appearance confirmed the urgency which had been represented to me. I tried to communicate with her, advising her again as to what the doctors had said. The only audible reply I could hear was "Against my will." It was obvious that the woman was not in a mental condition to make a decision. I was reluctant to press her because of the seriousness of her condition and because I felt that to suggest repeatedly the imminence of death without blood might place a strain on her religious convictions. I asked her whether she would oppose the blood transfusion if the court allowed it. She indicated, as best I could make out, that it would not then be her responsibility. . . .

[I] signed the order allowing the hospital to administer such transfusions as the doctors should determine were necessary to save her life. . . .

Before proceeding with this inquiry, it may be useful to state what this case does not involve. This case does not involve a person who, for religious or other reasons, has refused to seek medical attention. It does not involve a disputed medical judgment or a dangerous or crippling operation. Nor does it involve the delicate question of saving the newborn in preference to the mother. Mrs. Jones sought medical attention and placed on the hospital the legal responsibility for her proper care. In its dilemma, not of its own making, the hospital sought judicial direction. . . .

If self-homicide is a crime, there is no exception to the law's command for those who believe the crime to be divinely ordained. The Mormon cases in the Supreme Court establish that there is no religious exception to criminal laws, and state *obiter* the very example that a religiously inspired suicide attempt would be within the law's authority to prevent. . . . But whether attempted suicide is a crime is in doubt in some jurisdictions, including the District of Columbia.

The Gordian knot of this suicide question may be cut by the simple fact that Mrs. Jones did not want to die. Her voluntary presence in the hospital as a patient seeking medical help testified to this. Death, to Mrs. Jones, was not a religiously commanded goal, but an unwanted side effect of a religious scruple. . . . Nor are we faced with the question of whether the state should intervene to reweigh the relative values of life and death, after the individual has weighed them for himself and found life wanting. Mrs. Jones wanted to live.

A third set of considerations involved the position of the doctors and the hospital. Mrs. Jones was their responsibility to treat. The hospital doctors had the choice of administering the proper treatment or letting Mrs. Jones die in the hospital bed, thus exposing themselves, and the hospital, to the risk of civil and criminal liability in either case. It is not certain that Mrs. Jones had any authority to put the hospital and its doctors to this impossible choice. The normal principle that an adult patient directs her doctors is based on notions of commercial contract which may have less relevance to life-or-death emergencies. It is not clear just where a patient would derive her authority to command her doctor to treat her under limitations which would produce death. The patient's counsel suggests that this authority is part of constitutionally protected liberty. But neither the principle that life and liberty are inalienable rights, nor the principle of liberty of religion, provides an easy answer to the question whether the state can prevent martyrdom. Moreover, Mrs. Jones had no wish to be a martyr. And her religion merely prevented her consent to a transfusion. If the law undertook the responsibility of authorizing the transfusion without her consent, no problem would be raised with respect to her religious practice. Thus, the effect of the order was to preserve for Mrs. Jones the life she wanted without sacrifice of her religious beliefs.

The final, and compelling, reason for granting the emergency writ was that a life hung in the balance. There was no time for research and reflection. Death could have mooted the cause in a matter of minutes, if action were not taken to preserve the *status quo.* To refuse to act, only to find later that the law required action, was a risk I was unwilling to accept. I determined to act on the side of life.

From *In re Brooks Estate*

Emory C. Underwood

On and sometime before May 7, 1964, Bernice Brooks was in the McNeal General Hospital, Chicago, suffering from a peptic ulcer. She was being attended by Dr. Gilbert Demange, and had informed him repeatedly

Excerpted from the decision 32 Ill.2d 361, 205 N.E.2d 435 (1965). Reprinted as it appeared in *Experimentation with Human Beings,* ed. J. Katz (N.Y.: Russell Sage Foundation, 1972), pp. 559–60.

during a two-year period prior thereto that her religious and medical convictions precluded her from receiving blood transfusions. Mrs. Brooks, her husband and two adult children are all members of the religious sect commonly known as Jehovah's Witnesses. Among the religious beliefs adhered to by members of this group is the principle that blood transfusions are a violation of the law of God, and that transgressors will be punished by God.
. . .

Mrs. Brooks and her husband had signed a document releasing Dr. Demange and the hospital from all civil liability that might result from the failure to administer blood transfusions to Mrs. Brooks. The patient was assured that there would thereafter be no further effort to persuade her to accept blood.

Notwithstanding these assurances, however, Dr. Demange, together with several assistant State's attorneys, and the attorney for the public guardian of Cook County, Illinois, appeared before the probate division of the circuit court with a petition by the public guardian requesting appointment of that officer as conservator of the person of Bernice Brooks and further requesting an order authorizing such conservator to consent to the administration of whole blood to the patient. . . . Thereafter, the conservator of the person was appointed, consented to the administration of a blood transfusion, it was accomplished and apparently successfully so, although appellants now argue that much distress resulted from transfusions due to a "circulatory overload." . . .

Appellees argue that society has an overriding interest in protecting the lives of its citizens which justifies the action here taken. . . .

We believe Jefferson's fundamental concept that civil officers may intervene only when religious "principles break out into overt acts against peace and good order" has consistently prevailed. . . .

. . . It seems to be clearly established that the First Amendment of the United States Constitution, as extended to the individual States by the Fourteenth Amendment to that constitution, protects the absolute right of every individual to freedom in his religious belief and the exercise thereof, subject only to the qualification that the exercise thereof may properly be limited by governmental action where such exercise endangers, clearly and presently, the public health, welfare or morals. Those cases which have sustained governmental action as against the challenge that it violated the religious guarantees of the First Amendment have found the proscribed practice to be immediately deleterious to some phase of public welfare, health or morality. The decisions which have held the conduct complained of immune from proscription involve no such public injury and no danger thereof.

Applying the constitutional guarantees and the interpretations thereof heretofore enunciated to the facts before us we find a competent adult who has steadfastly maintained her belief that acceptance of a blood transfusion is a violation of the law of God. Knowing full well the hazards involved, she has firmly opposed acceptance of such transfusions, notifying the doctor and hospital of her convictions and desires, and executing documents releasing both the doctor and the hospital from any civil liability which might be thought to result from a failure on the part of either to administer such transfusions. No minor children are involved. No overt or affirmative act of appellants offers any clear and present danger to society—we have only a governmental agency compelling conduct offensive to appellant's religious principles. Even though we may consider appellant's beliefs unwise, foolish or ridiculous, in the absence of an overriding danger to society we may not permit interference therewith in the form of a conservatorship established in the waning hours of her life for the sole purpose of compelling her to accept medical treatment forbidden by her religious principles and previously refused by her with full knowledge of the probable consequences. In the final analysis, what has happened here involves a judicial attempt to decide what course of action is best for a particular individual, notwithstanding that individual's contrary views based upon religious convictions. Such action cannot be constitutionally countenanced. . . .

While the action of the circuit court herein was unquestionably well-meaning, and justified in the absence of decisions to the contrary, we have no recourse but to hold that it has interfered with basic constitutional rights.

Accordingly, the orders of the probate division of the circuit court of Cook County are reversed.

Status of the Law on Medical and Religious Conflicts in Blood Transfusions

Laurance T. Wren

Late one evening the quiet solitude of my home was shattered by an emergency call. A surgeon at the Flagstaff Community Hospital was on the phone. The problem he presented sent me racing to the County Law Library to research a knotty legal problem which I had never before encountered.

A patient on the operating table was hemorrhaging severely and only an immediate blood transfusion would save his life. He was, however, a member of the Jehovah's Witness Sect, and had, prior to the operation expressly refused consent to any such transfusion. Honestly believing additional blood would not be necessary, the doctor had assured him his religious beliefs would not be violated.

The attorney for the hospital staff joined me at the library, but a quick check of the authorities reflected no clear cut solution to a very enigmatic question. The doctor wanted very much to save a human life. He had taken the oath of Hippocrates to "follow that method of treatment which, according to his ability and judgment, he considered for the benefit of his patients."

Reprinted with permission of the author and publisher from *Arizona Medicine* 24, 970–73, October 1967.

But what were the consequences? Not only had the unconscious patient in a preoperative consultation expressly refused to consent, but his wife, contacted outside the operating room, also refused permission, even though told her spouse would not survive unless blood was transfused into his veins.

An order was entered on the physician's affidavit of necessity directing him to proceed with the administration of blood. To adopt the words of Judge J. Skelly Wright in a similar situation:

> I, admittedly, entered the order requiring the transfusion for the reason that death could have mooted the cause in a matter of minutes if action were not taken. To refuse to act only to find later that the law required action was a risk I was unwilling to accept. I determined to act on the side of life.

A patient's life had been saved. The doctor had lived up to his oath, but who was right and who was wrong? What would have been the consequences of a lawsuit had one been filed? A grateful wife later acknowledged her relief and gratitude to the tired surgeon. Her husband's life had been spared and her religious conscience was still clear.

Had I erred in putting the stamp of legality on what might be called a medical usurpation of the rights of an individual? A basic constitutional precept is that no person shall be deprived of life, liberty or property without due process of law. Had the court order here undermined the constitutional guarantees of due process of law and free exercise of religion? Because in the case of Jehovah's Witnesses the basic reason for rejection of blood transfusions is their worship. They believe that the Bible prohibits the use of blood from any creature to sustain life; that it was part of the law God gave to Noah. Hence, freedom of religion is involved. The First Amendment to the U.S. Constitution guarantees that "Congress shall make no law respecting the establishment of religion or prohibiting the free exercise thereof." And a basic right of every American is to "worship God according to the dictates of his own conscience."

The doctor involved later requested that I join him in co-authoring an article on this subject, and I promptly agreed. My interest had been fired by our bizarre and somewhat harrowing experience, and this time the good doctor allowed ample time to think and prepare.

The matter is not without judicial precedent. In fact, the Supreme Court of Illinois struck down a similar order to proceed with blood injection. In *Brooks Estate* v. *Brooks*,[1] the following questions were presented: Is it an infringement of the constitutional guarantee of freedom of worship to deny one the right to reject unwanted medical treatment? When one's action or refusal to act does no harm to the society of which he is a part can treatment that violated his religious beliefs properly be foisted on him?

The court responded with resounding support of the religious belief:

[1]32 Ill. 2d 361, 205 NE 2d 435 (1965).

Even though we may consider appellant's beliefs unwise, foolish and ridiculous, in the absence of an overriding danger to society we may not permit interference therewith. In the final analysis what has happened here involves a judicial attempt to decide what course of action is best for a particular individual notwithstanding that individual's contrary views based upon religious convictions. Such action cannot be constitutionally countenanced.

The Witnesses maintain in their literature that they are not religious fanatics, that they do not hate life, they love it, but are willing to give up a few years in this corrupt system in order to gain God's approval and everlasting life in a far, far better arrangement.[2] They liken their cause to the deification of early Christian martyrs who allowed their children to die in the lions' jaws rather than renounce their faith, and, therefore, condemn the courts for the modern day invasion of their religious beliefs that no foreign blood should enter the bodies of their children.

This belief finds some support in the profession. Dr. Arthur Kelly, Secretary of the Canadian Medical Association, has been quoted as saying:

> I believe that parents of minors and the next of kin of unconscious patients possess the right to interpret the will of the patient and that we should accept and respect their wishes.

What is the present status of our law? As a general proposition, a conscious adult patient who is mentally competent has the right to refuse medical treatment even when the best medical opinion deems it essential to save his life.[3]

Cases enunciating the rule that an emergency gives the physician a privilege to treat the patient without his consent involve those incapable of manifesting a refusal, either because of unconsciousness or minority. No case has applied the "emergency rule" in the face of a competent patient's express refusal to consent. Neither humanitarianism nor the skillful performance of treatment is a defense to a lawsuit for battery in such a case.

Into what category do we place the midnight case at the Flagstaff Hospital? Without the patient's consent, the surgeon would have refused to perform the operation if the need for a blood transfusion could have been anticipated. A sudden and completely unanticipated loss of blood threw the doctor into a dilemma not of his own making. Even without a court order, I submit that the administration of necessary treatment would have been legally proper under the emergency rule.

Normally a court order will insulate the physician from actionable responsibility. But the authorities, what few there are, are not uniform. In *Collins* v. *Davis*,[4] an application for an order permitting surgical operation on a patient was granted, where the patient was in a comatose state and could not give consent; his wife having refused consent, and evidence hav-

2"Awake," May 22, 1967.
3*Erickson* v. *Dilgard*, 252 NYS 2d 705, Sup. Crt. (1962).
4254 NYS 2d 666.

ing established that if the operation were not performed he would die. The court pointed out that the patient had sought medical attention from the hospital and had placed on the hospital the legal responsibility for his care. Without a consent the hospital doctors had the choice of performing the operation or letting him die. It cannot be reasonably said that the comatose patient and his wife should or could put the hospital to this impossible choice. Life hung in the balance. The opinion also pointed out that it did not involve a person who for religious or other reasons had refused to seek medical attention. The Brooks case, cited above, was decided the following year by the Supreme Court of Illinois.

Another Court[5] took the view that a judicially ordered blood transfusion could properly be administered to a pregnant patient, when such was necessary to save her life, even though she and her husband had refused to authorize transfusions because of their religious beliefs, upon the grounds that it would be justified in the interest of protecting the unborn child, and the woman had told the judge issuing the order that, if ordered, the transfusion would not be her responsibility. If the Court therefore undertook the responsibility, the sanctity of her religious convictions would not be violated.

Recently in New York[6] blood transfusions were ordered on the petition of a patient's husband that same were necessary to save her life following a Caesarian section. Again, the upper court commented on the fact that in the judge's view she was willing to accept such treatment although, because of her religious beliefs, she would not direct its use.

Clearly the Court, in each of these instances, was leaning over backwards to justify a means reasonably believed necessary to save life. Just as clearly, though, an ex parte order issued without a hearing or opportunity to be heard by the affected party overlooks procedural safeguards which form the barrier between rule by law and rule by whim or caprice.

It is seriously doubted, however, that the medical profession, or the law, in the case of minor children, will ever place the stamp of approval on the refusal of parents to permit blood transfusions believed medically necessary. Arizona, in fact, has a specific law on the subject. Sec. 44–133 A.R.S. reads:

Emergency consent for hospital care, medical attention or surgery by person in loco parentis

Notwithstanding any other provisions of the law, in cases of emergency in which a minor is in need of immediate hospitalization, medical attention or surgery and after reasonable efforts made under the circumstances, the parents of such minor cannot be located for the purpose of consenting thereto, consent for said emergency attention may be given by any person standing in loco parentis (in place of parent) to said minor.

[5] *In re:* Application of the President and Director of Georgetown College, Inc., 331 F. 2d 1000 (1964).

[6] *Powell* v. *Columbia Presbyterian Medical Center,* 267 NYS 2d 450 (1965).

Liability in transfusing a child member of the sect, despite the nonconsenting parent, is avoided generally by showing that a failure to do so would jeopardize the life of the child, and by a court appointed guardian authorized to give consent.[7] The consent of the minor himself, unless emancipated, would be held ineffective to relieve the doctor or hospital of responsibility.

Certain conclusions, therefore, appear sound. An adult person may refuse to receive a transfusion, however desperate the need in medical opinion, and his refusal, generally, must be honored. The attending physician or hospital may, however, seek an order authorizing the rejected treatment. This order if properly obtained will generally insulate them from legal responsibility. Without such it would quite accord with legal principles if a jury awarded damages for battery to a patient who refused his consent to a transfusion, even though the patient's life was saved thereby and the transfusion resulted in no injury to him. The insult to the person of a member of the Witnesses could support a recovery of "general" damages and the amount thereof lies largely in the discretion of the jury. It is, of course, unlikely that a jury would award more than nominal damages in such a case. Where harm resulted to the patient from a transfusion, however, a strong case for recovery would arise, no matter how careful the administration of blood.

It is recommended that no medical or surgical procedure be performed within the hospital in the face of a patient's refusal unless an order of the court is obtained. The refusal should be noted in the medical record and the physician should render the best care possible within the limits imposed by the patient's refusal. It is advisable in such case to secure a release to make it perfectly clear that the appropriate treatment would have been rendered had the patient not refused the treatment.

In the light of these decisions it is advisable that hospitals and physicians seek the advice of legal counsel when faced with a nonconsenting patient, and when a serious threat to health exists. Conceivably the risk of liability, such as it might be, for treatment which saves the life of a patient should be accepted where time does not permit resort to the courts. It is perhaps advisable that the hospital administrator, with the aid of legal counsel, formulate a policy regarding treatment when consent has been refused, and establish an administrative procedure to facilitate application for a court order when one is needed and time permits.

[7] *Wallace* v. *Labrenz*, 411 Ill. 618, 104 NE 2d 769 (1952).

From "Issues Involved with Surgery on Jehovah's Witnesses"

George Thomas, Robert W. Edmark, and Thomas Jones

... many courts have been asked to settle the issue of how free are we to decide our own fate. If matters of health are flagrantly disregarded or treatment refused, is this not a violation of a state's penal code laws which state that it is unlawful to take one's own life? In general, refusing medical care is not tantamount to "suicide." Jehovah's Witnesses seek medical attention but refuse only one facet of medical care. Refusal of medical care or parts thereof is not a "crime" committed on oneself by an overt act of the individual to destroy, as is suicide. Society, of course, has to have some protection and refusal, for example, to be hospitalized with active tuberculosis or institutionalized as a homicidal paranoiac is obviously unlawful. There is no difficulty in establishing unlawfulness when it involves public health and safety. Refusal to accept blood transfusion, as an adult considered mentally competent, is not unlawful.

Refusal of blood where an infant or child is involved is an entirely different matter. Society has generally responded where infants are concerned. In a case in Illinois early in 1952, which again has been used as legal precedent, the Superior Court of the State of Illinois rendered the following judgment: "Parents may be free to become martyrs themselves. It does not follow, however, that they are free in identical circumstances to make martyrs of their children before they have reached an age of full and legal discretion, when they can make that choice for themselves. Laws, while they cannot interfere with religious belief and opinion, may be constitutionally appropriate for interfering with religious practices."[1] If a child, for example, is born of parents of the Church of Jehovah's Witnesses and requires a blood transfusion such as in erythroblastosis fetalis or is involved in a serious accident, the current method of management for the physician is to notify the Juvenile Court of the problem. A writ of change of legal guardianship from the parents to a custodian, who is generally the administrator of the hospital or bailiff of the court, is obtained and blood transfusions are instituted. It has become apparent to many pediatricians on close questioning of some parents (decidedly in the minority) that strong registration of their religious beliefs against blood transfusions is important and eliminates guilt feelings when the court supervenes and takes over to save the life of their child. They feel better having objected to the practice, but approve of the judicial decision awarding these children to the custody of the court during the crisis. This relieves them of a practice contrary to their religious beliefs and they are happy for the continued health of their children. The Juvenile

Reprinted with permission of the authors and publisher from *The American Surgeon* 34:7, 542–43, July 1968.

[1]Muller, Albert: Meet Jehovah's Witnesses. Pp. 10–17. Franciscan Publishers, Pulaski, Wisc., copyright 1964.

Court of the State of Washington, as in most states, exercises the power of *parens patriae* over children not properly handled by their parents. In essence it is stated, "The principle applies that parents are under obligation to provide minor children with the necessities of life, which includes medical care deemed necessary to prevent children's deaths. If any or all of this is not performed, the principles of law override professed religious convictions of the parents."[2] In other words, although the First Amendment guarantees freedom of religion, it only truly guarantees religious belief, not religious acts, behavior or practices which may have certain martyrdom or reprehensible stigmata.

DISCUSSION

Many and all situations cannot possibly be mentioned here in this discussion. There are problem cases which will tax responsible physicians no end. Most prosecuting attorneys and Superior Court Judges, as well as many attorneys, are well versed in these situations and can be relied on to act quickly and justly in all cases and, of course, be of considerable help to all parties concerned.

Presented with a case, particularly an elective case, we submit some basic rules to be considered. First of all, physicians should have a definite respect for the religious beliefs of Jehovah's Witnesses when it concerns an adult. Chaplain Harris, of the University of Pennsylvania, when discussing this problem on a panel discussion including Drs. Isadore Ravdin, Francis Wood and Marshall Orloff, presents the key to the problem completely.[3] He states the following: "Spiritual integrity of the patient must be part of the picture, just as much as the physical well being is part of the picture. In other words, although a patient's religious conviction is one with which you and I may not agree and which may not make sense to us in terms of our own religious outlook, we must consider the fact that it is of central importance to the patient. It is not justifiable to cure a patient physically or give him what is technically the best medical treatment at the expense of his spiritual integrity. In the large sense, the best medical treatment is most simply that which is technically the most sufficient, but that which best ministers to the patient's total welfare. The patient's decision not to accept blood at all costs shows clearly that he is willing to sacrifice his life for the sake of something which he holds to be more precious than life and purpose greater than himself." It was partly on the basis of this philosophic viewpoint that we decided to operate upon these two patients and to provide continued good health for them. In essence, had massive hemorrhage occurred, all efforts short of administration of whole blood would have been used. If unsuccessful, there would have been no reproach.

[2]Holloway, J. W., Jr., LLB: Blood Transfusions—Jehovah's Witnesses. JAMA, *163:* 660, 1957.

[3]Fitts, W. T., Jr. and M. J. Orloff: Blood Transfusion and Jehovah's Witnesses. Surg. Gynec. Obstet., *108:* 502, 1959.

In contemplating the performance of major elective surgery, the surgeon should have a reasonably good chance of success. In the case of open-heart surgery, Beall and Cooley have published reports on the overall successes of this modality without blood transfusions in this religious group.

It would stand to reason that prior to undertaking elective operations, screening for coagulation disorders should be undertaken. Although the possibility of a Jehovah's Witness with a bleeding tendency might exist, the probability would be low. Nevertheless, it would be comforting to all concerned to have specifically ruled out unusual coagulation factor deficiencies. On advice of Hougie the following are ordered: (1) clotting time, (2) a one-stage prothrombin time, (3) a PTT test (partial thromboplastin time). If all are normal and combined with a good negative history for unusual clinical bleeding, no further testing is necessary.

It is important to have the best surgical help possible, which is intrinsic in working with another surgeon of equal talent and ability. Enough assistants to afford ideal exposure are likewise necessary to assure safe operating. Knowing there is no blood available, careful, meticulous surgery is paramount to the success and this fact is readily appreciated by the operating team. Even with blood losses in amounts normally replaced, saline and dextran replacement is often enough to avoid dangerous blood pressure falls and pulse elevations. Excessive blood losses unavoidably exist with certain procedures such as abdomino-perineal resections, hepatic lobe resections, radical pelvic operations and pneumonectomy. However anticipated, these can be modified or altered under prevailing operative conditions, with survival of the patient.

SUMMARY

It is hoped that in presenting some of the historical and theological background of the Jehovah's Witnesses the time-honored blood refusal problem might be more clearly understood. In dealing with members of this religious group it would appear to the authors that there are certain acceptable and currently practical courses of action that can be pursued. These have been outlined and discussed. One may avoid professional contretemps and ultimately provide good, safe surgical care to these people by adopting sound precedences established in the past. The success of the entire program, however, starts with an honorable respect for religious beliefs.

MORAL PROBLEMS CONCERNING LIFE AND DEATH

Chapter 3

INTRODUCTION

Every serious moral theory places a high value on life, supporting a *prima facie* duty to preserve life. None permits termination of life without strong moral justification. For instance, in Kant's theory, life is argued to be among each person's set of fundamental ends; utilitarians recognize that most persons want to live and that it is in the greatest general interest to protect this desire; and religious theories generally claim that there is a sanctity associated with life.

The value placed on life is so widespread and so fundamental that it does not demand justification. Rather, the burden of proof is always placed on those who would choose to disregard or override this value.

In this chapter, we are concerned with investigating what may count as sufficient justification for overriding the duty to preserve life. We need to know whether there are any values that can outweigh the value we place on life, and if so, when, if ever, we can be justified in ending an individual's life. It is not sufficient to note that there are circumstances under which persons choose death over life; we must still determine whether a person is morally justified in acting upon such a choice. By increasing our ability to save lives, modern medicine has put us in a position where we must frequently consider whether or not particular lives ought to be terminated.

Timothy Goodrich examines the range of attitudes popularly held toward life and the sanctions we place on killing. He notes that most people are inconsistent in their application of principles against killing, and demonstrates that there is a great deal of conceptual confusion associated with our feelings about life and death. Any claim to a fundamental sanctity of life needs clarification and defense, for example; such a claim is not intuitively self-evident, for we make no attempts to protect all life indiscriminately. We must, for instance, determine what it is about human life that justifies us in placing an extraordinarily high value on it.

Any defense of a right to life for some must also provide us with criteria by which to distinguish between those circumstances in which life must be protected and those in which it may be terminated. The problems Goodrich describes that are associated with any theory that values respect for life are elaborated on at length throughout the chapter; they present a challenge for all moral theories. An adequate ethical theory must be able to account for the moral distinctions we are called upon to draw in this area and must give guidance in situations when the value of life is challenged by other values.

Some standard of quality of life challenges the notion of an absolute human right to life. Many people believe that if a life is of poor quality, it may not be worth living and no individual should be made to continue living under such circumstances. It is argued that life is desirable only so long as it meets some standard of acceptable quality. And even though many persons choose to continue living when the quality of their lives seems to fall below any such minimal level, this evidence is not necessarily proof that they still view life as desirable, for their decision may be based on a feeling that it is wrong to deliberately end their lives.

There are several different questions to be resolved if we grant that the quality of a life may affect the value of that life. Under what circumstances can considerations of quality of life overrule the fundamental value placed on human life? Is anyone morally permitted to terminate his life when it seems to him that it can no longer achieve the minimal acceptable quality? When, if ever, is a person justified in deciding for another that the latter's life should be ended?

There are serious problems in allowing quality of life to be a criterion in decisions between life and death. With it, we seem to be moving from the realm of moral values into the area of tastes and preferences. Although we cannot provide empirical proofs for our ethical views, we can and do provide reasons and arguments on their behalf. Preferences, however, do not require defense. Deciding what constitutes a high or low quality of life may be just such a matter of taste. Many people uncomplainingly pursue life patterns others view as intolerable. Some take pleasure in ways of life that horrify and repulse others. How can we hope to make judgments on some general, universal standards of quality of life when we have such fundamental disagreements on the best ways to live?

It is most important that we move cautiously in such investigations. In decisions to end human life we must be certain that the criteria on which judgment is based are ethically relevant; that is, that we have ethically valid reasons for treating these cases differently from those in which life is protected.

There are two different sorts of conditions the presence of which may lead us to judge lives as being of such poor quality that it is questionable whether they are worth living, and hence, worth sustaining. The first is the *pain criterion:* if a life is devoid of any reasonable hope for happiness because of an incapacitating, misery-inducing condition, then the individual in question may want to cease living. Uncontrollable suffering seems always at least to call into question the value of the suffering life. The second criterion is some *standard of awareness:* the human being who is unconscious or unaware of his surroundings, who engages in no activity, and for whom there is no prospect of change in these respects, also challenges our notions of the absolute value of human life. Such a life seems scarcely human to us at all.

If it does seem clear that a life ought to be ended, is there any further moral problem in determining how to end it? In the first section, "Killing and Letting Die," the concern is with whether there is any moral difference between acts of killing and acts of letting die which makes one type of act less reprehensible than the other. In order to settle this question, we must determine if there is any general conceptual distinction to be drawn between acts of these types, such that we can readily identify acts as being of one type or another. Is turning off a respirator an act of killing or of letting die? Failure to administer antibiotics seems to be killing if it is a result of physician negligence and if the medication would have restored the patient to health; but it is generally thought to be an instance of letting the patient die when the patient is suffering from another terminal illness that cannot be controlled. Sometimes a solution is proposed in terms of distinguishing between ordinary and extraordinary means, but this distinction, too, is problematic.

In order to be useful in situations of moral decision-making, any distinction we draw must be based on some ethically relevant criterion by which we can recognize acts of letting die as morally different from acts of killing. Further, we must see if criteria that are plausible when death is viewed as an evil, as in the selections by Fletcher, Foot, Bennett, Dinello, and Fitzgerald, are the same as when death is thought to be the best outcome—as when choosing between active and passive euthanasia. Throughout, the authors in this section are concerned with determining whether or not the rightness or wrongness of ending a life depends on such distinctions at all.

In the section "Abortion," we begin to deal more concretely with the substantive issue of determining the particular sorts of circumstances under which human life may be taken. There is a vast literature on the moral problems of abortion and it is not possible to include even a representative survey of the variety of positions held on this issue within the spatial limits of this book. The three selections were chosen, not as comprehensive nor paradigmatic examples of the literature, but as interesting, important works on the subject.

There are several questions centering around the topic of abortion. Even if we could answer the most obvious question of whether or not abortion is morally acceptable, we must still decide what attitude to take toward it. Somewhat independent of the morality question per se is the social and legal question of whether it should be prohibited. (The U.S. Supreme Court made no judgment on the morality of abortion in 1973, but concluded that it was not a matter of legal policy.) In some contexts, the discussion focuses on whether the fetus is human and entitled to full human rights. Others argue that this is irrelevant, that even if the fetus is fully human, its parasitic relationship to the mother allows her the overriding right of terminating its life in exercising her right to control her own body. Even if we believe the fetus has a right to life, we still need to determine whether this is a *prima facie* or an absolute right.

John T. Noonan considers the problem of the morality of abortion from the perspective from which it has been most frequently discussed, that of the historical religious tradition. In this framework, he views the problem to be that of determining the humanity of a being. He claims that if the fetus is human, it deserves love since religion stresses the love of humanity; and, hence, it would follow that abortion is wrong.

Noonan's problem, then, is that of deciding at what point an organism becomes human and entitled to love and respect. He is concerned with finding some objectively identifiable criterion by which we may distinguish life deserving of full human rights from other life. His conclusion is stated in biological terms: whatever is conceived of human parents is human, and hence a fetus is human from the time of conception.

Michael Tooley is also concerned with providing a sound, morally significant criterion for determining who has a right to life. Tooley grants that a fetus is human, but not that this biological feature has moral significance. The relevant criterion rather, is that one has a right to life if one desires life or is at least "capable of desiring to continue existing as a subject of experiences and other mental states." Tooley argues that being a person, rather than simply being genetically human, is the significant feature. Neither fetuses nor very young infants fulfill this criterion, and hence, Tooley claims, they have no serious right to life. The point up to which we can morally kill human beings is, then, not conception, viability, or even birth, but some time after birth when self-awareness develops.

H. Tristram Engelhardt, Jr. also agrees that we must determine whether or not the fetus is a person in order to determine the general acceptability of abortion. He finds it conceptually unsatisfying to consider the fetus as a person, for it shows none of the characteristics he perceives us to associate with persons. It is true that fetuses are potential persons—that they normally develop into persons—but this does not make them persons. Still, it seems clear to him that infants have a right to life even though they, too, are not fully persons; they have some sorts of rights approaching those of persons. While Engelhardt's analysis of "personhood" is similar to Tooley's, his ethical intuitions demand a different conclusion from the one Tooley reached. Hence, he defines his task as that of constructing a theory that can account for the development of varying levels of significance associated with human life.

The key to the distinction, he claims, is that of social role. One acquires rights by virtue of one's membership in a social context. Because infants relate to persons by responding to their stimuli and by evoking responses in return, they are social members of the community and hence are entitled to protection. Because early-term fetuses (not yet viable) cannot even play this limited social role, their right to life is denied by this criterion as well as by that of personhood. And so Engelhardt concludes, as Noonan and Tooley claim it is not possible to do, that abortion is morally permissible up to the point of viability.

Even if we do not agree with Tooley that infanticide is generally permissible, we may still want to consider the question with respect to infants with serious birth defects. When infants are born with such severe defects that there is little or no hope of their achieving even a tolerable quality of life, it seems cruel to keep them alive. For many of these children, life seems to offer nothing but pain and suffering or perhaps permanent unconsciousness; for their families it may mean enormous emotional and financial hardship. In such cases, their speedy death seems to be in the interest of all, and yet there is a general prohibition against killing. Further, it is seldom possible for us to predict with perfect accuracy what any person's quality of life will actually be: Down's Syndrome (mongolism), for example, can be identified even before birth, but the degree of retardation and particular personality features relating to the afflicted individual's chances of happiness cannot be known for years. The personal experiences of the pediatrician Anthony Shaw bring out the problems such children pose and the awesome responsibility any decision entails.

The rest of the readings in the section on abortion all focus on one particular sort of birth defect known as spina bifida. Most children born with this condition either die within their first year or survive to experience a very unhappy life. Hence, the question arises whether or not we should approve vigorous medical treatment of such infants to improve their chances of survival. The problem is made all the more difficult by the uncertainty at birth of the individual's future quality of life. Spina bifida victims are physically handicapped, many are retarded, and almost all experience social difficulties; yet a few overcome these obstacles to live very worthwhile lives.

R. B. Zachary, Eliot Slater, John M. Freeman, and Robert E. Cooke are all physicians who have been involved in the treatment of spina bifida. The discussion amongst them concerns the nature of the responsibility of the physician and of society toward these children. Slater and Freeman argue that the humane and rational course is to help the hopeless amongst these infants to die quickly to save them suffering. Zachary and Cooke argue that there is indeed a responsibility to ease suffering, but that it should be fulfilled by more vigorous research and treatment rather than by the negative solution of death. All agree that at present, keeping all such infants alive will result in serious suffering for most of them.

The next paper in this section is a personal account of the experience of living with a severe birth defect. Karen Metzler is a young woman who was born with multiple birth defects including spina bifida; because of the severity of her handicaps, she has a special perspective on societal response to handicapped persons. Her essay is the transcript of a talk to a class in Moral Problems in Medicine.

In light of the empirical data, is it right to terminate the lives of these children? What sorts of criteria are relevant to this decision? R. M. Hare introduces a new factor in the decision-making process, for he directs us to resolve the problem by taking an impartial accounting of all interests at stake. He believes that this method should be used to settle all moral dilemmas, and claims that it is compatible with any moral theory; however, it does seem to conflict with Kant's demand to fulfill our duties independently of any particular interests at the time. In calculating the various interests of all concerned, Hare directs us to look not only at all persons currently affected by the outcome but also at possible future persons. In the case of the defective infant or fetus, we are to consider, among others, the interests of the child who will be born only if this one dies. He claims that we may be being unfair to this possible child we we deprive him of life by preserving the life of the defective, existent child who has such a poor chance for a decent life.

Derek Parfit challenges Hare's approach of considering possible persons in our calculations, for, as he demonstrates, there are serious conceptual problems in determining the interests of possible people. Parfit agrees that it is important to consider the interests of future persons in our moral calculations, at least to the extent that we take care not to harm those who will actually exist; however, he argues, it makes no sense to say we harm someone by preventing his existence because there is then no one to be harmed. But, Parfit concludes, we should nonetheless act to some extent as if possible people have interests.

In the section "Death and Dignity," the relation between quality of life and the value of life is again at issue, but with a significant difference. Here we are concerned with an individual's decision that his own life is not worth living, whereas the preceding section was concerned with making that decision for another. It is often argued that an individual has a special proprietorship over his own body—that he owns it and can do with it as he pleases. But there are other arguments to the effect that persons have special responsibilities toward their own bodies—that they have duties toward themselves that require protection of their bodies. Under what circumstances, if any, is a person justified in bringing about his own death?

Suicide has been a subject of special interest to physicians and philosophers through the ages. The section on suicide begins with a sampling of the philosophical literature on suicide going back to Seneca, who wrote in the first century A.D. Seneca addresses the question that has been central to this entire chapter: Is it living that matters or living well? Kant objects to this line of reasoning, for he thinks that it is a mistake to view happiness as the end of life. Such pursuit of pleasure, when frustrated, naturally leads to thoughts of suicide, but, Kant argues, we have no license to take our own lives. Suicide is not an act we could consistently will to be governed by a universal law, and hence it is not acceptable under the categorical imperative.

David Hume believes that persons naturally cherish life and only incline to suicide under desperate conditions. Further, he argues that there is nothing wrong with suicide even if it should be chosen: it is not a crime against God, other persons, or oneself. Of course, the question of whether suicide is wrong is separable from the question of whether the state can justifiably treat it as a crime, for the state can define as criminal acts that are otherwise morally neutral (for example, traveling at 60 miles per hour), and it can choose not to outlaw acts that are morally wrong (for example, being gratuitously insulting).

In the contemporary literature that follows we can perceive a radical change in emphasis. Classically, the debate has focused on whether or not the individual has a right to commit suicide, but now the issue has become whether or not it is *rational* to commit suicide. The underlying assumption is that if suicide is not rational, it should be prevented.

George Murphy, a psychiatrist, takes the position that most people who attempt suicide are psychiatrically ill and seeking treatment, and hence all should be treated. Glanville Williams takes a more moderate position, which allows that suicide may well be a rational choice, and, if so, should be allowed. But because there are cases where it is a result of irrationality, it is permissible to interfere with a suicide attempt in order to try to dissuade the person. This view is echoed by Jerome Motto, who tries to outline criteria by which to identify those who are properly (reasonably) exercising their right to suicide.

Throughout history there has always been the greatest sympathy for those who look to suicide as an escape from torturing illness. All but the most rigid opponents of suicide will approve of it when the person is experiencing extreme physical suffering. Mary Rose Barrington presents poignant examples in support of this view in her descriptions of persons whose quality of life has been made so poor by forces beyond their control that their lives are not worth living. How, she asks, can any humane person insist on keeping another alive under such circumstances? Our duty to respect life is in conflict with duties to minimize suffering and to respect an individual's decision in matters that affect primarily himself.

But it is not enough to grant these persons the right to suicide, for by the time they are so ill as to be ready to die they may not be able to exercise this right on their own. Thus the problems of euthanasia and assisted suicide are raised. Even if we decide that it is permissible for an individual to decide to end his own life, we need still to determine whether it is right for another to help. It may even be morally obligatory to help another die, if we adopt a moral principle that directs us to reduce suffering whenever possible.

If it is wrong to keep a particular individual alive, does it matter how we choose to end his life? Is there any moral difference between active and passive euthanasia? As we noted in the "Killing and Letting Die" section, it is difficult to distinguish between killing and letting die, and it is similarly difficult to make any perfect distinction between active and passive euthanasia. Fuzzy as the border may be, though, we can clearly identify many acts of euthanasia as either active or passive, and so the moral question is not meaningless. Generally in discussions of killing and letting die, the concern is with minimizing responsibility under regrettable circumstances; but it may be that the particular facts of a case of euthanasia require attention to different moral features. Because our aim is to reduce suffering, it may be that active euthanasia is more appropriate in that it is generally more efficient at achieving this end. Nonetheless, most people's moral intuitions see passive euthanasia as morally more acceptable than active euthanasia. Some people see neither as acceptable, and Yale Kamisar spells out some reasons for this attitude. His objections to euthanasia do not condemn it in principle, but rather warn against it as a social practice, for such a practice, he fears, would surely be open to abuses.

One of the most serious problems with euthanasia is that of obtaining informed consent. If suicide is to be permitted only when the individual has reached his decision rationally, it seems also that only those who have rationally chosen it should be subjects of euthanasia. But if we consider euthanasia appropriate only in conditions of extreme suffering, how can we expect the victim of such suffering to make a rational choice? He is surely depressed, probably heavily drugged, and perhaps out of his mind with pain. Is it appropriate to appeal to a decision he made at an earlier time when he did not really know what the experience would be like? With most people, we do not even have that information to go on, for few people carefully spell out their wishes on these matters while healthy. And what if the individual is unconscious and being kept alive, perhaps for years, by artificial means. Does anyone have a right to stop this life support? Who should have the power of making such decisions? And what if the patient is a child, not yet of the age of consent but still capable of personal decision-making, as was the girl described in "The Adolescent Patient's Decision to Die?"

It is the complexity of such issues that prompts Kamisar to object to legalizing euthanasia. It may well be a desirable alternative in some cases, but he doubts our ability to make the right decision generally in these matters and hence recommends not burdening anyone with such weighty moral responsibility. Even though euthanasia might on some occasions be morally permissible, it still may be that we are not competent to identify such occasions accurately—and hence should refrain from the practicing of euthanasia.

S.S.

KILLING AND LETTING DIE

From "The Morality of Killing"

Timothy Goodrich

At first sight there doesn't seem to be any problem about killing. Most people would say that it is wrong to kill and that's all there is to it. The same opinion is proclaimed by many members of the Christian religion. They say that "Thou shalt not kill" is an absolute command. But there are several issues involving the morality of killing where ordinary men, secular and religious alike, make judgements or evince perplexity which reveals that common sense morality is less clear about killing than it at first appears.

I want to elucidate these issues and to show that the usual ways of settling them are fallacious. At the same time I want to show how attention

Reprinted with permission of the author and publisher from *Philosophy* 44:168, 127–39, 1969. Copyright, the Royal Institute of Philosophy.

to these issues reveals the inadequacies of many philosophical theories about morals.

First of all there is a difficulty which frequently comes up in discussions of pacifism. Sometimes people object to military service just on the grounds that it is wrong to kill. (There are other grounds, but these are beside the point.) Against this the reply is often as follows. Suppose that by killing one person you can prevent more people being killed in the long run. Thus, if Hitler's assassins had succeeded, they might, in the long run, have prevented a great many other people from being killed. Are we to reproach them on the grounds that "It is wrong to kill"? Likewise the killings involved in the 1939–45 war were probably fewer than would have occurred if Hitler and his allies had gone unopposed. So, surely, "Killing is wrong" cannot be a valid reason for objecting to *any* sort of military service (although it might to some, depending on the nature of the action to be fought). How the difficulty is formulated will depend on whether we regard killing as just a physical act like shooting or stabbing or as also including actions which have as remote but foreseeable consequences that people will die. If we say that killing is just a physical act, then it follows at once that "killing is wrong" is not an absolute rule; the killing of Hitler is, e.g., an exception to it. If, on the other hand, we say that it includes actions which (knowingly) cause deaths in the long run, then it follows that there are moral questions about killing which "killing is wrong" does not cover. For, on this view, anyone who could have assassinated Hitler was a killer whatever he did—if he didn't kill Hitler then he killed the people who were killed as a result of Hitler's continuing to live. But if whatever a man does he is a killer, "killing is wrong" gives no guidance to action—yet most people would hold that in such a situation it is still true that some actions are better than others. Hence whichever view we take about the nature of killing, the common sense morality of killing cannot be summed up in the pristine simplicity of "killing is (absolutely) wrong."

The obvious next step is to say that, where there is an alternative, killing is wrong, but otherwise we should minimise the number of individuals killed. But so far the difficulties have only begun.

How far is this principle to be applied to animals? If we were to apply it completely to animals and there was a choice between the death of two animals and one man, then we would have to choose the death of the man, since the death of one man is a smaller number of deaths than the death of two animals. But few people would accept this consequence, so that common sense cannot regard animals as falling straightforwardly under the rule "minimise killing." In fact it seems generally to be held that human life is infinitely more valuable than animal life: there is no number of animals, however great, that is worth the sacrifice of even one human being.

But on what grounds is this huge bias in favour of human life based? Some say that the basis of the distinction is man's rationality. But it is certain that there are some human beings in mental institutions whose mental powers are inferior to those of an ape, so that rationality will not do as a defence of an absolute distinction between men and animals. Others say that what makes man special is the possession of a soul. But how can we tell if a creature has a soul? If the presence of a soul is signified by the possession of mental powers, then this is open to exactly the same objection as the first suggestion: some men have mental powers inferior to those of some animals, so either some men do not have souls or some animals do, and in either case we have not been provided with a basis for an absolute distinction between men and animals. If, on the other hand, the presence of a soul is not signified by the mental powers of its possessor, it is not clear how we are to discover whether a creature has a soul, and until some method is proposed, this suggestion is just useless. A third suggestion is that we regard all human life as sacred because unless we can be sure that *every* human life is regarded as equally valuable, no human being will feel safe. But this is to give up completely the idea that killing people is *just* wrong. It is now claimed to be wrong only in so far as it leads to insecurity. Killing is wrong not in itself but because of its consequences. Most men would be morally repelled by such a view. In any case, it is just false that unless every human life is respected no-one will feel safe. Evidently no-one feels insecure because the lives of animals are often held to be of little account. Likewise in slave-owning societies the slave-owning class felt no insecurity even though they held the lives of their slaves to be of little account. All that is necessary for security is that there should be respect for life in some class of individuals of which you are a member, and this need not be the class of human beings.

So it looks as if common sense knows of no grounds for the grand distinction it makes between men and animals.

Yet on the other hand people do on the whole seem to hold that we have *some* duties to animals.

Two kinds of view appear here. One is that it is wrong to kill animals, or at any rate some kinds of animals, as far as this is compatible with human life. The other is that we have a duty to prevent animal suffering. Where these seem to conflict—where an animal is suffering from an incurable disease, say, it is usually assumed that our duty to prevent the suffering outweighs our duty not to kill, and we should in fact kill it (i.e., have it "put to sleep").[1]

But there is a lot of moral diversity on this. Some people think that it is wrong to inflict suffering on animals, but not wrong to kill them. So they object to bullfighting, but not to the "putting down" of racehorses; to hunting, but not to the "humane killing" of cattle. (This shatters the notion that "common sense" says it is *always* wrong to kill.)

On the other hand there are some people who believe that *all* life should be respected (e.g., Dr. Schweitzer) and certainly most people seem to hold that we should have at least *some* respect for the lives of *some* animals.

Can any rational defence be put forward for any of these views? The one most frequently cited goes something like this: How would you like it if you were hunted by a pack of bloodthirsty hounds? According to Professor Hare, who is an influential philosopher, we must hold that this sort of

[1]But this is not the correct way of formulating the conflict. Cf. my conclusions on euthanasia.

question is made relevant by the very nature of moral language. Those who say that foxhunting is all right are committed to the universal judgment that anyone who inflicts suffering and death on another creature in this way is doing what is all right, and hence that, even if he were the creature in question, it would be all right. As Kant said: "So act that you may will the maxim of your action to the universal law." According to Hare, those who indulged in bear-baiting should have reasoned thus: "If we were bears we should suffer horribly if treated thus: therefore we cannot accept any maxim which permits bears to be treated thus; therefore we cannot say that it is all right to treat bears thus" ("Freedom and Reason").

But there is an obvious difficulty with this argument. I could conceive of myself as being considerably different from what I am while still being the same person. But could I be a bear or a fox and still be me? Does it make sense to say "What if you were the fox?" What could there be here to preserve my personal identity? This comes out even more clearly for those who believe that we should respect *all* (animal?) life. Could I conceive of myself as being a fly or a worm or an amoeba? It is difficult to see what sense there could be in saying "I happen to be a human, but I might have been a worm."

It might be suggested that I need only respect those individuals whom I could conceive myself as being. But this is far from self-evident. It certainly seems to make sense to say that I ought not to inflict suffering on a bear, even though I couldn't conceivably *be* a bear. (Kant did indeed say that his principle entailed (only) that we should treat *humanity* as an end. This was because he held that it was just humans (and angels) who were endowed with rationality. I hope I have shown that this view is doubly inadequate.)

A further difficulty with this argument is that, as far as killing goes, the question "How would you like it?" is not always a sensible one. To be able to like or dislike something, you must be aware of it. But sometimes animals may be killed without their knowing it: the household pet may be a nuisance and be taken to the vet where it is put in a comfortable basket and immersed in odourless lethal gas. If someone said "How would you like it, if you were that animal?" I could reply that the question did not arise, since if I were the animal, I wouldn't know anything about it.

This attempt to justify a certain moral attitude to animals fails, therefore—showing also, incidentally, an inadequacy of the philosophical theory associated with it.

There is another consequence of this way of justifying our attitudes to animals which is very curious. If it is said that "How would you like it, if you were that individual?" is just as relevant for animals as for men, then it seems to follow that animals are just as important as men, and this is in conflict with the common conviction that the lives of men are infinitely more valuable than the lives of animals.

If this consequence is accepted by those who advocate "respect for life," they will have to grapple with another. Is all non-human life equally valuable? Is the cow as important as the flies that buzz round its nose? If not, the animal kingdom will have to be graded in order of importance. Will this grading be done by species, or by the level of mental complexity, or what? What are the relevant grading criteria? If it is replied that animal life as such is valuable, irrespective of what kind of life, it will have to be conceded that the death of a monkey is to be preferred to the death of two earwigs. Furthermore, there is a smooth gradation of characteristics from the most complex forms of animal life, to the simple unicellular organisms and even to the bacteria and viruses. Where is "respect for life" to stop?

Clearly, then, there is *no* obviously correct moral attitude to the killing of animals. Again, common sense is less straightforward than it thinks it is.

Now I want to raise a number of new difficulties which come out particularly clearly in our consideration of animals, but, as we shall see, arise similarly for humans. If we say that we have duties to animals, or that we must respect their lives, this assumes that there are animals there to whom we have duties or whose lives must be respected. But if, say, we all decided to become vegetarians, the result would not be that all the livestock that we might have eaten would live long and happy lives and die at a ripe old age. Rather, farmers would simply cease to raise livestock. All those animals that we now feel sorry for would just never come into existence at all. Is it fulfilling our duty to these potential animals to prevent them from coming into existence? But we said just now that having a duty to an individual assumes that he exists. There is a logical objection to talking about a duty to a non-existent individual (which I shall go into later). We might try to overcome the difficulty by saying that our duties are to the animals that exist now, and we cannot start having duties to future animals until they are born. But this ignores the fact that, with farm animals, we can decide whether they reproduce or not, and the question is: Does the rule that we should minimise killing entail that, if we know for certain that an individual yet to be born will be killed, it is better that he should not be born?

We get similar puzzles if we introduce the idea of suffering. It is conceivable that we could know for certain that if an animal were born in certain circumstances, it would suffer all its life. In fact it may be that we can actually say this of animals born in some factory farms. We can ask, just as we did about killing: Does the rule that we should minimise suffering entail that, if we know for certain that an individual yet to be born will suffer all its life, it is better that it should not be born? Again, very often people even say that it is cruel to keep a suffering animal alive. We are thinking of ourselves, they say, not of the good of the animal, if we keep a pet with a painful and incurable disease instead of having it destroyed. But there is something odd in the idea that it is a kindness to an animal to end its existence. Just as it seems odd to say that it can be in an animal's interest not to begin to exist, so it seems odd to say that it can be in its interests to cease to exist.

These are logical puzzles, not moral ones. But logical confusion can lead to great moral confusion. Here the philosopher may make a humble contribution to enlightening the morals of our time. For these puzzles arise in a more exciting context. The questions we have just been considering in relation to animals reappear in relation to humans as questions about euthanasia, abortion and population control.

Consider euthanasia. Supporters of euthanasia sometimes say that it is cruel to keep an incurable and suffering person alive; that it would be an act of charity to end his life.

Yet while it seems obvious to the man of common sense that we should painlessly destroy animals suffering from incurable painful diseases, it does not seem equally obvious to him that this should be done to human beings. But he seems to have as much reason in the one case as the other. For it is generally held that we have a duty to minimise suffering among humans even more than among animals. However, there is a further factor in the case of humans which does not arise with animals. A man can give or withhold his assent to what is done to him. Common sense seems to recognize yet a third principle here: that a man should be free to make up his own mind about what concerns him alone (liberalism). And if anything concerns a man alone surely it is the question whether he should die. We might think, then, that the common sense view must be that the question of his death should be entirely up to the suffering man. This again would depart from the view that killing is always wrong. But matters are more complicated than this. Consider other kinds of suicide. Most people would think it their duty to try to stop a healthy person from committing suicide. So it seems that common sense does not hold that we have an absolute duty to leave people alone in all matters which concern themselves. Thus the relevance of the rule against interference in a man's private decision does not automatically decide the issue of euthanasia. We find, then, at least three rules that are considered to apply to euthanasia: minimise killing, minimise suffering ((Negative) Utilitarianism), and don't interfere in a man's private decisions (liberalism). But common sense does not obviously come down in favour of one rather than another. There does not seem to be any common sense view here at all. The Deontologist would say that we have to consider each situation on its merits with all of these rules in mind. "All we can do is consider all the appreciable advantages and disadvantages of which we can think in regard to each of the alternative actions between which we choose, and having done this see what the total impression is on our mind" (Ewing, *Ethics*). But, if we are to judge by the reports of doctors and nurses, the total impression produced by this exercise does not lead to any decisive result at all, and there seems no reason why it should. If the Deontologist holds that by bearing in mind all the morally significant features of a situation we will necessarily come to a decision about what is the right course of action, it is obvious that his is a false theory.

But perhaps the choice between killing and minimising suffering is not quite of the form that this view takes it to be. I have already claimed that there is something odd about saying that it is cruel to keep a suffering animal alive. The same, of course, will go for humans. It is a difficult logical problem whether it can make sense to say that it is in a man's interests to die. But this is better considered together with the questions of abortion and population control.

Perhaps it is worth pointing out that, again, appeal to the question "How would *you* like it? " will not settle this issue. Proponents of euthanasia are usually prepared to apply their prescriptions to themselves, and so are their opponents prepared to apply *their* prescription to *themselves.* And there hardly seems any ground for labelling one of these sides "fanatics."

A convenient way to start our discussion of the moral issue of abortion is by considering the conditions under which the bill to amend the law about abortion would make abortion permissible. They are:

> (a) that the continuance of the pregnancy would involve serious risk to the life or of grave injury to the health, whether physical or mental, of the pregnant woman whether before, at or after the birth of the child; or
>
> (b) that there is a substantial risk that if the child were born it would suffer from such physical or mental abnormalities as to be seriously handicapped; or
>
> (c) that the pregnant woman's capacity as a mother will be severely overstrained by the care of a child or of another child as the case may be (the 'Social clause'); or
>
> (d) that the pregnant woman is a defective or became pregnant while under the age of sixteen or became pregnant as a result of rape.[2]

In one case the reason for killing the foetus (=the human embryo) is that otherwise the mother is likely to die. If we say that the foetus is a living thing, this is a case where a man, the doctor, will cause a death whatever he does. If he does not kill the foetus, he kills the mother. This is a situation of the sort I mentioned first. Here again, "Killing is wrong" is not adequate to the situation. But we cannot make this choice on the basis of numbers, so even "Minimise killing" is inadequate. Most people think that in this situation, the foetus is to be killed. Why they think this is unclear. If it is because they think the mother, but not the foetus, deserves the title of "person," this should be borne in mind when we consider the view that abortion is murder. In all the other cases the reasons suggested for ending the existence of the embryo are connected with human suffering, either that of the mother or that of the potential child. Now we find that all the puzzles which seemed somewhat strained and ridiculous in our consideration of animals are actually propounded when people talk about abortion. It is reasonable to suppose that a child suffering from severe mental or physical abnormalities, or who is the unwanted child of a young girl, will be unhappy, to say the least. It is quite possible that it will suffer for the whole of its life. But is it obvious, as some people say it is, that, because we should minimise suffering, we should prevent these children from coming into existence? Some people say that we actually have the duty to these potential human beings, if we know they will suffer when they come into the world, of stopping them entirely from beginning their life. You will recognize these as essentially the same problems as we had before: "Can we have duties to non-existent individuals?" and "Does the rule that we should minimise suffering entail that, if we know an individual will suffer all its life, it is better

---

[2]"Medical Termination of Pregnancy Bill," 1966, presented by Mr. David Steel, M.P. (in its original form).

that it should not be born?" Then again, some people say that it is actually
in the interests of the unborn, sometimes, not to be born. This is of the same
type as the problem about euthanasia: just as there is something logically
odd about saying that it is being kind to someone, or in his interests, to cease
to exist, so it seems odd to say that it is kind to him or in his interests not
to let him begin to exist.

As a matter of fact, these questions are not special to abortion. They
arise whenever we consider the question of controlling the number of people to be born. What makes the question of abortion specially difficult is that
some people claim that the human embryo is a person and therefore that
to kill it is to commit murder. But let us consider the *general* problem first.

There are a great many miserable people in the world, and one of the
chief sources of misery is a lack of the basic necessities of life; food, drink,
clothing and shelter and so on. A great deal is done by charitable institutions
in providing these things, but, in spite of this, the problem gets no better.
This is because the population of the poor parts of the world, as a result of
the better life expectancy brought about by modern medicine, is expanding
at a colossal rate. By the end of the century, the population of the world will
have more than doubled. But the production of the material necessities of
life will scarcely have kept pace, even with all the help from such bodies as
Oxfam and Christian Aid. It is suggested, therefore, that the obvious thing
to do is to control the increase in population by the widespread application
of some form of contraception. And so it is. But it is worth asking on what
principle this suggestion is made. If the principle is that we should minimise
human suffering, are we saying that since we know that these individuals will
suffer all their lives, it is better that they should not be born? Are we saying
that we have duties to them, and that it is in their best interest not to exist?

The best way to sort out these puzzles is to go via a general consideration of utilitarianism. I will consider positive as well as negative utilitarianism; the same argument applies to both.[3]

Positive utilitarianism says that we should maximise happiness. It is
often held that this entails that we should produce as many children as
possible, so long as their happiness would exceed their misery, since this
increases the amount of happiness in the world. This assumes that we can
talk about a grand total of happiness. Now we certainly can say that a person
is not very happy, quite happy or very happy, so in a rough and ready way
we can talk about the amount of happiness of an individual. But can we talk
about the amount of happiness of a group? i.e., can we add up their individual happiness to make a sum total? If we put two pound weights together
we get a collection which has a weight of two pounds. But if we put two

---

[3]Jan Narveson deals with this subject in his "Utilitarianism and New Generations" in
Mind 1967. It will be seen that I do not follow his treatment. This is because he seems to accept
that we can talk of a sum of happiness or suffering. He is led to say that utilitarianism forbids
the bringing into the world of children who will on the whole suffer, but does not prescribe
bringing into the world children who will on the whole be happy. On my view utilitarianism
says nothing about either. It is very difficult to see how it can say something about the one and
not the other.

equally happy people together, do we get a group with twice their individual happiness? The same with suffering. If a room contains a miserable man, and he's joined by another equally miserable man, is there twice as much misery in the room? And if we put one fairly happy and one fairly miserable man together, do we have a collection that is neither miserable nor happy? Again, how happy would a man have to be for his happiness to equal the happiness of five slightly happy people together? Clearly it is just senseless to talk of adding up happiness as we add up weight or length. It follows, then, that there is no such thing as a grand total of happiness, and so we cannot sensibly be told to make this total as big as possible. Thus it makes no sense either to say that the more non-suffering people there are in the world, the more happiness there is in it. Nor does it make sense to say that the fewer suffering people there are in the world, the less suffering there is in it.

We can see then, that it is absurd to say, as so many philosophers have done, that "Happiness is good and suffering evil"—just so—since happiness and suffering cannot be talked about apart from individual people's experiencing them.[4] If utilitarianism is to make sense, it must include in it some reference to *whose* happiness is to be maximised. Let us take Bentham's "Everyone to count for one and no one for more than one" as our cue. We could reformulate utilitarianism now as "Everyone equally should be as happy as possible." Once we have said this, however, it follows that utilitarianism tells us nothing about how many individuals there should be. For "everyone" presupposes that we already have a class of humans, about which the principle goes on to assert something. Nothing can be made to follow from this about the number of members this class ought to contain; the class, i.e., the class with however members it contains, is presupposed from the start. It may be that the mistaken impression that this inference is valid has been fostered by an indecisive rendering of "the class of men." Suppose a radical reformer says: "There are now so many people that everyone is unhappy. So let us liquidate half the human population and then everyone will be happy." It is impossible to infer that the purge should be made via "Everyone should be happy." For "everyone" (i.e., the class of men) is not used univocally here: the first "everyone" may be expanded to "everyone now" and the second to "everyone after the purge." If "everyone" in the principle consists of the chosen people, then the fact about the first "everyone" is irrelevant to applying it. If it really means everyone, then so is the fact about the second "everyone." I think utilitarians have usually intended "everyone" in their principle to be what it says: everyone past, present and future. We may, indeed, raise a problem about "The class of men" since if it is in our choice how many men there are to be, the class, it might be said, is not well formed, because it has no definite number of

---

[4]Cp. G. E. Moore on pleasure: "Our question is: Is it the pleasure, as distinct from the consciousness of it, that we set value on? Do we think the pleasure valuable in itself, or must we insist that, if we are to think the pleasure good, we must have consciousness of it too?" (*Principia Ethica*, p. 88).

members. But all this would show is not that utilitarianism can tell us how many members it should have, but that "All men should be as happy as possible" is not a significant proposition.[5]

The upshot, then, is that decisions about population control cannot be based on the principle that we should maximise happiness (or at least minimise suffering). Now let us go back to our problems. One of our problems was this: "Does the rule that we should minimise suffering entail, if we know an individual will suffer all its life, it is better that it should not be born?" We can now see that the answer is "No." The rule "Minimise suffering" has to be formulated as "Everyone should suffer as little as possible," and nothing follows from this about how many people there should be. We may well want to adopt a further principle to the effect that the number of individuals should be such that each suffers as little as possible, or perhaps that the number of individuals should be such that each is as happy as possible. But it is important to see that these are completely different from the utilitarian principle and do not follow from it. Perhaps it is worth pointing out, by the way, that if we did adopt the latter principle, we would probably be committed to a very drastic reduction in the world's population indeed. It might be concluded, for instance, that the maximum happiness could only be obtained in a very few places, e.g., the South Sea Isles, so that ideally the population of the world should be scaled down to nothing elsewhere. . . .

Of course, once again we can say it would be a good thing if a couple had a child or if a man were to die. All I say is that these things cannot follow from saying that we should act benevolently to people. In particular, we cannot say that it would be *cruel* to bring an individual into the world, or that it would be *cruel* not to kill him. The concept of cruelty presupposes the applicability of utilitarian criteria, and this requirement is not met where the existence of an individual is in question.

To get back to abortion. I have considered the questions of suffering, but those who oppose abortion usually say this is not all there is to it. Abortion is (really) killing. So, in a Commons debate on the subject, Mrs. Jill Knight (M.P. for Edgbaston) said: "Babies are not like bad teeth to be jerked out just because they cause suffering. An unborn baby is a baby nevertheless. Would the sponsors of the Bill think it right to kill a baby they can see? Of course they would not. Why then do they think it right to kill one they cannot see? . . . I have come to believe that those who support abortion on demand do so because in all sincerity they cannot accept that an unborn baby is a human being. Yet surely it is. Its heart beats, it moves, it sleeps, it eats. Uninterfered with, it has a potential life ahead of it of 70 years or more; it may be a happy life, or a sad life; it may be a genius, or it may be just plain average; but surely as a healthy, living baby it has a right not to be killed simply because it may be inconvenient for a year or so to its mother." (Commons Debate, 22nd July, 1966.)

[5]The point in this paragraph has, of course nothing to do with the question of existential import. When I say that "All men should be as happy as possible" presupposes a class of men, I offer no opinion about what should be said if there were no men. Happily we do not have to consider this question, since the class of men is not the null class.

Is the foetus a person? The criteria offered by Mrs. Knight are that its heart beats, it moves, it sleeps and it eats. (The last two seem a bit doubtful.) But obviously these are very far from constituting *all* the criteria we use in applying the concept of "person." Mrs. Knight's criteria apply to a great many animals, which we do not normally describe as "people"—if we did, we could be charged with the grossest immorality in our actions towards them, since, as I observed earlier, we do not regard their lives as sacred.

Some people think that foetuses are people because they have souls. Actually, some of these people claim to know that God creates the soul just at the moment when the sperm fertilizes the ovum. But, as with animals, we may ask how we are to tell whether something has a soul? Doubtless I must accept this on faith. But how do I go about doing this? Either "soul" means "mind," or its meaning has not been explained. As to the second, I might as well be told to believe that the mome raths outgrabe. As to the first, all the normal tests for souls: thought, sensation, etc., fail, as far as we know, when applied to foetuses.

Now, contrary to these last two views of the matter, I maintain that the difficulty in deciding whether the foetus is a person is not that of hunting round till we find one crucial characteristic which will decide the question, for there is no such characteristic. The concept of a person is not that sort of concept. I will not be so adventurous as to say anything positive about "person"; I think it is enough to say that it is a concept with decidedly fuzzy edges, and that the foetus finds itself in the fuzz. The question "Is the foetus a person?" is like all those other borderline questions that philosophers have cited in the last 20 years: "Is a tomato a fruit or a vegetable?" "Is medicine a science?" "Are viruses living things?"

Supposing that what I have just said is correct, what follows about the rightness or wrongness of abortion? This depends on what view we take about how we establish the rightness or wrongness of *anything*. On the two most widely canvassed of such views, by intellectual apprehension and by committal, i.e., intuitionism and "existentialism," the results are extremely curious.

On the "existentialist" view we establish our moral principles by bare choice, by just committing ourselves to one principle rather than another. We are "self-legislating subjects in a kingdom of ends." But if this is so, our anxiety over whether the foetus is a person reveals a misunderstanding of our true position as moral agents. For to take it that the rule against killing people is already laid down and that our function is only to interpret this rule is to put ourselves in the position of judges applying an already promulgated law. Whereas, if we ourselves are the legislators there is no question of interpretation. If we laid down the law, we must have known what we intended by it—it would be absurd to say that someone said something and only later found out what he intended by it. If in some unclear case we want to legislate further, of course we *can*. But there is no question of agonising about it; there cannot be anything to agonise *about*. "To describe such ultimate decisions as arbitrary, because *ex hypothesi* everything which could be used to justify them has already been included in the decision, would be like saying that a complete description of the universe was utterly unfounded, because no further fact could be called upon in corroboration of it."[6]

The objection that may be felt here is that, after all, we *do* agonise. We know the effect of deciding one way or the other, but we still feel unable to make the *right* decision, or, as used to be said about Attitude Theories, we do not want merely to find out what *in fact* we approve of, but what is *worthy* of approval. The point is not that we lack feelings about the issue one way or the other. We feel that *some* attitude is appropriate, that some kind of behaviour is worthy of approval, but are unsure what it is.

Intuitionism does no better. Intuitionism claims that we know some moral statements just in the same way as we know some empirical statements. So "Abortion is wrong" is not merely rather like "Viruses are living creatures"; it is simply another example illustrating exactly the same thing—the only difference is that the one is about the moral world while the other is about the empirical world.

But in that case we must say exactly the same thing about both of them. We cannot straightforwardly answer the question "Are viruses living things?" We do not say: they *must* be either living or non-living, though perhaps we'll never know which. All we can say is: viruses satisfy *some* of the tests for living things, but not enough to make it unmisleading to say they *are* living things: "Say what you like." On analogy with this, the intuitionist is obliged to say that abortion is wrongish, though not wrong, and allright-ish, though not all right. If we *decide* to say that abortion is wrong, our decision is as arbitrary as the decision to say that viruses are living creatures. We are no longer making a simple report on the world of values. If someone says "We have *got* to decide, because we have to decide what to *do*," the intuitionist presumably replies that making a moral judgment is reporting on the world of values, what people *do* is another question. This is a neat example of that feature of intuitionism that prescriptivists have so long complained about.[7]

All this is rather unsettling. I would like now to give all the correct answers. Unfortunately I don't know them. However, it is something to have shown that arguments usually taken as valid are in fact fallacious. "We are in a better position in relation to a question if we not only do not know the answer, but do not even think we know."

[6] *Language of Morals,* p. 69.

[7] In case anyone should think that this difficulty can be surmounted by talking of "prima facie" duties, I should point out that this is not a conflict of duties but a doubtful application of one single duty.

Legal Aspects of the Decision Not to Prolong Life

George P. Fletcher

New medical techniques for prolonging life force both the legal and medical professions to re-examine their traditional attitudes toward life and death. The new set of problems emerges from the following recurrent situation: a comatose patient has a flat electroencephalogram reading; according to the best judgment, he has an infinitesimal chance of recovery; he can be sustained by intravenous therapy. What should his physician do? And in making his decision, how much weight should the physician give to the wishes of the family, to the financial condition of the family, and to the prospect that his time might be profitably used in caring for patients with a better chance for recovery?

It would be a mistake to think that our legal tradition contains clear answers to these questions. If this type of case demands moral sensitivity of the physician, it demands much more of the legal theorist and of the legislator. For, in confronting this type of case, the legal theorist must be concerned not only with situations in which the physician in the case is bestowed with sensitivity to the moral issues, but also with cases in which the physician and the family involved might be moved by lesser motives. The lawyer must be concerned about formulating legal norms that would permit a just resolution of the "clear" cases without providing an opportunity for abuse.

If one were to have a legal standard endorsing the physician's decision not to prolong life, should the standard be limited to the case of a doomed comatose patient with a flat EEG reading? Consider how this case blends so gradually into many related cases. First, there is the case of the doomed comatose patient who still shows some signs of brain activity. Does this patient *deserve* prolongation of life? Neither he nor his brother with a flat EEG reading can enjoy the beauties of life on earth. Why should we keep him alive? Secondly, compare the case of the doomed but conscious patient who can perceive the world about him but who suffers from excruciating pain. Is the fact of consciousness and the fact of an EEG reading sufficient to say that this man must be kept alive? In analyzing the physician's legal obligation to prolong a patient's life, we should keep in mind the infinitely graduated spectrum from the clear cases to the cases that are far from clear. The essential difficulty of approaching this problem as a lawyer is the difficulty of formulating standards for separating cases on one end of the spectrum from those on the other end.

There are a number of significant topics in the laws' relationship to the problem of prolonging life and to the more general problem of euthanasia. In recent years, we have seen a number of efforts toward legalizing voluntary euthanasia i.e., cases in which the patient is said to have consented to the termination of his life. And the literature abounds with vigorous debate for

Reprinted with permission of the publisher from the *Journal of the American Medical Association* 203:1, 119–22, January 1, 1968. Copyright 1968, American Medical Association.

and against these proposals. . . . Yet the term "prolongation of life" conveys slightly different meaning from that suggested by the term "euthanasia." The first term carries a suggestion of artificially lengthening a life that would otherwise end. In contrast, the latter term "euthanasia," sometimes called "mercy killing," suggests a beneficent termination of life that might otherwise continue. In speaking about voluntary euthanasia in particular, one has in mind cases in which the good of ending a man's suffering allegedly outweighs the wrong of intentionally terminating a life. The subject of euthanasia has received considerable comment in the legal literature. Thus, in this paper, I shall limit my remarks to the special problems posed by the term "prolongation of life."

ACTS AND OMISSIONS

One might begin legal analysis by considering one of the fundamental distinctions that runs through both the law of crimes and of torts. This is the distinction between acts and omissions, a distinction that has had a rich philosophical history as well. In acting, one intercedes to terminate life; one shoots and kills a man or one injects air in his veins. In omitting to act, one fails to intercede in order to preserve life and as a result, permits death to occur. It is the difference between active and passive behavior. It is also the difference between causing harm and permitting harm to occur. It is indisputably clear in the law that acting to terminate life is first-degree murder. This is true regardless of the motives of the actor. At one time in the evolution of the common law of murder, it might have made a difference whether a man was moved by emotions of spite or by emotions of mercy. One speaks of the element of "malice" in the common law definition of murder. Surely a man does not kill maliciously if he kills in order to save another man from unbearable suffering. But the concept of "malice" lost its force in the evolution of the common law; as early as the 16th and 17th centuries it came to mean nothing more significant than the requirement that the killing be intentional. Since a man killing for reasons of mercy does indeed kill intentionally, he kills maliciously—at least, according to the special dictionary of the law.

    Killing for reasons of mercy, like killing in order to rob one's victim, is murder. But one should recognize that this statement of the law is a statement of principle only. There is a gap between the law in theory and the law in practice. That the legal norm is severe and uncompromising does not mean that the people who administer the legal system are also severe and uncompromising. Prosecutors or grand juries may fail to indict someone who is clearly guilty of intentional euthanasia; judges or juries may acquit someone who is clearly guilty on the facts (and the acquittal is not appealable to a higher court); and even after conviction, judges often suspend the sentences of men who killed to end the suffering of their victim. . . . Despite these institutional checks against the severity of the law, some men guilty of killing for reasons of mercy are convicted and punished by imprisonment. But these cases of actual conviction and punishment do not include beneficent killings by medical practitioners. There is no case in the

Anglo-American tradition in which a doctor has been convicted of murder or manslaughter for having killed to end the suffering of his patient.

(In 1950, Dr. Herman Sander was brought to trial for injecting air into the veins of his cancer-stricken patient. He confessed the deed, and the attending nurse testified that the patient was still "gasping" when the doctor injected the air. Nonetheless, the motive of mercy prompted the jury of laymen to acquit Dr. Sanders [*Time,* March 6, 1950, p. 20; and *New York Times,* March 19, 1950, p. 1].)

The distinction between the law in theory and the law in action is critical when one turns to an examination of criminal or tort liability for omitting to render therapy and thus permitting a man to die. In this area, one can find no decided cases at all to support the theory of liability. Neither laymen nor doctors have been convicted of omitting to take steps that could have averted death. Yet it is clear as a matter of legal principle that a doctor would be liable for failing to take steps to save the life of his patient. One need only consider the following bizarre case. Dr. Brown is the family doctor of the Smith family and has been for several years. Tim Smith falls ill with pneumonia. Dr. Brown sees him once or twice at the family home and administers the necessary therapy. One evening, upon receiving a telephone call from the Smith family that Tim is in critical condition, Dr. Brown decides that he should prefer to remain at his bridge game than to visit the sick Smith child. In this case, Brown fails to render aid to the child. It is unquestionably clear that Brown would be liable criminally and civilly if death should ensue. That he has merely omitted to act, rather than asserted himself intentionally to end life, makes no difference in assessing his criminal and civil liability.

Of course, the doctor would not be under an obligation to respond to the call of a stranger who said that he needed help. But there is a difference between a stranger and someone who has put himself in the care of a physician. The factor of reliance and reasonable expectation that the doctor will render aid means that the doctor is legally obligated to do so. His failure to do so is then tantamount to an intentional infliction of harm. And as his motive, be it for good or ill, is irrelevant in analyzing his liability for intentional and assertive killing, his motive is also irrelevant in analyzing his liability for omitting to render aid when he is obligated to do so. Thus, it makes no difference whether a doctor omits to render aid because he prefers to continue playing bridge or if he does so in the hope that the patient's misery will come quickly to a natural end.

Thus, a doctor may be criminally and civilly liable either for intentionally taking life or for omitting to act and thus permitting death to occur. But the sources of these two legal prescriptions are different. And this difference in the source of the law may provide the key for the analysis of the doctor's liability in failing to prolong life in the cases discussed at the outset of this article. That a doctor may not actively kill is an application of the general principle that no man may actively kill a fellow human being. In contrast, the principle that a doctor may not omit to render aid to a patient justifiably relying upon him is a function of the special relationship that exists between doctor and patient. In cases of actions resulting in death, the doctor's duty arises from the simple fact that both he and his patients are human beings.

In cases of omissions resulting in death, the doctor's duty arises from the relationship between him and his patient. Thus, in analyzing the doctor's legal duty to his patient, one must take into consideration whether the question involved is an act or an omission. If it is an act, the relationship between the doctor and patient is irrelevant. If it is an omission, the relationship is all-controlling.

APPLYING THE DISTINCTION

With these theoretical distinctions in mind, we may turn to an analysis of specific aspects of medical decision not to prolong life. The first problem is to isolate the relevant medical activity. The recurrent pattern includes stopping cardiac resuscitation, turning off the respirator, removing the needle used in intravenous therapy. The problem, of course, is whether these activities are to be regarded as cases of acts terminating life or of omissions to render aid to sustain life. For, as we have seen, this initial decision of classification determines the subsequent legal analysis of the case. If turning off the respirator is an "act" under the law, then it is unequivocally forbidden: it is on a par with injecting air into the patient's veins. If, on the other hand, it is classified as an "omission," the analysis proceeds more flexibly. Whether it would be forbidden as an omission would depend on the demands imposed by the relationship between doctor and patient.

There are gaps in the law, and we are confronted with one of them. There is simply no way to bring to bear the legal authorities to determine whether the process of turning off the respirator is an act or an omission. It looks very much like an act, for it takes physical movement to turn off the respirator. But that fact need not be controlling. There might be "acts" without physical movement, as, for example, if one should sit motionless in the driver's seat as one's car heads toward an intended victim. That would surely be an act causing death; it would be first-degree murder regardless of the relationship between the victim and his assassin. Similarly, there might be cases of omissions involving physical exertions, perhaps even the effort required to turn off the respirator. The problem is not whether there is or there is not physical movement; there must be another test.

That other test, I should propose, is whether on all the facts we should be inclined to speak of the activity as one that causes harm or one merely that permits harm to occur. The usage of the verbs "causing" and "permitting" corresponds to the distinction in the clear cases between acts and omissions. If one injects air into the veins of a doomed patient, he is causing harm. On the other hand, if the doctor fails to stop on the highway to aid a stranger injured in an automobile accident, it is difficult to say that the doctor is causing harm; he surely is permitting harm to occur, and he might be morally blameworthy for that; but as the verb "cause" is ordinarily used, his failing to stop is not the cause of the harm.

As native speakers of English, we are equipped with a linguistic sensitivity for the distinction between causing harm and permitting harm to occur. And we should employ that sensitivity in classifying the hard cases arising in discussions of the prolongation of life. Is turning off the respirator an instance of causing death or permitting death to occur? If the patient is beyond recovery and on the verge of death, one balks at saying that the activity causes death. It is far more natural to speak of the case as one of permitting death to occur. It is significant that we are inclined to refer to the respirator as a means for prolonging life; we wouldn't speak of treatment for pneumonia in the same way. The use of the term "prolongation of life" builds on the same perception of reality that prompts us to say that turning off the respirator is an activity permitting death to occur, rather than causing death. And that basic perception is that using the respirator interferes artificially in the pattern of events. Of course, the perception of the natural and of the artificial is a function of time and culture. What may seem artificial today, may be a matter of course in ten years. Nonetheless, one *does* perceive many uses of the respirator today as artificial prolongations of life. And that sense of artificiality should be enough to determine the legal classification of the case. Because we are prompted to refer to the activity of turning off the respirator as activity permitting death to occur, rather than causing death, we may classify the case as an omission rather than as an act.

Let it be clear that using the label "omission" does not mean that the physician is free to do what he chooses. For he may be liable for omitting to do that which he is legally obligated to do. But moving from the arena of acts to the arena of omissions does yield some flexibility. Not all omissions are illegal; the problem is to determine which are and which are not. As we noted above, the legality of an omission to render aid depends on the relationship between the doctor and his patient. To take a clear case, let us suppose that prior to the onset of a terminal illness, the patient demands that his physician do everything to keep him alive and breathing as long as possible. And the physician responds, "Even if you have a flat EEG reading and there is no chance of recovery?" "Yes," the patient replies. If the doctor agrees to this bizarre demand, he does become obligated to keep the respirator going indefinitely. Thankfully, cases of this type do not occur in day-to-day medical practice. In the average case, the patient hasn't given a thought to the problem, and his physician is not likely to alert him to it. The problem then is whether there is an implicit understanding between physician and patient as to how the physician should proceed in the last stages of a terminal illness. An implicit understanding would be something akin to the expectation of a passenger on a bus that the driver plans to stop at the regular stops along the route. Might there be an understanding of that sort about what the physician should do if the patient is in a coma and dependent on a mechanical respirator? This is not the kind of thing regarding which the average man has expectations. And if he did, they would be expectations that would be based on the customary practices of the time. If he had heard about a number of cases in which patients had been sustained for long periods of time on respirators, he might (at least prior to going into the coma) expect that he would be similarly sustained.

Thus, the analysis leads us along the following path. The doctor's duty to prolong life is a function of his relationship with his patient, and, in the typical case, that relationship devolves into the patient's expectations of the treatment he will receive. Those expectations, in turn, are a function of the practices prevailing in the community at the time. And on what do those practices depend? Practices in the use of respirators to prolong life are no more and no less than what doctors actually do in the time and place. Thus, we have come full circle. We began the inquiry by asking: is it legally permissible for doctors to turn off respirators used to prolong the life of doomed patients? And the answer after our tortuous journey is simply this: it all depends on what doctors customarily do. The law is sometimes no more precise than that.

The moral of our circular journey is that doctors are in a position to fashion their own law to deal with cases of prolongation of life. By establishing customary standards, they may determine the expectations of their patients and thus regulate the understanding and the relationship between doctor and patient. And by regulating that relationship, they may control their legal obligations to render aid to doomed patients.

Thus the medical profession confronts the challenge of developing humane and sensitive customary standards for guiding decisions to prolong the lives of terminal patients. This is not a challenge that the profession may shirk. For the doctor's legal duties to render aid derive from his relationship with the patient. That relationship, along with the expectations implicit in it, is the responsibility of the individual doctor and the individual patient. With respect to problems not commonly discussed by the doctor with his patient, particularly the problems of prolonging life, the responsibility for the patient's expectations lies with the medical profession as a whole.

It will not do for the medical profession to demand that we lawyers devise a legal definition of death. There might be many uses of a legal definition of death; one might wish to know the time of death to apply rules on the disposition of the decedent's estate. But this is not what medical practitioners have in mind. It seems that they should like to have a clear standard for deciding when and when not to render aid to their dying patients. Sweden's Dr. Crafoord has proposed that a patient be declared legally dead when his EEG reading is flat. The standard is clear and easy to apply, but it is morally insensitive. Should one totally disregard all the other factors: the likelihood of recovery, the family's financial position, the patient's expressed wishes, other demands on hospital facilities and the attending physician's time? Even if we could formulate a just resolution of these conflicting factors today, would it be a resolution that would remain fair in the face of medical innovation? It surely would not. What one regards as excessive and extraordinary today might well become commonplace in a few years. A legal standard of death, which would define the limits of the doctor's duty to his patient, would be an overly rigid solution to a problem that changes dimensions with each medical innovation.

The Problem of Abortion and the Doctrine of the Double Effect

Philippa Foot

One of the reasons why most of us feel puzzled about the problem of abortion is that we want, and do not want, to allow to the unborn child the rights that belong to adults and children. When we think of a baby about to be born it seems absurd to think that the next few minutes or even hours could make so radical a difference to its status; yet as we go back in the life of the foetus we are more and more reluctant to say that this is a human being and must be treated as such. No doubt this is the deepest source of our dilemma, but it is not the only one. For we are also confused about the general question of what we may and may not do where the interests of human beings conflict. We have strong intuitions about certain cases; saying, for instance, that it is all right to raise the level of education in our country, though statistics allow us to predict that a rise in the suicide rate will follow, while it is not all right to kill the feeble-minded to aid cancer research. It is not easy, however, to see the principles involved, and one way of throwing light on the abortion issue will be by setting up parallels involving adults or children once born. So we will be able to isolate the "equal rights" issue, and should be able to make some advance.

I shall not, of course, discuss all the principles that may be used in deciding what to do where the interest or rights of human beings conflict. What I want to do is to look at one particular theory, known as the "doctrine of the double effect" which is invoked by Catholics in support of their views on abortion but supposed by them to apply elsewhere. As used in the abortion argument this doctrine has often seemed to non-Catholics to be a piece of complete sophistry. In the last number of the *Oxford Review* it was given short shrift by Professor Hart.[1] And yet this principle has seemed to some non-Catholics as well as to Catholics to stand as the only defence against decisions on other issues that are quite unacceptable. It will help us in our difficulty about abortion if this conflict can be resolved.

The doctrine of the double effect is based on a distinction between what a man foresees as a result of his voluntary action and what, in the strict sense, he intends. He intends in the strictest sense both those things that he aims at as ends and those that he aims at as means to his ends. The latter may be regretted in themselves but nevertheless desired for the sake of the end, as we may intend to keep dangerous lunatics confined for the sake of our safety. By contrast a man is said not strictly, or directly, to intend the foreseen consequences of his voluntary actions where these are neither the

Reprinted with the author's permission from the *Oxford Review*, No. 5, 5–15, (1967)
[1]H. L. A. Hart, "Intention and Punishment," *Oxford Review*, Number 4, Hilary 1967. I owe much to this article and to a conversation with Professor Hart, though I do not know whether he will approve of what follows.

end at which he is aiming nor the means to this end. Whether the word "intention" should be applied in both cases is not of course what matters: Bentham spoke of "oblique intention," contrasting it with the "direct intention" of ends and means, and we may as well follow his terminology. Everyone must recognize that some such distinction can be made, though it may be made in a number of different ways, and it is the distinction that is crucial to the doctrine of the double effect. The words "double effect" refer to the two effects that an action may produce: the one aimed at, and the one foreseen but in no way desired. By "the doctrine of the double effect" I mean the thesis that it is sometimes permissible to bring about by oblique intention what one may not directly intend. Thus the distinction is held to be relevant to moral decision in certain difficult cases. It is said for instance that the operation of hysterectomy involves the death of the foetus as the foreseen but not strictly or directly intended consequence of the surgeon's act, while other operations kill the child and count as the direct intention of taking an innocent life, a distinction that has evoked particularly bitter reactions on the part of non-Catholics. If you are permitted to bring about the death of the child, what does it matter how it is done? The doctrine of the double effect is also used to show why in another case, where a woman in labour will die unless a craniotomy operation is performed, the intervention is not to be condoned. There, it is said, we may not operate but must let the mother die. We foresee her death but do not directly intend it, whereas to crush the skull of the child would count as direct intention of its death.[2]

This last application of the doctrine has been queried by Professor Hart on the ground that the child's death is not strictly a means to saving the mother's life and should logically be treated as an unwanted but foreseen consequence by those who make use of the distinction between direct and oblique intention. To interpret the doctrine in this way is perfectly reasonable given the language that has been used; it would, however, make nonsense of it from the beginning. A certain event may be desired under one of its descriptions, unwanted under another, but we cannot treat these as two different events, one of which is aimed at and the other not. And even if it be argued that there are here two different events—the crushing of the child's skull and its death—the two are obviously much too close for an application of the doctrine of the double effect. To see how odd it would be to apply the principle like this we may consider the story, well known to philosophers, of the fat man stuck in the mouth of the cave. A party of potholers have imprudently allowed the fat man to lead them as they make their way out of the cave, and he gets stuck, trapping the others behind him. Obviously the right thing to do is to sit down and wait until the fat man grows thin; but philosophers have arranged that flood waters should be rising within the cave. Luckily (luckily?) the trapped party have with them a stick of dynamite with which they can blast the fat man out of the mouth

[2]For discussions of the Catholic doctrine on abortion see Glanville Williams, *The Sanctity of Life and the Criminal Law* (New York, 1957); also N. St. John Stevas, *The Right to Life* (London, 1963).

of the cave. Either they use the dynamite or they drown. In one version the fat man, whose head is *in* the cave, will drown with them; in the other he will be rescued in due course.[3] Problem: may they use the dynamite or not? Later we will find parallels to this example. Here it is introduced for light relief and because it will serve to show how ridiculous one version of the doctrine of the double effect would be. For suppose that the trapped explorers were to argue that the death of the fat man might be taken as a merely foreseen consequence of the act of blowing him up. ("We didn't want to kill him . . . only to blow him into small pieces" or even ". . . only to blast him out of the mouth of the cave.") I believe that those who use the doctrine of the double effect would rightly reject such a suggestion, though they will, of course, have considerable difficulty in explaining where the line is to be drawn. What is to be the criterion of "closeness" if we say that anything very close to what we are literally aiming at counts as if part of our aim?

Let us leave this difficulty aside and return to the arguments for and against the doctrine, supposing it to be formulated in the way considered most effective by its supporters, and ourselves bypassing the trouble by taking what must on any reasonable definition be clear cases of "direct" or "oblique" intention.

The first point that should be made clear, in fairness to the theory, is that no one is suggesting that it does not matter what you bring about as long as you merely foresee and do not strictly intend the evil that follows. We might think, for instance, of the (actual) case of wicked merchants selling, for cooking, oil they knew to be poisonous and thereby killing a number of innocent people, comparing and contrasting it with that of some unemployed gravediggers, desperate for custom, who got hold of this same oil and sold it (or perhaps *they* secretly gave it away) in order to create orders for graves. They strictly (directly) intend the deaths they cause, while the merchants could say that it was not part of their *plan* that anyone should die. In morality, as in law, the merchants, like the gravediggers, would be considered as murderers; nor are the supporters of the doctrine of the double effect bound to say that there is the least difference between them in respect of moral turpitude. What they are committed to is the thesis that *sometimes* it makes a difference to the permissibility of an action involving harm to others that this harm, although foreseen, is not part of the agent's direct intention. An end such as earning one's living is clearly not such as to justify *either* the direct or oblique intention of the death of innocent people, but in certain cases one is justified in bringing about knowingly what one could not directly intend.

It is now time to say why this doctrine should be taken seriously in spite of the fact that it sounds rather odd, that there are difficulties about the distinction on which it depends, and that it seemed to yield one sophistical conclusion when applied to the problem of abortion. The reason for its appeal is that its opponents have often *seemed* to be committed to quite indefensible views. Thus the controversy has raged around examples such

[3]It was Professor Hart who drew my attention to this distinction.

as the following. Suppose that a judge or magistrate is faced with rioters demanding that a culprit be found for a certain crime and threatening otherwise to take their own bloody revenge on a particular section of the community. The real culprit being unknown, the judge sees himself as able to prevent the bloodshed only by framing some innocent person and having him executed. Beside this example is placed another in which a pilot whose aeroplane is about to crash is deciding whether to steer from a more to a less inhabited area. To make the parallel as close as possible it may rather be supposed that he is the driver of a runaway tram which he can only steer from one narrow track on to another; five men are working on one track and one man on the other; anyone on the track he enters is bound to be killed. In the case of the riots the mob have five hostages, so that in both the exchange is supposed to be one man's life for the lives of five. The question is why we should say, without hesitation, that the driver should steer for the less occupied track, while most of us would be appalled at the idea that the innocent man could be framed. It may be suggested that the special feature of the latter case is that it involves the corruption of justice, and this is, of course, very important indeed. But if we remove that special feature, supposing that some private individual is to kill an innocent person and pass him off as the criminal we still find ourselves horrified by the idea. The doctrine of the double effect offers us a way out of the difficulty, insisting that it is one thing to steer towards someone foreseeing that you will kill him and another to aim at his death as part of your plan. Moreover there is one very important element of good in what is here insisted. In real life it would hardly ever be certain that the man on the narrow track would be killed. Perhaps he might find a foothold on the side of the tunnel and cling on as the vehicle hurtled by. The driver of the tram does not then leap off and brain him with a crowbar. This judge, however, needs the death of the innocent man for his (good) purposes. If the victim proves hard to hang he must see to it that he dies another way. To choose to execute him is to choose that this evil *shall come about,* and this must therefore count as a *certainty* in weighing up the good and evil involved. The distinction between direct and oblique intention is crucial here, and is of great importance in an uncertain world. Nevertheless this is no way to defend the doctrine of the double effect. For the question is whether the difference between aiming at something and obliquely intending it is *in itself* relevant to moral decisions; not whether it is important when correlated with a difference of certainty in the balance of good and evil. Moreover we are particularly interested in the application of the doctrine of the double effect to the question of abortion, and no one can deny that in medicine there are sometimes certainties so complete that it would be a mere quibble to speak of the "probable outcome" of this course of action or that. It is not, therefore, with a merely philosophical interest that we should put aside the uncertainty and scrutinize the examples to test the doctrine of the double effect. Why can we not argue from the case of the steering driver to that of the judge?

Another pair of examples poses a similar problem. We are about to give to a patient who needs it to save his life a massive dose of a certain drug in short supply. There arrive, however, five other patients each of whom could be saved by one-fifth of that dose. We say with regret that we cannot spare our whole supply of the drug for a single patient, just as we should say that we could not spare the whole resources of a ward for one dangerously ill individual when ambulances arrive bringing in the victims of a multiple crash. We feel bound to let one man die rather than many if that is our only choice. Why then do we not feel justified in killing people in the interests of cancer research or to obtain, let us say, spare parts for grafting on to those who need them? We can suppose, similarly, that several dangerously ill people can be saved only if we kill a certain individual and make a serum from his dead body. (These examples are not over fanciful considering present controversies about prolonging the life of mortally ill patients whose eyes or kidneys are to be used for others.) Why cannot we argue from the case of the scarce drug to that of the body needed for medical purposes? Once again the doctrine of the double effect comes up with an explanation. In one kind of case but not the other we aim at the death of the innocent man.

A further argument suggests that if the doctrine of the double effect is rejected this has the consequence of putting us hopelessly in the power of bad men. Suppose for example that some tyrant should threaten to torture five men if we ourselves would not torture one. Would it be our duty to do so, supposing we believed him, because this would be no different from choosing to rescue five men from his tortures rather than one? If so anyone who wants us to do something we think wrong has only to threaten that otherwise he himself will do something we think worse. A mad murderer, known to keep his promises, could thus make it our duty to kill some innocent citizen to prevent him from killing two. From this conclusion we are again rescued by the doctrine of the double effect. If we refuse, we foresee that the greater number will be killed but we do not intend it: it is he who intends (that is strictly or directly intends) the death of innocent persons; we do not.

At one time I thought that these arguments in favour of the doctrine of the double effect were conclusive, but I now believe that the conflict should be solved in another way. The clue that we should follow is that the strength of the doctrine seems to lie in the distinction it makes between what we do (equated with direct intention) and what we allow (thought of as obliquely intended). Indeed it is interesting that the disputants tend to argue about whether we are to be held responsible for what we allow as we are for what we do.[4] Yet it is not obvious that this is what they should be discussing, since the distinction between what one does and what one allows to happen is not the same as that between direct and oblique intention. To see this one has only to consider that it is possible *deliberately* to allow something to happen, aiming at it either for its own sake or as part of one's

[4]See, e.g., J. Bennett, "Whatever the Consequences," *Analysis,* January 1966, and G. E. M. Anscombe's reply in *Analysis,* June 1966. See also Miss Anscombe's "Modern Moral Philosophy" in *Philosophy,* January 1958.

plan for obtaining something else. So one person might want another person dead, and deliberately allow him to die. And again one may be said to *do* things that one does not aim at, as the steering driver would kill the man on the track. Moreover there is a large class of things said to be brought about rather than either done or allowed, and either kind of intention is possible. So it is possible to *bring about* a man's death by getting him to go to sea in a leaky boat, and the intention of his death may be either direct or oblique.

Whatever it may, or may not, have to do with the doctrine of the double effect, the idea of *allowing* is worth looking into in this context. I shall leave aside the special case of giving permission, which involves the idea of authority, and consider the two main divisions into which cases of allowing seem to fall. There is firstly the allowing which is forbearing to prevent. For this we need a sequence thought of as somehow already in train, and something that the agent could do to intervene. (The agent must be able to intervene, but does not do so.) So, for instance, he could warn someone, but *allows* him to walk into a trap. He could feed an animal but *allows* it to die for lack of food. He could stop a leaking tap but *allows* the water to go on flowing. This is the case of allowing with which we shall be concerned, but the other should be mentioned. It is the kind of allowing which is roughly equivalent to *enabling;* the root idea being the removal of some obstacle which is, as it were, holding back a train of events. So someone may remove a plug and *allow* water to flow; open a door and *allow* an animal to get out; or give someone money and *allow* him to get back on his feet.

The first kind of allowing requires an omission, but there is no other general correlation between omission and allowing, commission and bringing about or doing. An actor who fails to turn up for a performance will generally spoil it rather than allow it to be spoiled. I mention the distinction between omission and commission only to set it aside.

Thinking of the first kind of allowing (forbearing to prevent), we should ask whether there is any difference, from the moral point of view, between what one does or causes and what one merely allows. It seems clear that on occasions one is just as bad as the other, as is recognized in both morality and law. A man may murder his child or his aged relatives, by allowing them to die of starvation as well as by giving poison; he may also be convicted of murder on either account. In another case we would, however, make a distinction. Most of us allow people to die of starvation in India and Africa, and there is surely something wrong with us that we do; it would be nonsense, however, to pretend that it is only in law that we make a distinction between allowing people in the underdeveloped countries to die of starvation and sending them poisoned food. There is worked into our moral system a distinction between what we owe people in the form of aid and what we owe them in the way of non-interference. Salmond, in his *Jurisprudence*, expressed as follows the distinction between the two.

> A positive right corresponds to a positive duty, and is a right that he on whom the duty lies shall do some positive act on behalf of the person entitled. A negative right corresponds to a negative duty, and is a right that the person

bound shall refrain from some act which would operate to the prejudice of the person entitled. The former is a right to be positively benefited; the latter is merely a right not to be harmed."[5]

As a general account of rights and duties this is defective, since not all are so closely connected with benefit and harm. Nevertheless for our purposes it will do well. Let us speak of negative duties when thinking of the obligation to refrain from such things as killing or robbing, and of the positive duty, e.g., to look after children or aged parents. It will be useful, however, to extend the notion of positive duty beyond the range of things that are strictly called duties, bringing acts of charity under this heading. These are owed only in a rather loose sense, and some acts of charity could hardly be said to be *owed* at all, so I am not following ordinary usage at this point.

Let us now see whether the distinction of negative and positive duties explains why we see differently the action of the steering driver and that of the judge, of the doctors who withhold the scarce drug and those who obtain a body for medical purposes, of those who choose to rescue the five men rather than one man from torture and those who are ready to torture the one man themselves in order to save five. In each case we have a conflict of duties, but what kind of duties are they? Are we, in each case, weighing positive duties against positive, negative against negative, or one against the other? Is the duty to refrain from injury, or rather to bring aid?

The steering driver faces a conflict of negative duties, since it is his duty to avoid injuring five men and also his duty to avoid injuring one. In the circumstances he is not able to avoid both, and it seems clear that he should do the least injury he can. The judge, however, is weighing the duty of not inflicting injury against the duty of bringing aid. He wants to rescue the innocent people threatened with death but can do so only by inflicting injury himself. Since one does not *in general* have the same duty to help people as to refrain from injuring them, it is not possible to argue to a conclusion about what he should do from the steering driver case. It is interesting that, even where the strictest duty of positive aid exists, this still does not weigh as if a negative duty were involved. It is not, for instance, permissible to commit a murder to bring one's starving children food. If the choice is between inflicting injury on one or many there seems only one rational course of action; if the choice is between aid to some at the cost of injury to others, and refusing to inflict the injury to bring the aid, the whole matter is open to dispute. So it is not inconsistent of us to think that the driver must steer for the road on which only one man stands while the judge (or his equivalent) may not kill the innocent person in order to stop the riots. Let us now consider the second pair of examples, which concern the scarce drug on the one hand and on the other the body needed to save lives. Once again we find a difference based on the distinction between the duty to avoid injury and the duty to provide aid. Where one man needs a massive dose of the drug and we withhold it from him in order to save five men, we are

[5]J. Salmond, *Jurisprudence*, 11th edition, p. 283.

weighing aid against aid. But if we consider killing a man in order to use his body to save others, we are thinking of doing him injury to bring others aid. In an interesting variant of the model, we may suppose that instead of killing someone we deliberately let him die. (Perhaps he is a beggar to whom we are thinking of giving food, but then we say "No, they need bodies for medical research.") Here it does seem relevant that in allowing him to die we are aiming at his death, but presumably we are inclined to see this as a violation of negative rather than positive duty. If this is right, we see why we are unable in either case to argue to a conclusion from the case of the scarce drug.

In the examples involving the torture of one man or five men, the principle seems to be the same as for the last pair. If we are bringing aid (rescuing people about to be tortured by the tyrant), we must obviously rescue the larger rather than the smaller group. It does not follow, however, that we would be justified in inflicting the injury, or getting a third person to do so, in order to save the five. We may therefore refuse to be forced into acting by the threats of bad men. To refrain from inflicting injury ourselves is a stricter duty than to prevent other people from inflicting injury, which is not to say that the other is not a very strict duty indeed.

So far the conclusions are the same as those at which we might arrive following the doctrine of the double effect, but in others they will be different, and the advantage seems to be all on the side of the alternative. Suppose, for instance, that there are five patients in a hospital whose lives could be saved by the manufacture of a certain gas, but that this inevitably releases lethal fumes into the room of another patient whom for some reason we are unable to move. His death, being of no use to us, is clearly a side effect, and not directly intended. Why then is the case different from that of the scarce drug, if the point about that is that we foresaw but did not strictly intend the death of the single patient? Yet it surely is different. The relatives of the gassed patient would presumably be successful if they sued the hospital and the whole story came out. We may find it particularly revolting that someone should be *used* as in the case where he is killed or allowed to die in the interest of medical research, and the fact of *using* may even determine what we would decide to do in some cases, but the principle seems unimportant compared with our reluctance to bring such injury for the sake of giving aid.

My conclusion is that the distinction between direct and oblique intention plays only a quite subsidiary role in determining what we say in these cases, while the distinction between avoiding injury and bringing aid is very important indeed. I have not, of course, argued that there are no other principles. For instance it clearly makes a difference whether our positive duty is a strict duty or rather an act of charity: feeding our own children or feeding those in far away countries. It may also make a difference whether the person about to suffer is one thought of as uninvolved in the threatened disaster, and whether it is his presence that constitutes the threat to the others. In many cases we find it very hard to know what to say, and I have not been arguing for any general conclusion such as that we may never, whatever the balance of good and evil, bring injury to one for the sake of aid to others, even when this injury amounts to death. I have only tried to show that even if we reject the doctrine of the double effect we are not forced to the conclusion that the size of the evil must always be our guide.

Let us now return to the problem of abortion, carrying out our plan of finding parallels involving adults or children rather than the unborn. We must say something about the different cases in which abortion might be considered on medical grounds.

First of all there is the situation in which nothing that can be done will save the life of child and mother, but where the life of the mother can be saved by killing the child. This is parallel to the case of the fat man in the mouth of the cave who is bound to be drowned with the others if nothing is done. Given the certainty of the outcome, as it was postulated, there is no serious conflict of interests here, since the fat man will perish in either case, and it is reasonable that the action that will save someone should be done. It is a great objection to those who argue that the direct intention of the death of an innocent person is never justifiable that the edict will apply even in this case. The Catholic doctrine on abortion must here conflict with that of most reasonable men. Moreover we would be justified in performing the operation whatever the method used, and it is neither a necessary nor a good justification of the special case of hysterectomy that the child's death is not directly intended, being rather a foreseen consequence of what is done. What difference could it make as to how the death is brought about?

Secondly we have the case in which it is possible to perform an operation which will save the mother and kill the child or kill the mother and save the child. This is parallel to the famous case of the shipwrecked mariners who believed that they must throw someone overboard if their boat was not to founder in a storm, and to the other famous case of the two sailors, Dudley and Stephens, who killed and ate the cabin boy when adrift on the sea without food. Here again there is no conflict of interests so far as the decision to act is concerned; only in deciding whom to save. Once again it would be reasonable to act, though one would respect someone who held back from the appalling action either because he preferred to perish rather than do such a thing or because he held on past the limits of reasonable hope. In real life the certainties postulated by philosophers hardly ever exist, and Dudley and Stephens were rescued not long after their ghastly meal. Nevertheless if the certainty were absolute, as it might be in the abortion case, it would seem better to save one than none. Probably we should decide in favour of the mother when weighing her life against that of the unborn child, but it is interesting that, a few years later, we might easily decide it the other way.

The worst dilemma comes in the third kind of example where to save the mother we must kill the child, say by crushing its skull, while if nothing is done the mother will perish but the child can be safely delivered after her death. Here the doctrine of the double effect has been invoked to show that we may not intervene, since the child's death would be directly intended while the mother's would not. On a strict parallel with cases not involving the unborn we might find the conclusion correct though the reason given was wrong. Suppose, for instance, that in later life the presence of a child was certain to bring death to the mother. We would surely not think ourselves justified in ridding her of it by a process that involved its death. For in general we do not think that we can kill one innocent person to rescue another, quite apart from the special care that we feel is due to children once they have prudently got themselves born. What we would be prepared to do when a great many people were involved is another matter, and this is probably the key to one quite common view of abortion on the part of those who take quite seriously the rights of the unborn child. They probably feel that if *enough* people are involved one must be sacrificed, and they think of the mother's life against the unborn child's life as if it were many against one. But of course many people do not view it like this at all, having no inclination to accord to the foetus or unborn child anything like ordinary human status in the matter of rights. I have not been arguing for or against these points of view but only trying to discern some of the currents that are pulling us back and forth. The levity of the examples is not meant to offend.

From "Whatever the Consequences"

Jonathan Bennett

The following kind of thing can occur.[1] A woman in labour will certainly die unless an operation is performed in which the head of her unborn child is crushed or dissected; while if it is not performed the child can be delivered, alive, by post-mortem Caesarian section. This presents a straight choice between the woman's life and the child's.

In a particular instance of this kind, some people would argue for securing the woman's survival on the basis of the special facts of the case: the woman's terror, or her place in an established network of affections and dependences, or the child's physical defects, and so on. For them, the argument could go the other way in another instance, even if only in a very special one—e.g., where the child is well formed and the woman has cancer which will kill her within a month anyway.

Others would favour the woman's survival in the instance of the kind presented in my opening paragraph, on the grounds that women are human while unborn children are not. This dubious argument does not need to be attacked here, and I shall ignore it.

Others again would say, just on the facts as stated in my first paragraph, that the *child* must be allowed to survive. Their objection to any operation in which an unborn child's head is crushed, whatever the special features of the case, goes like this:

Reprinted with permission of the publisher from *Analysis* 26: 3, 83–97, 1966.

[1]J. K. Feeney and A. P. Barry in *Journal of Obstetrics and Gynaecology of the British Empire* (1954), p. 61. R. L. Cecil and H. F. Conn (eds.), *The Specialties in General Practice* (Philadelphia, 1957), p. 410.

To do the operation would be to kill the child, while to refrain from doing it would not be to kill the woman but merely to conduct oneself in such a way that—as a foreseen but unwanted consequence—the woman died. The question we should ask is not: "The woman's life or the child's?", but rather: "To kill, or not to kill, an innocent human?" The answer to *that* is that it is always absolutely wrong to kill an innocent human, even in such dismal circumstances as these.

This line of thought needs to be attacked. Some able people find it acceptable; it is presupposed by the Principle of Double Effect[2] which permeates Roman Catholic writing on morals; and I cannot find any published statement of the extremely strong philosophical case for its rejection. . . .

ACTING AND REFRAINING

Suppose the obstetrician does not operate, and the woman dies. He does not kill her, but he *lets her die.* The reproach suggested by these words is just an unavoidable nuisance, and I shall not argue from it. When I say "he lets her die," I mean only that he knowingly refrains from preventing her death which he alone could prevent, and he cannot say that her survival is in a general way 'none of my business' or "not [even *prima facie*] my concern." If my arguments so far are correct, then this one fact—the fact that the non-operating obstetrician *lets the woman die* but does not *kill her*—is the only remaining feature of the situation which the conservative can hope to adduce as supporting his judgment about what ought to be done in every instance of the obstetrical example.[3] Let us examine the difference between "X killed Y" and "X let Y die."

Some cases of letting-die are also cases of killing. If on a dark night X knows that Y's next step will take him over the edge of a high cliff, and he refrains from uttering a simple word of warning because he doesn't care or because he wants Y dead, then it is natural to say not only that X lets Y die but also that he kills him—even if it was not X who suggested the route, removed the fence from the cliff-top, *etc.* Cases like this, where a failure-to-prevent is described as a doing partly *because* it is judged to be wicked or indefensible, are beside my present point; for I want to see what difference there is between killing and letting-die which might be a *basis for* a moral judgment. Anyway, the letting-die which is also killing must involve malice or wanton indifference, and there is nothing like that in the obstetrical example. In short, to count these cases as relevant to the obstetrical example would be to suggest that not-operating would after all be killing the woman —a plainly false suggestion which I have disavowed. I wish to criticise the

[2]See G. Kelly, *Medico-Moral Problems* (Dublin, 1955), p. 20; C. J. McFadden, *Medical Ethics* (London, 1962), pp. 27–33; T. J. O'Donnell, *Morals in Medicine* (London, 1959), pp. 39–44; N. St. John-Stevas, *The Right to Life* (London 1963), p. 71.

[3]In a case where the child cannot survive anyway: "It is a question of the *direct taking* of one innocent life or merely *permitting* two deaths. In other words, there is question of one *murder* against two deaths . . ." Kelly, *op. cit.,* p. 181.

conservative's arguments, not to deny his premiss. So from now on I shall ignore cases of letting-die which are also cases of killing; and it will make for brevity to pretend that they do not exist. For example, I shall say that killing involves moving one's body—which is false of some of these cases, but true of all others.

One more preliminary point: the purposes of the present enquiry do not demand that a full analysis be given either of "X killed Y" or of "X let Y die." We can ignore any implications either may have about what X (a) expected, (b) should have expected, or (c) was aiming at; for the obstetrical example is symmetrical in all those respects. We can also ignore the fact that "X killed Y" loosely implies something about (e) immediacy which is not implied by "X let Y die," for immediacy in itself has no moral significance.

Consider the statement that *Joe killed the calf.* A certain aspect of the analysis of this will help us to see how it relates to *Joe let the calf die.* To say that Joe killed the calf is to say that

(1) Joe moved his body

and

(2) the calf died;

but it is also to say something about how Joe's moving was connected with the calf's dying—something to the effect that

(3) if Joe had not moved as he did, the calf would not have died.

How is (3) to be interpreted? We might take it, rather strictly, as saying

(3'): If Joe had moved in *any* other way, the calf would not have died.

This, however, is too strong to be a necessary condition of Joe's having killed the calf. Joe may have killed the calf even if he could have moved in other ways which would equally have involved the calf's dying. Suppose that Joe cut the calf's throat, but could have shot it instead: in that case he clearly killed it; but (3') denies that he killed it, because the calf might still have died even if Joe had not moved in just the way he did.

We might adopt a weaker reading of (3), namely as saying

(3"): Joe could have moved in *some* other way without the calf's dying.

But where (3') was too strong to be necessary, (3") is too weak to express a sufficient connexion between Joe's moving and the calf's dying. It counts Joe as having killed the calf not only in cases where we should ordinarily say that he killed it but also in cases where the most we should say is that he let it die.

The truth lies somewhere between (3'), which is appropriate to "Joe killed the calf in the only way open to him," and (3"), which is appropriate to "Joe killed the calf or let it die." Specifically, the connexion between Joe's moving and the calf's dying which is appropriate to "Joe killed the calf" but not to "Joe let the calf die" is expressed by

> (3'''): Of all the other ways in which Joe might have moved, *relatively few* satisfy the condition: if Joe had moved like that, the calf would have died.

And the connexion which is appropriate to "Joe let the calf die" but not to "Joe killed the calf" is expressed by

> (4): Of all the other ways in which Joe might have moved, *almost all* satisfy the condition: if Joe had moved like that, the calf would have died.

This brings me to the main thesis of the present section: apart from the factors I have excluded as already dealt with, the difference between "X killed Y" and "X let Y die" *is* the difference between (3''') and (4). When the killing/letting-die distinction is stripped of its implications regarding immediacy, intention, *etc.*—which lack moral significance or don't apply to the example—all that remains is a distinction having to do with where a set of movements lies on the scale which has "the only set of movements which would have produced that upshot" at one end and "movements other than the only set which would have produced that upshot" at the other.

This, then, is the conservative's residual basis for a moral discrimination between operating and not-operating. Operating would be killing: if the obstetrician makes movements which constitute operating, then the child will die; and there are very few other movements he could make which would also involve the child's dying. Not-operating would only be letting-die: if throughout the time when he could be operating the obstetrician makes movements which constitute not-operating, then the woman will die; but the vast majority of alternative movements he could make during that time would equally involve the woman's dying. I do not see how anyone doing his own moral thinking about the matter could find the least shred of moral significance in *this* difference between operating and not-operating.

Suppose you are told that X killed Y in the only way possible in the circumstances; and this, perhaps together with certain other details of the case, leads you to judge X's conduct adversely. Then you are told: "You have been misled: there is another way in which X could have killed Y." Then a third informant says: "That is wrong too: there are two other ways ... *etc.*" Then a fourth: "No: there are three other ways ... *etc.*" Clearly, these successive corrections put no pressure at all on your original judgment: you will not think it relevant to your judgment on X's killing of Y that it could have been carried out in any one of *n* different ways. But the move from "X killed Y in the only possible way" to "X killed Y in one of the only five possible ways" is of the same *kind* as the move from "X killed Y" to "X let Y die" (except for the latter's implications about immediacy); and the moral insignificance of the former move is evidence for the moral insignificance of the latter move also.

The difference between "X killed Y" and "X let Y die" is the sum-total of a vast number of differences such as that between "X killed Y in one of the only n possible ways" and "X killed Y in one of the only $n + 1$ possible ways." If the difference between "... n ..." and "... $n+1$ ..." were morally insignificant only because it was *too small* for any moral discrimination to be based upon it, then the sum-total of millions of such differences might still have moral significance. But in fact the differences in question, whatever their size, are of the *wrong kind* for any moral discrimination to be based upon them. Suppose you have judged X adversely, on the basis of the misinformation: "X killed Y in the only way possible in the circumstances"; and this is then replaced, in one swoop, by the true report: "X did not kill Y at all, though he did knowingly let Y die." Other things being equal, would this give you the slightest reason to retract your adverse judgment? Not a bit of it! It would be perfectly reasonable for you to reply: 'The fact remains that X chose to conduct himself in a way which he knew would involve Y's death. At first I thought his choice could encompass Y's death only by being the choice of some rather specific course of conduct; whereas the revised report shows me that X's choice could have encompassed Y's death while committing X to very little. At first I thought it had to be a choice to act; I now realize that it could have been a choice to refrain. What of it?'

There are several things a conservative is likely to say at this point—all equivalent. "When we know that the crucial choice could have been a choice to refrain from something, we can begin to allow for the possibility that it may have been a choice to refrain from doing something wrong, such as killing an innocent human." Or: "You say 'other things being equal,' but in the obstetrical example they aren't equal. By representing letting-die as a kind of wide-optioned killing you suppress the fact that the alternative to letting the woman die is killing the child."

Replies like these are available to the conservative only if he does not need them and can break through at some other point; for they assume the very point which is at issue, namely that in every instance of the obstetrical example it would be wrong to kill the child. I think that in some cases it would indeed be wrong—(I do not press for a blanket judgment on all instances of the example—quite the contrary); and in such a case the obstetrician, if he rightly let the woman die, could defend his doing so on the basis of the details of the particular case. Furthermore, he might wish to begin his defence by explaining: "I let the woman die, but I did not kill her"; for letting-die is in general likely to be more defensible than killing. My analysis incidentally shows one reason why: the alternatives to killing are always very numerous, and the odds are that at least one of them provides an acceptable way out of the impasse; whereas the alternative to letting-die is always some fairly specific course of conduct, and if there are conclusive objections to *that* then there's an end of the matter. All this, though, is a matter of likelihoods. It is no help in the rare cases where the alternatives to killing, numerous as they are, arguably do *not* include an acceptable way out of the impasse because they all involve something of the same order of gravity as a killing, namely a letting-die. The conservative may say: "Where innocent humans are in question, letting-die is not of the same order of gravity as killing: for one of them is not, and the other is, absolutely wrong in all possible circumstances." But this, like the rejoinders out of which this paragraph grew, assumes the very point which is at issue. All these conservative moves come down to just one thing: "At this point your argument fails; for the wrongness of killing the child, in any instance of the obstetrical example, *can* be defended on the basis of your own analysis of the acting/refraining distinction—plus the extra premiss that it would always be wrong to kill the child."

"On Killing And Letting Die"

Daniel Dinello

Jonathan Bennett in his paper, "Whatever the Consequences" attempts to refute what he refers to as the conservative position on the following problem:

> A woman in labour will certainly die unless an operation is performed in which the head of her unborn child is crushed or dissected; while if it is not performed the child can be delivered, alive, by post-mortem Caesarian section. This presents a straight choice between the woman's life and the child's.

The conservative position is as follows: The child's death is part of a killing; but, in the case of the mother, there is no killing and death occurs only as a consequence of what is done. Therefore, the principle, "It would always be wrong to kill an innocent human being whatever the consequences," when added to the premise, "operating involves the killing of an innocent human being," yields the conclusion: "it would be wrong to operate."

Part I of this paper is a brief exposition of Bennett's attempt to refute the conservative position; Part II consists of two counter-examples to Bennett's position; and, Part III is my analysis of the issue.

I

Bennett states correctly that, without an appeal to authority as ground for the principle, the conservative must argue that the premise: "In this case, operating would be killing an innocent human while not-operating would involve the death of an innocent human only as a consequence" gives some reason for the conclusion. The conservatives have drawn the action/consequence distinction correctly, namely, operating is killing while not-operat-

Reprinted with permission of the publisher from *Analysis* 31:3, 83–86, 1971.

ing is not. The questions are: By what criteria is the distinction drawn and
are the criteria morally significant in this case?

Bennett argues correctly that a number of criteria could support a
moral conclusion, but are irrelevant in this case. One criterion remains,
namely, not-operating is not killing-the-woman because it is not doing anything at all, but is merely refraining from doing something. This is the
conservative's final support. The question now is: Is there any moral significance in the acting/refraining (*i.e.,* killing/letting die) distinction?

Bennett suggests that the conditions for distinguishing between "x
killed y" and "x let y die" are the following:

(1) x kills y if (a) x moved his body
           (b) y died
           (c) there are relatively few other ways x could have moved which
               satisfy the condition: if x moved like that, y would have died.

(2) x lets y die if (a) x moved his body
              (b) y died
              (c) almost all the ways x could have moved satisfy the condi-
                 tion: if x moved like that, y would have died.

Bennett concludes that since the conservative position rests on there
being a morally significant difference between killing and letting die, and
since there is no moral significance in the distinction based on the number
of moves the agent can make, the conservative position has absolutely no
moral bite.

II

The following two counter-examples show that Bennett's conditions for
drawing the "killing/letting die" distinction are incorrect.

Case I: Jones and Smith are watching television. Jones intentionally
swallows a quantity of poison sufficient to kill himself. Smith, who knows the
antidote, pulls out a pistol, shoots, and *kills* Smith. But, according to Bennett's criteria, this would be a case of "letting die" since almost all the moves
Jones could make (*i.e.,* moves other than, e.g., forcing the antidote down
Smith's throat) would satisfy the condition "if Jones moved like that, y would
have died."

Case II: Jones and Smith are spies who have been captured by the
enemy. They have been wired to each other such that a movement by one
would electrocute the other. Jones moves and kills Smith. But, according to
Bennett's criteria, this too would be a case of "letting die" since almost all
the moves Jones could make, *etc.*

Bennett's conditions for drawing the distinction are clearly wrong, but
it remains to be seen whether his conclusion ("the conservative position has
no moral bite") is correct.

III

The following are what I take to be the conditions which distinguish "x killed y" from "x let y die":

(A) x killed y if x caused y's death by performing movements which affect y's body such that y dies as a result of these movements.

(B) x let y die if (a) there are conditions affecting y, such that if they are not altered, y will die.

 (b) x has reason to believe that the performance of certain movements will alter conditions affecting y, such that y will not die.

 (c) x is in a position to perform such movements.

 (d) x fails to perform these movements.

The following are clarification and justification of these conditions:

(1) Part (b) is necessary, in that we would not want to say that a person who knew no way of altering conditions that are affecting y had let y die. For example, suppose y is dying of an incurable disease and a doctor, x, has no choice, but to watch y die. It would not be true that x let y die.

(2) (c) is necessary because the other conditions could be fulfilled, and if y were incapable of performing the movements, we would not say that he had let y die. For example: y is dying. X knows what movements would alter the conditions affecting y, but he has been securely tied to a chair.

The "killing/letting die" distinction drawn in terms of the number of moves the agent could make clearly can have no moral significance. It is not obvious, though, that the distinction as I have now drawn it could have no moral significance. Consider the following example: Jones and Smith are in a hospital. Jones cannot live longer than two hours unless he gets a heart transplant. Smith, who had had one kidney removed, is dying of an infection in the other kidney. If he does not get a kidney transplant, he will die in about four hours. When Jones dies, his one good kidney can be transplanted to Smith, or Smith could be killed and his heart transplanted to Jones. Circumstances are such that there are no other hearts or kidneys available within the time necessary to save either one. Further, the consequences of either alternative are approximately equivalent, that is, heart transplants have been perfected, both have a wife and no children, *etc.* On Bennett's analysis, there is no morally significant difference between letting Jones die and killing Smith, the consequences of either alternative are equivalent and there is no moral distinction between killing and letting die. But, it seems clear that it would, in fact, be wrong to kill Smith and save Jones, rather than letting Jones die and saving Smith.

Further, suppose that Jones and Smith are in the same situation, but there is one difference between them: Jones has a wife and Smith does not.

Bennett would have to say that since killing and letting die are morally distinguishable only by reference to the consequences of each alternative, the doctor ought to kill Smith and save Jones (Jones' death would sadden his wife, but Smith has no wife and other things are equal). But, this also seems to be wrong.

Bennett argued that the conservative has absolutely no morally relevant factor to which he could appeal, *i.e.,* the "killing/letting die" distinction is not morally significant. The preceding two examples show this conclusion to be false: There are cases where consequences are equivalent and cases where the consequences of killing are preferable, yet still wrong to kill. The distinction as I have drawn it has some moral bite: it seems intuitively clear that causing a death is morally somewhat more reprehensible than knowingly refraining from altering conditions which are causing a death. Bennett has not refuted the conservative position because the question of whether an act is one of killing or letting die *is* relevant in determining the morality of the act. The conservative, though, gives this factor absolute status. In order to refute this position it must be shown that in many cases other factors outweigh this one. In other words, the question is not whether the conservative position has moral bite, but rather how much moral bite it has.

Acting and Refraining

P. J. Fitzgerald

Is it any worse to cause a man's death by doing something than by doing nothing? Or is it immaterial whether the death in question results from an act or an omission? J. Bennett ("Whatever the consequences"), has argued that the distinction between acting and refraining (on which reliance is sometimes placed by defenders of the "conservative" view in the mother-child controversy) is without moral significance. What I wish to contend (without necessarily supporting the "conservative" view) is that his analysis of the distinction is inadequate and that the distinction which he in fact describes is not devoid of moral significance.

I. First, Bennett's analysis. To develop this he compares the statements:

A. Joe killed the calf

and

B. Joe let the calf die.

Reprinted with permission of the publisher from *Analysis* 27: 4, 133–39, 1973.

In these, part of what is being said is

    (1) Joe moved his body[1]

and

    (2) The calf died.

According to Bennett the distinction between A and B lies in the difference in what connects (1) and (2) in the two statements. The connecting link appropriate to A but not to B is

> (3''') Of all the other ways in which Joe might have moved, *relatively few* satisfy the condition: if Joe had moved like that, the calf would have died.
> (In other words if Joe had moved in almost *any other way*, the calf would not have died.)

The connexion appropriate to B and not to A is

> (4) Of all the other ways in which Joe might have moved, *almost all* satisfy the condition: if Joe had moved like that, the calf would have died.
> (In other words unless Joe had moved in *one or two* particular ways, the calf would have died.)

But (1), (2) and (4) together do not describe what is being said by B. They add up to the statement "Joe did not prevent the calf's death," which is different from "Joe let the calf die." Refraining from preventing something is not the same as not preventing it. For refraining is not co-extensive with not doing; it is a species of it.

Take the following example. Joe's calf is dying for want of food. Joe does nothing about this. Neither does Bill, who owns the adjoining farm and who could, if he wishes, come and feed the calf. Now a proposition along the lines of (4) would be true both of Joe and of Bill, but in this example it is only Joe who lets the calf die. Bill does not let it die; he merely does nothing to save it.

At what point, then, does doing nothing become a case of refraining? When does doing nothing to prevent the calf's death amount to letting it die? At the point surely where there exists some other connexion between (1) and (2) over and above (4). This connexion Bennett indeed adverts to, if only to disregard it thereafter. He says:

> When I say "he lets her die," I mean only that he knowingly refrains from preventing her death which he alone could prevent, and he cannot say that her survival is in a general way "none of my business" or "not [even *prima facie*] my concern."

But this says both too much and too little. It says too much in stipulating that it must be a death which he *alone* could prevent. Take this example.

---

[1] In fact (1) could include in certain cases "Joe made no movements," though this would be more common in B than in A.

Several able-bodied adults watch a child drown, when any one of them could save him. Of none of them is it true that he alone could save the child, but of each of them it can be said that he lets the child die.

More important, it says too little. What we want is to be told more; for the crucial problem surely is what is meant by saying that it is his *business* or *concern*. If X's doing nothing to save Y amounts, not just to mere inactivity, but to refraining, by reason of the fact that it is X's business to save Y, then we shall want to know the criteria for saying that it is X's business.

In general, I suggest, we should say that X refrains from doing something if we should normally *expect* X to do it. If, for example, it leaves out some part of a routine procedure which most people normally put in, then he would generally be said to have refrained from doing it. Most motorists, say, start driving in bottom gear and change up through each gear to top gear. If X changes straight from second to fourth, he would be said to refrain from going into third. Now to describe X as refraining does not necessarily imply criticism; rather it implies surprise. Most people when attacked or criticised, retaliate. If X in fact refrains from retaliation, this is cause for commendation rather than blame, but still cause for surprise.

What is usual, however, often becomes the standard: what is expected comes to be required. This may be because the usual procedure has become usual simply because experience has shown it to be the best, surest or safest procedure. Or it may be because we like people to act according to our expectations, so that we may know where we are with them. Consequently to say that X refrained from doing something, though not necessarily implying criticism, may well carry a hint of blame.

But where blame becomes particularly appropriate is where it is X's *duty* to do a certain act and he refrains from doing it. Such a duty[2] might well arise if it is X's business in a literal sense to do the act: *e.g.*, if Joe, who lets the calf die, is the vet called in to save it. Or it may arise because of the special relationship between the agent and the victim: *e.g.* if the calf belongs to Joe. Or again, a duty to act may arise simply from the general relationship between human beings: *e.g.*, the bystanders who watched the child drown had a moral (though not in English law a legal) duty to save him.

Once this special connecting link is taken into account, it seems that refraining is in general no better and no worse than acting. If the result is morally indifferent (as, for argument, in the gear-changing example), then both acting and refraining to act are equally indifferent. If the result is not morally indifferent (*e.g.*, someone's death, as in the mother-child case where the obstetrician is faced with the choice of killing the unborn child to save the mother or refraining from operating so that the mother will die and the child survive) then both acting and refraining are equally open to criticism. It is as Bennett says, no justification of the 'conservative' view (*viz.* that killing the child will always be wrong) that the mother's death would be the result of refraining whereas the child's would be the result of a positive act.

Now the conservative view has one curious feature seldom noticed. Normally no one would suggest that it is permissible for a doctor to *refrain*

[2]On omissions in English criminal law see Smith and Hogan, *Criminal Law*, pp. 33–5.

from saving his patient's life, for we only talk in terms of refraining where not doing is at least unusual and in general wrong. Why then suggest that it is permissible in this case? Perhaps because of the lack of a simple term to describe not-doing. Mere non-performance of the operation (as opposed to refraining from performing it) would be permissible because non-performance applies precisely to those cases totally described by propositions of type (1), (2) and (4) without the addition of any further connecting link in the shape of a duty to act. Defenders of the conservative view then may be contending that if the obstetrician does not perform the operation, this is merely a case of not acting, and, as such, cannot be wrong. Their argument would then be: killing is wrong, but doing nothing is wrong unless there is a duty to save life, a duty which transforms doing nothing into refraining, and no such duty exists here. As against this the opponents of the conservative view can argue that non-performance of the operation in this case is wrong, since this is not a case of mere non-performance but one of refraining, because here there is a duty to act to save the mother. Their argument would be: agreed, killing is wrong, and so is refraining to save from death when there is a duty to save, and here there is such a duty.

II. This then points to one moral difference between acting and not-acting, where both will cause harm. Acting seems to start with a presumption against it: *e.g.*, killing is *prima facie* wrong. Not-acting starts without any such presumption, and it is only by establishing a duty to act that we show that not acting is wrong. Killing needs to be justified; not saving life does not.

Now the interesting feature of this is not that we sometimes do and sometimes do not expect a man to act, and that we use the term "refraining" to describe non-performance in the first type of case only. For it is only on certain occasions that a man's own previous conduct or general human behaviour leads us to expect him not to sit back and do nothing. The interesting question is why we do not invariably expect, and indeed require, a man to act in those cases where the result of his not acting would be that another will suffer harm. Why, in such cases, is it not always his "business or concern" to act so as to prevent harm to that other? For, as Bennett points out, the only difference between "Joe killed the calf" and "Joe did not prevent its death" is that in the first case most alternatives would have prevented its death whereas in the second most alternatives would not. And this is but a difference of degree.

At one end of the scale is (a) the case where *all* alternatives would have avoided death: X kills Y in the only way possible. At the other is the case (b) where all alternatives but one would not have avoided death: X does not do the only thing that would save Y. In between are:

(a') X kills Y in one of the five ways possible;
(a") X kills Y in one of the fifty ways possible;
(a"') X kills Y in one of the five hundred ways possible; *etc.*

But, so the argument runs, X is no less culpable in (a') than in (a), in (a") than in (a'), in (a"') than in (a") and so on. Accordingly he is no less culpable in (b) than in (a). Not saving is no less culpable than killing.

But if we concentrate on cases (a) and (b) and assume for the moment that X's culpability is equal in both, we can, I suggest, see certain differences between them which are morally relevant.

In the first place X will be equally exonerated in both (a) and (b) if he could not do otherwise than he did. But for this defence of impossibility to apply to (a) it must be necessary for X to be unable to *act otherwise, i.e.,* to avoid doing the very act he does. For it to apply to (b) it is only necessary for him to be unable *to do the act he does not do, i.e.,* the one thing that would save Y. X's inability to do this one act could arise from a variety of reasons, some of which may be in no way unusual, or peculiar to X: he may not have the necessary skill or strength or he may be too far away to do it. His inability to avoid doing the act he does in (a), by contrast, will be less usual, because to this one act there is not one but a whole range of alternatives, some of which may require no special skill, strength or proximity: doing nothing at all, for instance, in most cases, calls for no special ability. Impossibility in (a), therefore, will arise generally only from some special feature peculiar to X or his situation. He may be unable to avoid doing the act because of some physical compulsion: *e.g.,* if Z takes X's hand and therewith kills Y, this is not murder in X but in Z. Or he may be unable to avoid doing the act because of some inner compulsion: he may be acting under automatism due to disease or injury, for example.[3]

Impossibility, then, is more likely to be encountered in performing an act than in avoiding one. So, if we know nothing but the bare facts of (a) and (b), we at least know this, that a defence of impossibility is more on the cards in (b) than in (a). And this should make us keep a more open mind about (b) than about (a) and less ready to criticise X in (b) than in (a).

Secondly X's culpability will be partially reduced in both cases if it is very difficult for him to do otherwise in both instances. And here similar considerations apply as apply to the defence of impossibility. The act not done by X in (b) may be difficult for a variety of reasons connected not so much with X as with the act itself: it might require a great deal of effort, time or patience. By contrast, avoidance of the act done by X in (a) would in general only be difficult for reasons unusual and peculiar to X himself: he might be acting out of necessity, under provocation or because of some impulse difficult for X to resist.[4] Difficulty, like impossibility, is more probably to be met with in performing an act than in avoiding one. So, once again, if we know but the bare facts of (a) and (b) we should be more prepared to excuse and less ready to censure X in (b) than in (a).

Thirdly, there is the question how great a burden or inconvenience it would be for X to act otherwise in the two cases. Here again burden or inconvenience can play a greater part in (b) than in (a). To avoid doing what he does in (a) may be a burden to X in that he would prefer to do the act: but even if he does abstain from the act, there will remain a host of other

---

[3]See Smith and Hogan, *op. cit.,* pp. 30–31.

[4]Though irresistible impulse is not a defence in criminal law *per se,* it has found its way into the law in various connexions: in the defence of provocation, in the crime of infanticide, and in the defence of diminished responsibility.

actions which he can perform without producing any harmful effect. To avoid not doing the act in (b), *i.e.,* to perform it, will be much more of a burden for X, because it will mean that he can do *nothing else whatsoever* till he has done this act, whereas there may be many other things that he desires to do and which in a normal way he would have every right to do.

A requirement that he must not do the act in (a) merely closes off one avenue of activity; a requirement that he must do the act in (b) closes off all avenues but one.

How far we shall expect or require X to act in cases of type (b) and be his brother's keeper will depend partly on the degree of harm which Y is likely to suffer and partly on the value to X of being free to pursue his own activities. If Y were in danger of death, and a rescue operation would merely make X late for dinner, then we should generally expect X to rescue Y and consider it his duty to do so. If Y's horse were in danger of death and rescuing it would make X too late to perform an urgent medical operation, then we should neither expect nor require X to delay to rescue it. And if the harm to Y were trifling, *e.g.,* his wife's washing is hanging on the line and it is going to rain, then we should not consider that X, who may be sitting reading the paper next-door, had any duty to do anything about it; for after all there is a value in enjoying one's leisure and being free to do nothing at all, if one wishes.

And this surely is what lies behind the reluctance of the common law to attach liability to omissions—a reluctance which is a notable feature throughout the law. Crimes, for instance, consist more often of acts than omissions. Of this there are many examples besides the well-known failure-to-rescue cases referred to above. So, for example, a finder of a lost article commits the offence of larceny if he takes the article and keeps it for himself, but commits no offence by merely letting the article lie where it is, since the law does not require finders of property to drop everything in order to return it to its owner. In certain circumstances it may be a criminal or civil wrong to lie; but mere failure to speak the truth, *i.e.,* by remaining silent, will not normally amount to fraud, unless by virtue of some special relationship between the persons concerned, the law imposes a duty to reveal the truth. Although a contracting party can often avoid being bound by a contract which he entered into by reason of the other party's misrepresentations, mere silence does not generally amount in law to misrepresentation. In contracts of sale for instance the general rule is *caveat emptor:* the seller does not have to tell the buyer what is wrong with the goods. Again, the law of tort protects against intentional and negligent injury, and not in general against the non-performance of benefits. One may be liable in negligence for negligently injuring another, but not for not bothering to rescue that other.

And this reluctance to penalise omissions is justified by the fact that to prohibit an act (by making its commission a crime or civil wrong) leaves the subject free to do many alternative acts; to prohibit an omission (by requiring the act to be performed) leaves him free to do only *one* act, the act which he is forbidden to omit; and this is a more severe burden to place on the citizen than if he is merely forbidden to perform an act.

ABORTION

From "An Almost Absolute Value in History"

John T. Noonan, Jr.

What determines when a being is human? When is it lawful to kill? These questions are linked in any consideration of the morality of abortion. They are questions central to any morality for man.

In answering such moral questions the temptation to invoke historical determinism is not unknown. A species of behavior is said to be right because it inevitably will be practiced and accepted in the future. "Trends" are hypostatized into forces like older theological conceptions of the divine will; they are supposed to exist independently of human volition and to legitimate by necessity the human acts which they require.

Such use of history, I suppose, appears exploitative and dishonest to most men who have tried to discern the thought of the past. In looking at the data and documents of another age, one does not encounter irresistible trends moving with mysterious authority to foreordained results. Order in human history is the pattern made by the historian in his choice of categories and selection of events. What he encounters is a record of human thought with no greater necessity to it than the result of any meeting of human minds.

The rejection of necessity in human development is not a rejection of continuity, recurrences, and even direction in human experience. These philosophical notions, or something like them, appear as preconditions for the perception and organization of historical "facts." Something like organic behavior may be postulated in the experience of groups of men. Ideas do have implications which are sometimes worked out. No value can be pursued alone without its single-minded pursuit endangering other values, so that balance is the condition of stable phases. Human groups mature. To suppose that these characteristics of human behavior constitute suprahuman forces is to replace history with ideology. To ignore the organic character of human experience is to reduce history to chronology.

History can record insights gained by human beings, insights which once generalized by education are taken as a part of the mental outlook of the persons subject to such education. Such is the insight into the connection between being human and being free. Once men have seen that the determination of their own potential humanity can be injured by the domination of others, they insist on their freedom of action and of thought. The pursuit of freedom as a single absolute, however, is unworkable because the maximum conceivable freedom of action for one man necessarily involves the right to dispose of other men; and any society committed to freedom as a human good must move dynamically toward a balance where freedom for one man is not achieved at the expense of freedom for another.

In the conflict over abortion, the desire of many women to be free from restraints imposed by men and the desire of many contemporary human beings to be free from the domination of sexual codes established by others give dynamic power to any proposal to reject all limitations on abortion. In a society peculiarly conscious of the difference made by age, it is easy to define one class by age so that it is not regarded as even human, so that then there can be no objection to elimination of members of the class whenever a member of it interferes with the freedom of those who are human. In this case, then, there is no need to balance the gain in freedom of some humans by the loss to other humans.

The question remains, Can age be the determinant of humanity? Behind this question, the questions are repeated, What determines when a being is human? When can human freedom be vindicated by killing other human beings? In this chapter I propose to examine these questions as they have been answered in the context of a religious tradition concerned with them since its inception.

The impatience expressed by proponents of abortion with a view asserting the humanity of the fetus sometimes incorporates an elitism which assumes that everyone—that is, every enlightened person, everyone in the ruling group—knows who is human. The elite may become franker and say, Even if the embryo is human, we can distinguish between human lives. Some lives are more valuable than others. To sacrifice a poor, undeveloped life for a rich developed life is a decision which morally can and should be made. More probably, the expedient of the rulers of *Animal Farm* will be adopted, and some lives will be recognized as more equal than others. To any variety of this viewpoint, a religious teaching which asserts the basic equality of men must seem irrelevant; but it is difficult to extricate the aspirations of the modern world from the assumption of basic equality. A teaching anchored in this assumption may be stronger than the very strong attraction to believe that some lives are more valuable than others.

The teaching of a religious body may invoke revelation, claim authority, employ symbolism, which make the moral doctrine it teaches binding for believers in the religion but of academic concern to those outside its boundaries. The moral teaching of a religious body may also embody insights, protect perceptions, exemplify values, which concern humanity. The teaching of the moralists of the Catholic Church on abortion is particularly rich in interaction between specifically supernatural themes—for example, the Nativity of the Lord and the Immaculate Conception of Mary—and principles of a general ethical applicability. In its full extent, the teaching depends on the self-sacrificing example of the Lord—to the Greeks, foolishness. In its basic assumption of the equality of human lives, it depends on a stoic, democratic contention which any man might embrace and Western humanism has hitherto embraced. In its reliance on ecclesiastical authority to draw a line, it withdraws from the sphere of debate with all men of goodwill; in its casuistic examination of principle, it offers instances where the common tools of moral analysis may be observed industriously employed. The teaching in its totality cannot be detached from the religious tradition which has borne it. The teaching in its fundamental questions about the meaning of love and humanity cannot be disregarded by those who would meet the needs of man humanly. . . .

The most fundamental question involved in the long history of thought on abortion is: How do you determine the humanity of a being? To phrase the question that way is to put in comprehensive humanistic terms what the theologians either dealt with as an explicitly theological question under the heading of "ensoulment" or dealt with implicitly in their treatment of abortion. The Christian position as it originated did not depend on a narrow theological or philosophical concept. It had no relation to theories of infant baptism. It appealed to no special theory of instantaneous ensoulment. It took the world's view on ensoulment as that view changed from Aristotle to Zacchia. There was, indeed, theological influence affecting the theory of ensoulment finally adopted, and, of course, ensoulment itself was a theological concept, so that the position was always explained in theological terms. But the theological notion of ensoulment could easily be translated into humanistic language by substituting "human" for "rational soul"; the problem of knowing when a man is a man is common to theology and humanism.

If one steps outside the specific categories used by the theologians, the answer they gave can be analyzed as a refusal to discriminate among human beings on the basis of their varying potentialities. Once conceived, the being was recognized as man because he had man's potential. The criterion for humanity, thus, was simple and all-embracing: if you are conceived by human parents, you are human.

The strength of this position may be tested by a review of some of the other distinctions offered in the contemporary controversy over legalizing abortion. Perhaps the most popular distinction is in terms of viability. Before an age of so many months, the fetus is not viable, that is, it cannot be removed from the mother's womb and live apart from her. To that extent, the life of the fetus is absolutely dependent on the life of the mother. This dependence is made the basis of denying recognition to its humanity.

There are difficulties with this distinction. One is that the perfection of artificial incubation may make the fetus viable at any time: it may be removed and artificially sustained. Experiments with animals already show that such a procedure is possible. This hypothetical extreme case relates to an actual difficulty: there is considerable elasticity to the idea of viability. Mere length of life is not an exact measure. The viability of the fetus depends on the extent of its anatomical and functional development. The weight and length of the fetus are better guides to the state of its development than age, but weight and length vary. Moreover, different racial groups have different ages at which their fetuses are viable. Some evidence, for example, suggests that Negro fetuses mature more quickly than white fetuses. If viability is the norm, the standard would vary with race and with many individual circumstances.

The most important objection to this approach is that dependence is not ended by viability. The fetus is still absolutely dependent on someone's care in order to continue existence; indeed a child of one or three or even five years of age is absolutely dependent on another's care for existence; uncared for, the older fetus or the younger child will die as surely as the early fetus detached from the mother. The unsubstantial lessening in dependence at viability does not seem to signify any special acquisition of humanity.

A second distinction has been attempted in terms of experience. A being who has had experience, has lived and suffered, who possesses memories, is more human that one who has not. Humanity depends on formation by experience. The fetus is thus "unformed" in the most basic human sense.

This distinction is not serviceable for the embryo which is already experiencing and reacting. The embryo is responsive to touch after eight weeks and at least at that point is experiencing. At an earlier stage the zygote is certainly alive and responding to its environment. The distinction may also be challenged by the rare case where aphasia has erased adult memory: has it erased humanity? More fundamentally, this distinction leaves even the older fetus or the younger child to be treated as an unformed inhuman thing. Finally, it is not clear why experience as such confers humanity. It could be argued that certain central experiences such as loving or learning are necessary to make a man human. But then human beings who have failed to love or to learn might be excluded from the class called man.

A third distinction is made by appeal to the sentiments of adults. If a fetus dies, the grief of the parents is not the grief they would have for a living child. The fetus is an unnamed "it" till birth, and is not perceived as personality until at least the fourth month of existence when movements in the womb manifest a vigorous presence demanding joyful recognition by the parents.

Yet feeling is notoriously an unsure guide to the humanity of others. Many groups of humans have had difficulty in feeling that persons of another tongue, color, religion, sex, are as human as they. Apart from reactions to alien groups, we mourn the loss of a 10-year-old boy more than the loss of his one-day-old brother or his 90-year-old grandfather. The difference felt and the grief expressed vary with the potentialities extinguished, or the experience wiped out; they do not seem to point to any substantial difference in the humanity of baby, boy, or grandfather.

Distinctions are also made in terms of sensation by the parents. The embryo is felt within the womb only after about the fourth month. The embryo is seen only at birth. What can be neither seen nor felt is different from what is tangible. If the fetus cannot be seen or touched at all, it cannot be perceived as man.

Yet experience shows that sight is even more untrustworthy than feeling in determining humanity. By sight, color became an appropriate index for saying who was a man, and the evil of racial discrimination was given foundation. Nor can touch provide the test; a being confined by sickness, "out of touch" with others, does not thereby seem to lose his humanity. To the extent that touch still has appeal as a criterion, it appears to be a survival of the old English idea of "quickening"—a possible mistranslation of the

Latin *animatus* used in the canon law. To that extent touch as a criterion seems to be dependent on the Aristotelian notion of ensoulment, and to fall when this notion is discarded.

Finally, a distinction is sought in social visibility. The fetus is not socially perceived as human. It cannot communicate with others. Thus, both subjectively and objectively, it is not a member of society. As moral rules are rules for the behavior of members of society to each other, they cannot be made for behavior toward what is not yet a member. Excluded from the society of men, the fetus is excluded from the humanity of men.

By force of the argument from the consequences, this distinction is to be rejected. It is more subtle than that founded on an appeal to physical sensation, but it is equally dangerous in its implications. If humanity depends on social recognition, individuals or whole groups may be dehumanized by being denied any status in their society. Such a fate is fictionally portrayed in *1984* and has actually been the lot of many men in many societies. In the Roman empire, for example, condemnation to slavery meant the practical denial of most human rights; in the Chinese Communist world, landlords have been classified as enemies of the people and so treated as nonpersons by the state. Humanity does not depend on social recognition, though often the failure of society to recognize the prisoner, the alien, the heterodox as human has led to the destruction of human beings. Anyone conceived by a man and a woman is human. Recognition of this condition by society follows a real event in the objective order, however imperfect and halting the recognition. Any attempt to limit humanity to exclude some group runs the risk of furnishing authority and precedent for excluding other groups in the name of the consciousness or perception of the controlling group in the society.

A philosopher may reject the appeal to the humanity of the fetus because he views "humanity" as a secular view of the soul and because he doubts the existence of anything real and objective which can be identified as humanity. One answer to such a philosopher is to ask how he reasons about moral questions without supposing that there is a sense in which he and the others of whom he speaks are human. Whatever group is taken as the society which determines who may be killed is thereby taken as human. A second answer is to ask if he does not believe that there is a right and wrong way of deciding moral questions. If there is such a difference, experience may be appealed to; to decide who is human on the basis of the sentiment of a given society has led to consequences which rational men would characterize as monstrous.

The rejection of the attempted distinctions based on viability and visibility, experience and feeling, may be buttressed by the following considerations: Moral judgments often rest on distinctions, but if the distinctions are not to appear arbitrary fiat, they should relate to some real difference in probabilities. There is a kind of continuity in all life, but the earlier stages of the elements of human life possess tiny probabilities of development. Consider for example, the spermatozoa in any normal ejaculate: There are about 200,000,000 in any single ejaculate, of which one has a chance of developing into a zygote. Consider the oocytes which may become ova: there are 100,000 to 1,000,000 oocytes in a female infant, of which a maximum of 390 are ovulated. But once spermatozoon and ovum meet and the conceptus is formed, such studies as have been made show that roughly in only 20 percent of the cases will spontaneous abortion occur. In other words, the chances are about 4 out of 5 that this new being will develop. At this stage in the life of the being there is a sharp shift in probabilities, an immense jump in potentialities. To make a distinction between the rights of spermatozoa and the rights of the fertilized ovum is to respond to an enormous shift in possibilities. For about twenty days after conception the egg may split to form twins or combine with another egg to form a chimera, but the probability of either event happening is very small.

It may be asked, What does a change in biological probabilities have to do with establishing humanity? The argument from probabilities is not aimed at establishing humanity but at establishing an objective discontinuity which may be taken into account in moral discourse. As life itself is a matter of probabilities, as most moral reasoning is an estimate of probabilities, so it seems in accord with the structure of reality and the nature of moral thought to found a moral judgment on the change in probabilities at conception. The appeal to probabilities is the most commonsensical of arguments, to a greater or smaller degree all of us base our actions on probabilities, and in morals, as in law, prudence and negligence are often measured by the account one has taken of the probabilities. If the chance is 200,000,000 to 1 that the movement in the bushes into which you shoot is a man's, I doubt if many persons would hold you careless in shooting; but if the chances are 4 out of 5 that the movement is a human being's, few would acquit you of blame. Would the argument be different if only one out of ten children conceived came to term? Of course this argument would be different. This argument is an appeal to probabilities that actually exist, not to any and all states of affairs which may be imagined.

The probabilities as they do exist do not show the humanity of the embryo in the sense of a demonstration in logic any more than the probabilities of the movement in the bush being a man demonstrate beyond all doubt that the being is a man. The appeal is a "buttressing" consideration, showing the plausibility of the standard adopted. The argument focuses on the decisional factor in any moral judgment and assumes that part of the business of a moralist is drawing lines. One evidence of the nonarbitrary character of the line drawn is the difference of probabilities on either side of it. If a spermatozoon is destroyed, one destroys a being which had a chance of far less than 1 in 200 million of developing into a reasoning being, possessed of the genetic code, a heart and other organs, and capable of pain. If a fetus is destroyed, one destroys a being already possessed of the genetic code, organs, and sensitivity to pain, and one which had an 80 percent chance of developing further into a baby outside the womb who, in time, would reason.

The positive argument for conception as the decisive moment of humanization is that at conception the new being receives the genetic code.

It is this genetic information which determines his characteristics, which is the biological carrier of the possibility of human wisdom, which makes him a self-evolving being. A being with a human genetic code is man.

This review of current controversy over the humanity of the fetus emphasizes what a fundamental question the theologians resolved in asserting the inviolability of the fetus. To regard the fetus as possessed of equal rights with other humans was not, however, to decide every case where abortion might be employed. It did decide the case where the argument was that the fetus should be aborted for its own good. To say a being was human was to say it had a destiny to decide for itself which could not be taken from it by another man's decision. But human beings with equal rights often come in conflict with each other, and some decision must be made as whose claims are to prevail. Cases of conflict involving the fetus are different only in two respects: the total inability of the fetus to speak for itself and the fact that the right of the fetus regularly at stake is the right to life itself.

The approach taken by the theologians to these conflicts was articulated in terms of "direct" and "indirect." Again, to look at what they were doing from outside their categories, they may be said to have been drawing lines or "balancing values." "Direct" and "indirect" are spatial metaphors; "line-drawing" is another. "To weigh" or "to balance" values is a metaphor of a more complicated mathematical sort hinting at the process which goes on in moral judgments. All the metaphors suggest that, in the moral judgments made, comparisons were necessary, that no value completely controlled. The principle of double effect was no doctrine fallen from heaven, but a method of analysis appropriate where two relative values were being compared. In Catholic moral theology, as it developed, life even of the innocent was not taken as an absolute. Judgments on acts affecting life issued from a process of weighing. In the weighing, the fetus was always given a value greater than zero, always a value separate and independent from its parents. This valuation was crucial and fundamental in all Christian thought on the subject and marked it off from any approach which considered that only the parents' interests needed to be considered.

Even with the fetus weighed as human, one interest could be weighed as equal or superior: that of the mother in her own life. The casuists between 1450 and 1895 were willing to weigh this interest as superior. Since 1895, that interest was given decisive weight only in the two special cases of the cancerous uterus and the ectopic pregnancy. In both of these cases the fetus itself had little chance of survival even if the abortion were not performed. As the balance was once struck in favor of the mother whenever her life was endangered, it could be so struck again. The balance reached between 1895 and 1930 attempted prudentially and pastorally to forestall a multitude of exceptions for interests less than life.

The perception of the humanity of the fetus and the weighing of fetal rights against other human rights constituted the work of the moral analysts. But what spirit animated their abstract judgments? For the Christian community it was the injunction of Scripture to love your neighbor as yourself. The fetus as human was a neighbor; his life had parity with one's own. The commandment gave life to what otherwise would have been only rational calculation.

The commandment could be put in humanistic as well as theological terms: Do not injure your fellow man without reason. In these terms, once the humanity of the fetus is perceived, abortion is never right except in self-defense. When life must be taken to save life, reason alone cannot say that a mother must prefer a child's life to her own. With this exception, now of great rarity, abortion violates the rational humanist tenet of the equality of human lives.

For Christians the commandment to love had received a special imprint in that the exemplar proposed of love was the love of the Lord for his disciples. In the light given by this example, self-sacrifice carried to the point of death seemed in the extreme situations not without meaning. In the less extreme cases, preference for one's own interests to the life of another seemed to express cruelty or selfishness irreconcilable with the demands of love.

Abortion and Infanticide[1]

Michael Tooley

This essay deals with the question of the morality of abortion and infanticide. The fundamental ethical objection traditionally advanced against these practices rests on the contention that human fetuses and infants have a right to life. It is this claim which will be the focus of attention here. The basic issue to be discussed, then, is what properties a thing must possess in order to have a serious right to life. My approach will be to set out and defend a basic moral principle specifying a condition an organism must satisfy if it is to have a serious right to life. It will be seen that this condition is not satisfied by human fetuses and infants, and thus that they do not have a right to life. So unless there are other substantial objections to abortion and infanticide, one is forced to conclude that these practices are morally acceptable ones. In contrast, it may turn out that our treatment of adult members of other species—cats, dogs, polar bears—is morally indefensible. For it is quite possible that such animals do possess properties that endow them with a right to life.

I. ABORTION AND INFANTICIDE

One reason the question of the morality of infanticide is worth examining is that it seems very difficult to formulate a completely satisfactory liberal

Reprinted with permission of the author and publisher from *Philosophy and Public Affairs* 2:1, 37–65, 1972. Copyright © 1972 by Princeton University Press.

[1] I am grateful to a number of people, particularly the Editors of *Philosophy & Public Affairs*, Rodelia Hapke, and Walter Kaufmann, for their helpful comments. It should not, of course, be inferred that they share the views expressed in this paper.

position on abortion without coming to grips with the infanticide issue. The problem the liberal encounters is essentially that of specifying a cutoff point which is not arbitrary: at what stage in the development of a human being does it cease to be morally permissible to destroy it? It is important to be clear about the difficulty here. The conservative's objection is not that since there is a continuous line of development from a zygote to a newborn baby, one must conclude that if it is seriously wrong to destroy a newborn baby it is also seriously wrong to destroy a zygote or any intermediate stage in the development of a human being. His point is rather that if one says it is wrong to destroy a newborn baby but not a zygote or some intermediate stage in the development of a human being, one should be prepared to point to a *morally relevant* difference between a newborn baby and the earlier stage in the development of a human being.

Precisely the same difficulty can, of course, be raised for a person who holds that infanticide is morally permissible. The conservative will ask what morally relevant differences there are between an adult human being and a newborn baby. What makes it morally permissible to destroy a baby, but wrong to kill an adult? So the challenge remains. But I will argue that in this case there is an extremely plausible answer.

Reflecting on the morality of infanticide forces one to face up to this challenge. In the case of abortion a number of events—quickening or viability, for instance—might be taken as cutoff points, and it is easy to overlook the fact that none of these events involves any morally significant change in the developing human. In contrast, if one is going to defend infanticide, one has to get very clear about what makes something a person, what gives something a right to life.

One of the interesting ways in which the abortion issue differs from most other moral issues is that the plausible positions on abortion appear to be extreme positions. For if a human fetus is a person, one is inclined to say that, in general, one would be justified in killing it only to save the life of the mother.[2] Such is the extreme conservative position.[3] On the other hand, if the fetus is not a person, how can it be seriously wrong to destroy it? Why would one need to point to special circumstances to justify such

[2]Judith Jarvis Thomson, in her article "A Defense of Abortion," *Philosophy & Public Affairs* 1, no. 1 (Fall 1971): 47–66, has argued with great force and ingenuity that this conclusion is mistaken. I will comment on her argument later in this paper.

[3]While this is the position conservatives tend to hold, it is not clear that it is the position they ought to hold. For if the fetus is a person it is far from clear that it is permissible to destroy it to save the mother. Two moral principles lend support to the view that it is the fetus which should live. First, other things being equal, should not one give something to a person who has had less rather than to a person who has had more? The mother has had a chance to live, while the fetus has not. The choice is thus between giving the mother more of an opportunity to live while giving the fetus none at all and giving the fetus an opportunity to enjoy life while not giving the mother a further opportunity to do so. Surely fairness requires the latter. Secondly, since the fetus has a greater life expectancy than the mother, one is in effect distributing more goods by choosing the life of the fetus over the life of the mother.

The position I am here recommending to the conservative should not be confused with the official Catholic position. The Catholic Church holds that it is seriously wrong to kill a fetus directly even if failure to do so will result in the death of *both* the mother and the fetus. This perverse value judgment is not part of the conservative's position.

action? The upshot is that there is no room for a moderate position on the issue of abortion such as one finds, for example, in the Model Penal Code recommendations.[4]

Aside from the light it may shed on the abortion question, the issue of infanticide is both interesting and important in its own right. The theoretical interest has been mentioned: it forces one to face up to the question of what makes something a person. The practical importance need not be labored. Most people would prefer to raise children who do not suffer from gross deformities or from severe physical, emotional, or intellectual handicaps. If it could be shown that there is no moral objection to infanticide the happiness of society could be significantly and justifiably increased.

Infanticide is also of interest because of the strong emotions it arouses. The typical reaction to infanticide is like the reaction to incest or cannibalism, or the reaction of previous generations to masturbation or oral sex. The response, rather than appealing to carefully formulated moral principles, is primarily visceral. When philosophers themselves respond in this way, offering no arguments, and dismissing infanticide out of hand, it is reasonable to suspect that one is dealing with a taboo rather than with a rational prohibition.[5] I shall attempt to show that this is in fact the case.

II. TERMINOLOGY: "PERSON" VERSUS "HUMAN BEING"

How is the term "person" to be interpreted? I shall treat the concept of a person as a purely moral concept, free of all descriptive content. Specifically, in my usage the sentence "X is a person" will be synonymous with the sentence "X has a (serious) moral right to life."

This usage diverges slightly from what is perhaps the more common way of interpreting the term "person" when it is employed as a purely moral term, where to say that X is a person is to say that X has rights. If everything that had rights had a right to life, these interpretations would be extensionally equivalent. But I am inclined to think that it does not follow from acceptable moral principles that whatever has any rights at all has a right to life. My reason is this. Given the choice between being killed and being tortured for an hour, most adult humans would surely choose the latter. So it seems plausible to say it is worse to kill an adult human being than it is to torture him for an hour. In contrast, it seems to me that while it is not seriously wrong to kill a newborn kitten, it is seriously wrong to torture one for an hour. This *suggests* that newborn kittens may have a right not to be tortured without having a serious right to life. For it seems to be true that an individual has a right to something whenever it is the case that, if he wants

[4] Section 230.3 of the American Law Institute's *Model Penal Code* (Philadelphia, 1962). There is some interesting, though at times confused, discussion of the proposed code in *Model Penal Code—Tentative Draft No. 9* (Philadelphia, 1959), pp. 146–162.

[5] A clear example of such an unwillingness to entertain seriously the possibility that moral judgments widely accepted in one's own society may nevertheless be incorrect is provided by Roger Wertheimer's superficial dismissal of infanticide on pages 69–70 of his article "Understanding the Abortion Argument," *Philosophy & Public Affairs* 1, no. 1 (Fall 1971): 67–95.

that thing, it would be wrong for others to deprive him of it. Then if it is wrong to inflict a certain sensation upon a kitten if it doesn't want to experience that sensation, it will follow that the kitten has a right not to have sensation inflicted upon it.[6] I shall return to this example later. My point here is merely that it provides some reason for holding that it does not follow from acceptable moral principles that if something has any rights at all, it has a serious right to life.

There has been a tendency in recent discussions of abortion to use expressions such as "person" and "human being" interchangeably. B. A. Brody, for example, refers to the difficulty of determining "whether destroying the foetus constitutes the taking of a human life," and suggests it is very plausible that "the taking of a human life is an action that has bad consequences for him whose life is being taken."[7] When Brody refers to something as a human life he apparently construes this as entailing that the thing is a person. For if every living organism belonging to the species homo sapiens counted as a human life, there would be no difficulty in determining whether a fetus inside a human mother was a human life.

The same tendency is found in Judith Jarvis Thomson's article, which opens with the statement: "Most opposition to abortion relies on the premise that the fetus is a human being, a person, from the moment of conception."[8] The same is true of Roger Wertheimer, who explicitly says: "First off I should note that the expressions 'a human life,' 'a human being,' 'a person' are virtually interchangeable in this context."[9]

The tendency to use expressions like "person" and "human being" interchangeably is an unfortunate one. For one thing, it tends to lend covert support to antiabortionist positions. Given such usage, one who holds a liberal view of abortion is put in the position of maintaining that fetuses, at least up to a certain point, are not human beings. Even philosophers are led astray by this usage. Thus Wertheimer says that "except for monstrosities, every member of our species is indubitably a person, a human being, at the very latest at birth."[10] Is it really *indubitable* that newborn babies are persons? Surely this is a wild contention. Wertheimer is falling prey to the confusion naturally engendered by the practice of using "person" and "human being" interchangeably. Another example of this is provided by Thomson: "I am inclined to think also that we shall probably have to agree that the fetus has already become a human person well before birth. Indeed, it comes as a surprise when one first learns how early in its life it begins to acquire human characteristics. By the tenth week, for example, it already has a face, arms and legs, fingers and toes; it has internal organs, and brain

---

[6]Compare the discussion of the concept of a right offered by Richard B. Brandt in his *Ethical Theory* (Englewood Cliffs, N.J., 1959), pp. 434–441. As Brandt points out, some philosophers have maintained that only things that can *claim* rights can have rights. I agree with Brandt's view that "inability to claim does not destroy the right" (p. 440).

[7]B. A. Brody, "Abortion and the Law," *Journal of Philosophy*, LXVIII, no. 12 (17 June 1971): 357–369. See pp. 357–358.

[8]Thomson, "A Defense of Abortion," p. 47.

[9]Wertheimer, "Understanding the Abortion Argument," p. 69.

[10]*Ibid.*

activity is detectable."[11] But what do such physiological characteristics have to do with the question of whether the organism is a person? Thomson, partly, I think, because of the unfortunate use of terminology, does not even raise this question. As a result she virtually takes it for granted that there are some cases in which abortion is "positively indecent."[12]

There is a second reason why using "person" and "human being" interchangeably is unhappy philosophically. If one says that the dispute between pro- and anti-abortionists centers on whether the fetus is a human, it is natural to conclude that it is essentially a disagreement about certain facts, a disagreement about what properties a fetus possesses. Thus Wertheimer says that "if one insists on using the raggy fact-value distinction, then one ought to say that the dispute is over a matter of fact in the sense in which it is a fact that the Negro slaves were human beings."[13] I shall argue that the two cases are not parallel, and that in the case of abortion what is primarily at stake is what moral principles one should accept. If one says that the central issue between conservatives and liberals in the abortion question is whether the fetus is a person, it is clear that the dispute may be either about what properties a thing must have in order to be a person, in order to have a right to life—a moral question—or about whether a fetus at a given stage of development as a matter of fact possesses the properties in question. The temptation to suppose that the disagreement must be a factual one is removed.

It should now be clear why the common practice of using expressions such as "person" and "human being" interchangeably in discussions of abortion is unfortunate. It would perhaps be best to avoid the term "human" altogether, employing instead some expression that is more naturally interpreted as referring to a certain type of biological organism characterized in physiological terms, such as "member of the species Homo sapiens." My own approach will be to use the term "human" only in contexts where it is not philosophically dangerous.

III. THE BASIC ISSUE: WHEN IS A MEMBER OF THE SPECIES HOMO SAPIENS A PERSON?

Settling the issue of the morality of abortion and infanticide will involve answering the following questions: What properties must something have to be a person, i.e., to have a serious right to life? At what point in the development of a member of the species Homo sapiens does the organism possess the properties that make it a person? The first question raises a moral issue. To answer it is to decide what basic[14] moral principles involving the ascription of a right to life one ought to accept. The second question

[11]Thomson, "A Defense of Abortion," pp. 47–48.

[12]*Ibid.*, p. 65.

[13]Wertheimer, "Understanding the Abortion Argument," p. 78.

[14]A moral principle accepted by a person is *basic for him* if and only if his acceptance of it is not dependent upon any of his (nonmoral) factual beliefs. That is, no change in his factual beliefs would cause him to abandon the principle in question.

raises a purely factual issue, since the properties in question are properties of a purely descriptive sort.

Some writers seem quite pessimistic about the possibility of resolving the question of the morality of abortion. Indeed, some have gone so far as to suggest that the question of whether the fetus is a person is in principle unanswerable: "we seem to be stuck with the indeterminateness of the fetus' humanity."[15] An understanding of some of the sources of this pessimism will, I think, help us to tackle the problem. Let us begin by considering the similarity a number of people have noted between the issue of abortion and the issue of Negro slavery. The question here is why it should be more difficult to decide whether abortion and infanticide are acceptable than it was to decide whether slavery was acceptable. The answer seems to be that in the case of slavery there are moral principles of a quite uncontroversial sort that settle the issue. Thus most people would agree to some such principle as the following: No organism that has experiences, that is capable of thought and of using language, and that has harmed no one, should be made a slave. In the case of abortion, on the other hand, conditions that are generally agreed to be sufficient grounds for ascribing a right to life to something do not suffice to settle the issue. It is easy to specify other, purportedly sufficient conditions that will settle the issue, but no one has been successful in putting forward considerations that will convince others to accept those additional moral principles.

I do not share the general pessimism about the possibility of resolving the issue of abortion and infanticide because I believe it is possible to point to a very plausible moral principle dealing with the question of *necessary* conditions for something's having a right to life, where the conditions in question will provide an answer to the question of the permissibility of abortion and infanticide.

There is a second cause of pessimism that should be noted before proceeding. It is tied up with the fact that the development of an organism is one of gradual and continuous change. Given this continuity, how is one to draw a line at one point and declare it permissible to destroy a member of Homo sapiens up to, but not beyond, that point? Won't there be an arbitrariness about any point that is chosen? I will return to this worry shortly. It does not present a serious difficulty once the basic moral principles relevant to the ascription of a right to life to an individual are established.

Let us turn now to the first and most fundamental question: What properties must something have in order to be a person, i.e., to have a serious right to life? The claim I wish to defend is this: An organism possesses a serious right to life only if it possesses the concept of a self as a continuing subject of experiences and other mental states, and believes that it is itself such a continuing entity.

My basic argument in support of this claim, which I will call the self-consciousness requirement, will be clearest, I think, if I first offer a simplified version of the argument, and then consider a modification that seems

[15]Wertheimer, "Understanding the Abortion Argument," p. 88.

desirable. The simplified version of my argument is this. To ascribe a right to an individual is to assert something about the prima facie obligations of other individuals to act, or to refrain from acting, in certain ways. However, the obligations in question are conditional ones, being dependent upon the existence of certain desires of the individual to whom the right is ascribed. Thus if an individual asks one to destroy something to which he has a right, one does not violate his right to that thing if one proceeds to destroy it. This suggests the following analysis: "A has a right to X" is roughly synonymous with "If A desires X, then others are under a prima facie obligation to refrain from actions that would deprive him of it."[16]

Although this analysis is initially plausible, there are reasons for thinking it not entirely correct. I will consider these later. Even here, however, some expansion is necessary, since there are features of the concept of a right that are important in the present context, and that ought to be dealt with more explicitly. In particular, it seems to be a conceptual truth that things that lack consciousness, such as ordinary machines, cannot have rights. Does this conceptual truth follow from the above analysis of the concept of a right? The answer depends on how the term "desire" is interpreted. If one adopts a completely behavioristic interpretation of "desire," so that a machine that searches for an electrical outlet in order to get its batteries recharged is described as having a desire to be recharged, then it will not follow from this analysis that objects that lack consciousness cannot have rights. On the other hand, if "desire" is interpreted in such a way that desires are states necessarily standing in some sort of relationship to states of consciousness, it will follow from the analysis that a machine that is not capable of being conscious, and consequently of having desires, cannot have any rights. I think those who defend analyses of the concept of a right along the lines of this one do have in mind an interpretation of the term "desire" that involves reference to something more than behavioral dispositions. However, rather than relying on this, it seems preferable to make such an interpretation explicit. The following analysis is a natural way of doing that: "A has a right to X" is roughly synonymous with "A is the sort of thing that is a subject of experiences and other mental states, A is capable of desiring X, and if A does desire X, then others are under a prima facie obligation to refrain from actions that would deprive him of it."

The next step in the argument is basically a matter of applying this analysis to the concept of a right to life. Unfortunately the expression "right to life" is not entirely a happy one, since it suggests that the right in question concerns the continued existence of a biological organism. That this is incorrect can be brought out by considering possible ways of violating an individual's right to life. Suppose, for example, that by some technology of the future the brain of an adult human were to be completely reprogrammed, so that the organism wound up with memories (or rather, apparent memories), beliefs, attitudes, and personality traits completely different from those associated with it before it was subjected to reprogramming. In such a case one would surely say that an individual had been destroyed, that

---

[16]Again, compare the analysis defended by Brandt in *Ethical Theory*, pp. 434–441.

an adult human's right to life had been violated, even though no biological organism had been killed. This example shows that the expression "right to life" is misleading, since what one is really concerned about is not just the continued existence of a biological organism, but the right of a subject of experiences and other mental states to continue to exist.

Given this more precise description of the right with which we are here concerned, we are now in a position to apply the analysis of the concept of a right stated above. When we do so we find that the statement "A has a right to continue to exist as a subject of experiences and other mental states" is roughly synonymous with the statement "A is a subject of experiences and other mental states, A is capable of desiring to continue to exist as a subject of experiences and other mental states, and if A does desire to continue to exist as such an entity, then others are under a prima facie obligation not to prevent him from doing so."

The final stage in the argument is simply a matter of asking what must be the case if something is to be capable of having a desire to continue existing as a subject of experiences and other mental states. The basic point here is that the desires a thing can have are limited by the concepts it possesses. For the fundamental way of describing a given desire is as a desire that a certain proposition be true.[17] Then, since one cannot desire that a certain proposition be true unless one understands it, and since one cannot understand it without possessing the concepts involved in it, it follows that the desires one can have are limited by the concepts one possesses. Applying this to the present case results in the conclusion that an entity cannot be the sort of thing that can desire that a subject of experiences and other mental states exist unless it possesses the concept of such a subject. Moreover, an entity cannot desire that it itself *continue* existing as a subject of experiences and other mental states unless it believes that it is now such a subject. This completes the justification of the claim that it is a necessary condition of something's having a serious right to life that it possess the concept of a self as a continuing subject of experiences, and that it believe that it is itself such an entity.

Let us now consider a modification in the above argument that seems desirable. This modification concerns the crucial conceptual claim advanced about the relationship between ascription of rights and ascription of the corresponding desires. Certain situations suggest that there may be exceptions to the claim that if a person doesn't desire something, one cannot violate his right to it. There are three types of situations that call this claim into question: (i) situations in which an individual's desires reflect a state of emotional disturbance; (ii) situations in which a previously conscious indi-

---

[17]In everyday life one often speaks of desiring things, such as an apple or a newspaper. Such talk is elliptical, the context together with one's ordinary beliefs serving to make it clear that one wants to eat the apple and read the newspaper. To say that what one desires is that a certain proposition be true should not be construed as involving any particular ontological commitment. The point is merely that it is sentences such as "John wants it to be the case that he is eating an apple in the next few minutes" that provide a completely explicit description of a person's desires. If one fails to use such sentences one can be badly misled about what concepts are presupposed by a particular desire.

vidual is temporarily unconscious; (iii) situations in which an individual's desires have been distorted by conditioning or by indoctrination.

As an example of the first, consider a case in which an adult human falls into a state of depression which his psychiatrist recognizes as temporary. While in the state he tells people he wishes he were dead. His psychiatrist, accepting the view that there can be no violation of an individual's right to life unless the individual has a desire to live, decides to let his patient have his way and kills him. Or consider a related case in which one person gives another a drug that produces a state of temporary depression; the recipient expresses a wish that he were dead. The person who administered the drug then kills him. Doesn't one want to say in both these cases that the agent did something seriously wrong in killing the other person? And isn't the reason the action was seriously wrong in each case the fact that it violated the individual's right to life? If so, the right to life cannot be linked with a desire to live in the way claimed above.

The second set of situations are ones in which an individual is unconscious for some reason—that is, he is sleeping, or drugged, or in a temporary coma. Does an individual in such a state have any desires? People do sometimes say that an unconscious individual wants something, but it might be argued that if such talk is not to be simply false it must be interpreted as actually referring to the desires the individual *would* have if he were now conscious. Consequently, if the analysis of the concept of a right proposed above were correct, it would follow that one does not violate an individual's right if one takes his car, or kills him, while he is asleep.

Finally, consider situations in which an individual's desires have been distorted, either by inculcation or irrational beliefs or by direct conditioning. Thus an individual may permit someone to kill him because he has been convinced that if he allows himself to be sacrificed to the gods he will be gloriously rewarded in a life to come. Or an individual may be enslaved after first having been conditioned to desire a life of slavery. Doesn't one want to say that in the former case an individual's right to life has been violated, and in the latter his right to freedom?

Situations such as these strongly suggest that even if an individual doesn't want something, it is still possible to violate his right to it. Some modification of the earlier account of the concept of a right thus seems in order. The analysis given covers, I believe, the paradigmatic cases of violation of an individual's rights, but there are other, secondary cases where one also wants to say that someone's right has been violated which are not included.

Precisely how the revised analysis should be formulated is unclear. Here it will be sufficient merely to say that, in view of the above, an individual's right to X can be violated not only when he desires X, but also when he *would* now desire X were it not for one of the following: (i) he is in an emotionally unbalanced state; (ii) he is temporarily unconscious; (iii) he has been conditioned to desire the absence of X.

The critical point now is that, even given this extension of the conditions under which an individual's right to something can be violated, it is still true that one's right to something can be violated only when one has the conceptual capability of desiring the thing in question. For example, an individual who would now desire not to be a slave if he weren't emotionally unbalanced, or if he weren't temporarily unconscious, or if he hadn't previously been conditioned to want to be a slave, must possess the concepts involved in the desire not to be a slave. Since it is really only the conceptual capability presupposed by the desire to continue existing as a subject of experiences and other mental states, and not the desire itself, that enters into the above argument, the modification required in the account of the conditions under which an individual's rights can be violated does not undercut my defense of the self-consciousness requirement.[18]

To sum up, my argument has been that having a right to life presupposes that one is capable of desiring to continue existing as a subject of experiences and other mental states. This in turn presupposes both that one has the concept of such a continuing entity and that one believes that one is oneself such an entity. So an entity that lacks such a consciousness of itself as a continuing subject of mental states does not have a right to life.

It would be natural to ask at this point whether satisfaction of this requirement is not only necessary but also sufficient to ensure that a thing has a right to life. I am inclined to an affirmative answer. However, the issue is not urgent in the present context, since as long as the requirement is in fact a necessary one we have the basis of an adequate defense of abortion and infanticide. If an organism must satisfy some other condition before it has a serious right to life, the result will merely be that the interval during which infanticide is morally permissible may be somewhat longer. Although the point at which an organism first achieves self-consciousness and hence the capacity of desiring to continue existing as a subject of experiences and other mental states may be a theoretically incorrect cutoff point, it is at least a morally safe one: any error it involves is on the side of caution.

IV. SOME CRITICAL COMMENTS ON ALTERNATIVE PROPOSALS

I now want to compare the line of demarcation I am proposing with the cutoff points traditionally advanced in discussions of abortion. My fundamental claim will be that none of these cutoff points can be defended by appeal to plausible, basic moral principles. The main suggestions as to the point past which it is seriously wrong to destroy something that will develop into an adult member of the species Homo sapiens are these: (a) conception;

---

[18]There are, however, situations other than those discussed here which might seem to count against the claim that a person cannot have a right unless he is conceptually capable of having the corresponding desire. Can't a young child, for example, have a right to an estate, even though he may not be conceptually capable of wanting the estate? It is clear that such situations have to be carefully considered if one is to arrive at a satisfactory account of the concept of a right. My inclination is to say that the correct description is not that the child now has a right to the estate, but that he will come to have such a right when he is mature, and that in the meantime no one else has a right to the estate. My reason for saying that the child does not now have a right to the estate is that he cannot now do things with the estate, such as selling it or giving it away, that he will be able to do later on.

(b) the attainment of human form; (c) the achievement of the ability to move about spontaneously; (d) viability; (e) birth.[19] The corresponding moral principles suggested by these cutoff points are as follows: (1) It is seriously wrong to kill an organism, from a zygote on, that belongs to the species Homo sapiens. (2) It is seriously wrong to kill an organism that belongs to Homo sapiens and that has achieved human form. (3) It is seriously wrong to kill an organism that is a member of Homo sapiens and that is capable of spontaneous movement. (4) It is seriously wrong to kill an organism that belongs to Homo sapiens and that is capable of existing outside the womb. (5) It is seriously wrong to kill an organism that is a member of Homo sapiens that is no longer in the womb.

My first comment is that it would not do *simply* to omit the reference to membership in the species Homo sapiens from the above principles, with the exception of principle (2). For then the principles would be applicable to animals in general, and one would be forced to conclude that it was seriously wrong to abort a cat fetus, or that it was seriously wrong to abort a motile cat fetus, and so on.

The second and crucial comment is that none of the five principles given above can plausibly be viewed as a *basic* moral principle. To accept any of them as such would be akin to accepting as a basic moral principle the proposition that it is morally permissible to enslave black members of the species Homo sapiens but not white members. Why should it be seriously wrong to kill an unborn member of the species Homo sapiens but not seriously wrong to kill an unborn kitten? Difference in species is not per se a morally relevant difference. If one holds that it is seriously wrong to kill an unborn member of the species Homo sapiens but not an unborn kitten, one should be prepared to point to some property that is morally significant and that is possessed by unborn members of Homo sapiens but not by unborn kittens. Similarly, such a property must be identified if one believes it seriously wrong to kill unborn members of Homo sapiens that have achieved viability but not seriously wrong to kill unborn kittens that have achieved that state.

What property might account for such a difference? That is to say, what *basic* moral principles might a person who accepts one of these five principles appeal to in support of his secondary moral judgment? Why should events such as the achievement of human form, or the achievement of the ability to move about, or the achievement of viability, or birth serve to endow something with a right to life? What the liberal must do is to show that these events involve changes, or are associated with changes, that are morally relevant.

Let us now consider reasons why the events involved in cutoff points (b) through (e) are not morally relevant, beginning with the last two: viability and birth. The fact that an organism is not physiologically dependent upon another organism, or is capable of such physiological independence,

---

[19]Another frequent suggestion as to the cutoff point not listed here is quickening. I omit it because it seems clear that if abortion after quickening is wrong, its wrongness must be tied up with the motility of the fetus, not with the mother's awareness of the fetus' ability to move about.

is surely irrelevant to whether the organism has a right to life. In defense of this contention, consider a speculative case where a fetus is able to learn a language while in the womb. One would surely not say that the fetus had no right to life until it emerged from the womb, or until it was capable of existing outside the womb. A less speculative example is the case of Siamese twins who have learned to speak. One doesn't want to say that since one of the twins would die were the two to be separated, it therefore has no right to life. Consequently it seems difficult to disagree with the conservative's claim that an organism which lacks a right to life before birth or before becoming viable cannot acquire this right immediately upon birth or upon becoming viable.

This does not, however, completely rule out viability as a line of demarcation. For instead of defending viability as a cutoff point on the ground that only then does a fetus acquire a right to life, it is possible to argue rather that when one organism is physiologically dependent upon another, the former's right to life may conflict with the latter's right to use its body as it will, and moreover, that the latter's right to do what it wants with its body may often take precedence over the other organism's right to life. Thomson has defended this view: "I am arguing only that having a right to life does not guarantee having either a right to the use of or a right to be allowed continued use of another person's body—even if one needs it for life itself. So the right to life will not serve the opponents of abortion in the very simple and clear way in which they seem to have thought it would."[20] I believe that Thomson is right in contending that philosophers have been altogether too casual in assuming that if one grants the fetus a serious right to life, one must accept a conservative position on abortion.[21] I also think the only defense of viability as a cutoff point which has any hope of success at all is one based on the considerations she advances. I doubt very much, however, that this defense of abortion is ultimately tenable. I think that one can grant even stronger assumptions than those made by Thomson and still argue persuasively for a semiconservative view. What I have in mind is this. Let it be granted, for the sake of argument, that a woman's right to free her body of parasites which will inhibit her freedom of action and possibly impair her health is stronger than the parasite's right to life, and is so even if the parasite has as much right to life as an adult human. One can still argue that abortion ought not to be permitted. For if A's right is stronger than B's, and it is impossible to satisfy both, it does not follow that A's should be satisfied rather than B's. It may be possible to compensate A if his right isn't satisfied, but impossible to compensate B if his right isn't satisfied. In such a case the best thing to do may be to satisfy B's claim and to compensate A. Abortion may be a case in point. If the fetus has a right to life and the right is not satisfied, there is certainly no way the fetus can be compensated. On the other hand, if the woman's right to rid her body of harmful and annoying parasites is not satisfied, she can be compensated. Thus it would

[20]Thomson, "A Defense of Abortion," p. 56.
[21]A good example of a failure to probe this issue is provided by Brody's "Abortion and the Law."

seem that the just thing to do would be to prohibit abortion, but to compensate women for the burden of carrying a parasite to term. Then, however, we are back at a (modified) conservative position.[22] Our conclusion must be that it appears unlikely there is any satisfactory defense either of viability or of birth as cutoff points.

Let us now consider the third suggested line of demarcation, the achievement of the power to move about spontaneously. It might be argued that acquiring this power is a morally relevant event on the grounds that there is a connection between the concept of an agent and the concept of a person, and being motile is an indication that a thing is an agent.[23]

It is difficult to respond to this suggestion unless it is made more specific. Given that one's interest here is in defending a certain cutoff point, it is natural to interpret the proposal as suggesting that motility is a necessary condition of an organism's having a right to life. But this won't do, because one certainly wants to ascribe a right to life to adult humans who are completely paralyzed. Maybe the suggestion is rather that motility is a sufficient condition of something's having a right to life. However, it is clear that motility alone is not sufficient, since this would imply that all animals, and also certain machines, have a right to life. Perhaps, then, the most reasonable interpretation of the claim is that motility together with some other property is a sufficient condition of something's having a right to life, where the other property will have to be a property possessed by unborn members of the species Homo sapiens but not by unborn members of other familiar species.

The central question, then, is what this other property is. Until one is told, it is very difficult to evaluate either the moral claim that motility together with that property is a sufficient basis for ascribing to an organism a right to life or the factual claim that a motile human fetus possesses that property while a motile fetus belonging to some other species does not. A conservative would presumably reject motility as a cutoff point by arguing that whether an organism has a right to life depends only upon its potentialities, which are of course not changed by its becoming motile. If, on the other hand, one favors a liberal view of abortion, I think that one can attack this third suggested cutoff point, in its unspecified form, only by determining what properties are necessary, or what properties sufficient, for an individual to have a right to life. Thus I would base my rejection of motility as a cutoff point on my claim, defended above, that a necessary condition of an organism's possessing a right to life is that it conceive of itself as a continuing subject of experiences and other mental states.

The second suggested cutoff point—the development of a recognizably human form—can be dismissed fairly quickly. I have already remarked that membership in a particular species is not itself a morally relevant property. For it is obvious that if we encountered other "rational animals," such as Martians, the fact that their physiological makeup was very different

---

[22]Admittedly the modification is a substantial one, since given a society that refused to compensate women, a woman who had an abortion would not be doing anything wrong.

[23]Compare Wertheimer's remarks, "Understanding the Abortion Argument," p. 79.

from our own would not be grounds for denying them a right to life.[24] Similarly, it is clear that the development of human form is not in itself a morally relevant event. Nor do there seem to be any grounds for holding that there is some other change, associated with this event, that is morally relevant. The appeal of this second cutoff point is, I think, purely emotional.

The overall conclusion seems to be that it is very difficult to defend the cutoff points traditionally advanced by those who advocate either a moderate or a liberal position on abortion. The reason is that there do not seem to be any basic moral principles one can appeal to in support of the cutoff points in question. We must now consider whether the conservative is any better off.

V. REFUTATION OF THE CONSERVATIVE POSITION

Many have felt that the conservative's position is more defensible than the liberal's because the conservative can point to the gradual and continuous development of an organism as it changes from a zygote to an adult human being. He is then in a position to argue that it is morally arbitrary for the liberal to draw a line at some point in this continuous process and to say that abortion is permissible before, but not after, that particular point. The liberal's reply would presumably be that the emphasis upon the continuity of the process is misleading. What the conservative is really doing is simply challenging the liberal to specify the properties a thing must have in order to be a person, and to show that the developing organism does acquire the properties at the point selected by the liberal. The liberal may then reply that the difficulty he has meeting this challenge should not be taken as grounds for rejecting his position. For the conservative cannot meet this challenge either; the conservative is equally unable to say what properties something must have if it is to have a right to life.

Although this rejoinder does not dispose of the conservative's argument, it is not without bite. For defenders of the view that abortion is always wrong have failed to face up to the question of the basic moral principles on which their position rests. They have been content to assert the wrongness of killing any organism, from a zygote on, if that organism is a member of the species Homo sapiens. But they have overlooked the point that this cannot be an acceptable *basic* moral principle, since differences in species is not in itself a morally relevant difference. The conservative can reply, however, that it is possible to defend his position—but not the liberal's— *without* getting clear about the properties a thing must possess if it is to have a right to life. The conservative's defense will rest upon the following two claims: first, that there is a property, even if one is unable to specify what it is, that (i) is possessed by adult humans, and (ii) endows any organism

---

[24]This requires qualification. If their central nervous systems were radically different from ours, it might be thought that one would not be justified in ascribing to them mental states of an experiential sort. And then, since it seems to be a conceptual truth that only things having experiential states can have rights, one would be forced to conclude that one was not justified in ascribing any rights to them.

possessing it with a serious right to life. Second that if there are properties which satisfy (i) and (ii) above, at least one of those properties will be such that any organism potentially possessing that property has a serious right to life even now, simply by virtue of that potentiality, where an organism possesses a property potentially if it will come to have that property in the normal course of its development. The second claim—which I shall refer to as the potentiality principle—is critical to the conservative's defense. Because of it he is able to defend his position without deciding what properties a thing must possess in order to have a right to life. It is enough to know that adult members of Homo sapiens do have such a right. For then one can conclude that any organism which belongs to the species Homo sapiens, from a zygote on, must also have a right to life by virtue of the potentiality principle.

The liberal, by contrast, cannot mount a comparable argument. He cannot defend his position without offering at least a partial answer to the question of what properties a thing must possess in order to have a right to life.

The importance of the potentiality principle, however, goes beyond the fact that it provides support for the conservative's position. If the principle is unacceptable, then so is his position. For if the conservative cannot defend the view that an organism's having certain potentialities is sufficient grounds for ascribing to it a right to life, his claim that a fetus which is a member of Homo sapiens has a right to life can be attacked as follows. The reason an adult member of Homo sapiens has a right to life, but an infant ape does not, is that there are certain psychological properties which the former possesses and the latter lacks. Now, even if one is unsure exactly what these psychological properties are, it is clear that an organism in the early stages of development from a zygote into an adult member of Homo sapiens does not possess these properties. One need merely compare a human fetus with an ape fetus. What mental states does the former enjoy that the latter does not? Surely it is reasonable to hold that there are no significant differences in their respective mental lives—assuming that one wishes to ascribe any mental states at all to such organisms. (Does a zygote have a mental life? Does it have experiences? Or beliefs? Or desires?) There are, of course, physiological differences, but these are not in themselves morally significant. *If* one held that potentialities were relevant to the ascription of a right to life, one could argue that the physiological differences, though not morally significant in themselves, are morally significant by virtue of their causal consequences they will lead to later psychological differences that are morally relevant, and for this reason the physiological differences are themselves morally significant. But if the potentiality principle is not available, this line of argument cannot be used, and there will then be no differences between a human fetus and an ape fetus that the conservative can use as grounds for ascribing a serious right to life to the former but not to the latter.

It is therefore tempting to conclude that the conservative view of abortion is acceptable if and only if the potentiality principle is acceptable. But to say that the conservative position can be defended if the potentiality principle is acceptable is to assume that the argument is over once it is granted that the fetus has a right to life, and, as was noted above, Thomson has shown that there are serious grounds for questioning this assumption. In any case, the important point here is that the conservative position on abortion is acceptable *only if* the potentiality principle is sound.

One way to attack the potentiality principle is simply to argue in support of the self-consciousness requirement—the claim that only an organism that conceives of itself as a continuing subject of experiences has a right to life. For this requirement, when taken together with the claim that there is at least one property, possessed by adult humans, such that any organism possessing it has a serious right to life, entails the denial of the potentiality principle. Or at least this is so if we add the uncontroversial empirical claim that an organism that will in the normal course of events develop into an adult human does not from the very beginning of its existence possess a concept of a continuing subject of experiences together with a belief that it is itself such an entity.

I think it best, however, to scrutinize the potentiality principle itself, and not to base one's case against it simply on the self-consciousness requirement. Perhaps the first point to note is that the potentiality principle should not be confused with principles such as the following: the value of an object is related to the value of the things into which it can develop. This "valuation principle" is rather vague. There are ways of making it more precise, but we need not consider these here. Suppose now that one were to speak not of a right to life, but of the value of life. It would then be easy to make the mistake of thinking that the valuation principle was relevant to the potentiality principle—indeed, that it entailed it. But an individual's right to life is not based on the value of his life. To say that the world would be better off if it contained fewer people is not to say that it would be right to achieve such a better world by killing some of the present inhabitants. *If* having a right to life were a matter of a thing's value, then a thing's potentialities, being connected with its expected value, would clearly be relevant to the question of what rights it had. Conversely, once one realizes that a thing's rights are not a matter of its value, I think it becomes clear that an organism's potentialities are irrelevant to the question of whether it has a right to life.

But let us now turn to the task of finding a direct refutation of the potentiality principle. The basic issue is this. Is there any property J which satisfies the following conditions: (1) There is a property K such that any individual possessing property K has a right to life, and there is a scientific law L to the effect that any organism possessing property J will in the normal course of events come to possess property K at some later time. (2) Given the relationship between property J and property K just described, anything possessing property J has a right to life. (3) If property J were not related to property K in the way indicated, it would not be the case that anything possessing property J thereby had a right to life. In short, the question is whether there is a property J that bestows a right to life on an organism *only because* J stands in a certain causal relationship to a second property K, which is such that anything possessing that property ipso facto has a right to life.

My argument turns upon the following critical principle: Let C be a causal process that normally leads to outcome E. Let A be an action that initiates process C, and B be an action involving a minimal expenditure of energy that stops process C before outcome E occurs. Assume further that actions A and B do not have any other consequences, and that E is the only morally significant outcome of process C. Then there is no moral difference between intentionally performing action B and intentionally refraining from performing action A, assuming identical motivation in both cases. This principle, which I shall refer to as the moral symmetry principle with respect to action and inaction, would be rejected by some philosophers. They would argue that there is an important distinction to be drawn between "what we owe people in the form of aid and what we owe them in the way of non-interference."[25] and that the latter, "negative duties," are duties that it is more serious to neglect than the former, "positive" ones. This view arises from an intuitive response to examples such as the following. Even if it is wrong not to send food to starving people in other parts of the world, it is more wrong still to kill someone. And isn't the conclusion, then, that one's obligation to refrain from killing someone is a more serious obligation than one's obligation to save lives?

I want to argue that this is not the correct conclusion. I think it is tempting to draw this conclusion if one fails to consider the motivation that is likely to be associated with the respective actions. If someone performs an action he knows will kill someone else, this will usually be grounds for concluding that he wanted to kill the person in question. In contrast, failing to help someone may indicate only apathy, laziness, selfishness, or an amoral outlook: the fact that a person knowingly allows another to die will not normally be grounds for concluding that he desired that person's death. Someone who knowingly kills another is more likely to be seriously defective from a moral point of view than someone who fails to save another's life.

If we are not to be led to false conclusions by our intuitions about certain cases, we must explicitly assume identical motivations in the two situations. Compare, for example, the following: (1) Jones sees that Smith will be killed by a bomb unless he warns him. Jones's reaction is: "How lucky, it will save me the trouble of killing Smith myself." So Jones allows Smith to be killed by the bomb, even though he could easily have warned him. (2) Jones wants Smith dead, and therefore shoots him. Is one to say there is a significant difference between the wrongness of Jones's behavior in these two cases? Surely not. This shows the mistake of drawing a distinction between positive duties and negative duties and holding that the latter impose stricter obligations than the former. The difference in our intuitions about situations that involve giving aid to others and corresponding situations that involve not interfering with others is to be explained by reference to probable differences in the motivations operating in the two situations,

---

[25]Philippa Foot, "The Problem of Abortion and the Doctrine of the Double Effect," *The Oxford Review* 5 (1967): 5–15.

and not by reference to a distinction between positive and negative duties. For once it is specified that the motivation is the same in the two situations, we realize that inaction is as wrong in the one case as action is in the other.

There is another point that may be relevant. Action involves effort, while inaction usually does not. It usually does not require any effort on my part to refrain from killing someone, but saving someone's life will require an expenditure of energy. One must then ask how large a sacrifice a person is morally required to make to save the life of another. If the sacrifice of time and energy is quite large it may be that one is not morally obliged to save the life of another in that situation. Superficial reflection upon such cases might easily lead us to introduce the distinction between positive and negative duties, but again it is clear that this would be a mistake. The point is not that one has a greater duty to refrain from killing others than to perform positive actions that will save them. It is rather that positive actions require effort, and this means that in deciding what to do a person has to take into account his own right to do what he wants with his life, and not only the other person's right to life. To avoid this confusion, we should confine ourselves to comparisons between situations in which the positive action involves minimal effort.

The moral symmetry principle, as formulated above, explicitly takes these two factors into account. It applies only to pairs of situations in which the motivations are identical and the positive action involves minimal effort. Without these restrictions, the principle would be open to serious objection; with them, it seems perfectly acceptable. For the central objection to it rests on the claim that we must distinguish positive from negative duties and recognize that negative duties impose stronger obligations than positive ones. I have tried to show how this claim derives from an unsound account of our moral intuitions about certain situations.

My argument against the potentiality principle can now be stated. Suppose at some future time a chemical were to be discovered which when injected into the brain of a kitten would cause the kitten to develop into a cat possessing a brain of the sort possessed by humans, and consequently into a cat having all the psychological capabilities characteristic of adult humans. Such cats would be able to think, to use language, and so on. Now it would surely be morally indefensible in such a situation to ascribe a serious right to life to members of the species Homo sapiens without also ascribing it to cats that have undergone such a process of development: there would be no morally significant differences.

Secondly, it would not be seriously wrong to refrain from injecting a newborn kitten with the special chemical, and to kill it instead. The fact that one could initiate a causal process that would transform a kitten into an entity that would eventually possess properties such that anything possessing them ipso facto has a serious right to life does not mean that the kitten has a serious right to life even before it has been subjected to the process of injection and transformation. The possibility of transforming kittens into persons will not make it any more wrong to kill newborn kittens than it is now.

Thirdly, in view of the symmetry principle, if it is not seriously wrong to refrain from initiating such a causal process, neither is it seriously wrong to interfere with such a process. Suppose a kitten is accidentally injected with the chemical. As long as it has not yet developed those properties that in themselves endow something with a right to life, there cannot be anything wrong with interfering with the causal process and preventing the development of the properties in question. Such interference might be accomplished either by injecting the kitten with some "neutralizing" chemical or simply by killing it.

But if it is not seriously wrong to destroy an injected kitten which will naturally develop the properties that bestow a right to life, neither can it be seriously wrong to destroy a member of Homo sapiens which lacks such properties, but will naturally come to have them. The potentialities are the same in both cases. The only difference is that in the case of a human fetus the potentialities have been present from the beginning of the organism's development, while in the case of the kitten they have been present only from the time it was injected with the special chemical. This difference in the time at which the potentialities were acquired is a morally irrelevant difference.

It should be emphasized that I am not here assuming that a human fetus does not possess properties which in themselves, and irrespective of their causal relationships to other properties, provide grounds for ascribing a right to life to whatever possesses them. The point is merely that if it is seriously wrong to kill something, the reason cannot be that the thing will later acquire properties that in themselves provide something with a right to life.

Finally, it is reasonable to believe that there are properties possessed by adult members of Homo sapiens which establish their right to life, and also that any normal human fetus will come to possess those properties shared by adult humans. But it has just been shown that if it is wrong to kill a human fetus, it cannot be because of its potentialities. One is therefore forced to conclude that the conservative's potentiality principle is false.

In short, anyone who wants to defend the potentiality principle must either argue against the moral symmetry principle or hold that in a world in which kittens could be transformed into "rational animals" it would be seriously wrong to kill newborn kittens. It is hard to believe there is much to be said for the latter moral claim. Consequently one expects the conservative's rejoinder to be directed against the symmetry principle. While I have not attempted to provide a thorough defense of that principle, I have tried to show that what seems to be the most important objection to it—the one that appeals to a distinction between positive and negative duties—is based on a superficial analysis of our moral intuitions. I believe that a more thorough examination of the symmetry principle would show it to be sound. If so, we should reject the potentiality principle, and the conservative position on abortion as well.

VI. SUMMARY AND CONCLUSIONS

Let us return now to my basic claim, the self consciousness requirement: An organism possesses a serious right to life only if it possesses the concept of a self as a continuing subject of experiences and other mental states, and believes that it is itself such a continuing entity. My defense of this claim has been twofold. I have offered a direct argument in support of it, and I have tried to show that traditional conservative and liberal views on abortion and infanticide, which involve a rejection of it, are unsound. I now want to mention one final reason why my claim should be accepted. Consider the example mentioned in section II—that of killing, as opposed to torturing, newborn kittens. I suggested there that while in the case of adult humans most people would consider it worse to kill an individual than to torture him for an hour, we do not usually view the killing of a newborn kitten as morally outrageous, although we would regard someone who tortured a newborn kitten for an hour as heinously evil. I pointed out that a possible conclusion that might be drawn from this is that newborn kittens have a right not to be tortured, but do not have a serious right to life. If this is the correct conclusion, how is one to explain it? One merit of the self-consciousness requirement is that it provides an explanation of this situation. The reason a newborn kitten does not have a right to life is explained by the fact that it does not possess the concept of a self. But how is one to explain the kitten's having a right not to be tortured? The answer is that a desire not to suffer pain can be ascribed to something without assuming that it has any concept of a continuing self. For while something that lacks the concept of a self cannot desire that a self not suffer, it can desire that a given sensation not exist. The state desired—the absence of a particular sensation, or of sensations of a certain sort—can be described in a purely phenomenalistic language, and hence without the concept of a continuing self. So long as the newborn kitten possesses the relevant phenomenal concepts, it can truly be said to desire that a certain sensation not exist. So we can ascribe to it a right not to be tortured even though, since it lacks the concept of a continuing self, we cannot ascribe to it a right to life.

This completes my discussion of the basic moral principles involved in the issue of abortion and infanticide. But I want to comment upon an important factual question, namely, at what point an organism comes to possess the concept of a self as a continuing subject of experiences and other mental states, together with the belief that it is itself such a continuing entity. This is obviously a matter for detailed psychological investigation, but everyday observation makes it perfectly clear, I believe, that a newborn baby does not possess the concept of a continuing self, any more than a newborn kitten possesses such a concept. If so, infanticide during a time interval shortly after birth must be morally acceptable.

But where is the line to be drawn? What is the cutoff point? If one maintained, as some philosophers have, that an individual possesses concepts only if he can express these concepts in language, it would be a matter of everyday observation whether or not a given organism possessed the concept of a continuing self. Infanticide would then be permissible up to the time an organism learned how to use certain expressions. However, I think the claim that acquisition of concepts is dependent on acquisition of language is mistaken. For example, one wants to ascribe mental states of a conceptual sort—such as beliefs and desires—to organisms that are incapable of learning a language. This issue of prelinguistic understanding is clearly outside the scope of this discussion. My point is simply that *if* an organism can acquire concepts without thereby acquiring a way of expressing those concepts linguistically, the question of whether a given organism possesses the concept of a self as a continuing subject of experiences and other mental states, together with the belief that it is itself such a continuing entity, may be a question that requires fairly subtle experimental techniques to answer.

If this view of the matter is roughly correct, there are two worries one is left with at the level of practical moral decisions, one of which may turn out to be deeply disturbing. The lesser worry is where the line is to be drawn in the case of infanticide. It is not troubling because there is no serious need to know the exact point at which a human infant acquires a right to life. For in the vast majority of cases in which infanticide is desirable, its desirability will be apparent within a short time after birth. Since it is virtually certain that an infant at such a stage of its development does not possess the concept of a continuing self, and thus does not possess a serious right to life, there is excellent reason to believe that infanticide is morally permissible in most cases where it is otherwise desirable. The practical moral problem can thus be satisfactorily handled by choosing some period of time, such as a week after birth, as the interval during which infanticide will be permitted. This interval could then be modified once psychologists have established the point at which a human organism comes to believe that it is a continuing subject of experiences and other mental states.

The troubling worry is whether adult animals belonging to species other than Homo sapiens may not also possess a serious right to life. For once one says that an organism can possess the concept of a continuing self, together with the belief that it is itself such an entity, without having any way of expressing that concept and that belief linguistically, one has to face up to the question of whether animals may not possess properties that bestow a serious right to life upon them. The suggestion itself is a familiar one, and one that most of us are accustomed to dismiss very casually. The line of thought advanced here suggests that this attitude may turn out to be tragically mistaken. Once one reflects upon the question of the *basic* moral principles involved in the ascription of a right to life to organisms, one may find himself driven to conclude that our everyday treatment of animals is morally indefensible, and that we are in fact murdering innocent persons.

The Ontology of Abortion

H. Tristram Engelhardt, Jr.

Abortion as an ethical issue involves the sense in which the fetus is a person to whom one has obligations. Beyond that, abortion involves other issues of various degrees of severity. There are legal and economic conditions which compel a woman to continue an unwanted pregnancy or which limit resources for its termination.[1] There are gynecological problems of perfecting techniques to reduce mortality and morbidity[2] and psychological problems with respect to the mental sequelae of an abortion.[3] There are also sociological problems insofar as abortion can alter the birth rate[4] and change the number of defective births as well as, perhaps, changing certain attitudes toward sexual activity, including the use of contraceptives.[5] Further, one must assess the significance of the change in the role of the physician implied by his now being not only the preserver, but also the destroyer of human life.[6] If it is resolved that the fetus is not a human person, there still remain unaddressed issues concerning the proper treatment of subpersonal human animals.[7] Finally, there are problems concerning the husband-father's rights and interest in the conceptus.[8] The focus of this paper is meant to deny none of these problems, but it does presuppose that the issue of the possible taking of the life of an innocent person holds precedence; it will, then, begin with its focus upon the ontological status of the fetus. By this is meant the quandary of determining whether or to what extent the fetus is a person. Thus, by ontological status I shall mean certain general categories of being, such as being an inanimate object, being a mere animal, being a fully developed self-conscious human person. With regard to the question of abortion, this is the issue of whether the fetus shows itself to be something to which one owes obligations in the sense one owes

Reprinted by permission of the author and the University of Chicago Press from *Ethics* 84, 217–34, April 1974.

[1] Kathryn G. Milman, "Abortion Reform: History, Status, and Prognosis," *Case Western Reserve Law Review* 21 (April 1970): 521–48; Garrett Hardin, "Abortion—or Compulsory Pregnancy," *Journal of Marriage and the Family* 30 (May 1968): 246–51.

[2] New techniques are, for example, being developed to allow abortion early in pregnancy without the need for cervical dilation, thus further decreasing the incidence of complications (Sadja Goldsmith and Allan J. Margolis, "Aspiration Abortion without Cervical Dilation," *American Journal of Obstetrics and Gynecology,* June 15, 1971, pp. 580–82).

[3] Bengt Jansson, "Mental Disorders after Abortion," *Acta Psychiatrica Scandinavica* 41 (1965): 88–110.

[4] Richard J. Endres, "Abortion in Perspective," *American Journal of Obstetrics and Gynecology* 111 (October 1971): 436–39.

[5] Harold Frederiksen and James W. Brackett, "Demographic Effects of Abortion," *Public Health Reports* 83 (December 1968): 999–1010.

[6] Ian Donald, "Abortion and the Obstetrician," *Lancet,* June 12, 1971, p. 1233.

[7] James S. Scott, "The Abortion Law Reform Debate, United Kingdom, 1966–67: A Gynaecological Viewpoint," *Social Science and Medicine* 1 (January 1968): 390–91.

[8] Leroy Augenstein, *Come, Let Us Play God* (New York: Harper & Row, 1969), p. 121.

obligations to persons. Resolution of other issues, such as the rights of women over their own bodies and the interest of society in more liberal abortion laws,[9] depends first upon whether the fetus is a person, an entity which can claim rights. It is this question of the significance of the status of the fetus which will be the crux of this paper's examination.

The centrality of this ontological quandary is implicit in the conclusion of B. A. Brody in a recent article on abortion. Starting from the premise that questions concerning "the status of the fetus and of whether destroying the fetus constitutes the taking of a human life . . . seem difficult, if not impossible, to resolve upon rational grounds,"[10] he infers that without resolution of this issue it is impossible to justify "liberal" abortion laws.[11] As long as the status of the fetus is unresolved and the clear possibility remains that the fetus enjoys the status of a human person, Brody holds that one is obliged to diminish the incidence of abortions and, therefore, the possible taking of innocent lives. The issue of abortion resolutely leads to the ontological question of when a fetus enjoys the status of a human person.[12] It is in this guise that the issue of the substantiality of the soul or subject reappears (i.e., what counts as the substance, essence, or core of human personhood, and when can this be said to appear in human ontogeny?). The question when fully adumbrated has two poles: ontological and operational. The ontological issue is the meaning of "human person" vis-à-vis "human life"—the issue of distinguishing the significance of two categories: one ethical, the other biological. The operational question arises in deciding what measurable criteria justify the statement that a person now exists where none existed previously. In this question, more is involved than a clarification of the categories of reality. Analogously to the proof of the existence of the immortal soul in medieval philosophy, here a proof or disproof of the presence or absence of at least a mortal human soul is required for the identification of the existence of psychological (or personal), not merely biological, "reality." Unlike Brody, I will be more optimistic with regard to a rational solution of the question of the status of the fetus. This essay will attempt to adduce rational grounds for deciding the status of the fetus and for thus allowing a positive stance with regard to the reform of abortion laws.

I. DISTINCTIONS: ORDINARY AND NEUROLOGICAL

In ordinary circumstances, one distinguishes with ease between things and persons. One distinguishes between those organisms which are persons— subjects of self-consciousness vis-à-vis those organisms which, though they may be the subjects of feelings (and, indeed, perhaps of consciousness),

[9]Judith Jarvis Thomson, "A Defence of Abortion," *Philosophy and Public Affairs* 1 (Fall 1971): 47–66.
[10]B. A. Brody, "Abortion and the Law," *Journal of Philosophy*, June 17, 1971, p. 357.
[11]Ibid., p. 368.
[12]Ibid., p. 369.

show no indication of being self-conscious. That is, one distinguishes between rational animals and brute animals, those that are persons and those that are not. The problem is one of the concepts involved in or the language used to describe substantial change in man. The issue of substance or substantiality with regard to the fetus involves identifying what or who the fetus is and whether this "what" or "who" is the same as the adult "who" which develops out of the fetus.[13] Who is it, as a fetus, who will grow into an adult human? Can one speak in terms of a "who" when referring to the zygote or the fetus in anything but a metaphorical sense? These questions concerning the use of language focus on the issue of whether it is better to describe the appearance of the fully developed person as the emergence of a new level of substantiality. Wittgenstein remarked that "essence is expressed by grammar"[14] and the "grammar tells us what kind of object anything is."[15] I by no means wish to suggest that the problem can be reduced to one of the use of language. But at least the use of language suggests the significance of objects so that syntactically deviant statements can indicate the limits of a type of meaning.[16] That is, when one recognizes that it is nonsensical to speak of stones having pains, one realizes something about the kind of objects stones are—what falls within and what exceeds the sense of their type.[17] Here, the problem is the extent to which it makes sense to speak of the fetus as a person, as a rational animal. The problem is to explicate the sense of "human person," to see the extent to which fetuses fall within the type, "person." This can be indicated at least to a point by what can be spoken of and make sense.

One already has a general idea of what counts as a person or what has the sense of a personal predicate. Of a clubfooted man, one says he is clubfooted, but at death this loses its sense. Of the body of a person who has been pronounced dead but whose functions are being sustained awaiting a transplant operation, does one say he is clubfooted, or that the body has a clubfoot? Moving to our question at the opposite end of the spectrum, how does one speak of the fetus? It would seem to be somewhat metaphorical to speak in the case of the fetus of "he" or "she" doing anything. The use of the personal pronouns "he" and "she" is truncated, for *in utero* there are neither sexual roles nor personal roles to be played by the fetus. If the fetus is more than an "it," "it" surely does not show itself as a person. At

[13]Many philosophers and theologians have held that the fetus was substantially the same from the moment of conception: "What the theologians maintained . . . and what I maintain in following them, is that everyone is human who is conceived by a human being; that human beings may not be discriminated by their varying potentials" (John T. Noonan, Jr., "Deciding Who Is Human," *Natural Law Forum* 13 [1968]: 134).

[14]Ludwig Wittgenstein, *Philosophical Investigations*, trans. G. E. M. Anscombe (Oxford: Basil Blackwell, 1963), par. 371, p. 116.

[15]Ibid., par. 373, p. 116.

[16]The limits of language form the limits of knowledge and, in that sense, grammar is often similar to Kant's transcendental conditions (see Stanley Cavell, "The Availability of Wittgenstein's Later Philosophy," in *Wittgenstein: The Philosophical Investigations*, ed. George Pitcher [Garden City, N.Y.: Doubleday & Co., 1966], pp. 172–82).

[17]Wittgenstein, pars. 282–86, pp. 97–98.

most, the fetus is an animal with great promise of becoming more than just an animal. One speaks more of what the fetus will do or will be as a person, rather than what it is. For example, it is nonsensical to ask someone what he was doing as an embryo or a fetus. This nonsense is closely analogous to that involved in asking someone who has signed papers to donate his body upon death what he will be doing after being pronounced dead while his body is being prepared for a transplant operation. Such discourse appears metaphorical because there is no personal action or personal deportment to which one can refer. Similarly, there is no immediate sense to be made of personal language with reference to the fetus if one restricts oneself to the present state of the fetus. Yet, description of the fetus in frankly personal fashion would have to be appropriate if the fetus were considered a person. In that case, it would make sense to talk about what one did as a fetus. The metaphorical character of such speech suggests that its object does not fall within the usual limits of personal life, that there may be merely human life present but not a person. Again, one is attempting to find the limits of personal life and to establish when there is not merely human life but a person present.

Some might object, though, that there is a paradigm for such talk offered by the case of sleep. In what respect is there a "who" present during sleep, especially dreamless sleep? In what fashion is one to understand one's obligations to sleeping persons, or to understand what it means to talk of a sleeping person, as a person? If nothing of what one is doing while asleep is personal, what sense does it make to speak of a person being present in any but a merely potential or metaphorical fashion? Should one die while asleep, there may very well be merit in saying that one's last presence in the world occurred prior to his sleep. In that case, the only sense that can be made of one's status while asleep is in terms of the expected future, one's potential of awaking. This introduces all the very complex issues of potentiality and their relationship to the continuity of personal life through time. In particular, there is the question whether there is any difference at all between the potentiality of the fetus and the potentiality of the sleeping person.

The difference is suggested by the fact that the potentiality of the sleeping person is concrete and real in the sense of being based upon the past development of a full-blown human person. Unlike the fetus, the sleeping person has secured the capability of being fully human and has exercised it in the world. Far from a promissory note, the potentiality of the sleeping person to awaken is presented in concrete actuality in the physical substratum of that person, in his intact and functioning neocortex. In this case, the concept of person and personal presence depends heavily upon an intact normally developed brain; it presupposes some doctrine of the concomitance of mental personal life with an appropriate physical substratum.[18]

[18]Terence Penelhum, *Survival and Disembodied Existence* (New York: Humanities Press, 1970).

Further, it requires recognizing the singular role of this intact substratum in weaving together the otherwise discontinuous life of the mind.[19] This is completed in a phenomenological basis for distinction between the fetus and the sleeping person. One goes to sleep expecting to awake, and upon awaking, the life that one was leading prior to sleep is felt to continue again.[20] That is, unlike the fetus, the sleeping person had an active conscious life beforehand, rich in protensions of the future which will be woven together in the retentions of the past, in the future when he has awakened. The discontinuity of sleep, in other words, is bridged and woven together in mental life. A physical sign of this is the fact that a sleeping person, unlike the fetus, has a well-developed physical substratum of consciousness—an intact normal brain which can be recognized as the usual basis for presence in the world.

This difference is presented in the issue of brain death. The Ad Hoc Committee of the Harvard Medical School to Examine the Definition of Brain Death[21] and the Ad Hoc Committee of the American Electroencephalographic Society on EEG Criteria for Determination of Cerebral Death[22] have argued that (1) the brain is the physical substratum of conscious life and (2) one can consequently decide when death occurs by appropriate operational parameters which indicate the destruction of the brain as an intact functioning organ. It was decided that a prolonged flat electroencephalograph (in the absence of particular distorting conditions) is a true index of the destruction of the higher central nervous system and, thus, indicates that death has occurred. Importantly, the crucial level of life is more than the mere continuance of biological life. Biological life, in the sense of the integrated function of all the other organs and the lower elements of the central nervous system, continues even in the presence of brain death.[23] Also, for example, a decorticate male who continues to produce sperm would be identifiable as a living member of his species (i.e., as being cross-fertile with other members), and thus would satisfy a minimum definition

[19]John Hughlings Jackson (1835–1911), the father of modern neurology who forwarded a doctrine of the concomitance of mental life and its physical substructure, realized that the continuity of mental life from one period of consciousness to another depends upon the permanence in the interval of the physical substrata of consciousness ("Evolution and Dissolution of the Nervous System" [Croonian Lectures], in *John Hughlings Jackson: Selected Writings*, ed. James Taylor [London: Staples Press, 1958], pp. 45–75).

[20]Alfred Schutz and Thomas Luckmann, *The Structures of the Life-World*, trans., with introduction, R. M. Zaner and H. T. Engelhardt, Jr. (Evanston, Ill.: Northwestern University Press, 1973), p. 47.

[21]Ad Hoc Committee of the Harvard Medical School to Examine the Definition of Brain Death, "A Definition of Irreversible Coma," *Journal of the American Medical Association*, August 5, 1968, pp. 85–88.

[22]Daniel Silverman, Michael G. Saunders, Robert S. Schwab, and Richard L. Masland, "Cerebral Death and the Electroencephalogram," *Journal of the American Medical Association*, September 8, 1968, pp. 1505–10.

[23]Task Force on Death and Dying of the Institute of Society, Ethics, and the Life Sciences, "Refinements in Criteria for the Determination of Death, an Appraisal," *Journal of the American Medical Association*, July 3, 1972, pp. 48–53.

of human biological life.[24] The question of whether a comatose man is dead is the question of whether the actual basis for his being personally present in the world and having rights (i.e., his embodiment in his brain) has been lost. The measurement of the activity of the brain is an attempt to answer the question whether the actual basis for personal presence in the world has been destroyed and the presence of personal human life has, thus, ceased.

The significance of the presence or absence of a flat EEG is different here (i.e., with respect to an unconscious man) than with respect to a fetus.[25] The presence of more than a flat EEG indicates a level of activity of the brain which is a necessary—though not sufficient—condition for personal human life. In the absence of the necessary basis for presence in the world, the issue is resolved and the judgment can be made that personal life has ended: the patient is dead. But presence of more than an active EEG is required to indicate the presence of a human person. In short, the difference lies in the fact that, unlike the sleeping or comatose man, the fetus has not established in the world an actually developed physical basis for personal presence whose loss can then be indicated. It is this physical aspect or dimension of personality, absent in the case of the fetus and present in the case of the sleeping person, which suggests a clear and obvious distinction. The potentiality of the sleeping man is concrete and already established in the world; that of the fetus is abstract and yet to be accomplished. In talking of the sleeping man, one knows of whom one speaks, for the who has been present. In talking of the fetus, one has no idea of whom one speaks, for that who has not yet been present and has not yet, so to speak, laid claim to a body in the world.

In short, everyday decisions have led to a more refined appreciation of what it means to be present in the world. In the distinction between personal human life and biological human life, it is the first not the second which has been recognized as a person before the law. This suggests that one can make similar distinctions at the other end of the developmental scale—namely, with regard to when the fetus becomes a person. Medicine has made a decision concerning a change in the ontological status of a human with regard to death (i.e., it has begun to distinguish between a human person and merely human life). The distinction would appear to involve a judgment that if something can perform none of the actions of a rational being, then it is not one: essence is manifested in existence.[26] It is inviting to apply this criterion to the problem of distinguishing fetuses from children. As in the case of death where one recognizes degeneration from personal human life to merely biological human life, can one not in the case

[24]That is, a criterion for membership in a species is the ability to have fertile mating with its members (Theodosius Dobzhansky, *Genetics of the Evolutionary Process* [New York and London: Columbia University Press, 1970], pp. 359–60).

[25]Recordable electrical activity can be measured from the fetal brain as early as eight weeks of gestation (see D. Goldblatt, "Nervous System and Sensory Organs," in *Intrauterine Development,* ed. A. C. Barnes [Philadelphia: Lea & Febiger, 1968], p. 168).

[26]As Saint Thomas put it, the new perfection of intellectual versus animal existence, in the case of the fetus, is an essential change (*S. T.* I, 118, art. 2, reply to objection 2).

of the fetus recognize a development from merely human biological life to human personal life?

II. SUBSTANTIALITY, POTENTIALITY, AND CONTINUITY

Many who talk about the fetus as a person do so because of its potentiality to become an adult, rational human.[27] This may suggest that there is one substance present throughout the history of the being involved, and, since this being is later rational, the substance itself must be a rational substance *ab initio.*[28] This argument contrasts with the interpretations suggested by this paper: that human ontogeny begins with the body as a "what" or, at most a "who" in the sense that an animal is a who, which then, because of the development or new properties, becomes a who in a personal sense. This, again, brings us forthrightly to the construal of potentiality. If one holds that the fetus is already a person, one is in a sense holding that something is what it will be; that is, since the fetus will be a human person, it already is one. If this is not a claim that future predicates are present predicates, it is at least the position that anything which would in the future have the properties of being a person is already a person. This argument presupposes that only that which already is a human person can in the future acquire the properties of a person, that since it will be a who that will be rational, then the bearer of the potentiality to be a who, a person, must itself be that person. This, though, presupposes what is at issue: whether there is substantial continuity from conception to death. The argument begins with the quandary introduced by an object (i.e., the fetus—child—mature adult) which, though continuous, possesses materially different properties during its development. In an attempt to account for the continuity, the more significant personal predicates which the object will possess in the future are held to be internalized in the present and are made "essentially" part of the object. The object is then said to possess them "potentially" from the beginning. Apart from the concern for continuity, this move is made to account for one's valuing this object because of its promise to have striking and singular significance (i.e., personal significance) in the future. Yet if the potential has the significance and value of the actual, one loses the ability to distinguish between the value of the future and the value of the present. It would seem that one can account for the value of human fetuses vis-à-vis other fetuses as one does with other objects, in terms of their promise, without assuming that their promise is already fulfilled. The value of a potential future state endows an object with value, but not the actual value of that future state. Again, one is back to the question of making sense of potential persons having actual personal status and rights.

[27]John F. Monagle, "The Ethics of Abortion," *Social Justice Review* 65 (July–August 1972): 112–19.

[28]Germaine Grisez, *Abortion: The Myth, the Realities and the Argument* (New York: Corpus Books, 1970); see also Rudolph J. Gerber's comments on Grisez's arguments in "Abortion: Parameters for Decision," *International Philosophical Quarterly* 11 (December 1971): 568.

To account for continuity and future value through a metaphysical doctrine of potentiality or substance (i.e., one in which the potential has real status and defines the "substance" of an object *ab initio*) involves serious difficulties. One runs the risk of conflating properties with the unity of properties. The properties of a bearer are distinguished in order to isolate discrete aspects of a unity. But, as Locke concluded, there is very little one can say about the bearer of the predicates apart from its properties.[29] At most, one can say that the substance is that which bears properties or is the unity of properties.[30] Similarly, Kant held that the unity of the properties apart from unity and permanence is nothing[31] and that to look for a real substance is to mistake what is a unity in appearance for something material in itself.[32] Dealing with substantiality as if it were a thing involves one in talking about superfluous entities, structures imputed to reality though not ingredient in its actual appearance or presented significance. In contrast, in everyday life, one can distinguish a live dog from a dead one and recognize an "essential" change while still recognizing continuity. One need no more ask "where" the potentiality of being a grown dog came from with reference to a fetal dog than to ask "where" the "dogness" went when the dog died. The "dogness" came from where the "dogness" went; the same holds for men. The future properties of an object are not tucked away in its substantiality waiting to be unveiled—the potentiality to have certain properties is not the same as having those properties. To be of the type of object which can in the future have personal predicates does not mean that the object is already a person.

One is faced with adequately categorizing the real distinction in the world between biological and personal life. This is the motive in the choice between various conceptual or ontological systems: one wants to capture and portray adequately the unities and distinctions in the world. It is precisely on this issue that holding a fetus to be a person fails: it is easier to construe the situation as a development from biological properties to personal properties with a consequent essential and substantial change in the significance of the bearer of the properties. An organism changes in significance when it encompasses not merely biological but also personal characteristics, just as it changes in death; though the "matter" remains, the significance is altered. One is forced to consider distinct levels of development with distinct significance.

[29]"So that if any one will examine himself concerning his notion of pure substance in general, he will find he has no other idea of it at all, but only a supposition of he knows not what support of such qualities which are capable of producing simple ideas in us; which qualities are commonly called accidents" (John Locke, *An Essay concerning Human Understanding* [Oxford: Clarendon Press, 1950], bk. 2, chap. 23, p. 155).

[30]"Yet because we cannot conceive how they should subsist alone, nor one in another, we suppose them existing in, and supported by, some common subject; which support we denote by the name substance" (ibid., p. 157).

[31]"The unity of experience would never be possible if we were willing to allow that new things, that is, new *substances*, could come into existence. . . . This permanence is, however, simply the mode in which we represent to ourselves the existence of things in the [field of] appearance" (Immanuel Kant, *Critique of Pure Reason*, trans. Norman Kemp Smith [New York: St. Martin's Press, 1964], p. 216, A 186–B 230).

[32]Ibid., A 277–B 333.

III. ARISTOTLE AND SAINT THOMAS

Unlike his neo-Thomistic descendants, Aristotle conceived of human ontogeny in developmental, even in discontinuous terms. He attempted to
distinguish via formal principles between the significance of organization at
a vegetative level vis-à-vis that at an animal level vis-à-vis that at a rational
level.[33] By distinguishing between various entelechies, actually perfected
structures of being, Aristotle introduced conceptual distinctions allowing
the identification of discrete stages in human ontogeny. One might very well
want to contest his description of the early stages of the fetus as vegetative,
but there is very little to suggest that the fetus is a rational animal as opposed
to merely an animal. The crucial distinction remains between animal life and
personal life. Some have attempted to erode this distinction on the basis of
the evidence for genetic continuity acquired since Aristotle's time. They
argue that genetic endowment at conception implies substantial continuity
and, therefore, personal continuity from that moment.[34] Yet, the significance of continuity in this regard is obscure. Both biological life and genetic
continuity remain after personal death, a distinction implicit in the Kansas
Law of 1970.[35] Further, in the absence of a distinction between personal and
biological life, one would have difficulty in accounting for certain limiting
cases. For example, if one engaged in a thought experiment and imagined
taking a somatic cell and, by cloning, developing it into a second human
individual, one would have difficulty in deciding when there is a second
person and not merely a cell. There is genetic continuity from the first
moment when the cell is removed from the original individual; yet just as
surely one would not want to hold that every cell removed from an individual was another person. When does it become another person? Genetic
continuity is not enough. In fact, strict genetic continuity is not a necessary
condition for personal identity, for one undergoes mutations in a number
of his cells during the course of his life, many such occurring in germ
tissue.[36] It is not surprising, though, that the genetic fact of biological
continuity neither counts for nor against the obvious differences in the
stages of human development. Purely biological facts, as such, have no
implications concerning psychological or personal reality. The genetic basis
for the development of the physiological substratum of consciousness is not
yet that substratum. In Aristotelian language, the genetic endowment would
be part of the matter of human life, and an Aristotelian would have no need
to consider the object (i.e., the human organism) substantially the same
throughout its history. At most, it would be materially the same.

Interestingly, Saint Thomas followed Aristotle in holding for a se-

[33]Aristotle *De Generatione Animalium* 2. 3. 736a and b.

[34]David Granfield, *The Abortion Decision* (Garden City, N.Y.: Doubleday & Co., 1969),
pp. 31–35.

[35]*Kansas Statutes Annotated, Section 77–202.* As William J. Curran noted, this allows the
patient to be pronounced legally dead even though his vital organs are still sustained ("Legal
and Medical Death—Kansas Takes the First Step," *New England Journal of Medicine*, February
4, 1971, pp. 260–61).

[36]M. W. Strickberger, *Genetics* (New York: Macmillan Co., 1968), pp. 523–26.

quence of three souls, the rational soul following the appearance first of the vegetative and then the animal soul.[37] Saint Thomas's doctrine of mediate animation was influenced by Aristotle's observation that "in the case of male children, the first movement usually occurs . . . about the fortieth day, but if the child be a female . . . about the ninetieth day."[38] Aristotle was in error with regard to how early fetal movements could be felt. This passage, though, in conjunction with similar ones of other authors—including a passage in the Septuagint translation of Exodus 21:22—had a significant impact on subsequent thought concerning abortion.[39] This criterion influenced Catholic doctrine, and canon law evolved a distinction between abortion of an ensouled versus abortion of an unensouled fetus. The former was held to be murder, the latter tantamount to birth control.[40] The final shift in Catholic doctrine from mediate to immediate animation (the doctrine that ensoulment takes place at the moment of conception) developed under the pressure of the Catholic dogma of the Immaculate Conception. Since there was already a feast for the birthday of the Blessed Virgin, this raised the issue of what relation the date of the Immaculate Conception should have to the birthday. Following Aristotle, Mary's date of conception as a person should have fallen six months prior to her birth, since she was female. Not unexpectedly, the date of the conception varied from December 8 to the first week in May.[41] But in 1708, Pope Clement XI set the date (i.e., December 8) as an observance for the whole church nine months prior to the date set for her birth (i.e., September 8).[42] This fateful decision suggested that her conception as a person occurred nine months prior to her birth and presupposed the doctrine of immediate animation. Consistently,

[37] *S. T.* I, 118, art. 2.

[38] Aristotle, *The Works of Aristotle Translated into English,* J. A. Smith and W. D. Ross, vol. 4, *Historia Animalium,* trans. D'Arcy W. Thompson (Oxford: Clarendon Press, 1910), 7. 3. 583 b.

[39] The passage in the Septuagint translation distinguished between a formed and an unformed embryo, i.e., between an ensouled and unensouled fetus (see John T. Noonan, Jr., "An Almost Absolute Value in History," in *The Morality of Abortion,* ed. John T. Noonan, Jr. [Cambridge, Mass.: Harvard University Press, 1971], p. 6).

[40] A distinction was made in canon law between the crime of murder and the destruction of an unformed, i.e., an unensouled fetus (*Corpus Juris Canonici Emendatum et Notis Illustratum, cum Glossae: Decretalium d. Gregorii Papae Noni Compilatio* [Rome, 1585], *Glossa ordinaria* at bk. 5, title 12, chap. 20, p. 1713).

[41] C. A. Bouman, "The Immaculate Conception in the Liturgy," in *The Dogma of the Immaculate Conception,* ed. E. D. O'Connor (Notre Dame, Ind.: University of Notre Dame Press, 1958), pp. 125–26. One must be sensitive to the ambiguity of "conception" and "immaculate conception" given a doctrine of mediate animation. "The fetus, being not yet animated by a spiritual soul, cannot be a subject of grace—or of sin either, for that matter. . . . Human nature does not even exist yet in this embryo, which contains human nature only in germ. . . . Before the creation of Mary's soul, that which was to become her body shared the common lot; but before the creation of her soul, *Mary* did not yet exist" (Marie-Joseph Nicolas, "The Meaning of the Immaculate Conception in the Perspectives of St. Thomas," in ibid., p. 333).

[42] Commentary on Section 1400 *Enchiridion Symbolorum Definitionum et Declarationum de Rebus Fidei et Morum,* ed. H. Denziner, rev. A. Schön-Metzer, 33d ed. (Barcelona: Herder, 1965), p. 348. The fact of this decision is explicitly mentioned, for example, in a daily missal which was widely used until the establishment of the vernacular mass (Gaspar Lefebvre, *St. Andrew Daily Missal* [Saint Paul, Minn.: E. M. Lohmann, 1953], p. 866).

Pope Pius IX, who proclaimed the doctrine of the Immaculate Conception in 1854, also was the pope who established the doctrine of immediate animation. On the one hand, he held that Mary was free from original sin "from the first instant of her conception" ("in primo instanti suae conceptionis"),[43] and on the other hand in 1869 he removed from canon law the distinction between an ensouled and unensouled fetus.[44] In so doing, he reversed the trends in canon law which had been in accord with Saint Thomas's doctrine and established the present canonical position.[45] Undoubtedly, this was influential in causing Thomists to reconstrue their Aristotelian account of the substantial unity of man and to attempt to undercut a doctrine of substantial development. They wanted to hold instead that a human was a human person from the moment of conception.[46] One is struck, though, by some possible curious theological consequences inasmuch as at least 28 percent if not 50 percent of all conceptions may end in unnoticed early spontaneous abortions.[47] One would have to hold that a third of humanity entered "eternal life" directly from uterine life. Given the doctrine of original sin, perhaps one would have to take Tristram Shandy's reflections concerning intrauterine baptism more seriously.[48]

IV. SOME CONCLUSIONS
CONCERNING ONTOLOGICAL STATUS

In summary, there are serious difficulties in holding that personal life begins with conception, that the embryo or fetus is a human person. (1) If the human person is characterized as a rational animal, the significance of this with respect to the fetus is mysterious. The fetus shows none of these characteristics. It has no marks of rationality nor of the deportment of a person. (2) To assert that the fetus is a rational animal, a person, because it will be rational and will show the deportment of a person is (*a*) to confuse present and future states, or (*b*) to presuppose a doctrine of substance for which there is no ready warrant in appearance. (3) Some doctrine of mediate animation, analogous to Aristotle's and Saint Thomas's, does better service to the actual ontogeny of humans by categorizing the widely different developmental stages. (4) Further, the possibility of twinning, which exists

---

[43]Pope Pius IX, Bulla "Ineffabilis Deus," December 8, 1854, *Enchiridion Symbolorum Definitionum et Declarationum de Rebus Fidei et Morum,* par. 2803, p. 562.

[44]John T. Noonan, Jr., "An Almost Absolute Value in History," p. 39.

[45]The present canon of the Roman Catholic church makes no distinction between abortion in the early stages vis-à-vis later stages of gestation. It treats them all as if they were instances of homicide (*Codex Juris Canonici* [Vatican: Typis Polyglottis Vaticanis, 1965], canons 985, n. 4, and 2350, sec. 1).

[46]E.g., "If the fetus were not animated by a rational soul from the first moment of conception, it would not develop into a human being" (John P. Kenney, *Principles of Medical Ethics,* 2d ed. [Westminster, Md.: Newman Press, 1962], p. 185).

[47]Arthur T. Hertig, "Human Trophoblast: Normal and Abnormal," *American Journal of Clinical Pathology* 47 (March 1967): 249–68.

[48]Laurence Sterne, *The Life and Opinions of Tristram Shandy, Gentleman* (New York: Holt, Rinehart & Winston, 1962), 1: 51–54.

through the second or third week of gestation would seem to preclude true human individuation until after this period.[49] If one held strictly to the doctrine of immediate animation, one would have a serious dilemma in the case of monozygous twins: would there be splitting of the person or soul, or would one have to hold that there were *ab initio* two persons present (i.e., since in the future there would be two persons present)? Such solutions are conceptually very expensive.[50] In other words, it is difficult to hold that an embryo or fetus is a person, beyond there being no good evidence for holding this. What is proposed here is to start anew with an attempt (1) to account for the development of different levels of significance in human life, and (2) to see what implications this has for the practice of abortion.

V. THE CRITERION OF VIABILITY

In starting from this point, one is faced with the difficulty of adducing criteria to distinguish between merely biological human life and personal human life, between fetuses and persons. Human life is an unbroken continuum which not only extends from one person to another but to the very origin of terrestrial life. Along this continuum, there are significant qualitative differences, but they are tied to quantitative increments which grade one into the other. That is, the qualitative differences are spread over a spectrum so that there is a progression of one into the other: no particular increment of quantitative changes is crucial. Yet, there are differences. Adult intact mature humans have a significance, and they command one's moral acknowledgment in a fashion quite different from ova and sperm. When does a human individual develop, then, to a stage at which one can recognize it as a person to whom one has obligations? This is the problem of identifying where quantitative changes become of qualitative significance, of categorizing a qualitative change along a spectrum manifesting only gradual quantitative progression. In the case of a human being, one has a continuum beginning with the formation of the zygote at conception, progressing to the development of a rational human being, and ending after cerebral death in mere biological existence. When focusing on the continuum between the zygote and the mature person, the ends of the spectrum appear qualitatively distinct, though no particular quantitative change identified a development of a status different in kind.

Following Hegel, one could recognize that this complexity is integral to the category of measure, here the measure of being truly human.[51] Resolving this issue involves clarifying both the conceptual and operational

[49]Frank O. Allan, *Essentials of Human Embryology*, 2d ed. (London: Oxford University Press, 1969), pp. 33–34.

[50]For discussion of splitting persons, see John Perry, "Can the Self Divide?" *Journal of Philosophy*, September 7, 1972, pp. 463–88; also Derek Parfit, "Personal Identity," *Philosophical Review* 80 (January 1971): 3–27.

[51]"Measure is the qualitative quantum, in the first place as immediate—a quantum, to which a determinate being or a quality is attached" (G. W. F. Hegel, *The Logic of Hegel*, trans. William Wallace [London: Oxford University Press, 1965], sec. 107, p. 201).

definitions of being a human person. On the one hand, one must decide what is integral to the concept of human person. On the other, one must decide which quantitative, operational measurements can be used to identify instances of this concept. As a point of departure, the definition of a human person as a rational animal will be accepted: only that which is rational, self-conscious, and embodied in an animal organism counts as a human person. Aristotle's use of fetal movements as an indication of ensoulment is an example of an operational definition. This operational criterion of ensoulment is also found in the common-law criterion of quickening. At common law, abortion appears to have been licit as long as the woman was not yet "quick with child." Prior to that point, she was simply pregnant.[52] This concept lives on in the 1970 State of Washington Law which allows the termination of "a pregnancy of a woman not quick with child."[53] A similar criterion exists in other recent laws which either have chosen a period of gestation taken to preclude viability or simply allow the termination of "the pregnancy of a non-viable fetus," as in the statutes of Alaska and Hawaii.[54] In each case, viability has played a role similar to that of quickening: it is taken to distinguish that level of development at which destruction of fetal life, merely at the desire of the mother, is no longer licit.

The problem is to specify the difference between a fetus and an infant —when is merely a fetus present and when a helpless infant who can claim our obligation to help? Furthermore, as techniques with artificial placentae are developed, will they blur the criterion of viability and involve one in negative infanticide?[55] Presumably, the criterion of viability is employed to identify when there is an obligation to a patient, infants being considered persons who can be patients, vis-à-vis fetuses to which such obligations do not exist. But to understand obligations, more is requisite than just biological criteria, and viability is simply a biological fact. In the case of the fetus, "viability" is used to identify a stage at which the stability of certain basic physiological processes allows for extrauterine life without extraordinary measures tantamount to a surrogate womb. Viability or self-maintenance, as such, implies no social status or level of personal interaction, which could be the basis for the context of physician-patient obligations. To borrow from G. E. Moore's concept of the naturalistic fallacy, biological facts simply as such do not imply ethical obligations.[56] The problem here is central to understanding the nature of human medicine which, unlike veterinary medicine, is caught up with immediate obligation to equals, to other fellow humans. Therefore, the problem is whether the fetus is such an equal, a

[52]*American Law Reports*, annotated, 5th ed. (Rochester, N.Y.: Lawyers Cooperative Publishing Co., 1956), 46: 1396.

[53]*1970 Session Laws of the State of Washington*, chap. 3, sec. 1.

[54]*Alaska Statutes, 1970*, sec. 11.15.060 (a); *Hawaii Revised Statutes 1970 Supplement*, sec. 453–16 (a).

[55]Geoffrey Chamberlain, "An Artificial Placenta," *American Journal of Obstetrics and Gynecology*, March 1, 1968, pp. 615–26.

[56]I.e., purely biological observations, in that they prescind from any other notes of significance, cannot imply anything of nonbiological significance such as ethical obligations.

fellow human person. The character of medicine depends upon the ontological status of the subjects with which it is concerned. To appreciate the fetus
ethically, it must fall within a social category. The ethical significance of a
person, as an object which is an end in itself, is a significance appreciated
socially (i.e., as a value to be respected individually and by the community).
A useful social criterion is needed to set the fetus or infant apart from other
objects and subjects as a person, or at least as a member of human society.
Yet, as Joshua Lederberg has suggested, the only prima facie criterion
appears late in infancy. "An operationally useful point of divergence of the
developing [human] organism would be at approximately the first year of
life when the human infant continues his intellectual development, proceeds
to the acquisition of language, and then participates in a meaningful cognitive interaction with his mother and with the rest of society. At this point
only does he enter into the cultural tradition which has been the special
attribute of man by which he is set apart from the rest of the species."[57]
Thus, the state of affairs is problematic.

VI. VIABILITY AS A SOCIAL CRITERION

If a stringent definition of "human person" is accepted, one would have to
allow not only abortion but infanticide as well. Unlike abortion, however,
infanticide would involve the destruction of members of the species who had
begun to play an explicit role within the social structure of the family and
society, even though they had not yet assumed a full personal life. If nothing
else, such destruction would erode the status of the individual within society
by undermining the status of a positive active social role and relation. To
make sense of the significance of the role "child" and the relation "mother-
child," one needs a point earlier than the acquisition of language as a
criterion for being a human person. Although in early infancy a human
person is not actually present, the child is appreciated socially as an individual to whom one has actual—not potential—obligations in a fashion quite
different from the fetus in the mother-fetus relationship. The newborn
infant, unlike the fetus, can elicit a series of regular responses and activities
from rational humans even though the infant is not itself rational. Even

---

[57]Joshua Lederberg, "A Geneticist Looks at Contraception and Abortion," *Annals of
Internal Medicine* 67 (September 1967): 26–27. I do not mean to suggest that Lederberg advocates infanticide. For a discussion and defense of infanticide see Michael Tooley, "Abortion
and Infanticide," *Philosophy and Public Affairs* 2 (Fall 1972): 37–65. Tooley argues for a strict
concept of person. For him, only that which has the concept of a continuing subject of experiences, and believes itself to be such, has a right to life (pp. 45–47). He holds that infants fail
to satisfy these conditions and thus do not possess a right to life. He suggests, though, that
animals may satisfy these conditions (pp. 62–65). By this last suggestion, he deserts the intuitive
distinction between persons as self-conscious, moral agents, and animals as conscious, nonmoral agents. I identify self-consciousness as a condition for being a person and hold that only
self-conscious agents fall within our ordinary use of person. Only self-conscious subjects can
value themselves, and, thus, be ends in themselves, and, consequently, themselves make claims
against us. It is this which is the intrinsic value of persons. Cf. I. Kant, *Grundlegung zur Metaphysik
der Sitten*, Akademie Textausgabe (Berlin: Walter de Gruyter & Co., 1968), 4: 430.

within primitive social contexts, its crying appears as a demand for food, etc., and initiates a series of activities directed to the infants as if it were a person. That is, even in cultures where full personhood is not accorded until later in childhood, the child plays a role socially and qualitatively distinct from that of the fetus. It is this new social richness which distinguishes the role "child." The biological fact of viable extrauterine life allows a new social level of interaction and significance which contrasts with the lack of regular and usual social communication of need between the fetus and the mother. The infant, in being able to assume the role "child," is socialized in virtue of this role, and the social significance "person" is imputed to it. Although the infant is arational and not yet actually a human person, it can play a relatively independent role in a social matrix which is rational. A relation of obligation is then granted because the infant can engage in crude interactions with others and, thus, play the role "child." A social structure not simply a biological structure is available, namely, the "mother-child" relationship.

At stake is neither a new level of feelings nor even feelings of obligation, but the opportunity for a socially qualitatively different relationship than the mother-fetus relation. Unlike the mother-fetus relationship which is primarily biological and occurs automatically without active involvement of the mother, the mother-child relation is actively and explicitly social. The difference lies in the social schema, the well-developed social role "child," in which the infant can be acted upon as if it were a person and in which it acts back. It is in virtue of this explicit role that the infant is construed as a human person and appreciated as someone to whom one is obliged, especially within the social context of medicine. The biological fact of viability is translated into social terms. Before it is viable without supplying what would be tantamount to a surrogate womb, the fetus remains isolated from the socialization of family life and, in short, has not reached a sufficient level of humanity to be easily recognized within the social category "child." In that the social criterion of viability is not a quantitative category, exact quantitative discriminations are not available. As more can be done for the survival of premature infants, social action can obscure even more of the moment when the fetus becomes socialized and appreciated as a "child." New avenues for sustaining aborted fetuses in a sense will bring the fetus within the social context of the hospital, even if not within that of the family. Thus, the time for acknowledging the fetus as a human person falls within an uncertain range made more uncertain. But the exact time fails to be crucial, for in a strict sense there is not a rational animal present. One need be concerned only that the role "child," when established, not be eroded. Viable (i.e., without special medical intervention, on a par with a term baby) near-term fetuses, if aborted, should be sustained. Beyond that, the period of gestation allowable before an abortion is arbitrary. With that stipulation, though, one finally possesses a quantitative operational criterion. That is, to avoid with a certain degree of certainty the abortion of an otherwise viable fetus, one establishes periods of gestation as the upper limit for abortion on demand. Put in other terms, by setting a particular period of gestation as a criterion, one decides how few such instances there will be. Surely, if by

viability one means viable without any more assistance than required by a
healthy term baby, then in the very early weeks of gestation (under twenty
weeks if the ascertainment of the period of gestation of the mother has been
accurate) the probability approaches zero.

The question of the time of the emergence of a human person has,
thus, received two answers. First, a human person in the strict sense of a
self-conscious rational animal is not present until somewhat late in infancy.
Second, there is a social category of child into which one allows newborn
infants to enter as one brings them within the social context and schema of
the family. The identification of the first instances in human ontogeny of
personal human life (i.e., the "metaphysical pole" of the issue in the sense
of giving a proof in particular cases for the existence of a person) is, thus,
approached through a social construal of the biological criterion of viability.[58] This has the virtue of preserving social values, such as the dignity and
integrity of the role and office of human person, while allowing latitude for
the stipulation of exact quantitative criteria. Further, the social criterion of
viability places the fetus with regard to the obligations of medicine and sets
a time in the ontogeny of man for the infant to emerge as a person to whom
medicine has obligations. In that man is a social animal and medicine a social
enterprise or even a social science as Rudolf Virchow characterized it,[59] it
is not surprising that medicine should employ such a social category. This
criterion has the advantage of preserving the social values ingredient in the
dignity of the human person and preserving the role of the physician as the
guardian of personal human life without recourse to inaccessible metaphysical principles. In short, the first answer concerning the strict definition of
a person establishes the rationale for liberal abortion laws, and the second
answer concerning the social category "child" gives a basis for the proscription of abortion on demand beyond the point when viable birth is possible.

VII. OTHER ISSUES AND CONCLUSIONS

In closing, certain general issues and problems in abortion need mention.
The rights of the mother regarding abortion are paramount. After all, she
is the only actual person involved. As a fully actual, developed rational
human, it is she, surely, who has prima facie rights over her own body.
Consequently, it is to her that one owes overriding obligations. Medicine
must be acutely concerned that the pregnant woman's rights be satisfied
before those of another (namely, the rights of the fetus) emerge to challenge
hers. Further, one should strive in all cases to perform abortions as early in
gestation as possible, because from the mother's point of view it would
reduce mortality and morbidity. Another reason for following this course is
consideration of the fetus. As Dr. James S. Scott has emphasized, evidence

[58]It might be worth remarking here that there is a difference between inferring ethical
consequences from biological facts and identifying the usual biological substrata or of conditions for ethical interactions.

[59]Rudolf Virchow, "Die naturwissenschäftliche Methode und die Standpunkte in der
Therapie," *Archive für pathologische Anatomie und Physiologie und für klinische Medizin* 2 (1849): 36.

shows that the fetus is sensitive to pain, and the more developed the fetus becomes, the more acutely the pain of abortion is perceived.[60] If one is concerned about the pain of subhuman animals, one should also be attentive to the pain of subpersonal human animals.

The examination of the ontological status of the fetus, then, has led to certain conclusions. It has proved impossible to establish a basis for holding the fetus is a human person. Everyday distinctions between nonpersonal organisms and persons, between biological life and personal life in the case of death, between the abstract promissory potentiality of fetuses vis-à-vis the meaning of potentiality when referring to concrete, actual persons (even sleeping men) all point to a distinction between fetuses and other humans based on the distinction between biological life and personal life. Though the fetus is obviously an example of human life, it is in no way suggestive of personal life. In choosing categories with which to think and talk of the fetus's status, those suggested by Aristotle and Saint Thomas coincide to a great extent with the available evidence: human ontogeny is marked by a series of stages in which the human progressively acquires greater worth, moving from mere biological life to full personal existence. It has been noted that the discovery of genetic continuity from the point of conception in no way alters these conclusions. The result is, then, the recognition of two categories of human life: biological and personal. In short, the ontological status of the fetus is found to be nonpersonal, or merely biological.

The conclusion is, therefore, that one can prosecute the establishment of liberal abortion laws and support the recent United States Supreme Court decisions[61] on the prima facie ground of a woman's right to control her own body. No one else's personal rights are intimately involved; the fetus has no personal rights. Further, the role of medicine as caretaker of human life is preserved, or, at most, refined: medicine serves human persons, not merely human life. The role of the physician in the termination of fetal life in no way erodes his traditional position as defendant of human persons through the vicissitudes of nature but rather sustains it. In short, the problem of abortion hinges upon the philosophical problem of clarifying the definition of "human." Ultimately, such distinctions are of immense moment for the practice of medicine and the future of medical technology. The abilities of medicine to support mere human biological life are immense, but resources for such support are limited. The distinction between human biological and personal life is central to an understanding which can focus technology on the enhancement of human personal life. Here in particular it means not compelling a woman to have an unwanted pregnancy, a family to have unwanted children, or families and societies to have defective children whose emergence as persons can be prevented by abortion. In each instance, this enhancement of personal life is sought not through the limitation of the life of other persons, but only of nonpersonal, human biological life. Being clear about the ontological status of fetuses focuses medicine more clearly on the value of persons.

[60]Scott (n. 7 above), pp. 390–91.
[61]Roe v. Wade, 93 S.CT.705 (1973), and Doe v. Bolton 93 S.CT.739 (1973).

From "Dilemmas of 'Informed Consent' in Children"

Anthony M. Shaw and Iris A. Shaw

Numerous articles have been written about "rights" of patients. We read about "right to life" of the unborn, "right to die" of the elderly, "Bill of Rights" for the hospitalized, "Declaration of Rights" for the retarded, "right of privacy" for the pregnant and, of course, "right to medical care" for us all.

Whatever the legitimacy of these sometimes conflicting "rights" there is at present general agreement that patients have at least one legal right: that of "informed consent"—i.e., when a decision about medical treatment is made, they are entitled to a full explanation by their physicians of the nature of the proposed treatment, its risks and its limitations. Once the physician has discharged his obligation fully to inform* an adult, mentally competent patient, that patient may then accept or reject the proposed treatment, or, indeed, may refuse any and all treatment, as he sees fit. But if the patient is a minor, a parental decision rejecting recommended treatment is subject to review when physicians or society disagree with that decision.

The purpose of this paper is to consider some of the moral and ethical dilemmas that may arise in the area of "informed consent" when the patient is a minor. The following case reports, all but two from my practice of pediatric surgery, raise questions about the rights and obligations of physicians, parents and society in situations in which parents decide to withhold consent for treatment of their children.

Instead of presenting a full discussion of these cases at the end of the paper, I have followed each case presentation with a comment discussing the points I wish to make, relating the issues raised by that case to those raised in some of the other cases, and posing the very hard questions that I had to ask myself in dealing with the patients and parents. At present the questions are coming along much faster than the answers.

CASE REPORTS

A. Baby A was referred to me at 22 hours of age with a diagnosis of esophageal atresia and tracheoesophageal fistula. The infant, the firstborn of a professional couple in their early thirties, had obvious signs of mongolism, about which they were fully informed by the referring physician. After explaining the

Reprinted with permission of the authors and publishers from *The New England Journal of Medicine*, 289:17, 885–890, October 25, 1973. Copyright, Massachusetts Medical Society.

*I agree with Ingelfinger that "educate" is a better concept here than "inform."

nature of the surgery to the distraught father, I offered him the operative consent. His pen hesitated briefly above the form and then as he signed, he muttered, "I have no choice, do I?" He didn't seem to expect an answer, and I gave him none. The esophageal anomaly was corrected in routine fashion, and the infant was discharged to a state institution for the retarded without ever being seen again by either parent.

Comment

In my opinion, this case was mishandled from the point of view of Baby A's family, in that consent was not truly informed. The answer to Mr. A's question should have been, "You *do* have a choice. You might want to consider not signing the operative consent at all." Although some of my surgical colleagues believe that there is no alternative to attempting to save the life of every infant, no matter what his potential, in my opinion, the doctrine of informed consent should, under some circumstances, include the right to withhold consent. If the parents do have the right to withhold consent for surgery in a case such as Baby A, who should take the responsibility for pointing that fact out to them—the obstetrician, the pediatrician or the surgeon?

Another question raised by this case lies in the parents' responsibility toward their baby, who has been saved by their own decision to allow surgery. Should they be obligated to provide a home for the infant? If their intention is to place the baby after operation in a state-funded institution, should the initial decision regarding medical or surgical treatment for their infant be theirs alone?

B. Baby B was referred at the age of 36 hours with duodenal obstruction and signs of Down's syndrome. His young parents had a 10-year-old daughter, and he was the son they had been trying to have for 10 years; yet, when they were approached with operative consent, they hesitated. They wanted to know beyond any doubt whether the baby had Down's syndrome. If so, they wanted time to consider whether or not to permit the surgery to be done. Within 8 hours a geneticist was able to identify cells containing 47 chromosomes in a bone-marrow sample. Over the next 3 days the infant's gastrointestinal tract was decompressed with a nasogastric tube, and he was supported with intravenous fluids while the parents consulted with their ministers, with family physicians in their home community and with our geneticists. At the end of that time the B's decided not to permit surgery. The infant died 3 days later after withdrawal of supportive therapy.

Comment

Unlike the parents of Baby A, Mr. and Mrs. B realized that they did have a choice—to consent or not to consent to the intestinal surgery. They were afforded access to a wide range of resources to help them make an informed decision. The infant's deterioration was temporarily prevented by adequate intestinal decompression and intravenous fluids.

Again, some of the same questions are raised here as with Baby A. Do the parents have the right to make the decision to allow their baby to die without surgery?

Can the parents make a reasonable decision within hours or days after the birth of a retarded or brain-damaged infant? During that time they are overwhelmed by feelings of shock, fear, guilt, horror and shame. What is the proper role of the medical staff and the hospital administration? Can parents make an intelligent decision under these circumstances, or are they simply reacting to a combination of their own instincts and fears as well as to the opinions and biases of medical staff? Rickham has described the interaction of physician and parents in such situations as follows:

> Every conscientious doctor will, of course, give as correct a prognosis and as impartial an opinion about the possible future of the child as he can, but he will not be able to be wholly impartial, and, whether he wants it or not, his opinion will influence the parents. At the end it is usually the doctor who has to decide the issue. It is not only cruel to ask the parents whether they want their child to live or die, it is dishonest, because in the vast majority of cases, the parents are consciously or unconsciously influenced by the doctor's opinion.

I believe that parents often *can* make an informed decision if, like the B's, they are afforded access to a range of resources beyond the expertise and bias of a single doctor and afforded sufficient time for contemplation of the alternatives. Once the parents have made a decision, should members of the medical staff support them in their decision regardless of their own feelings? (This support may be important to assuage recurrent feelings of guilt for months or even years after the parents' decision.)

When nutritional and fluid support was withdrawn, intestinal intubation and pain medication were provided to prevent suffering. To what extent should palliative treatment be given in a case in which definitive treatment is withheld? The lingering death of a newborn infant whose parents have denied consent for surgery can have a disastrous effect on hospital personnel, as illustrated . . . by the well publicized Johns Hopkins Hospital case, which raised a national storm of controversy. In this case, involving an infant with mongoloidism and duodenal atresia, several of the infant's physicians violently disagreed with the parents' decision not to allow surgery. The baby's lingering death (15 days) severely demoralized the nursing and house staffs. In addition, it prolonged the agony for the parents, who called daily to find out if the baby was still alive. Colleagues of mine who have continued to keep such infants on gastrointestinal decompression and intravenous fluids for weeks after the parents have decided against surgery have told me of several cases in which the parents have finally changed their minds and given the surgeon a green light! Does such a change of heart represent a more deliberative decision on the part of the parents or merely their capitulation on the basis of emotional fatigue?

After the sensationalized case in Baltimore, Johns Hopkins Hospital established a committee to work with physicians and parents who are confronted by similar problems. Do such medical-ethics committees serve as a useful resource for physicians and families, or do they, in fact, further complicate the decision-making process by multiplying the number of opinions?

Finally, should a decision to withhold surgery on an infant with Down's syndrome or other genetically determined mental-retardation states be allowed on clinical grounds only, without clear-cut chromosomal evidence?

> C. I was called to the Newborn Nursery to see Baby C, whose father was a busy surgeon with 3 teen-age children. The diagnoses of imperforate anus and microcephalus were obvious. Doctor C called me after being informed of the situation by the pediatrician. "I'm not going to sign that op permit," he said. When I didn't reply, he said, "What would you do, doctor, if he were your baby?" "I wouldn't let him be operated on either," I replied. Palliative support only was provided, and the infant died 48 hours later.

Comment

Doctor C asked me bluntly what I would do were it my baby, and I gave him my answer. Was my response appropriate? In this case I simply reinforced his own decision. Suppose he had asked me for my opinion before expressing his own inclination? Should my answer in any case have simply been, "It's not my baby"—with a refusal to discuss the subject further? Should I have insisted that he take more time to think about it and discuss it further with his family and clergy, like the parents of Baby B? Is there a moral difference between withholding surgery on a baby with microcephalus and withholding surgery on a baby with Down's syndrome?

Some who think that all children with mongolism should be salvaged since many of them are trainable, would not dispute a decision to allow a baby with less potential such as microcephalic Baby C to die. Should, then, decisions about life and death be made on the basis of IQ? . . .

> E. A court order *was* obtained for Baby E. . . . This infant, with Down's syndrome, intestinal obstruction and congenital heart disease, was born in her mother's car on the way to the hospital. The mother thought that the retarded infant would be impossible for her to care for and would have a destructive effect on her already shaky marriage. She therefore refused to sign permission for intestinal surgery, but a local child-welfare agency, invoking the state child-abuse statute, was able to obtain a court order directing surgery to be performed. After a complicated course and thousands of dollars worth of care, the infant was returned to the mother. The baby's continued growth and development remained markedly retarded because of her severe cardiac disease. A year and a half after the baby's birth, the mother felt more than ever that she had been done a severe injustice.

Comment

Is the crux of this case parental rights versus the child's right to life? Can the issue in this case be viewed as an extension of the basic dilemma in the abortion question? Does this case represent proper application of child-abuse legislation—i.e., does the parents' refusal to consent to surgery constitute neglect as defined in child-abuse statutes? If so, under these statutes does a physician's concurrence in a parental decision to withhold treatment constitute failure to report neglect, thereby subjecting him to possible prosecution?

Baby E's mother voluntarily took the baby home, but had she not done so, could the state have forced her to take the baby? Could the state have required her husband to contribute to the cost of medical care and to the subsequent maintenance of the infant in a foster home or institution?

If society decides that the attempt must be made to salvage every human life, then, as I have written, ". . . society *must* provide the necessary funds and facilities to meet the continuing medical and psychological needs of these unfortunate children."

> F. Baby F was conceived as the result of an extramarital relation. Mrs. F had sought an abortion, which she had been denied. F was born prematurely, weighing 1600 g and in all respects normal except for the presence of eso-phageal atresia and tracheoesophageal fistula. Mrs. F signed the operative consent, and the surgery was performed uneventfully. Mrs. F fears that her husband will eventually realize that the baby is not his and that her marriage may collapse as a result of this discovery.

Comment

Like those of Mrs. E, Mrs. F's reasons for not wanting her baby were primarily psychosocial. However, Mrs. F never raised the question of with-holding consent for surgery even though the survival of her infant might mean destruction of her marriage. Does the presence of mental retardation or severe physical malformation justify withholding of consent for psychoso-cial reasons (Babies B, C, . . ., and E), whereas the absence of such conditions does not (Baby F)? If she had decided to withhold consent there is no doubt in my mind that I would have obtained a court order to operate on this baby, who appeared to be normal beyond her esophageal anomaly. Although I personally would not have objected to an abortion in this situation for the sociopsychologic reasons, I would not allow an otherwise normal baby with a correctable anomaly to perish for lack of treatment for the same reasons. Although those who believe that all life is sacred, no matter what its level of development, will severely criticize me for the apparent inconsistency of this position, I believe it to be a realistic and humane approach to a situation in which no solution is ideal.

Although my case histories thus far have dealt with the forms of mental retardation most common in my practice, similar dilemmas are encountered by other physicians in different specialties, the most obvious being in the spectrum of hydrocephalus and meningomyelocele. Neurosurgeons are still grappling unsuccessfully and inconsistently with indications for surgery in this group, trying to fit together what is practical, what is moral, and what is humane. If neurosurgeons disagree violently over criteria for operability on infants with meningomyelocele, how can the parents of such a child decide whether to sign for consent? Who would say that they *must* sign if they don't want a child whose days will be measured by operations, clinic visits and infections? I have intentionally omitted from discussion in this paper the infant with crippling deformities and multiple anomalies who does not have rapidly lethal lesions. Infants with such lesions may survive for long periods and may require palliative procedures such as release of limb contractures, ventriculoperitoneal shunts, or colostomies to make their lives more tolerable or to simplify their management. The extent to which these measures are desirable or justifiable moves us into an even more controversial area.

I must also point out that the infants discussed in the preceding case reports represent but a small percentage of the total number of infants with mental-retardation syndromes on whom I have operated. Once the usual decision to operate has been made I, of course, apply the same efforts as I would to any other child. . . .

DISCUSSION

If an underlying philosophy can be gleaned from the vignettes presented above, I hope it is one that tries to find a solution, humane and loving, based on the circumstances of each case rather than by means of a dogmatic formula approach. ([Joseph] Fletcher has best expressed this philosophy in his book, *Situation Ethics,* and in subsequent articles.) This outlook contrasts sharply with the rigid "right-to-life" philosophy, which categorically opposes abortion, for example. My ethic holds that all rights are not absolute all the time. As Fletcher points out, ". . .all rights are imperfect and may be set aside if human *need* requires it." My ethic further considers quality of life as a value that must be balanced against a belief in the sanctity of life.

Those who believe that the sanctity of life is the overriding consideration in all cases have a relatively easy time making decisions. They say that all babies must be saved; no life may be aborted from the womb, and all attempts to salvage newborn life, whatever its quality and whatever its human and financial costs to family and society, must be made. Although many philosophies express the view that "heroic" efforts need not be made to save or prolong life, yesterday's heroic efforts are today's routine procedures. Thus, each year it becomes possible to remove yet another type of malformation from the "unsalvageable" category. All pediatric surgeons, including myself, have "triumphs"—infants who, if they had been born 25 or even five years ago, would not have been salvageable. Now with our team approaches, staged surgical technics, monitoring capabilities, ventilatory support systems and intravenous hyperalimentation and elemental diets, we can wind up with "viable" children three and four years old well below the third percentile in height and weight, propped up on a pillow, marginally tolerating an oral diet of sugar and amino acids and looking forward to another operation.

Or how about the infant whose gastrointestinal tract has been removed after volvulus and infarction? Although none of us regard the insertion of a central venous catheter as a "heroic" procedure, is it right to insert a "lifeline" to feed this baby in the light of our present technology, which can support him, tethered to an infusion pump, for a maximum of a year and some months?

Who should make these decisions? The doctors? The parents? Clergymen? A committee? As I have pointed out, I think that the parents must participate in any decision about treatment and that they must be fully informed of the consequences of consenting and of withholding consent. This is a type of informed consent that goes far beyond the traditional presentation of possible complications of surgery, length of hospitalization, cost of the operation, time lost from work, and so on.

It may be impossible for any general agreement or guidelines for making decisions on cases such as the ones presented here to emerge, but I believe we should bring these problems out into public forum because whatever the answers may be, they should not be the result of decisions made solely by the attending physicians. Or should they?

Spina Bifida

The Editors

Spina bifida is the result of faulty embryological development of the spinal cord and the vertebral column. In serious cases of spina bifida, the infant is born with a meningomyelocele (also called myelomeningocele), a protruding sac filled with cerebrospinal fluid and containing a defective spinal cord. The sac is not usually covered by anything resembling normal skin and may leak fluid. These lesions occur most commonly at the small of the back, but may be higher or lower.

As a consequence of the spinal cord deformity, the child is paralyzed below the level of the lesion. This always involves loss of bladder and bowel control and, depending on the level of the sac, paraplegia. The kidneys may also be dysfunctional. There is usually impairment of normal circulation of cerebrospinal fluid, leading to hydrocephalus—an accumulation of excess fluid in the brain which can result in mental retardation. Without this complication the child may have normal or above average intelligence.

The incidence of spina bifida with a meningomyelocele is about two per 1000 live births. One pediatric surgeon estimates that years of spina bifida treatment will cost $250,000 or $300,000 per patient. For a family with one child with spina bifida, the chances of having another damaged child are about 9%.

Treatment of these infants involves immediate closure of the defect to prevent infection and further rapid neurologic loss. A surgical shunt may be necessary to alleviate the hydrocephalus. Efforts at correcting orthopedic problems may include putting the legs in casts. Later, incontinence may be modified surgically or with devices. Even with vigorous therapy, the results are seldom very good. In a study of 323 "vigorously attended" children, British physician John Lorber found that 134 were still alive after 8 to 12

Reprinted from *Teaching Medical Ethics: A Report on One Approach,* Moral Problems in Medicine Project, Department of Philosophy, Case Western Reserve University, Cleveland, 1973, pp. 29–30.

years. But most lived pitiful lives. About half had shunts draining their hydrocephalus (many of these with an IQ below 80), 40% were totally incontinent, 43% had chronic urinary infections, and only 17 of the 134 survivors could walk unaided. Although the advent of new drugs and new therapies has enabled physicians to treat these children more actively, Lorber feels that it has not improved the quality of their lives, but instead has kept alive a larger percentage of more severely handicapped retarded children. He has proposed that the worst cases not be treated, citing studies that over 90% of untreated cases are dead by their first birthday.

Dr. John Freeman, of Johns Hopkins Medical School, who has also treated many spina bifida children, is concerned about these untreated survivors, some of whom live for years, whose quality of life is worse than if they had been treated initially. Therefore, given the choice of treating or not treating, he feels that one is compelled to give maximum treatment.

Ethical and Social Aspects of Treatment of Spina Bifida

R. B. Zachary

In our society the actions of one individual towards another are not without their effect on the rest of the community. Our plans of action in the treatment of myelomeningocele and their attainment are directed in the first place to the patient, but there are also important and significant effects on the family and on the community. Although we acknowledge and accept these wider effects of our treatment, we have always thought that our primary duty is to the patient, and that the most important decision is to do what is right and best for him.

I shall therefore consider first the question of the treatment of the patient and afterwards the important social implications of this treatment.

THE CHILD

The first and the most serious ethical problem arising in the case of a child with myelomeningocele is whether he should receive medical treatment or not. The relative merits of early operation, secondary operation, or no operation at all, can only be decided when this basic principle has been established.

When a baby is born with a serious spina bifida (i.e., a myelomeningocele with a plaque of neural tissue exposed on the surface and with all the associated complications) there are three possible lines of thought: (1) he

Reprinted with permission of author and publisher from *The Lancet*, 274–76, August 3, 1968.

should be killed; (2) he should be encouraged to die, either by giving no treatment at all (e.g., no feeding) or by not treating complications (e.g., no treatment of infection by antibiotics); or (3) he should be encouraged to live.

The ethical principle that the direct and deliberate killing of a human being is wrong is widely accepted on a religious and philosophical basis, and has been the basis of medical practice since the time of Hippocrates, and even earlier. (I am talking of medical matters here, not of crime and war.) The second alternative has no better justification. To leave a child without food is to kill it as deliberately and directly as if one was cutting its throat. Even the prescribing of antibiotics for infection, such as pneumonia, must now be considered as ordinary care of patients.

Once the principle has been established that the child should be encouraged to live, we are then in a position to consider which method of management gives the child the best chance to live, and secondly, which method of treatment will reduce the handicap to a minimum.

There is a widely held but mistaken view that the purpose of early operation in myelomeningocele is to save the child's life—that if operation is undertaken the child will live, and if operation is not undertaken the child will die. Pediatric surgeons will at once recognize that this is untrue, and that it contrasts with the treatment of many other congenital abnormalities. For example, in esophageal atresia we know for certain that the child will die unless a neonatal operation is undertaken, but quite a number of patients with myelomeningocele survive without any operation at all on the back, and some die as a direct result of operation when otherwise they might have survived.

In other words, there is no necessary connection between early operation and survival. It is true that in a large series of cases treated with and without operation, the results favour surgery as far as mortality is concerned. Yet this is probably not a valid reflection of the effect of operation on survival-rates. Surgical patients are receiving active treatment from all points of view: infections are treated vigorously whether they are local infections, systemic infections, or ventriculitis, and the child will probably be getting better attention to the renal tract than those who are receiving no treatment at all. I do not think it has been proved, from a concurrent study of two large series of cases, that the mortality is less in those receiving early operation than in those who do not have early operation but, in every other respect, receive the same care and attention as the surgical series.

The question at issue is whether there are advantages of early operation which outweigh any possible extra risks that such operation might have for the life of the child.

The surgeon who operates on such a child in the neonatal period has a continuing concern for the fullest development of the child; and I think it is right to emphasize the maximum development of the child, rather than the reduction of handicaps to the minimum, for this will influence the whole attitude to the child and his future.

The doctor who accepts the responsibility for the early treatment of the child, whether he be pediatrician, or pediatric surgeon, or neurosurgeon, has a duty to see that the long-term total development of the child is always kept in mind. The treatment of the hydrocephalus is only a part of the total care of these children, and we have no hesitation in calling upon other specialists to help in those aspects of the total care of the child in which we ourselves are not competent. The amount of outside help required will vary from one centre to another, but we must be quite certain that the child's orthopedic difficulties, those of the lower limbs and the spine, his renal-tract problems, and his ophthalmic problems, are dealt with competently.

What will be the effect of this treatment on the child himself? Most of the survivors who have had a severe myelomeningocele will still remain severely handicapped—they will have considerable weakness of the lower limbs and will probably be wearing callipers. About 10% will be permanently in a wheelchair, but others may use a wheelchair for most of the time, but will be able to walk a little. Few will have normal renal tracts, either because of poor control of the bladder or because of renal-tract infection and renal damage, and there will be many with urinary diversions. In most cases the hydrocephalus will be well controlled, but even as the children approach school age it may still be necessary for revision operations on the ventriculocaval shunt.

As the child grows up, therefore, his disabilities are mainly those of the lower part of the body—his arms are normal, and his head circumference will usually be within the normal range or only slightly above, and 90% of the children will be educable. In fact it is likely that between two-thirds and three-quarters of them will have an intelligence quotient within the normal range, and from this point of view be capable of receiving normal education.

THE FAMILY

But the child is not going to develop in vacuo, he is going to be brought up in a family as part of a community, and his prospects will depend very much on his integration into the life of the family and the possibility of the community supplying any special needs.

We should consider first the effect on the family of the birth of a seriously handicapped child such as one with serious myelomeningocele. Such an event is not merely a disappointment after nine months of pregnancy, it is a shattering blow to the confidence of the parents in themselves, and one which we must understand if we are to be able to help. It is strange that in these days of equality of the sexes, there is a very common and frequent feeling among the mothers that they have failed their husbands by producing a baby who is not perfect, and there is an immediate searching back in the memory for any event in the early part of pregnancy which could have contributed to this catastrophe. Later comes the recognition on the part of each parent that this may be not entirely due to them, that perhaps the other partner is partly or mainly to blame, and I think it is very important to foresee these doubts, particularly when the parents ask whether there is an hereditary factor concerned with the deformity. If parents ask me whether it is likely that another child in the family will also have spina bifida my immediate answer is that it is most unlikely to happen. If they would like some further information on this point, I give them the figures that we have used for a long time as the basis of our advice, namely, that there is, perhaps, a 5–10% chance of another child having this congenital anomaly. This is, of course, about 20–30 times the incidence in the rest of the community, and such a risk would deter some parents from having further children. However, I think it should be pointed out to them that this means that there is perhaps a 90–95% chance of a subsequent child being normal in this respect: strangely, this alternative way of expressing the same facts seems much more promising to them (indeed, compared with the odds that they get on the football pools, the prospects seem very good indeed).

Parents are entitled to have this information, but it can produce a serious rift in domestic harmony unless some further explanation is given. Very soon you will find that the wife's knowledge about her husband's ancestors is only equalled by that of the husband's knowledge of the wife's ancestors, and I think it is vital to make clear two aspects of family incidence: firstly, that there is a genetic factor which is almost certainly derived from both sides of the family and, secondly, that the genetic factor is not the only one, there must be some environmental factor which may be of great importance. The clearest way of explaining this to the parents is to tell them that it is possible for one of a pair of identical twins to have spina bifida and the other to be perfectly normal; indeed, there is some evidence to show that the incidence among twins is less than the incidence among non-twin siblings.

A most important step in integrating the handicapped child into the life of the family is the acceptance of the child back home by the parents at the earliest possible moment. In many cases the child will only have been shown to the mother for a brief moment and the father may not have seen him at all before he is sent to a special centre for treatment. This may involve a child travelling a long distance from home, and separation from the mother at this stage will do harm unless special efforts are made to prevent it. Firstly, the mere fact of the child going to a special centre for treatment should in itself give the parents some hope that the child can be helped to overcome his disability. If there is no attempt to send the child for special treatment, if the parents are told that the case is hopeless, that the baby will not survive, that he will be mentally defective, or that he will never be able to walk or go to school or earn his living, the parents are left without any hope at all and their morale drops to zero.

If, on the other hand, they are told that their child is seriously handicapped but active treatment is to be undertaken to help the child to develop himself more fully, and to reduce the handicaps to the minimum, they look forward to having the child back home to do what they can to help him. The child should not be kept in hospital any longer than is absolutely necessary, and if there are to be delays of even two or three weeks between operations it is most important that he should be allowed home. Moreover, if at all possible, the mother should be encouraged to visit the child in hospital, and to learn how to feed him and take care of him under the supervision of the sister. With this attitude of optimistic realism, with the encouragement of visiting by the mother and the early discharge of the patient, it is very seldom indeed that the child is rejected by the parents, no matter how serious his disabilities. The rejection-rate is far greater in those areas where there is no policy of active treatment, and, even if the child is not left for months in the hospital or in an institution, the family has a heavy burden of unhappiness because they have been given no hope.

Besides the anxieties which the parents have about the survival of their child, his disabilities, and their feelings of guilt, there are also other heavy burdens which they must bear. During infancy the task of the mother may not be very much greater than with a normal child, but as he grows older there is considerable extra work which the parents accept so very willingly. They find themselves tied to the household very much more than the parents of normal children, for they feel a grave responsibility which will not permit them to leave the child in the care of a baby-sitter, so that free evenings and even holidays become very difficult indeed, unless the parents get help from outside.

There is also a considerable financial burden which is sometimes overlooked. Although apparatus and special shoes may be supplied by the Health Service, the wear and tear on clothing is very much greater than with other children, as a result of the apparatus and appliances which they wear. In addition, the frequent admissions to hospital for the various operations which are going to be required mean that the parents have to spend quite a lot of money on travelling to the hospital, for which they may have to give up some of the ordinary dangerous habits such as smoking.

As the children grow the anxiety of the parents does not diminish, and they are extremely worried about the prospects of education for their children, and about their chances of being accepted by the community.

THE COMMUNITY

What are the responsibilities of the community in the care of the children with myelomeningocele? I think the health authorities in Britain are only now becoming aware of the size of this problem and of its gravity. It has taken a considerable time to obtain a clear idea of the incidence of serious spina bifida in our country, and of the survival-rates to be expected. We know that there is a considerable variation in incidence from one country to another, and even in different parts of the same country—for example, in South Wales and in the area around Liverpool the incidence is about twice as great as in some other parts of England. For the country as a whole it seems likely that a figure approaching 2 per 1000 live births is not very far off the mark. Survival-rates are even more difficult to assess, but when all cases are accepted for treatment it seems likely that at least 70% will be surviving at the end of one year, and probably between 50% and 60% will be alive at five years of age.

In the first place the health authorities should make themselves aware of the extent of the problem. It will be necessary to provide treatment centres, and we have found in this special type of neonatal surgery that there are very great advantages in operations being undertaken in special units designed for neonatal surgery, where the whole hospital is geared to the special needs of seriously ill neonates and infants. There are also many advantages in concentrating this work so that not merely 5 or 6 cases are done in the course of a year, but perhaps a minimum of 20 or 30. I think the maximum that we have had has been 170 in a year, and I think this is too many, and we have now persuaded other centres to undertake this work and we do about 120 a year at present.

An adult who sustains a spinal injury causing paraplegia has already received his education, and in many countries there are opportunities for retraining of the adult paraplegic. The child paraplegic, the child with a serious myelomeningocele, has many handicaps in his struggle to obtain even a basic education.

How can these children be fitted into the educational system of the country? In the first place, if the intelligence quotient of a child is normal, he should go to an ordinary school if at all possible. His two major problems are difficulty in walking and incontinence. Many modern schools are built on one floor and have no steps, and so children can attend them even though they spend most of their time in a wheelchair or use callipers; but if there are many steps in a school, it is quite impossible for the child to attend.

A more serious barrier to attendance at a normal school is incontinence, and it is largely for this reason that special day-schools are needed, where frequent attention can be given to the children and, most important, where the child does not feel embarrassed and become emotionally disturbed by being the only incontinent child in the class.

A small number of residential schools for the seriously handicapped are important when parents live too far away from a day-school for handicapped children, or when the child's condition needs very frequent supervision, and I think there are advantages in having such a residential school closely related to a centre for treatment.

We must also look forward to the time when they are about to leave school and consider in what way they are going to make their living. Education is even more important than for those children who have no handicap at all, and vocational training should be specially directed towards the needs of the seriously handicapped.

They will have to rely on their brains and their arms and hands to earn a living, and I think it is most important that the vocational training should not be narrow, simply learning how to undertake mechanical procedures with the hands; it should also have a wide scope, with the possibilities of developing the talents and abilities of these young people in many directions. Simple clerical and manual mechanical work is well within the capacity of most of these young people, but there must be many who are potentially great authors, artists, linguists, musicians, scientists, and philosophers, and yet they may have no opportunity to advance themselves in this way because of the lack of educational opportunities and the lack of vocational training.

It is here, I think, that the parents' associations have proved most valuable. These associations are now scattered widely throughout Great

Britain, and although their aim at first was to provide moral support for the parents in the management and care of their children, it has now become clear that a major concern of the parents is education.

In helping these children the community is helping itself. If it provides adequate treatment these children will be less handicapped than they would otherwise be: if it provides adequate educational and vocational training, they will be able to earn their living. In simple economic terms the potential for a child with myelomeningocele must be very much greater than that of the old person with carcinoma of the lung or stomach. Let us be fair to children born with myelomeningocele. Let us plan their treatment so that their handicap is minimal. Let us develop their minds and bodies so as to compensate for their serious disability, and give them education and vocational training to fit them for a career.

Ethical and Social Aspects of Treatment of Spina Bifida

Sir,—I feel that the ethical justification given by Mr. Zachary for the treatment of children with severe spina bifida is shallow and cruel. It is no longer accepted that the preservation of life as such is the doctor's most important task. We now consider the patient's wellbeing and happiness to be equally at stake. It is now an accepted principle that we treat terminal patients in a way that makes for comfort rather than long survival. Surely we should apply the same sort of principles to children whose prognosis is despairingly poor? If long-term survival entails many operations, much pain and disfigurement, an inability to lead a normal life because of incontinence and paraplegia, and mental strain and distress to parents, should we always attempt it?

R. C. Sanders

This letter has been shown to Mr. Zachary, whose reply follows.—Ed. L.

Sir,—The whole point of my paper has been missed by Dr. Sanders. I would have thought that the three main premises of the argument were abundantly clear: (1) babies with spina bifida should not be killed; (2) the main purpose of all treatment is not to save the child's life, but to improve his function and reduce his handicaps to the minimum; (3) the child with spina bifida deserves that every effort should be made to improve his wellbeing and happiness. If Dr. Sanders thinks these babies should be killed he should say so. If not he should encourage efforts to enable the child to walk, to

Reprinted with permission from *The Lancet,* August 24, 1968, September 9, 1968, October 12, 1968, November 2, 1968, and November 9, 1968, respectively.

help his mental development, and to overcome the problems of incontinence.

Dr. Sanders is welcome to visit our follow-up clinic any Tuesday afternoon, when we see 40–70 patients. He will see for himself whether our outlook is "shallow and cruel" and whether we have a real concern for "the patient's wellbeing and happiness."

R. B. Zachary

Sir,—In his well-written and beguiling paper Mr. Zachary makes out a good case for treating all babies with severe spina bifida surgically, yet Dr. Sanders describes this as "shallow and cruel," to which Mr. Zachary retorts that the alternative is to kill these babies. Clearly this is a highly emotional subject. There is, of course, a third approach—namely, to let Nature take its course. Over the years without any active intervention on my part, over 90% of the untreated babies I have seen have died before their first birthday.

Now that surgical treatment is available for such babies, the easiest way out for the doctor is to transfer the neonates to a unit where all such babies are operated upon without delay. The parents, in their confused and highly disappointed state, will gladly clutch at any offer to help, fervently hoping that the miracle of modern surgery will put the baby right. It will take time before the awful truth dawns upon them and by then it will be too late to step back. Then their only course is to put on a brave face—one that warms the heart of the surgeon in the follow-up clinic. The advent of such a severely handicapped child into a family will transform the lives of all its members—in some cases permanently and completely. That some parents gain fulfilment by dedicating their lives to the care of such children is one of the saving graces of this tragic story, but who can be sure that their lives would have been emptier with a healthy replacement?

The haste that is recommended in order to get the best surgical results often precludes careful consideration of the implications for the family as a whole if the neonate survives. Whenever possible, I try to put the argument for and against surgery to the parents as objectively as I can—a difficult task in the emotionally charged atmosphere that surrounds the birth of any baby, let alone a seriously deformed one. Some down-to-earth parents have no hesitation in letting Nature solve the problem so that they can try again, knowing that the risk of a recurrence is not very great. In such cases we offer to keep the baby in the ward indefinitely should they so wish. Others are grateful for the hope which surgery offers and here there is no problem. But it is the waverers, who can be swayed either way according to the views of the doctor interviewing them, who constitute the heart of the problem—which is most easily, though not necessarily correctly, dealt with by the unquestioning committal of the baby to surgery. One can argue that this is the baby's fundamental right, but have we forgotten that parents and their living children also have rights? Should they not also be considered and consulted?

Ian G. Wickes

Sir,—Every chronic and disabling condition in medicine necessarily presents an emotional problem to the patient's family. Except in this sense, and certainly at professional level, discussion of the management of the severe forms of spina bifida should be kept to the facts.

Dr. Wickes claims that a policy of "letting Nature take its course"—he does not define that phrase though it is highly ambiguous—achieves, if that is the word, a mortality of more than 90% of such cases in the first year of life. What is the alternative? It is difficult to compare figures without knowing the criteria on which Dr. Wickes judges that a case is only suitable for expectant treatment; but even restricting the discussion to the most severe form of the disorder, that in which without treatment anything short of complete paraplegia is unusual and the incidence of hydrocephalus 96%—namely, open thoracolumbar myelocele—we find that with adequate surgical treatment 35% survive to the age of 16 years, and that 70% of these are of normal intelligence. Moreover there is, at the time of birth, an important group among these (48%) which can be detected by clinical methods and in which immediate operation gives an even chance of preserving useful function in the legs. Similar findings have been reported by Zachary and his colleagues in Sheffield and from other centres.

We believe that it is doubt about the realities of the prognosis which causes parents (and physicians) to be "waverers." No reasonable person would advise "the unquestioning committal of the baby to surgery." Instead one can and should tell the parents of a baby born with severe spina bifida, as defined above:

1. Whether with immediate operation there is a good chance that he will achieve natural ambulation. If not, then the haste which Dr. Wickes deplores is unnecessary. More conservative methods can be used.

2. That there is a serious risk of hydrocephalus, but that this can be surgically controlled with a reasonable mortality and morbidity.

3. That orthopædic and urological treatment will be required also, but that there is a better than even chance that, if he survives, the baby will grow up as a normally intelligent human being.

Whether these results are to be preferred to Dr. Wickes' 90% mortality within the first year (we trust that at least he encourages treatment of hydrocephalus in the survivors), is a matter for personal judgment. But parents are not interested in percentages: they want to know what we can do for their own individual children.

A. A. Fernandez-Serrats
A. N. Guthkelch
S. A. Parker

Sir,—Pediatricians cannot possibly assess the prognosis of individual cases unless they have themselves been involved in the operative treatment. By his attitude Dr. Wickes is denying neonates their right to a surgical opinion. No-one would quarrel with his expressions of dismay over handicapped survivors, but what of the many metabolic disorders and known mental defects obvious at birth? Dr. Wickes should have the courage to publish the progress of his 10% untreated survivors. They probably have brain damage which could have been spared and paralysis more extensive than it need have been. Dr. Wickes is extending the principles of social abortion into the neonatal period. This influence is unhealthy in the nurseries of maternity units.

D. F. Ellison Nash

Sir,—Dr. Wickes is by no means the only pediatrician who prefers to let Nature take its course in cases of severe thoracolumbar myelocele with paraplegia. I, for one, have not been impressed by the long-term results of surgical treatment, and after a period of treating these with immediate operation have now returned to a conservative approach to this problem. As Dr. Fernandez-Serrats and his colleagues themselves admit, 65% of surgically treated patients will be dead by the age of sixteen anyway. In the meantime, however, the care of such a child will have been an intolerable strain on the family, especially the mother. In the vast majority of cases she will forego her chances of having further normal children. As for the survivors, only two-thirds of whom are of normal intelligence, they have to find their place in society as paraplegics with incontinence, subject to repeated urinary infections and bedsores.

Mr. Ellison Nash surely exaggerates when he talks of "social abortion" in the neonatal period. The old dictum we were taught as medical students, "Thou shalt not kill; but need'st not strive officiously to keep alive," is a very different principle from that of abortion, which means the active physical destruction of a presumably healthy, normal fetus. I should like to assure Mr. Ellison Nash that spina bifida is not the only state in neonatal pediatrics in which non-interference is the kinder course of action if one considers the well-being of the family as a whole. I personally never see the problem of the untreated survivor with severe thoracolumbar myelocele, hydrocephalus, and paraplegia. Nature if left alone will always correct its own mistakes in these cases.

L. Haas

Sir,—Dr. Wickes and Dr. Haas last week probably command more support amongst pediatricians than is evident in your columns. It is comforting that a surgeon also has doubts about current approaches.

Dr. Fernandez-Serrats and his colleagues appreciate only half the problem when they suggest a detailed conference with the parents before an infant is submitted to operation. Current surgical advice insists that immediate transfer to a surgical unit is imperative. How is this compatible with the careful conference? A half-anaesthetised mother and a distraught father are in no position to make rational decisions. In any case it is doubtful whether they should be allowed to take part in a decision at this stage. Whether the results are death, or handicapped survival, they are likely to feel some guilt if the decision has been theirs.

Mr. Ellison Nash says that by selecting some children (and accepting the responsibility ourselves) we are denying infants the right to a surgical opinion. But it is not the infant who needs the opinion—it is his parents. In how many cases would it be possible to say that the parents have read and *understood* the operation consent-form which they sign? This refers to an operation "the effect and nature of which have been explained to me." All too often the referral for surgical opinion means that the infant will be swept up into the machinery of a first-rate specialist hospital which is operation-oriented. In how many cases has the consultant surgeon, before operation, fully explained the intended programme and the odds against complete normality? Has he explained about the likelihood of urinary diversion, and the prospects of education—and of life as an independent citizen? Has he waited for the question " . . . and if he survives will he have children of his own, and will they also be affected?" It is the very essence of the problem that these questions are often neither asked nor answered, and make the operation consent-form a blank cheque. It is partly because of this that some pediatricians have some doubts.

Some of us think that as well as the right to live there is also the right to die. This has been well stated for the sick and for the aged. It is well that this view should also be aired by pediatricians, who are increasingly involved both with the initial decisions and with the aftermath.

R. M. Forrester

From "Health Service or Sickness Service?"

Eliot Slater

PERINATAL RISKS

The processes of meiosis and mitosis, of spermatogenesis and oogenesis, and after them of the development of the embryo through all its stages are very delicately controlled. But they are extremely complex and have no margin for error; any error, however minor, has cumulative effects. Nevertheless, the defective embryos are progressively eliminated. Out of every 1,000 conceptuses 120 to 150 die in the first four weeks of life. Probably all of them are seriously abnormal. They cause no more disturbance in the mother than perhaps an unusually heavy menstrual bleeding. Between the end of the first four weeks and the seventh month of pregnancy there will be a further 100 to 150 miscarriages. More than half of these spontaneously aborted fetuses can be seen to be abnormal, even on superficial examination. These are nature's discards.

Reprinted with permission by author and publisher from *The British Medical Journal,* 4, 734–35, December 18, 1971.

Of the babies who come to term some 2% are stillborn and a further 4% or so have gross defects. The save-all policy has become the rule in our obstetric and pediatric services, with results which could become grave in terms of human suffering. About three in every 1,000 babies born are affected by spina bifida, in a high proportion of cases to a moderate or severe degree. When I was a student and no treatment was known the usual course was put the little mistake of nature in a cool spot while attention was diverted to the mother. The baby died, the mother wept. But a few months later she would be entering on another pregnancy with every chance of having a normal healthy child.

Then came the time when these damaged babies were given their chance of surviving and got the same support as any other baby. Then the life span was somewhat longer, though only the very mildest cases ever reached adolescence. The most heavily handicapped babies died off rapidly, and four out of five were gone in the first year.

Nowadays pediatric surgery proceeds stage by stage to ward off all the dangers. There is operation after operation, always new adjustments having to be made as the child grows. Attention is needed because the child is spastic and paralysed and incontinent. There has to be special education to help him to adjust to the combination of defects, among which there is often superadded mental subnormality.

It appears that the proportion of spina bifida babies now having an immediate operation is rising. So too no doubt are the numbers of severely handicapped survivors; and so too the medical, educational, social, and family burdens. In the first five years of life most survivors spend an average of two years in hospital, mainly in spells of one to two weeks. Admissions are numbered in dozens, and the child is hardly out of hospital before the time is nearing for him to go back again. Special schooling can usually enable these children to walk and to get their incontinence under a socially acceptable degree of control. But if Britain were to provide special schools for every spina bifida child who is now being salvaged Leach estimated that it would have to build one with 50 places, and staff it with about 10 skilled people, each and every month for the next 15 years.

These children are now beginning to come into puberty and adolescence, when their sufferings will really begin. Only the most miserably impaired social life will be open to them; they will be equipped with normal sex drive but no normal sex function; all around them they will see the normal, the vigorous, and the healthy. Will they really be grateful to the fates, the all too human fates, but for whose intervention they would have died before their miseries began?

Perhaps the whole procedure is mistaken. If this is one of the necessary consequences of the sanctity-of-life ethic perhaps our formulation of the principle should be revised. The spina bifida baby is a mistake of nature not equipped to survive. Who suffers if he dies at birth? Certainly not the child, though if he is forced to survive he faces years of suffering. Do the parents suffer if he dies? Yes, in the disappointment of not having a baby when they had hoped for a normal little boy or girl; but in a few months they can try

again. If the child survives, however, they have years of servitude, of tortured love, trying to make up to him for all his disadvantages. And society,
the community? The death costs nothing; the life costs not only money but
the pre-emption of precious medical, nursing, social, and educational resources.

It is sometimes said that the handicapped child has the same right as
the normal child to a normal family life. But the mentally subnormal and the
severely handicapped child cannot have a normal family life. The abnormal
child causes emotional reactions in his parents and sibs that distort normal
relationships, and these families suffer severely. . . . The true ethic is, I
believe, that normal parents have a right to a normal child. It is their first
duty to preserve the normality of their home, the welfare of their marriage,
their mutual relationship, and their family life. They should think it wrong
to inflict an abnormal sib on their other normal children, who cannot defend
themselves against this trauma. Sometimes parents do reject the abnormal
baby when he is born, but if so it is in the face of strong emotional pressures
from everyone—doctors, nurses, and neighbours. Yet common sense and
humanity are on the side of rejection. The spina bifida baby, the mongol,
the phenylketonuric are not babies so much as attempts at babyhood that
misfired. If as a community we impose on our medical services the duty of
keeping them alive, then through these and other State services we should
bear the whole burden. It is one for specialists. We should not shuffle it off
on to untrained women and men of only average ability and stability, who
by their relationship with the abnormal infant are put under particular
strain.

Is There a Right to Die—Quickly?

John M. Freeman

A child born with a meningomyelocele has a readily and accurately diagnos-
able lesion at birth. The degree of neurologic deficit is ascertainable and
irreversible; the risks of hydrocephalus and mental retardation are largely
predictable, as is the risk of bladder involvement and urinary incontinence.
While 10 to 15 years ago few physicians were enthusiastic about treating
children with meningomyeloceles, under the leadership of the English
groups there has been an increasing interest in early, vigorous, and comprehensive treatment. Dr. John Lorber, one of the leading exponents of early
and vigorous intervention in these children, has recently assessed his long-
term results, with some second thoughts. After careful analysis of his data,
Lorber states that not all children with meningomyeloceles should be
treated. He states that depending on the level of the lesion, the presence

of hydrocephalus, and other factors, certain children should be left unoperated—to die. He quotes from the few available studies of untreated meningomyeloceles to show that untreated, a large percentage (60 to 80 per cent) die within the first year of life. While some might interpret the quoted studies differently, the significant factor is that many do not die quickly, but slowly over months or years, dying of meningitis, hydrocephalus, or renal disease. However, of equal importance is the fact that many survive, and the quality of their survival after drying and infection of the spinal cord, hydrocephalus, and renal decompensation is poorer than if they had had early, vigorous—optimal—treatment.

We are thus between the Scylla of treating all children with meningomyeloceles with resultant increase in the number of survivors with severe handicapping conditions, and the Charybdis of not treating some children and permitting nature to take its often long, lingering course. There are all gradients of this latter position: One could not feed the child and allow him to starve to death; one could feed, but not treat meningitis or infection if they occur; one could close the back so that the child is aesthetically more desirable and could be cared for at home, but not treat the hydrocephalus; one could close the back and shunt the hydrocephalus, but allow the child to die later of renal disease, with or without orthopedic treatment. In short, when one decides not to treat, or to treat only partially, patients survive. It is not the patient or the problem that goes away—it is the physician who goes away from the problem, leaving the family and the patient to suffer.

One of the recent "advances" in medicine is prenatal diagnosis. By this technique, we can now detect certain genetic or metabolic diseases before birth and "allow the family to have only normal children." This is the current euphemism used for abortion on fetal indication. Physicians, to a large extent backed by society, have decided that it may not only be permissible, but laudable, to kill at 20 weeks a fetus who might die of Tay-Sachs disease at 2 years, or one with mongolism who might lead an impaired life for many years. Indeed, if there were mechanisms for the diagnosis of meningomyeloceles at 20 to 24 weeks of gestation, would we not encourage parents to request termination of pregnancy? If it is permissible to kill a fetus at 20 to 24 weeks, should it not also be permissible to kill such an infant at 40 weeks of gestation?

A discussion of killing is an anathema to most of us who are trained and dedicated to saving lives. However, physicians should admit that in deciding that some children with meningomyeloceles should not be operated upon, as Lorber has done, they are making a decision between life and death. The unoperated infant is being condemned to death, sooner or later, by less than optimal care—what might be termed passive euthanasia. The physician does not take into account the increased pain and suffering to both child and parent attendant to "letting nature take its course." If we make that decision for a given child, should we not then, as physicians, also have the opportunity to alleviate the pain and suffering by accelerating that death? This conversion from passive euthanasia to active euthanasia is not an easy one for society or for the individual physician faced with the decisions and with their consequences. Having seen children with unoperated meningomyeloceles lie around the ward for weeks or months untreated, waiting to die, one cannot help but feel that the highest form of medical ethic would have been to end the pain and suffering, rather than wishing that the patient would go away.

It is time that society and medicine stopped perpetuating the fiction that withholding treatment is ethically different from terminating life. It is time that society began to discuss mechanisms by which we can alleviate the pain and suffering for those individuals whom we cannot help.

People will ask: If we are to kill some children with meningomyeloceles, then where will we draw the line? At children with mongolism who may have a long, if impaired life? At children with muscular dystrophy who have a shorter life, but a number of normal years? At the severely retarded child? At the mildly retarded child? At the child with phocomelia, or with a congenital amputation? These are areas where I do not believe euthenasia should be considered, but which physicians and society can and should discuss. However, in those rare instances where the decision has been made to avoid "heroic" measures and to allow "nature to take its course," should society not allow physicians to alleviate the pain and suffering and help nature to take its course—quickly?

Whose Suffering?

Robert E. Cooke

In an accompanying editorial, "Is there a right to die—quickly?," Dr. John Freeman raises old issues concerning a new problem. New dilemmas are being created with the advances of science. Before meningomyeloceles could be repaired, the physician had no options. Now that a poor prognosis is no longer a certainty new dilemmas arise—who should be operated upon, when should antibiotics be given, and at what stage should the physician admit defeat in his efforts to prolong life?

The comments in this editorial are not addressed to the issue of operating or not operating, but to the handling of the case not operated upon. Dr. Freeman adequately states the case for the infant's suffering. In so doing, he adopts understandable, commonplace, yet to my mind erroneous, reasoning. He applies what may loosely be called the anthropomorphic approach to the infant, attributing to it perceptions and emotions characteristic of the mature adult. Yet the infants that Dr. Freeman says, "lie around the ward for weeks or months untreated, *waiting to die*" are not fully conscious in adult terms, not capable of abstraction, and respond only to relatively simple stimuli with relatively simple internal as well as external

Reproduced with permission of author and publisher from *J. Pediatr.* 80, 906–908, 1972; copyright by The C. V. Mosby Company, St. Louis, Missouri.

behavior. Quite simply, "waiting to die," is a nonexistent thought of the infant.

Dr. Freeman refers to the "suffering of society." It is an unfortunate fact that society suffers very little: So many competing pains and pleasures exist that only a small percentage of society is even aware that the unoperated hydrocephalic patient exists. One aspect of suffering may be fiscal hardship. If that is the case, all of us should suffer the tortures of the damned as billions go to the Defense Department. Only a small portion of this fiscal hardship could result if all such children were cared for for a lifetime.

The word "suffering" is often appropriate to the parents. Yet how many of us in pediatrics have seen love and devotion, not misery, come at least occasionally to the parents of the handicapped. Surely all of us know of many cases in which even a severely handicapped child has brought great joy to a family. How much the hopelessly handicapped infant or the unoperated-upon patient decreases or augments the humanity of the doctors or the parents about him cannot readily be measured. In an indirect way at least, he makes a contribution to our heritage—primarily personal—but occasionally public, and this qualifies him as human, according to Monod's definition. "Unwanted by both family and society" might apply as a criterion for termination of life, but let us be careful since much of the pediatrician's "heroics," such as intensive care for the 1,200 Gm. offspring of the 13-year-old unmarried girl from the ghetto, would come to an end.

Medicine is the science of care, not the science of cure, and in caring, we as physicians must suffer. Such difficult experiences are part of the fabric of medicine that bring humane people to medicine, not drive them away. Medicine would change for the worse if the physician joined too fully the new discomfort-free society.

Lest the reader consider the author a harbinger of the ethic of suffering, let us examine another aspect of Dr. Freeman's argument. If it is acceptable to kill the defective fetus by abortion before birth, why not the infant with noncorrectable serious abnormalities after birth? Dr. Freeman is correct that biologically there is little difference between fetus and infant; the birth process or viability conveys few new biological properties. In the newborn infant, the respiratory system is adequately developed and no functioning umbilical cord is necessary. But without external support, i.e., feeding, every human new born infant would die. The potential for humanity in the fetus and neonate is the same. The newborn infant directly contributes little more or benefits little more than the fetus from the heritage of our culture. Yet I cannot agree with Dr. Freeman. There is indeed a vast difference, in a large part of our society, between the fetus and the neonate. The neonate is perceived as human, giving and receiving and inspiring love. The differences are psychological, but nevertheless real in both the public and the private mind. Individuals in most societies see in the infant's face and appearance human goodness and love; yet it would be difficult for them to imagine the fetus in these terms. The public mind also views the fetus and the neonate differently. The law regards termination of the fetus' life as "abortion"—considered acceptable by many in society, and desirable by many in some circumstances. Yet infanticide is "murder." The difference in attitude toward the fetus and neonate does not exist because of the law, rather the law exists because of the attitude of the public. Whether abortion is condoned or condemned is irrevelant—the difference still exists between it and infanticide. We do not know if these differences will persist or disappear in generations to come, but the fact is that at the moment they do exist.

I can only conclude that pediatricians must accept the suffering and offer corrective measures as needed to all who have a probability of response, as long as it is impossible to predict with a high degree of precision the outcome in an individual case. Therapy without cure, if it contributes to *care,* is a necessary part of medicine in spite of the fact that the physician must sometimes suffer. Death of the unoperated patient is an unacceptable means of alleviating this suffering.

Human and Handicapped

Karen M. Metzler

In preparing these remarks, I was undecided as to whether I should use lecture form to give you my experience of society's attitudes toward handicappedness, or should continue by allowing both of us to do our questioning, searching, and experiencing out loud together. I have decided to begin by sharing my experience with you so that you can know how deeply I am willing to probe into being aware of and understanding myself, you, our encounters, and life itself.

I am a humanist—I see life, growth, and potential in every human circumstance. I also see the pain, sorrow, and grief in them. But I work towards choosing to empathize the former qualities. Such an attitude is truly me. It is real. It is no pretense. But I do know that I learned at an early age that if I wanted to be praised and accepted I had to smile. And smile I did, always, even when the pain inside wanted to howl like a pack of wolves in the dark. And I smiled and people said, "Look at Karen, how she's always smiling. Boy, she's strong. She's accepted her handicap. She never complains." I wanted to be strong, to be healthy. But most of all, I wanted to be accepted by others. And it appeared to me that the rules were that in order to be accepted, I had to keep to myself any of the negative aspects of being handicapped, because society had to deny them in order for society to be free of discomfort. I am taking, now, a big risk in being honest and open about my feelings and perceptions, which means that I do not sugarcoat any which may need it for social acceptability. The risk is of being accused, by both the able-bodied and the disabled persons in society, of not

This article was presented originally to an undergraduate course on Moral Problems in Medicine at Case Western Reserve University. It is published here by permission of the author.

having accepted being handicapped. Knowing my own life process, I believe that it was not until I was able to begin to accept myself that I was able to speak honestly not only to myself, but to others as well. When I speak out against what I perceive as injustices, though they often be unintentional, in such areas as education, employment, and even daily living, I am not complaining, but confronting. To complain means just to express undirected, immature hostility with no goal in mind except the mere release of inner tension caused by the abrasion of one's personal existence against Existence itself. But to confront means that I have as my goal the bringing about of awareness and action upon that awareness.

Let me allow you to become aware of what it is like to be me—a white, female, middle-class handicapped person. Not a black or an upper-class or a male handicapped person, but me. Though there are commonalities among persons who are handicapped, there are differences, because we are all individuals. I do not presume to say that my feelings, perceptions, and experiences are the way it is for all. I can only say that it is the way it is for me.

I think that the underlying emotion behind my total experience of being a person with a handicap is that because I am imperfect in one way, I *must* be perfect in all other ways. Admittedly, this comes from a need within me to compensate. But you, as a society and as individuals, also help to create this need, because you—as a society and as individuals—become fixated to the fact that I am different and unable to do certain things, and then generalize this fixation into a belief that I am unable to do anything at all. It is this generalization which leads you to discriminate against allowing me to do those things which I am in fact capable of doing. It would or should not be as important to me that I am unable to do certain things. After all, isn't that part of being human?

But am I human? Am I less human as a person because my body is not like that of other humans? Are my feelings, thoughts, needs, and desires different from theirs because my body is? Is the development of my potential distorted, or just in some ways delayed? It is my belief that the development of a person with a handicap should not be considered abnormal, and need not be abnormal. His or her development, just like that of any other person, has meaning and consistency within itself. For instance, when I was sixteen my emotional energies were invested in dealing with an unknown blood disorder and the impending loss of a leg. How, emotionally, could I have been at the same place it is expected that sixteen-year-olds be, for instance in regard to social development—e.g., dating? For my situation, I was normal, but for the hypothetical or average situation, I was abnormal. But consider this. What would you think about a sixteen-year-old who had come to grips with the concept and reality of death? You would call her mature for her age or situation, would you not? But the hypothetical or average situation of a sixteen-year-old does not include the achievement of that particular developmental task. In this sense, he or she is not being "normal" but "abnormal." Why then do we make such distinctions and value judgments about the direction in which a person can deviate from the developmental norms? It is because we make comparisons of persons, rather than accepting them as they are and where they are.

However, even those individuals who are able to accept the handicapped person as he is—that is, as handicapped—are often unable to accept where the handicapped person is emotionally in dealing with his handicappedness. The individuals around him and society in general expect him to have reached the stage of acceptance, while emotionally and behaviorally they are only willing to allow him to go through the first stage—denial of the existence of his or her handicap—in his struggle towards acceptance. They often will not even let him talk about it. But there are intermediate and succeeding stages which are just as necessary and valid for the handicapped person to go through if he is ever to reach the stage of acceptance. These stages consist of such emotional reactions as anger, self-pity, and self-rejection. To allow a handicapped person to experience and express such emotions threatens other people, particularly those who are deeply involved with him or her, because their own feelings of anger, pity, and rejection may become surfaced. What people must realize, particularly if they are professionally or personally involved, is that there are ways of showing respect for a handicapped person's need to be at a certain stage without having necessarily to reinforce him or her so that he or she never grows beyond the earlier stages to that of acceptance.

Some people are able to recognize the existence of and need for this process more easily in situations involving a person who becomes handicapped after having lived as a non-handicapped person. But a child born with a birth defect must also go through the same process. The difference is that the onset of the process is undatable. Any one of the stages may become his mode of personality, since they are occurring during his formative years, and he has not established a prior personality on which to build or with which to buffer against any permanent adoption of the emotional responses (i.e., hostility, self-rejection, denial, etc.).

And for some persons, like myself, even though we have gone through the process before, since our bodies and body-images continue to undergo repeated trauma and mutilation, the process must be gone through again each time. But people do not easily recognize this. For instance, when I told people that my leg was going to be amputated, some responded by saying that since I had gone through so much already, I should be able to handle this easily. It was as though they were saying that it was less of a trauma for me than it would be for someone else! This only complicated the guilt feelings I had later about my having to go through the less socially acceptable stages in the process of acceptance.

One element of acceptance is the ability to feel a positive regard towards oneself and to feel that others hold one in positive regard as well. One source in our society of positive regard is through the achievement of expectations and goals as set for one by himself or others. The fulfillment of these expectations or goals constitutes, in the general mind, success. But one like myself wonders if he or she has truly achieved success, when its acknowledgement is accompanied by such statements as, "For someone handicapped like yourself," or "Despite your handicaps." It makes me wonder if what I have done would be only mediocre, or less, if I were ablebodied, but because I am not, it deserves praise. To assure myself that when I succeed, I truly succeed, I set out towards goals that would be difficult for anyone, whether or not he had a handicap. I do not want the left-overs or what might only be the spoils after everyone else's victories.

In my case, goals and success centered around my mind, my intellect. But even though my mind earned me recognition and respect, I still felt insecure about it. I had grown up from birth hearing the words, "And you should have been retarded, but you are not." Well, with such an expectation as that, even mediocrity would seem praiseworthy. But whether or not I was the genius that I thought I had to be, I did at least have enough intelligence. I felt compelled to use what I had because I was concerned about what might have happened if I had not had a mind which was capable of compensating for my imperfect body. What would have given my life value so that people would want me? I wondered often about those children who were not as lucky as myself. I am bothered when I see a documentary about a handicapped boy which ends by saying that he can be a physicist someday. What if he becomes a plumber instead? Would his success as a handicapped person be any less?

Putting myself in the place of the other person has always been something which I have tried to do. But I have never liked to be compared with another person—that was something only I could do in my perennial profession as self-criticizer. It bothered me, though I understood their good intentions, to have people always telling me about some other handicapped person they knew who was able to do this, that, or the other thing. My initial response would be that they were not really listening to me. I was not that person, but me! I was an individual, separate from the other to whom I was being compared, with a different set of problems and potentialities whether or not they were greater or less than someone else's—for in the end they were mine, and only mine. Comparisons tend to imply at an unconscious level a test of one's adequacy. And at some level within me, it made me feel inadequate. For instance, I knew that amputees could swim, but I had not always been an amputee. Instead, I had spent my life with my legs in casts, unable to go in water. If I had had the opportunity, I would have learned. And when the opportunity did arise, I did learn. Still, if I had never been able to learn to swim, knowing that it was something which amputees could in fact do, there would have been a part of me asking, "Have I failed? Am I less well-adjusted than others?"

A successful handicapped person is one who has not only gained his own acceptance of himself, but the acceptance of himself from others as well. But from whom and how does a handicapped person gain his acceptance? His parents, who have been trained by society to react towards handicappedness with rejection, discomfort, and denial add to these feelings those of guilt and anger. They have also incorporated from society a set of expectations about their child's behavior and potential. Thus, they are given the difficult task of re-educating their emotions so that they may become compassionate and accepting facilitators of their child's development. They are often left to do this alone, unaided by professional or non-professional help and support while they are attempting to re-educate the emotions of other people in order that their child eventually be accepted as the human being he is. His parents must also supply him with what he needs to be successful in life as a handicapped person, while they themselves do not know the experience of being handicapped. Other children will see the child who is handicapped as something to be feared and ridiculed, because they are learning from unenlightened adults the same old attitudes. And because he is a handicapped child, adults will see him as someone to be pitied and babied. When he becomes a handicapped teenager or adult, people will choose to ignore his existence in order not to have to deal with their own feelings.

Relationships with people then, become the responsibility of the handicapped person, if for no other reason than that he is the only person who has the experience of dealing with such encounters where there is included an added negative element to be overcome—that is, his or her handicap. His encounters with persons who will be able to become his friends are subject to the same filteration process that all peoples' possibilities must go through, but his handicap forces some possibilities to go through a filter once more. Thus, a handicapped person can not afford to have any further obstacles to his having relationships with other people, particularly any placed before him by his personality. I, for instance, have felt pressures against being the quiet and shy person I believe myself naturally to be. Since people are most often deterred from wanting to know me because of my first impression—that is, my disfigured body—I am forced to become the initiator. Also, oftentimes quietness on my part has led people to think that I was withdrawn and inhibited due to my handicap. The problem is that sometimes this is true and sometimes it is not. Thus, I do not have the freedom to be a quiet person in circumstances where other people might be allowed to be. Yet, I also learned that I must move with caution and not reach out to people too eagerly, for there are those people who feel uncomfortable having attention called to them in my presence. If people are staring at me, that means that they are staring at those who are with me as well.

I might also include here my feelings about the matter of staring. In our culture, people are not supposed to look directly at other people—which adds to the discomfort people have about staring. There is also the problem that the person doing the staring feels guilty about doing it and the person being stared at feels attacked. The attitude that I have tried to maintain, since I have been older, is that staring is a way of making familiar something which is unfamiliar. Such reasoning came out of my examination of my own reaction to when I see another handicapped person. I want to stare, too; but I do it out of curiosity and not attack. Still, there are those times when I feel attacked by stares and want to attack back.

But it is acceptance, not attack, which is going to bridge the gap between handicapped and non-handicapped persons. Yet, there are those individuals whose attitude, implicit if not explicit, remains one of rejection of me because I am handicapped. I strive, however, to accept even those who reject me. For I have realized that in essence I reject others when I do not accept their own rejection of me. Therefore, I do not think that it was best for people to console me by saying, "They're just small-minded people, or ignorant," etc. Such a condemning attitude is ineffective, both for me and those to whom it is directed. It unrightfully places me in a position of superiority and also makes me defensive. If I am defensive, I am walled within my own experience and feelings. And thus, I have no empathy for the person rejecting me. But if I do not allow myself to become defensive, I am open to the rejecting person's experience, and thus I am able not only to learn from him, but to help him to deal with his own feelings. Although I see him as an individual, I also see the context within which he is an individual. He is a member of a society in which handicappedness is not a universal, but a uniqueness—a stigmatized one. Knowing this, I can not condemn nor judge him, for he has not actively sought such personal attitudes. Thus when one of my peers says to me, "When I first saw you, I decided then that I did not want to get to know you. I guess this is bad and that I should not feel this way. I'm sorry." I ask him not to apologize or feel guilty, but to accept his feelings without judgment. I assure him that I do not judge or criticize his feelings. After we both have accepted his feelings, it is up to me to help him come to understand them so that in the future they need not be in the way of him and other handicapped people. For I realize that I and others like me are not seen as individuals, but as a stereotype or category. Thus, in order to gain acceptance I must compete against that stereotype. Yet, since I am seen as a stereotype, anything which I may be or do is added to that generalized image. Thus, I have always felt a responsibility to insure that I do not become a detriment to those who may come after me.

It is my hope then, that I have enabled you to feel more comfortable and willing to deal with the emotions surrounding handicappedness for both sides. It is my hope to facilitate honest acceptance and healthy support. As I discussed the handicapped person, I wanted to impress upon you the reality that although he is handicapped, he is as human as those who are not, although while he is human, he is also handicapped. The "humanness" and the "handicappedness" of the person are not separate, for they are integrated throughout his entire existence. Just as man's soul may be surrounded by his body, so is his humanness by his handicaps, whether physical or otherwise.

Survival of the Weakest

Richard M. Hare

THE ABNORMAL CHILD—MORAL DILEMMAS OF DOCTORS AND PARENTS

I was asked to make a philosophical contribution to our discussions; and any philosopher who tries to do this sort of thing is up against a serious difficulty. If he is content to act merely as a kind of logical policeman and pick up bad arguments that are put forward by other people, he will be unpopular, but may (if he is competent at his trade) establish for himself a fairly strong negative position. But if he wants to do something more constructive than that, and is going to rely on something more solid than his own intuitions and more stable than the received opinions on the subject, he will have to start from some general theory about how one argues on questions like this; and then at once he is on much shakier ground, because there is no general theory about moral argument that is universally accepted. All I can do in this situation is to tell you in outline the theory that I accept myself and then argue from that.

However, I have perhaps made my position sound shakier than it actually is; for the theory that I shall be using is one which ought to be acceptable to most of the main schools of ethics, because it relies only on certain formal characteristics of the moral words or concepts which we use in these arguments. I *think* (though obviously I shall have no time to argue) that this theory is consonant with the Christian principles that we should do to others as we wish that they should do to us, and that we should love our neighbour as ourselves; with the Kantian principle that we should act in such a way that we can will the maxim of our action to be a universal law; and with the utilitarian principle that everybody is to count as one and nobody as more than one (that is to say, that their interests are to be equally regarded). Other approaches to the theory of moral argument which lead to the same kind of principle are the so-called Ideal Observer theory, according to which what we ought to do is what a person would prescribe who was fully acquainted with the facts and impartially benevolent to all those affected; and the so-called Rational Contractor theory which says that the principles we ought to follow are those which a rational self-interested person would agree to if he did not know which end of the stick *he* was going to receive in any of the situations to be adjudicated by the principles.

All these methods come really to the same thing, that when faced with a decision which affects the interests of different people, we should treat the interests of all these people (including ourselves if we are affected) as of equal weight, and do the best we can for them. This is the fundamental

This article was first given in lecture form to the London Medical Group. It is printed here by permission of the author. © R. M. Hare 1973.

principle. There are a great many other principles, some of them of great importance, which occupy a different level from this fundamental principle, and may appear to conflict with it, as they certainly do conflict on occasion with one another. I mean principles like those which forbid lying or promise-breaking or murder; or that (very important to doctors) which demands loyalty to those to whom one is under some special obligation owing to a particular relation one stands in to them (for example one's wife or one's child or one's patient).

However, I think it is right to subordinate all these principles to the fundamental one, because in cases of conflict between these different principles, it is only the fundamental principle that can give us any secure answer as to what we should do. The fundamental principle is the law and the prophets; although particular laws (and particular prophecies for that matter) are no doubt very important, they take their origin from the need to preserve and to do justice between the interests of people (that is, to secure to them their rights); and when there is a conflict between the principles— or even some doubt about the application of a particular principle—it is this fundamental principle which has to be brought in to resolve it.

An example that may occur to you after having heard what has been said is this: granted that the obstetrician has a special duty to his patient, the mother, and that the pediatrician has a special duty to *his* patient, the child, surely what they ought all in all to do when the interests of mother and child conflict should be governed by equal consideration for these interests and not by what branch of the profession each of them happens to have specialized in.

I am going therefore, in the hope of shedding some light on the dilemmas of doctors and parents, to ask, first of all, what are the different interests involved in the sort of case we are considering. There is first the interest of the child; but what *is* this? We can perhaps illuminate this question by asking "What if it were ourselves in that child's position—what do we prescribe for *that* case?" On the one hand it may be presumed to be in the child's interest to live, if this is possible; but if the life is going to be a severely handicapped one, it is possible that this interest in living may be at least greatly diminished. Then there is the interest of the mother, in whose interest also it is to live, and whose life may be in danger; and it is also in her interest not to have an abnormal child, which might prevent or severely impair the normal development of the rest of the family. The other members of the family have a similar interest. Against this, it is said that good sometimes comes to a family through having to bring up an abnormal child; and I can believe that this is so in some cases.

Then there are the interests (not so great individually but globally very great) which belong to those outside the family: first of all those of doctors and nurses who are concerned; then those of the rest of the staffs of hospitals, homes and other services which will be involved in looking after the child and the family. There are also the interests of all those people who *would* be looked after, or looked after better, by all these services if they did not already have too much on their hands; and there are the interests of the taxpayers who pay for it all. And lastly, there is another interest which is commonly ignored in these discussions, and which is so important that it often, I think, ought to tip the balance; but what this other interest is I shall not reveal until I have talked about those I have mentioned so far.

When I said that equal consideration ought to be given to all the interests affected, I did not mean that we should treat as equal the interest of the mother in continuing to live and that of the doctor in not being got out of bed in the middle of the night. As individuals, these people are entitled to equal consideration; but because life matters more to one than sleep to the other, that makes it right for the doctor to get out of bed and go and look after the mother. If the doctor had a car smash outside the mother's front door and she could save *his* life by getting out of bed in the middle of the night, then by the same principle she should do so. As individuals, they are equipollent; the difference is introduced by the differing importance to each of them of the various outcomes.

The number of those affected can also be important; if a G.P. can save a patient from a sleepless and distressful night by going along in the evening and providing a pain-killer, he will often do it, even in these days; but if a pill were not enough, and it were necessary for a whole team of nurses and an ambulance to turn out, he might decide to wait till the morning unless there were a real danger of a grave deterioration in the patient's condition. A very large number of people each of whom is affected to a small degree may outweigh one person who is affected to a greater degree. So even the fact that 60 million taxpayers will have to pay an average of 20 pence extra each a year to improve or extend the Health Service is of some moral, as well as political, importance. But I agree on the whole with those who ask us not to attach too much importance to these economic arguments; although I totally failed recently to get from an economist a straight answer to the question of the order of size of the sums involved in looking after handicapped children, I am prepared to accept for the sake of argument that they are relatively small. So let us leave the taxpayer out of it, and the rival claimants for care, and just consider the interests of the immediate family.

Here, however, we must notice the other important interest that I mentioned just now—that of the next child in the queue. For some reason that I cannot understand this is seldom considered. But try looking at the problem with hindsight. The example I am going to use is oversimplified, and I am deliberately not specifying any particular medical condition, because if I do I shall get my facts wrong. Suppose the child with the abnormality was not operated on. It had a substantial chance of survival, and, if it survived, it had a large chance of being severely handicapped. So they didn't operate, and what we now have is not that child, but young Andrew who was born two years later, perfectly normal, and leaves school next summer. Though not brilliant, he is going probably to have a reasonably happy life and make a reasonably useful contribution to the happiness of others. The choice facing the doctors and the family was really a choice between (if they didn't operate) a very high probability of having Andrew (who would not have been contemplated if they had a paralysed child in the family) and on the other hand (if they did operate) a combination of probabilities depending on the precise prognosis (shall we say a 10% chance of a living normal child, a 40% chance of a living but more or less seriously handicapped child, and a 50% chance of a dead child plus the possibility of Andrew in the future).

If we agree with most people that family planning is right, and that therefore this family is justified in limiting its children to a predetermined number (however large), then that is the kind of choice it will be faced with, and in the situation I have imagined *was* faced with. We should try discussing with Andrew himself whether they made the right choice.

If I have characterized the choice correctly, then nearly everything is going to depend on what the prognosis was, and on our estimates of the value *to the persons concerned* of being alive and normal, and, by contrast, of being alive and defective or handicapped in some specified way. In making these value-judgments I do not see that we can do better than put ourselves imaginatively in the places of those affected, and judge as if it were our own future that was at stake. Since a sensitive doctor is bound constantly, in the course of his practice, to make this sort of imaginative judgment about what is for the best for other people, looking at it from their point of view, I do not think that it can be said that it raises any difficulties of principle; but it obviously raises very great difficulties in practice, which the sensitive and experienced doctor is as likely as anybody to be able to overcome in consultation with parents and others affected.

But the problems mostly arise from the difficulty of prognosis. That is why the work reported by Professor Smithells is so crucial. In principle it might be possible to put a numerical value upon the probabilities of the various outcomes, and having estimated how the various outcomes for the people involved affect their interests, to make a utilitarian calculation and choose the course that gives the best prospect of good and the least prospect of harm for those concerned, all in all. In practice we are bound to rely a lot on guesswork; but when guessing, it is an advantage to have a clear idea of what you are guessing *at,* and I have suggested that what we should be guessing at is what is for the best for all the parties taken together.

The prognosis, however, is always going to be pretty uncertain, and the question therefore arises of *when* the decision should be made. I suppose that it would be agreed that if there is doubt in the very early stages of pregnancy, it might be advisable to wait until the fetus had developed sufficiently to make the prognosis more certain. A hard-headed utilitarian might try to extend this principle and say that in cases of suspected abnormality we should let the child be born, operate if appropriate, and then kill the child if the operation resulted in a very severe handicap, and have another child instead. In this way we should maximize the chances of bringing into the world a human being with a high prospect of happiness. If the medical profession finds this suggestion repugnant, as it almost certainly does, and does not *want* the law changed; or if it is thought (perhaps rightly) to inflict too much mental suffering on the mother, then we shall have to be content with a far less certain procedure—that of either terminating or, if we don't terminate and then the child is born, estimating the chances *before* deciding whether to operate, and (if we do decide to operate) taking the risk, however small, of being left with a dreadfully handicapped child.

If we imagine our possible Andrew and his possible brother (the former existing only as a possible combination of sperm and ovum, the latter already existing as a foetus)—if, I say, we imagine them carrying out a prenatal dialogue in some noumenal world (and of course the supposition is just as fantastic in one case as it is in the other) and trying to arrive at a solution which will give them, taken together, the best chance of happy existence, the dialogue might go like this. Andrew points out that if the foetus is not born there is a high probability that he, Andrew, will be born and will have a normal and reasonably happy life. There is of course a possibility that the parents will change their minds about having any more children, or that one of them will die; but let us suppose that this is rather unlikely, and that there is no particular fear that the next child will be abnormal.

To this the foetus might reply "At least I have got this far; why not give me a chance?" But a chance of what? They then do the prognosis as best they can and work out the chances of the various outcomes if the present pregnancy is not terminated. It turns out that there is a slim chance, but only a slim chance, that the foetus will, if born and operated on, turn into a normal and, let us hope, happy child; that there is a considerable chance on the other hand that it will perish in spite of the operation; and that there is a far from negligible chance of its surviving severely handicapped. In that case, I think Andrew, the later possible child, can claim that he is the best bet, because the chance of the parents dying or changing their minds before he is born is pretty small, and certainly far less than the chance that the present foetus, if born, will be very seriously handicapped.

In order for the foetus to prevent Andrew winning the argument in this way, there is one move it can make. It can say, "All right, we'll make a bargain. We will say that I am to be born and operated on, in the hope of restoring me to normality. If the operation is successful, well and good. If it isn't, then I agree that I should be scrapped and make way for Andrew." I think you will see if you look at the probabilities that this compromise gives the best possible chance of having a healthy baby, and at the same time gives the foetus all the chance that it ever had of itself being that baby. But it does this at the cost of abolishing the substantial chance that there was of having this particular child, albeit in a seriously handicapped condition. I call this a *cost*, because many will argue (though I am not sure that I want to follow them) that life with a severe handicap is preferable, for the person who has it, to no life at all. Of course it depends on the severity of the handicap. And of course this policy involves so much distress for the mother that we might rule it out on that score alone, and terminate instead.

Perhaps I should end by removing what might be an obstacle to understanding. In order to expound the argument, I asked you to imagine Andrew and the foetus having a discussion in some noumenal world (and, by the way, it needn't bother you if you don't know what "noumenal" means; I only used it in order to keep my philosophical end up in the face of all your no doubt necessary medical jargon). This way of dramatizing the argument is perhaps useful though not necessary; and it carries with it one danger. We have to imagine the two possible children conducting this very rational discussion, and therefore we think of them being in a sense already grown up enough to conduct it; and that may lead us to suppose that, for either of them, to be deprived of the possibility of adulthood *after* having had this taste of it would be a very great evil. People (most of them) cling tenaciously to life (though it is a matter for argument, at what age they start to do this); and therefore to deprive a person of life is thought of as *normally* an evil. This certainly does not apply to Andrew, since he is not alive yet and so cannot be *deprived* of life in the relevant sense, though it can be *withheld* from him. I do not think it applies to the foetus as such, since it has as yet no conscious life (which is what we are talking about) and therefore cannot feel the loss of it or even the fear of that loss. If anybody thinks that foetuses *do* have conscious feelings sufficient to be put in this balance, I ask him to agree at least that their intensity is relatively small, and likewise of those of the newborn infant. So I do not think that the harm you are doing to the foetus or the unsuccessfully operated upon newborn infant by killing them is greater than that which you are doing to Andrew by stopping him from being conceived and born. In fact I think it is much less, because Andrew, unlike them, has a high prospect of a normal and happy life.

In my view as a philosopher, these are the sorts of considerations that doctors, surgeons and parents ought to be looking at when they are faced with these dilemmas.

Rights, Interests, and Possible People[1]

Derek Parfit

Do possible people have rights and interests? Professor Hare has argued that they do. I shall claim that, even if they don't, we should often act *as if* they do.

We can start with future people. Suppose that the testing of a nuclear weapon would, through radiation, cause a number of deformities in the people who are born within the next ten years. This would be against the interests of these future people. These people will exist whether or not the weapon is tested, and, if it is, they will be affected for the worse—they will be worse off than they would otherwise have been. We can harm these people though they don't live *now*, just as we can harm foreigners though they don't live *here*.

What about *possible* people? The difference between these and future people can be defined as follows. Suppose that we must act in one of two ways. "Future people" are the people who will exist whichever way we act.

Presented as a lecture at Case Western Reserve University. Reprinted by permission of the author.
[1] *This essay is a portion of an address written in 1973 as a companion piece to R. M. Hare's "Survival of the Weakest," above.*   Eds.

"Possible people" are the people who will exist if we act in one way, but who won't exist if we act in the other way. To give the simplest case: if we are wondering whether to have children, the children that we *could* have are possible people.

Do they have rights and interests? Suppose, first, that we decide to have these children. Can this affect their interests? We can obviously re-phrase this question so that it no longer asks about possible people. We can ask: can it be in, or be against, an *actual* person's interests to have been conceived? I shall return to this.

Suppose, next, that we decide not to have children. Then these possi-ble people never get conceived. Can *this* affect their interests? Can it, for instance, harm these children?

The normal answer would be "No." Professor Hare takes a different view. We can simplify the example he discussed. We suppose that a child is born with some serious handicap or abnormality, which is incurable, and would probably make the child's life, though still worth living, less so than a normal life. We next suppose that unless we perform some operation the child will die; and that, if it does, the parents will have another normal child, whom they wouldn't have if this child lives. The question is, should we operate?

Hare suggests that we should not. He first assumes that we ought to do what is in the best interests of all the people concerned. He then claims that among these people is "the next child in the queue"—the normal child whom the parents would later have only if the handicapped child dies. The interests of this possible child may, he thinks, "tip the balance." The possi-ble child, unlike the actual child, "has a high prospect of a normal and happy life"; Hare would therefore claim that we do *less* harm to the actual child by failing to save his life than we do to the possible child "by stopping him from being conceived and born."

In this particular case, many would agree with Hare that we shouldn't operate, but for different reasons. They may think that a new-born child is not yet a full person, with rights and interests;[1] or they may doubt whether life with a serious handicap would be worth living.

The implications of Hare's view can be better seen in another case. Take a couple who—we assume—live in an age before the world was over-populated, and who are wondering whether to have children. Suppose next that, if they do, their children's lives would probably be well worth living. Then, on Hare's view, if the couple choose not to have these children they would be doing them serious harm. Since there is no over-population, it would seem to follow that their choice is morally wrong. Most of us, I think, would deny this. We believe that there can be nothing wrong in deciding to remain childless. And if we also ask what Hare would count as over-population, his conclusion would again be widely disputed. This is another subject to which I shall return.

What I have called "Hare's view" is that we can harm people by

---

[1] Cf. Michael Tooley, "Abortion and Infanticide," *Philosophy and Public Affairs,* 2, No. 1 (Fall 1972).

preventing their conception. There are precedents for this view. The Talmud says that when Amram decided not to beget children, he was admonished for denying them the World to Come.[2] But, as Hare admits, his view is unusual. He would argue that it can be justified by an appeal to the logic of moral reasoning.[3] I shall not discuss whether this is so; but instead take a complementary path. I shall assume that we cannot harm those we don't conceive. Even so, I shall argue, it is hard to avoid Hare's conclusions.

The principle with which Hare works is that we should do what is in the best interests of those concerned. Most of us accept some principle of this kind. We may believe that other principles are often more important; but we accept, as one of our principles, something to do with interests, with preferences, or with happiness and misery. As this list suggests, such a principle can take different forms. We need only look at a single difference. The principle can take what I call an "impersonal" form: for example, it can run

(1) We should do what most reduces misery and increases happiness.

It can instead take a "person-affecting" form: for example

(2) We should do what harms people the least and benefits them most.

When we can only affect actual people, those who do or will exist, the difference between these forms of the principle makes, in practice, no difference. But when we can affect *who* exists, it can make a great difference.

Return, for instance, to the childless couple in the uncrowded world. According to principle (1)—the "impersonal" principle—they should do what most increases happiness. One of the most effective ways of increasing the quality of happiness is to increase the number of happy people. So the couple ought to have children; their failure to do so is, according to (1), morally wrong.

Most of us would say: "This just shows the absurdity of the impersonal principle. What we ought to do is make people happy, not make happy people. The right principle is (2), the 'person-affecting' principle. If the couple don't have children, there is no-one whom they've harmed, or failed to benefit. That is why they have done nothing wrong."

This reply involves the rejection of Hare's view. It assumes that we cannot harm people by preventing their conception. If we *can*, the childless couple would be doing wrong even on the person-affecting principle.

We can generalize from this example. Most of us hold a person-affecting, not an impersonal, principle. If we reject Hare's view, there are cases where this makes a great practical difference. But if we accept Hare's view,

[2]Quoted in G. Tedeschi, "On Tort Liability for 'Wrongful Life,'" *Israel Law Review,* October 1966, p. 514, footnote 3.

[3]The logic he describes in his books, *The Language of Morals,* O.U.P. 1952, and *Freedom and Reason,* O.U.P. 1963.

it makes no difference. The person-affecting principle, when combined with Hare's view, leads to the same conclusions as the impersonal principle.

Some of these conclusions are, as I said, striking. I shall now begin to argue towards them. We can avoid these conclusions only if we *both* accept what I shall call "the restriction of our principles to acts which affect people" *and* claim that our acts cannot affect possible people. Hare denies the latter; I shall be denying the former. The person-affecting restriction seems to me, at least in any natural form, unacceptable.

We can start with one of the two questions that I postponed. Can it be in our interests to have been conceived? Can we benefit from receiving life?

If we can, the childless couple are again at fault, even on person-affecting grounds—for if they have children they will be benefitting people, as principle (2) tells them to do.

We might say: "But we can only benefit if we are made better off than we would otherwise have been. This couple's children wouldn't otherwise have been—so they cannot benefit from receiving life." I have doubts about this reasoning. For one thing, it implies that we cannot benefit people if we *save* their lives, for here too they wouldn't otherwise have been. True, there are problems in comparing life with non-existence. But if we assume that a person's life has been well worth living, should we not agree that to have saved this person's life many years ago would be to have done this person a great benefit? And if it can be in a person's interests to have had his life prolonged, even, say, just after it started, why can it not be in his interests to have had it started?

Here is a second problem. If we cannot benefit a person by conceiving him, then we cannot harm him either. But suppose we know that any child whom we could conceive will have an abnormality so severe that it will live for only a few years, will never develop, and will suffer fairly frequent pain. It would seem to be clearly wrong to go ahead, knowingly, and conceive such a child.[4] And the main reason why it would be wrong is that the child will suffer. But if we cannot *harm* a child by giving it a life of this kind, then this reason why the act is wrong cannot be stated in "person-affecting" terms. We shall have to say, "It is wrong because it increases suffering." We should then be back with half of the impersonal principle; and it will be hard, in consistency, to avoid the other half. (We might perhaps claim that only suffering matters morally—that happiness is morally trivial. But this position, though superficially attractive, collapses when we think it through.)

We have been asking whether the act of conceiving a child can affect this child, for better or worse. If we answer "Yes," the person-affecting restriction makes no difference; principle (2) leads to the same conclusions as principle (1). We may therefore wish to answer "No"—but to this we have found objections.

The problem here can, I think, be solved. We can state the person-affecting principle in a different form:

[4]For a legal discussion of related issues, see "A Cause of Action for 'Wrongful Life,'" *Minnesota Law Review*, 55, No. 1 (November 1970).

(3) It is wrong to do what, of the alternatives, affects people for the worse.

We interpret (3) so that if people fail to receive possible benefits, they count as affected for the worse. If we adopt principle (3), we can afford to allow that conceiving someone is a case of affecting him. Since failing to receive benefits counts as being affected for the worse, principle (3) still tells us—like principle (2)—to do what benefits people most. But there is one exception. To the one benefit of receiving life (3)—unlike (2)—gives no weight. For when we fail to give this benefit, there isn't an actual person who fails to receive it—who is thus affected for the worse. (I am now assuming, you remember, that we cannot affect possible people.)

Most of us, I claimed, think there is nothing wrong in *not* having children, even if they would have been very happy. But we think that having children who are bound to suffer is wrong. Principle (3) supports this asymmetrical pair of judgments. It supports our view that the Childless Couple did no wrong; but it also supports our view about "wrongful conception" —for the child here is an actual person affected for the worse.

In the move from (2) to (3), a natural principle is revised in a somewhat artificial way. But this revision does not seem to drain the principle of its plausibility. All the revision does is this. When we are choosing what to do, we are told to aim, not to achieve the outcome where people are better off, but to avoid the outcome where they are worse off. This procedure, adding up the "minuses," seems to be just as general and as plausible as the other, adding up the "pluses." So we are not, in moving to (3), "tailoring" our principles in an *ad-hoc* way. And the justification for the move is that only principle (3) (combined with the assumption that conceiving is affecting) gives support to the asymmetrical judgments that we find plausible.[5]

So far, so good. But I shall now argue that the person-affecting principle needs to be more drastically revised. This *may* drain it of its plausibility.

Consider the following case, which involves two women. The first is one month pregnant, and is told by her doctor that, unless she takes a simple treatment, the child she is carrying will develop a certain handicap. We suppose again that life with this handicap would probably be worth living, but less so than a normal life. It would obviously be wrong for the mother not to take the treatment, for this will handicap her child. And the person-affecting principle tells us that this would be wrong. (Note that we need not assume that a one-month old foetus is a person, for there *will be* a person whom the woman has affected for the worse.)

We next suppose that there is a second woman, who is about to stop taking contraceptive pills so that she can have another child. She is told that she has a temporary condition such that any child she conceives now will have just the same handicap; but that if she waits three months she will then conceive a normal child. It seems clear that it would be wrong for this second woman, by not waiting, to deliberately have a handicapped rather

[5]This asymmetry is discussed in Jan Narveson's two articles: "Utilitarianism and New Generations," *Mind*, January 1967, and "Moral Problems of Population," *The Monist*, January 1973. I have learned much from both of these.

than a normal child. And it seems (at least to me) clear that this would be just *as* wrong as it would be for the first woman to deliberately handicap her child.

But if the second woman does deliberately have a handicapped child, has she harmed him—affected him for the worse? We must first ask: "Could he truly claim, when he grows up, 'If my mother had waited, I would have been born three months later, as a normal child'?" The answer is, "No." If his mother had waited, he would not have been born at all; she would have had a different child. When I claim this, I need not assume that the time of one's conception, or the particular cells from which one grew, are essential to one's identity. *Perhaps* we can suppose that *I* might have been conceived a year later, if we are supposing that my parents had no child when they in fact had me, but a year later had a child who was exactly or very much *like* me. But in our case the child the woman would have if she waits would be as unlike the child she would have now as any two of her actual children would be likely to be. Given this, we cannot claim that they would have been the same child. (To argue this in another way. Suppose that I am in fact my mother's first child and eldest son. And suppose that things had gone like this: she had no child when I was in fact born, then had a girl, then a boy. Can I claim that I, her first child, would have been that girl? Why not claim that I, her eldest son, would have been that boy? Both claims are equally good, and so, since they cannot both be true, equally bad. So, if she *had* waited before having children, I would not have been born at all.)[6]

The second woman's handicapped child is, then, not worse off than he would otherwise have been, for he wouldn't otherwise have been. Might we still claim that in deliberately conceiving a handicapped child, the woman harms this child? We might perhaps claim this if the child's life would be not worth living—would be worse than nothing; but we have assumed that it would be worth living. And in this case being handicapped is the only way in which this child can receive life. So the case is like that in which a doctor removes a person's limb to save his life. It would not be true, at least in a morally relevant sense, that the doctor harmed this person, or affected him for the worse. We seem bound to say the same about my second woman.

I conclude, then, that if the second woman deliberately conceives a handicapped rather than a normal child, she would not be harming this child. The first woman, if she deliberately neglects the treatment, would be harming her child. Notice next that in every other way the two acts are exactly similar. The side-effects on other people should be much the same. These side-effects would provide *some* person-affecting grounds for the claim that the second woman's act would be wrong. But it is obvious that if we judge the two acts on person-affecting principles, the first woman's act must be considerably *more* wrong. In her case, there are not just side-effects —her child is seriously harmed. The second woman's child is *not* harmed. Since this is the only difference between the two acts, the case provides a

---

[6]For a different view, take a remark in Gwen Raverat's *Period Piece,* Faber and Faber 1952, "It is always a fascinating problem to consider who we would have been if our mother (or our father) had married another person."

test for person-affecting principles. The impersonal principle tells us to reduce misery and increase happiness, whether or not people are affected for better or worse. If there is any plausibility in the restriction to acts which affect people, it must be worse to *harm* someone than to cause equivalent unhappiness in a way which harms no-one. The second woman's act must, in other words, be less wrong than the first's. If we think that it is not less wrong, we cannot accept the restriction to acts which affect people.

The acts which I have described are of course unusual. But this does not make them a worse test for the person-affecting restriction. On the contrary, they are unusual because they are designed as a test. The two women's acts are designed to be as similar as they could be, except in one respect. Each woman deliberately brings it about that she has a handicapped rather than a normal child. The only difference is that in one case the handicapped and the normal child are the same child, while in the other they are not. This is precisely the difference which, on the person-affecting principle, matters. If we think that the two acts would be just as wrong, we cannot believe that it does matter.

Some of you may think that the person-affecting principle survives this test. You may think: "Since the second woman doesn't harm her child, what she does *is* less wrong." But there are other cases where such implications seem harder to accept. Take genetic counseling. We could not advise the dominant carriers of diseases to accept genetic counseling *for the sake* of their children, for if they reject this counseling, and marry other dominant carriers, it will not be true that their children will have been harmed, or affected for the worse. Or again, Dr. Kass has argued that it would be wrong to use certain kinds of artificial fertilization, on the ground that if children are conceived in these ways, rather than in normal ways, they run greater risks of certain deformities.[7] But these particular children cannot be conceived in normal ways. For them, the alternatives are artificial fertilization, or nothing. So we can only claim that we would be harming them, or affecting them for the worse, if the risks of deformities were so great that their lives would probably be not worth living.

When we turn to population policy, the implications become much harder to accept. . . .

[Editorial note: the rest of Parfit's talk is not reprinted here. His more recent thoughts about the problems discussed in this talk, and the larger problems of population policy, will appear in a future issue of the journal, *Philosophy & Public Affairs,* under the title "Overpopulation."]

[7]"Making babies—the new biology and the 'old' morality," Leon Kass, *The Public Interest,* Winter, 1972.

DEATH AND DIGNITY

From *Epistula Morales,* "On Suicide"

Seneca

. . . life has carried some men with the greatest rapidity to the harbour, the harbour they were bound to reach even if they tarried on the way, while others it has fretted and harassed. To such a life, as you are aware, one should not always cling. For mere living is not a good, but living well. Accordingly, the wise man will live as long as he ought, not as long as he can. He will mark in what place, with whom, and how he is to conduct his existence, and what he is about to do. He always reflects concerning the quality, and not the quantity, of his life. As soon as there are many events in his life that give him trouble and disturb his peace of mind, he sets himself free. And this privilege is his, not only when the crisis is upon him, but as soon as Fortune seems to be playing him false; then he looks about carefully and sees whether he ought, or ought not, to end his life on that account. He holds that it makes no difference to him whether his taking-off be natural or self-inflicted, whether it comes later or earlier. He does not regard it with fear, as if it were a great loss; for no man can lose very much when but a driblet remains. It is not a question of dying earlier or later, but of dying well or ill. And dying well means escape from the danger of living ill.

Duties Towards the Body in Regard to Life

Immanuel Kant

What are our powers of disposal over our life? Have we any authority of disposal over it in any shape or form? How far is it incumbent upon us to take care of it? These are questions which fall to be considered in connexion with our duties towards the body in regard to life. We must, however, by way of introduction, make the following observations. If the body were related to life not as a condition but as an accident or circumstance so that we could at will divest ourselves of it; if we could slip out of it and slip into

Reprinted from *Ethical Choice,* eds. R.N. Beck and J. B. Orr (New York: The Free Press, 1970), p. 54, with permission of the publisher and The Loeb Classical Library, from *Epistula Morales* Vol. II, trans. R. M. Gumere (Cambridge: Harvard University Press, 1920).

Reprinted by permission of the publisher from Immanuel Kant, *Lectures on Ethics,* trans. Louis Infield (New York: Harper & Row, 1963), pp. 147–48.

another just as we leave one country for another, then the body would be subject to our free will and we could rightly have the disposal of it. This, however, would not imply that we could similarly dispose of our life, but only of our circumstances, of the movable goods, the furniture of life. In fact, however, our life is entirely conditioned by our body, so that we cannot conceive of a life not mediated by the body and we cannot make use of our freedom except through the body. It is, therefore, obvious that the body constitutes a part of ourselves. If a man destroys his body, and so his life, he does it by the use of his will, which is itself destroyed in the process. But to use the power of a free will for its own destruction is self-contradictory. If freedom is the condition of life it cannot be employed to abolish life and so to destroy and abolish itself. To use life for its own destruction, to use life for producing lifelessness, is self-contradictory. These preliminary remarks are sufficient to show that man cannot rightly have any power of disposal in regard to himself and his life, but only in regard to his circumstances. His body gives man power over his life; were he a spirit he could not destroy his life; life in the absolute has been invested by nature with indestructibility and is an end in itself; hence it follows that man cannot have the power to dispose of his life.

Suicide

Immanuel Kant

Suicide can be regarded in various lights; it might be held to be reprehensible, or permissible, or even heroic. In the first place we have the specious view that suicide can be allowed and tolerated. Its advocates argue thus. So long as he does not violate the proprietary rights of others, man is a free agent. With regard to his body there are various things he can properly do; he can have a boil lanced or a limb amputated, and disregard a scar; he is, in fact, free to do whatever he may consider useful and advisable. If then he comes to the conclusion that the most useful and advisable thing that he can do is to put an end to his life, why should he not be entitled to do so? Why not, if he sees that he can no longer go on living and that he will be ridding himself of misfortune, torment and disgrace? To be sure he robs himself of a full life, but he escapes once and for all from calamity and misfortune. The argument sounds most plausible. But let us, leaving aside religious considerations, examine the act itself. We may treat our body as we please, provided our motives are those of self-preservation. If, for instance, his foot is a hindrance to life, a man might have it amputated. To preserve his person he has the right of disposal over his body. But in taking his life he does not preserve his person; he disposes of his person and not

Reprinted by permission of the publisher from Immanuel Kant, *Lectures on Ethics*, trans. Louis Infield (New York: Harper & Row, 1963), pp. 148–154.

of its attendant circumstances; he robs himself of his person. This is contrary to the highest duty we have towards ourselves, for it annuls the condition of all other duties; it goes beyond the limits of the use of free will, for this use is possible only through the existence of the Subject.

There is another set of considerations which make suicide seem plausible. A man might find himself so placed that he can continue living only under circumstances which deprive life of all value; in which he can no longer live conformably to virtue and prudence, so that he must from noble motives put an end to his life. The advocates of this view quote in support of it the example of Cato. Cato knew that the entire Roman nation relied upon him in their resistance to Caesar, but he found that he could not prevent himself from falling into Caesar's hands. What was he to do? If he, the champion of freedom, submitted, every one would say, "If Cato himself submits, what else can we do?" If, on the other hand, he killed himself, his death might spur on the Romans to fight to the bitter end in defence of their freedom. So he killed himself. He thought that it was necessary for him to die. He thought that if he could not go on living as Cato, he could not go on living at all. It must certainly be admitted that in a case such as this, where suicide is a virtue, appearances are in its favour. But this is the only example which has given the world the opportunity of defending suicide. It is the only example of its kind and there has been no similar case since. Lucretia also killed herself, but on grounds of modesty and in a fury of vengeance. It is obviously our duty to preserve our honour, particularly in relation to the opposite sex, for whom it is a merit; but we must endeavour to save our honour only to this extent, that we ought not to surrender it for selfish and lustful purposes. To do what Lucretia did is to adopt a remedy which is not at our disposal; it would have been better had she defended her honour unto death; that would not have been suicide and would have been right; for it is no suicide to risk one's life against one's enemies, and even to sacrifice it, in order to observe one's duties towards oneself.

No one under the sun can bind me to commit suicide; no sovereign can do so. The sovereign can call upon his subjects to fight to the death for their country, and those who fall on the field of battle are not suicides, but the victims of fate. Not only is this not suicide; but the opposite, a faint heart and fear of the death which threatens by the necessity of fate, is no true self-preservation; for he who runs away to save his own life, and leaves his comrades in the lurch, is a coward; but he who defends himself and his fellows even unto death is no suicide, but noble and high-minded; for life is not to be highly regarded for its own sake. I should endeavour to preserve my own life only so far as I am worthy to live. We must draw a distinction between the suicide and the victim of fate. A man who shortens his life by intemperance is guilty of imprudence and indirectly of his own death; but his guilt is not direct; he did not intend to kill himself; his death was not premeditated. For all our offences are either *culpa* or *dolus*. There is certainly no *dolus* here, but there is *culpa;* and we can say of such a man that he was guilty of his own death, but we cannot say of him that he is a suicide. What constitutes suicide is the intention to destroy oneself. Intemperance and excess which shorten life ought not, therefore, to be called suicide; for if we raise intemperance to the level of suicide, we lower suicide to the level of intemperance. Imprudence, which does not imply a desire to cease to live, must, therefore, be distinguished from the intention to murder oneself. Serious violations of our duty towards ourselves produce an aversion accompanied either by horror or by disgust; suicide is of the horrible kind, *crimina carnis* of the disgusting. We shrink in horror from suicide because all nature seeks its own preservation; an injured tree, a living body, an animal does so; how then could man make of his freedom, which is the acme of life and constitutes its worth, a principle for his own destruction? Nothing more terrible can be imagined; for if man were on every occasion master of his own life, he would be master of the lives of others; and being ready to sacrifice his life at any and every time rather than be captured, he could perpetrate every conceivable crime and vice. We are, therefore, horrified at the very thought of suicide; by it man sinks lower than the beasts; we look upon a suicide as carrion, whilst our sympathy goes forth to the victim of fate.

Those who advocate suicide seek to give the widest interpretation to freedom. There is something flattering in the thought that we can take our own life if we are so minded; and so we find even right-thinking persons defending suicide in this respect. There are many circumstances under which life ought to be sacrificed. If I cannot preserve my life except by violating my duties towards myself, I am bound to sacrifice my life rather than violate these duties. But suicide is in no circumstances permissible. Humanity in one's own person is something inviolable; it is a holy trust; man is master of all else, but he must not lay hands upon himself. A being who existed of his own necessity could not possibly destroy himself; a being whose existence is not necessary must regard life as the condition of everything else, and in the consciousness that life is a trust reposed in him, such a being recoils at the thought of committing a breach of his holy trust by turning his life against himself. Man can only dispose over things; beasts are things in this sense; but man is not a thing, not a beast. If he disposes over himself, he treats his value as that of a beast. He who so behaves, who has no respect for human nature and makes a thing of himself, becomes for everyone an Object of freewill. We are free to treat him as a beast, as a thing, and to use him for our sport as we do a horse or a dog, for he is no longer a human being; he has made a thing of himself, and, having himself discarded his humanity, he cannot expect that others should respect humanity in him. Yet humanity is worthy of esteem. Even when a man is a bad man, humanity in his person is worthy of esteem. Suicide is not abominable and inadmissible because life should be highly prized; were it so, we could each have our own opinion or how highly we should prize it, and the rule of prudence would often indicate suicide as the best means. But the rule of morality does not admit of it under any condition because it degrades human nature below the level of animal nature and so destroys it. Yet there is much in the world far more important than life. To observe morality is far more important. It is better to sacrifice one's life than one's morality. To live is not a necessity; but to live honourably while life lasts is a necessity. We can at all times go on living and doing our duty towards ourselves without having to do violence to ourselves. But he who is prepared to take his own life is no longer worthy to live at all. The pragmatic ground of impulse to live is happiness. Can I then take my own life because I cannot live happily? No! It is not necessary that whilst I live I should live happily; but it is necessary that so long as I live I should live honourably. Misery gives no right to any man to take his own life, for then we should all be entitled to take our lives for lack of pleasure. All our duties towards ourselves would then be directed towards pleasure; but the fulfilment of those duties may demand that we should even sacrifice our life.

Is suicide heroic or cowardly? Sophistication, even though well meant, is not a good thing. It is not good to defend either virtue or vice by splitting hairs. Even right-thinking people declaim against suicide on wrong lines. They say that it is arrant cowardice. But instances of suicide of great heroism exist. We cannot, for example, regard the suicides of Cato and of Atticus as cowardly. Rage, passion and insanity are the most frequent causes of suicide, and that is why persons who attempt suicide and are saved from it are so terrified at their own act that they do not dare to repeat the attempt. There was a time in Roman and in Greek history when suicide was regarded as honourable, so much so that the Romans forbade their slaves to commit suicide because they did not belong to themselves but to their masters and so were regarded as things, like all other animals. The Stoics said that suicide is the sage's peaceful death; he leaves the world as he might leave a smoky room for another, because it no longer pleases him; he leaves the world, not because he is no longer happy in it, but because he disdains it. It has already been mentioned that man is greatly flattered by the idea that he is free to remove himself from this world, if he so wishes. He may not make use of this freedom, but the thought of possessing it pleases him. It seems even to have a moral aspect, for if man is capable of removing himself from the world at his own will, he need not submit to any one; he can retain his independence and tell the rudest truths to the cruellest of tyrants. Torture cannot bring him to heel, because he can leave the world at a moment's notice as a free man can leave the country, if and when he wills it. But this semblance of morality vanishes as soon as we see that man's freedom cannot subsist except on a condition which is immutable. This condition is that man may not use his freedom against himself to his own destruction, but that, on the contrary, he should allow nothing external to limit it. Freedom thus conditioned is noble. No chance or misfortune ought to make us afraid to live; we ought to go on living as long as we can do so as human beings and honourably. To bewail one's fate and misfortune is in itself dishonourable. Had Cato faced any torments which Caesar might have inflicted upon him with a resolute mind and remained steadfast, it would have been noble of him; to violate himself was not so. Those who advocate suicide and teach that there is authority for it necessarily do much harm in a republic of free men. Let us imagine a state in which men held as a general opinion that they were entitled to commit suicide, and that there was even merit and honour in so doing. How dreadful everyone would find them. For he who does not respect his life even in principle cannot be restrained from the most dreadful vices; he recks neither king nor torments.

But as soon as we examine suicide from the standpoint of religion we immediately see it in its true light. We have been placed in this world under certain conditions and for specific purposes. But a suicide opposes the purpose of his Creator; he arrives in the other world as one who has deserted his post; he must be looked upon as a rebel against God. So long as we remember the truth that it is God's intention to preserve life, we are bound to regulate our activities in conformity with it. We have no right to offer violence to our nature's powers of self-preservation and to upset the wisdom of her arrangements. This duty is upon us until the time comes when God expressly commands us to leave this life. Human beings are sentinels on earth and may not leave their posts until relieved by another beneficent hand. God is our owner; we are His property; His providence works for our good. A bondman in the care of a beneficent master deserves punishment if he opposes his master's wishes.

But suicide is not inadmissible and abominable because God has forbidden it; God has forbidden it because it is abominable in that it degrades man's inner worth below that of the animal creation. Moral philosophers must, therefore, first and foremost show that suicide is abominable. We find, as a rule, that those who labour for their happiness are more liable to suicide; having tasted the refinements of pleasure, and being deprived of them, they give way to grief, sorrow, and melancholy.

From "Essay on Suicide"

David Hume

One considerable advantage that arises from Philosophy consists in the sovereign antidote which it affords to superstition and false religion. All other remedies against that pestilent distemper are vain, or at least uncertain. Plain good sense and the practice of the world, which alone serve most purposes of life, are here found ineffectual: History as well as daily experience furnish instances of men endowed with the strongest capacity for business and affairs, who have all their lives crouched under slavery to the grossest superstition. Even gaiety and sweetness of temper, which infuse a balm into every other wound, afford no remedy to so virulent a poison; as we may particularly observe of the fair sex, who, though commonly possest of these rich presents of nature, feel many of their joys blasted by this importunate intruder. But when sound Philosophy has once gained possession of the mind, superstition is effectually excluded; and one may fairly affirm that her triumph over this enemy is more complete than over most of the vices and imperfections incident to human nature. Love or anger, ambition or avarice, have their root in the temper and affections, which the

Reprinted with permission from *Ethics and Metaethics*, ed. R. Abelson, (New York: St. Martin's Press, 1963) pp. 108–16.

soundest reason is scarce ever able fully to correct; but superstition being founded on false opinion, must immediately vanish when true philosophy has inspired juster sentiments of superior powers. The contest is here more equal between the distemper and the medicine, and nothing can hinder the latter from proving effectual, but its being false and sophisticated.

It will here be superfluous to magnify the merits of philosophy by displaying the pernicious tendency of that vice of which it cures the human mind. The superstitious man, says Tully, is miserable in every scene, in every incident of life; even sleep itself, which banishes all other cares of unhappy mortals, affords to him matter of new terror; while he examines his dreams, and finds in those visions of the night prognostications of future calamities. I may add, that though death alone can put a full period to this misery, he dares not fly to this refuge, but still prolongs a miserable existence from a vain fear lest he offend his maker by using the power with which that beneficent being has endowed him. The presents of God and nature are ravished from us by this cruel enemy; and notwithstanding that one step would remove us from the regions of pain and sorrow, her menaces still chain us down to a hated being, which she herself chiefly contributes to render miserable.

'Tis observed by such as have been reduced by the calamities of life to the necessity of employing this fatal remedy, that if the unseasonable care of their friends deprive them of that species of Death which they proposed to themselves, they seldom venture upon any other, or can summon up so much resolution a second time, as to execute their purpose. So great is our horror of death that when it presents itself, under any form, besides that to which a man has endeavoured to reconcile his imagination, it acquires new terrors and overcomes his feeble courage: But when the menaces of superstition are joined to this natural timidity, no wonder it quite deprives men of all power over their lives, since even many pleasures and enjoyments, to which we are carried by a strong propensity, are torn from us by this inhuman tyrant. Let us here endeavour to restore men to their native liberty by examining all the common arguments against Suicide, and shewing that that action may be free from every imputation of guilt or blame, according to the sentiments of all the ancient philosophers.

If Suicide be criminal, it must be a transgression of our duty either to God, our neighbour, or ourselves. To prove that suicide is no transgression of our duty to God, the following considerations may perhaps suffice. In order to govern the material world, the almighty Creator has established general and immutable laws by which all bodies, from the greatest planet to the smallest particle of matter, are maintained in their proper sphere and function. To govern the animal world, he has endowed all living creatures with bodily and mental powers; with senses, passions, appetites, memory and judgment, by which they are impelled or regulated in that course of life to which they are destined. These two distinct principles of the material and animal world continually encroach upon each other, and mutually retard or forward each other's operations. The powers of men and of all other animals are restrained and directed by the nature and qualities of the surrounding bodies; and the modifications and actions of these bodies are incessantly altered by the operation of all animals. Man is stopt by rivers in his passage over the surface of the earth; and rivers, when properly directed, lend their force to the motion of machines, which serve to the use of man. But though the provinces of material and animal powers are not kept entirely separate, there results from thence no discord or disorder in the creation; on the contrary, from the mixture, union and contrast of all the various powers of inanimate bodies and living creatures, arises that surprising harmony and proportion which affords the surest argument of supreme wisdom. The providence of the Deity appears not immediately in any operation, but governs everything by those general and immutable laws, which have been established from the beginning of time. All events, in one sense, may be pronounced the action of the Almighty; they all proceed from those powers with which he has endowed his creatures. A house which falls by its own weight is not brought to ruin by his providence more than one destroyed by the hands of men; nor are the human faculties less his workmanship than the laws of motion and gravitation. When the passions play, when the judgment dictates, when the limbs obey; this is all the operation of God, and upon these animate principles, as well as upon the inanimate, has he established the government of the universe. Every event is alike important in the eyes of that infinite being, who takes in at one glance the most distant regions of space and remotest periods of time. There is no event, however important to us, which he has exempted from the general laws that govern the universe, or which he has peculiarly reserved for his own immediate action and operation. The revolution of states and empires depends upon the smallest caprice or passion of single men; and the lives of men are shortened or extended by the smallest accident of air or diet, sunshine or tempest. Nature still continues her progress and operation; and if general laws be ever broke by particular volitions of the Deity, 'tis after a manner which entirely escapes human observation. As, on the one hand, the elements and other inanimate parts of the creation carry on their action without regard to the particular interest and situation of men; so men are entrusted to their judgment and discretion, in the various shocks of matter, and may employ every faculty with which they are endowed, in order to provide for their ease, happiness, or preservation. What is the meaning then of that principle that a man, who, tired of life, and haunted by pain and misery, bravely overcomes all the natural terrors of death and makes his escape from this cruel scene; that such a man, I say, has incurred the indignation of his Creator by encroaching on the office of divine providence, and disturbing the order of the universe? Shall we assert that the Almighty has reserved to himself in any peculiar manner the disposal of the lives of men, and has not submitted that event, in common with others, to the general laws by which the universe is governed? This is plainly false; the lives of men depend upon the same laws as the lives of all other elements; and these are subjected to the general laws of matter and motion. The fall of a tower, or the infusion of poison, will destroy a man equally with the meanest creature; an inundation sweeps away every thing without distinction that comes within the reach of its fury. Since therefore the lives of men are for ever dependent on the general laws of matter and motion, is a man's disposing of his life criminal, because in every case it is criminal to encroach upon these laws, or disturb their operation? But this seems absurd; all animals are entrusted to their own prudence and skill for their conduct in the world, and have full authority, as far as their power extends, to alter all the operations of nature. Without the exercise of this authority they could not subsist a moment; every action, every motion of a man, innovates on the order of some parts of matter, and diverts from their ordinary course the general laws of motion. Putting together, therefore, these conclusions, we find that human life depends upon the general laws of matter and motion, and that it is no encroachment on the office of providence to disturb or alter these general laws: Has not everyone, of consequence, the free disposal of his own life? And may he not lawfully employ that power with which nature has endowed him? In order to destroy the evidence of this conclusion, we must shew a reason why this particular case is excepted; is it because human life is of so great importance, that 'tis a presumption for human prudence to dispose of it? But the life of a man is of no greater importance to the universe than that of an oyster. And were it of ever so great importance, the order of nature has actually submitted it to human prudence, and reduced us to a necessity in every incident of determining concerning it. Were the disposal of human life so much reserved as the peculiar province of the Almightly that it were an encroachment of his right for men to dispose of their own lives; it would be equally criminal to act for the preservation of life as for its destruction. If I turn aside a stone which is falling upon my head, I disturb the course of nature, and I invade the peculiar province of the Almighty by lengthening out my life beyond the period which by the general laws of matter and motion he had assigned it.

A hair, a fly, an insect is able to destroy this mighty being whose life is of such importance. Is it an absurdity to suppose that human prudence may lawfully dispose of what depends on such insignificant causes? It would be no crime in me to divert the Nile or Danube from its course, were I able to effect such purposes. Where then is the crime of turning a few ounces of blood from their natural channel? Do you imagine that I repine at providence or curse my creation, because I go out of life, and put a period to a being, which, were it to continue, would render me miserable? Far be such sentiments from me; I am only convinced of a matter of fact, which you yourself acknowledge possible, that human life may be unhappy, and that my existence, if further prolonged, would become ineligible: but I thank providence, both for the good which I have already enjoyed, and for the power with which I am endowed of escaping the ill that threatens me. To you it belongs to repine providence, who foolishly imagine that you have no such power, and who must still prolong a hated life, though loaded with pain and sickness, with shame and poverty. Do you not teach that when any ill befalls me, though by the malice of my enemies, I ought to be resigned to providence, and that the actions of men are the operations of the Almighty as much as the actions of inanimate beings? When I fall upon my own sword, therefore, I receive my death equally from the hands of the Deity as if it had proceeded from a lion, a precipice, or a fever. The submission which you require to providence in every calamity that befalls me excludes not human skill and industry, if possibly by their means I can avoid or escape the calamity: And why may I not employ one remedy as well as another? If my life be not my own, it were criminal for me to put it in danger, as well as to dispose of it; nor could one man deserve the appellation of *hero* whom glory or friendship transports into the greatest dangers, and another merit the reproach of *wretch* or *miscreant* who puts a period to his life for like motives. There is no being which possesses any power or faculty that it receives not from its Creator, nor is there any one which by ever so irregular an action can encroach upon the plan of his providence, or disorder the universe. Its operations are his works equally with that chain of events which it invades, and whichever principle prevails, we may for that very reason conclude it to be most favoured by him. Be it animate, or inanimate, rational, or irrational; 'tis all a case: Its power is still derived from the supreme creator, and is alike comprehended in the order of his providence. When the horror of pain prevails over the love of live; when a voluntary action anticipates the effects of blind causes; 'tis only in consequence of those powers and principles which he has implanted in his creatures. Divine providence is still inviolate and placed far beyond the reach of human injuries. 'Tis impious, says the old Roman superstition, to divert rivers from their course, or invade the prerogatives of nature. 'Tis impious, says the French superstition, to inoculate for the small-pox, or usurp the business of providence, by voluntarily producing distempers and maladies. 'Tis impious, says the modern European superstition, to put a period to our own life, and thereby rebel against our creator; and why not impious, say I, to build houses, cultivate the ground, or sail upon the ocean? In all these actions we employ our powers of mind and body to produce some innovation in the course of nature; and in none of them do we any more. They are all of them therefore equally innocent, or equally criminal. *But you are placed by providence, like a sentinel in a particular station, and when you desert it without being recalled, you are equally guilty of rebellion against your almighty sovereign, and have incurred his displeasure.* I ask, why do you conclude that providence has placed me in this station? For my part I find that I owe my birth to a long chain of causes, of which many depend upon voluntary actions of men. *But Providence guided all these causes, and nothing happens in the universe without its consent and cooperation.* If so, then neither does my death, however voluntary, happen without its consent; and whenever pain or sorrow so far overcome my patience as to make me tired of life, I may conclude that I am recalled from my station in the clearest and most express terms. 'Tis Providence surely that has placed me at this present moment in this chamber: But may I not leave it when I think proper, without being liable to the imputation of having deserted my post or station? When I shall be dead, the principles of which I am composed will still perform their part in the universe, and will be equally useful in the grand fabric, as when they composed this individual creature. The difference to the whole will be no greater than betwixt my being in a chamber and in the open air. The one change is of more importance to me than the other; but not more so to the universe.

'Tis a kind of blasphemy to imagine that any created being can disturb the order of the world or invade the business of providence! It supposes that

that being possesses powers and faculties which it received not from its creator, and which are not subordinate to his government and authority. A man may disturb society no doubt, and thereby incur the displeasure of the Almighty: But the government of the world is placed far beyond his reach and violence. And how does it appear that the Almighty is displeased with those actions that disturb society? By the principles which he has implanted in human nature, and which inspire us with a sentiment of remorse if we ourselves have been guilty of such actions, and with that of blame and disapprobation, if we ever observe them in others. Let us now examine, according to the method proposed, whether Suicide be of this kind of actions, and be a breach of our duty to our *neighbour* and to *society.*

A man who retires from life does no harm to society: He only ceases to do good; which, if it is an injury, is of the lowest kind. All our obligations to do good to society seem to imply something reciprocal. I receive the benefits of society and therefore ought to promote its interests, but when I withdraw myself altogether from society, can I be bound any longer? But, allowing that our obligations to do good were perpetual, they have certainly some bounds; I am not obliged to do a small good to society at the expense of a great harm to myself; why then should I prolong a miserable existence, because of some frivolous advantage which the public may perhaps receive from me? If upon account of age and infirmities I may lawfully resign any office, and employ my time altogether in fencing against these calamities, and alleviating as much as possible the miseries of my future life: Why may I not cut short these miseries at once by an action which is no more prejudicial to society? But suppose that it is no longer in my power to promote the interest of society; suppose that I am a burthen to it; suppose that my life hinders some person from being much more useful to society. In such cases my resignation of life must not only be innocent but laudable. And most people who lie under any temptation to abandon existence are in some such situation; those who have health, or power, or authority, have commonly better reason to be in humour with the world.

A man is engaged in a conspiracy for the public interest; is seized upon suspicion; is threatened with the rack; and knows from his own weakness that the secret will be extorted from him: Could such a one consult the public interest better than by putting a quick period to a miserable life? This was the case of the famous and brave Strozi of Florence. Again, suppose a malefactor is justly condemned to a shameful death; can any reason be imagined why he may not anticipate his punishment, and save himself all the anguish of thinking on its dreadful approaches? He invades the business of providence no more than the magistrate did, who ordered his execution; and his voluntary death is equally advantageous to society by ridding it of a pernicious member.

That suicide may often be consistent with interest and with our duty to ourselves, no one can question who allows that age, sickness, or misfortune may render life a burthen, and make it worse even than annihilation. I believe that no man ever threw away life while it was worth keeping. For such is our natural horror of death that small motives will never be able to reconcile us to it; and though perhaps the situation of a man's health or fortune did not seem to require this remedy, we may at least be assured that any one who, without apparent reason, has had recourse to it, was curst with such an incurable depravity or gloominess of temper as must poison all enjoyment, and render him equally miserable as if he had been loaded with the most grievous misfortunes. If suicide be supposed a crime 'tis only cowardice can impel us to it. If it be no crime, both prudence and courage should engage us to rid ourselves at once of existence, when it becomes a burthen. 'Tis the only way that we can then be useful to society, by setting an example, which, if imitated, would preserve to everyone his chance for happiness in life and would effectually free him from all danger or misery.

Suicide and the Right to Die

George E. Murphy

At least one recent court case has upheld a patient's right to freedom from unwanted intervention in the process of dying. Medical societies across the country are publicly supporting carefully considered decisions to limit intervention in terminal illness. Excesses of therapeutic zeal, bred of a burgeoning life-support technology, are giving way to a more careful consideration of the patient's humanity. At the same time, euthanasia receives little public support. The deliberate induction of death is foreign to the spirit of medicine. But we are once again becoming aware of the mortally ill individual's right to die with dignity.

Physicians know full well they cannot prevent death. They can only postpone it. Where death is imminent—and every clinician knows that judgment is fugitive at times—the questions are when and how, not whether. Suicide, or the threat of it, raises the question of *whether,* in the sense that death is not otherwise near. Symposia, panel discussions, and debates have been held on the question of the individual's right to suicide. But the assertion of such a "right" leaves out of consideration what is known about those who have taken their lives. So-called "rational" suicide is a rarity. Only a few persons who commit suicide are suffering from a terminal illness (and may perhaps be excluded from the discussion that follows). The descriptive facts are that most persons who commit suicide are suffering from clinically recognizable psychiatric illnesses often carrying an excellent prognosis; that the majority have sought help from physicians for their symptoms; and that few have received the indicated treatment. To say that this person is exercising a right is to mock him in his frustration at failing to find the understanding and the technical skill he sought.

To be sure, there are those who condemn any effort to interfere with an individual's behavior against his wishes. But their grounds are philosoph-

Reprinted from the *American Journal of Psychiatry*, 130, No. 4, 472–473, April 1973. Copyright by the American Psychiatric Association, 1973.

ical, not clinical, and foreign to our concerns as physicians. Others, in the hope of de-stigmatizing suicide, would establish "thanatoria" to facilitate, regulate, and sanitize the act. This idea seems to be the intellectual toy of frustrated would-be suicide preventers. There is much to be frustrated about. Our ability to predict suicide is still crude. Our ability to prevent suicide is at best unproven. The loss of federal support for research in these vital areas coincides with an unprecedented rise in suicide among the young. But suicide is not a topic on which to take the position: "If you can't beat them, join them!"

From our knowledge of the natural history of the psychiatric disorders underlying the suicidal urge, we can confidently predict recovery from that urge in the great majority of cases, when other symptoms of depression lift. The desire to terminate one's life is usually transient. The "right" to suicide is a "right" desired only temporarily. Every physician should feel the obligation to support the desire for life, which will return even in a patient who cannot believe that such a change can occur. To cooperate in the patient's hopelessness violates an important responsibility of the physician.

From "The Right to Commit Suicide"

Glanville Williams

. . . I want to consider first the right to commit suicide and secondly the position of persons other than the suicide himself.

The act of 1961, which declared that suicide should no longer be a crime, legalized suicide as such. For no legal purpose does the self-killer commit a crime.

It is still not fully recognized that everyone has not merely a legal but a moral right to drink the hemlock, so far as society in general is concerned. Of course there are many personal obligations of which suicide would be a dereliction: chief among them the duties of consideration that young people owe to their parents, parents to their young children, and spouses to each other. These are moral arguments that one would naturally urge upon any acquaintance who was contemplating a premature departure from life. What I deny is that the individual owes any duty *to society* to stay alive. It has been said that life itself would be insupportable were it not for the prospect of death, and in some miserable situations one may be comforted in the knowledge that one's distress is voluntarily accepted to the extent that one chooses to stay alive.

Some favourite methods of suicide are being taken from us: most of our gas is no longer lethal, and barbiturates are harder to obtain. But the

Reprinted with permission of author and publisher from the *Medico-Legal Journal* 41, 26–29, 1973.

plastics industry has come to the rescue with what seems to be an acceptable means of self annihilation.

I mention these practical and macabre details for the purpose of pointing out that people who are living normally do not need a protected right to commit suicide. It is a decision that they can execute for themselves, if they feel strongly enough, whether society chooses to acknowledge their right or not. But the point is important for those who have lost their liberty, in prisons or hospitals or geriatric homes, or who are simply too ill to take any action.

A prisoner who tries to starve himself to death, whether by way of protest or otherwise, is sometimes forcibly fed and this has been held to be legal by our courts. I hold that forcibly feeding anyone is wrong, and I do not know how medical practitioners feel able to take part in it. . . . It may be embarrassing for the authorities if a hunger-strike by a prisoner fortifies criticism of the prisons in general or of a particular instance of imprisonment, but this embarrassment is, to my mind, quite irrelevant to the right of the individual to decide whether he wishes to continue to exist or not.

As regards hospitals, I have never forgotten a heartrending novel called *The Rack,* by A. E. Ellis, which gave a strong impression of being partly autobiographical, though I hope it was not. It appeared just before the advent of antibiotics, which revolutionized the outlook of patients with tuberculosis. The story opened with a patient entering a Swiss sanatorium for treatment; and it proceeded to chronicle the slow destruction of hope as one remedy after another lost its efficacy. There were rumours of patients who had escaped from suffering by jumping out of an upper window or dragging themselves out into the winter night. The patient whose tale is told planned an easier exit by trying to accumulate sufficient of his sleeping tablets to amount to a fatal dose; but on each occasion his secret hoard was discovered and confiscated by the nursing staff. The book closes with our patient lying in bed contemplating the open window.

The opinion I hold as to the patient's rights applies also to mental hospitals. I reject the argument that mental patients as a class are unable to form a competent decision to commit suicide. This may be the one rational decision that they are able to make. Many years ago a well-known broadcaster killed his wife while his mind was disturbed. He was put on trial and sent to Broadmoor. From the moment of his arrival he spent his time looking for some place in this carefully-arranged hospital where he could hang himself. After some weeks he succeeded. It seems to be deeply pathetic that an utterly miserable man who forms a decision that he does not want to live is forced to carry his intention out in this horrible and lonely way.

WHEN IS THERE A RIGHT TO PREVENT AN ACT OF SUICIDE?

If one suddenly comes upon another person attempting suicide, the natural and humane thing to do is to try to stop him, for the purpose of ascertaining the cause of his distress and attempting to remedy it, or else of attempting moral dissuasion if it seems that the act of suicide shows lack of consideration for others, or else again for the purpose of trying to persuade him to accept psychiatric help if this seems to be called for. Whatever the strict law may be (and authority is totally lacking), no one who intervened for such reasons would thereby be in danger of suffering a punitive judgment. But nothing longer than a temporary restraint could be defended. I would gravely doubt whether a suicide attempt should be a factor leading to a diagnosis of psychosis or to compulsory admission to hospital. Psychiatrists are too ready to assume that an attempt to commit suicide is the act of a mentally sick person. I am aware that the Mental Health Act 1959, sections 25 and 26, authorize compulsory admission for treatment of mentally disordered patients where, *inter alia*, this is necessary in the interests of the patient's safety, but this course appears to me to be more justifiable where the fear is that the patient will injure himself than where it is that he will make away with himself in a reasonably efficient way. Admittedly, it is not easy to make this distinction in practice.

Even if the suicidal patient is already in hospital, I would deny the right of the hospital authorities, in the last resort, to prevent an act of suicide. I say "in the last resort" partly because of the matters just considered, partly because of the right of the hospital (or nursing home) to protect its own property and other persons using the premises (self-inflicted death may be messy, dangerous or upsetting to others), and partly perhaps because of the duty of a hospital to save a mentally abnormal patient from injuring himself in an abortive suicide attempt.[1] Subject to these considerations, I hold with Thomas Szasz, R. D. Laing and their followers that mental patients are people, who are entitled to their liberty and right of self-determination like anyone else, except to the extent that the requirements of society dictate otherwise.

The case for letting would-be suicides alone cannot be more eloquently put than it was in a letter to *New Society* (5 September 1963).

> I am one of those who has made an unsuccessful attempt at suicide, and will, at some time, have to go to the trouble of making another. "Most would have benefited from psychiatric treatment," says Professor Stengel sweepingly, and he goes on to talk of "depressive illness." I do not deny that depressive illness could, in some cases, be helped by treatment, but I detect a curious eagerness on the part of such writers as Professor Stengel to dismiss as easily curable the sorrow of loss and the pain of loneliness, as "mental illness." The assumption is that the world is such an agreeable place that no one who was *not* mentally ill could possibly wish to leave it, and that if grief, or a mere sense of having

---

[1]This last consideration may explain the decision in *Selfe* v. *Ilford and District Hospital Management Committee, The Times,* 26 Nov., 1970, where a paraplegic who was in hospital and was known to be a suicide risk was insufficiently watched by the nurses. He climbed out of the window, into the grounds, and then climbed on to a roof, from which he threw himself, suffering serious injuries. The hospital was held liable in damages. Would it have been held liable if the patient had succeeded in committing suicide? The plaintiff was apparently a voluntary patient, so the hospital had no right to restrain him from walking out.

had enough of life, persuades a man to contemplate suicide, he ought to be bullied into living a little longer by psychiatric treatment. Since treatment can hardly be expected to remove the *cause* of his grief, it is presumably applied merely in order to make a man capable of enduring his miserable state a little longer. This seems to me to equate psychiatry with drink and drugs as nerve-deadeners, but perhaps Professor Stengel would accept this.

The question which is never asked is: to what purpose? Why should one be coerced into living if one does not wish to? We are coerced enough in this life as it is. To die is almost only the absolutely free choice we have, and Pliny observed that it gave us superiority over the gods: *Deus non sibi potest mortem consciscere si velit, quod homini dedit optimum in tantis vitae paenis.* To what purpose, in particular, should the old and sick and frail be induced to prolong their lives? The fact that the incidence of suicide greatly increases among the elderly of all classes (hurrah for statistics!) should warn the medical profession of the signal disservice that modern drugs perform in interfering with the natural processes of death, at least among the old. Let us be thankful at least that the barbiturates provide a counter-measure against enforced life. Of course, it is possible that in time old age may become a pleasanter state but too frequently it is as miserable as imprisonment, as painful as torture. Why does Professor Stengel think it an admirable thing to persuade people to endure it? To go on living into dotage, and risk not only that desire will fail, and the windows be darkened in the streets, but that the will both to make a decision to die, and to carry it into effect, may well fail too? If anyone can view this prospect with complacency, he must, I think, be very insensible of the horrors of old age, both to himself and to those who must support him and bear with him. . . .

While I regret the Hippocratic conscience which leads doctors to resuscitate if possible those who attempt suicide (an intolerable interference, to my mind), I agree with Professor Stengel that there are some who make the attempt only in order to be rescued. If it were clearly recognized that doctors would make no effort to revive them, I suspect that there would at once be an appreciable drop in the number of attempted suicides, and a consequent release of many hospital beds for more deserving cases. But it is not likely any of us, doctors or not, will lose the irrational desire to save life.

I cannot really agree, however, with his statement that suicide is "an act of aggression directed against the self, particularly those aspects of the self which the individual hates and wants to destroy." This is typical rule-of-thumb psychiatry, and a most dangerous generalization. Reasons for suicide must be infinite since man's nature, as Whitman said of himself, is huge. It contains multitudes. Moreover, even if this aggressive "death-wish" does exist, it is still obvious that many who commit suicide are in full command of their reason when they do so, and far from being impelled by some dark unrecognized urge in their psyche, make use of it rationally to strengthen their will and support their courage in the attempt. For, *pace* Doctor Stephen Ward, it *does* take courage to attempt one's life, and I hope this much-quoted letter will not encourage any would-be suicides to embark on the business thoughtlessly. . . .

For obvious reasons, I prefer not to sign my name, but will use that of Arria, the stoic wife who, when her husband Paetus faltered, drove the dagger into her own breast with the inspiring words: "Paete, non dolet" ["Paetus, it does not hurt."]

                                                                                        Arria

From "The Right to Suicide: A Psychiatrist's View"

Jerome A. Motto

To speak as a psychiatrist may suggest to some that psychiatrists have a certain way of looking at things. This would be a misconception, though a common one. I know of no professional group with more diverse approaches to those matters concerning it than the American psychiatric community. All physicians, however, including psychiatrists, share a tradition of commitment to both the preservation and the quality of human life. With this one reservation, I speak as a psychiatrist strictly in the singular sense.

The emergence of thoughts or impulses to bring an end to life is a phenomenon observed in persons experiencing severe pain, whether that pain stems from physical or emotional sources. Thus physicians, to whom persons are inclined to turn for relief from suffering, frequently encounter suicidal ideas and impulses in their patients. Those who look and listen do, at least.

From a psychiatric point of view, the question as to whether a person has the right to cope with the pain in his world by killing himself can be answered without hesitation. He does have that right. With a few geographical exceptions the same can be said from the legal and social point of view as well. It is only when philosophical or theological questions are raised that one can find room for argument about the right to suicide, as only in these areas can restrictions on behavior be institutionalized without requiring social or legal support.

The problem we struggle with is not whether the individual *has* the right to suicide; rather, we face a twofold dilemma stemming from the fact that he does have it. Firstly, what is the extent to which the exercise of that right should be subject to limitations? Secondly, when the right is exercised, how can we eliminate the social stigma now attached to it?

LIMITATIONS ON THE INDIVIDUAL'S RIGHT TO SUICIDE

Putting limitations on rights is certainly not a new idea, since essentially every right we exercise has its specified restrictions. It is generally taken for granted that certain limitations must be observed. In spite of this, it is inevitable that some will take the position that unless the right is unconditional it is not "really" granted.

I use two psychological criteria as grounds for limiting a person's exercise of his right to suicide: (*a*) the act must be based on a realistic assessment of his life situation, and (*b*) the degree of ambivalence regarding

Reprinted with permission of author and publisher from *Life-Threatening Behavior*, 2, No. 3 (Fall 1972), 183–88. Copyright 1972 by Behavioral Publications, Inc. 72 Fifth Ave., New York, N.Y. 10011.

the act must be minimal. Both of these criteria clearly raise a host of new questions.

Realistic Assessment of Life Situation

What is reality? Who determines whether a realistic assessment has been made? Every person's perception is reality to *him*, and the degree of pain experienced by one can never be fully appreciated by another, no matter how empathic he is. Differences in capacity to *tolerate* pain add still another crucial yet unmeasurable element.

As formidable as this sounds, the psychiatrist is obliged to accept this task as his primary day-to-day professional responsibility, whether or not the issue of suicide is involved. With an acute awareness of how emotions can —like lenses—distort perceptions which in turn shape one's thoughts and actions, and with experience in understanding and dealing with this underlying substrate of emotion, he is constantly working with his patients on the process of differentiating between what is realistic and what is distorted. The former must be dealt with on a rational level; the latter must be explored and modified till the distortion is reduced at least to the point where it is not of handicapping severity. He is aware of the nature and extent of his own tendency to distort ("Physician, heal thyself"), and realizes that the entire issue is one of degree. Yet he must use his own perception of reality as a standard, shortcomings notwithstanding, realizing full well how much information must be carefully considered in view of the frailty of the human perceptual and reality-testing apparatus.

Some persons have a view of reality so different from mine that I do not hesitate to interfere with their right to suicide. Others' perceptions are so like mine that I cannot intercede. The big problem is that large group in between.

In the final analysis, then, when a decision has to be made, what a psychiatrist calls "realistic" is whatever looks realistic to *him*. At the moment of truth, that is all any person can offer. This inherent human limitation in itself is a reality that accounts for a great deal of inevitable chaos in the world; it is an article of faith that not to make such an effort would create even greater chaos. On a day-to-day operational level, one contemporary behavioral scientist expressed it this way: "No doubt the daily business of helping troubled individuals, including suicides, gives little time for the massive contemplative and investigative efforts which alone can lead to surer knowledge. And the helpers are not thereby to be disparaged. They cannot wait for the best answers conceivable. They must do only the best they can *now*."

Thus if I am working with a person in psychotherapy, one limitation I would put on his right to suicide would be that his assessment of his life situation be realistic as *I* see it.

A related concept is that of "rational suicide," which has enjoyed a certain vogue since at least the seventeenth century, when the "Rationalist Era" saw sharp inroads being made into the domination of the church in determining ethical and social values. According to one contemporary philosopher, "the degree of rationality of the [suicidal] act would depend on the degree of rationality of the philosophy which was guiding the person's deliberations." Rationality is defined as a means of problem solving, using "methods such as logical, mathematical, or experimental procedures which have gained men's confidence as reliable tools for guiding instrumental actions." The rationality of one's philosophy is determined by the degree to which it is free of mysticism. Further, "A person who is considering how to act in an intensely conflicting situation cannot be regarded as making the most rational decision, unless he has been as critical as possible of the philosophy that is guiding his decision. If the philosophy is institutionalized as a political ideology or a religious creed, he must think critically about the institution in order to acquire maximum rationality of judgment. This principle is clear enough, even if in practice it is enormously difficult to fulfill."

The idea of "rational suicide" is a related yet distinctly different issue from the "realistic assessment of one's life situation" referred to above. Making this assessment involves assembling and understanding all the facts clearly, while the idea of a "rational suicide" can only be entertained after this assessment is done and the question is "what to do" in the light of those facts.

The role of the psychiatrist and the thinking of the rationalist tend to merge, at one point, however. In the process of marshaling all the facts and exploring their meaning to the person, the psychiatrist must ensure that the patient does indeed critically examine not only his perception of reality but his own philosophy. This often entails making that philosophy explicit for the first time (without ever using the term "philosophy"), and clarifying how it has influenced his living experience. The implication is clear that modification of the person's view of his world, with corresponding changes in behavior, may lead to a more satisfying life.

The rationalist concedes that where one's philosophy is simply an "intellectual channeling of emotional forces," rational guidelines have severe limitations, since intense emotional conflicts cut off rational guidance. These circumstances would characterize "irrational" grounds for suicide and would identify those persons whose suicide should be prevented.

The argument for "rational suicide" tends to apply principally to two sets of circumstances: altruistic self-sacrifice for what is perceived as a noble cause; and the severe, advanced physical illness with no new therapeutic agents anticipated in the foreseeable future. This does not help us very much because these circumstances generate relatively little real controversy among behavioral scientists. The former situations are not usually recognized till after the act, and the latter at present are receiving a great deal of well-deserved attention from the point of view of anticipating (and sometimes hastening) the foreseeable demise in comfort and dignity.

Our most difficult problem is more with the person whose pain is emotional in origin and whose physical health is good, or at most constitutes a minor impairment. For these persons, the discussion above regarding "rational" and "irrational" distinctions seems rather alien to the clinical situation. This is primarily due to the rationalist's emphasis on intellectual processes, when it is so clear (at least to the psychiatrist) that it is feelings of worthiness of love, of relatedness, of belonging, that have the strongest stabilizing influence on the suicidal person.

I rarely hear a patient say, "I've never looked at it that way," yet no response is more frequently encountered than, "Yes, I understand, but I don't feel any differently." It is after a continuing therapeutic effort during which feelings of acceptance and worthiness are generated that emotional pain is reduced and suicidal manifestations become less intense. Either exploring the philosophy by which one lives or carefully assessing the realities of one's life can provide an excellent means of accomplishing this, but it is rarely the influence of the philosophy or the perception of the realities per se that brings it about. Rather, it is through the influence of the therapeutic relationship that the modified philosophy or perception develops, and can then be applied to the person's life situation.

Manifestations of Ambivalence

The second criterion to be used as the basis for limiting a person's exercise of his right to suicide is minimal ambivalence about ending his life. I make the assumption that if a person has no ambivalence about suicide he will not be in my office, nor write to me about it, nor call me on the telephone. I interpret, rightly or wrongly, a person's calling my attention to his suicidal impulses as a request to intercede that I cannot ignore.

At times this call will inevitably be misread, and my assumption will lead me astray. However, such an error on my part can be corrected at a later time; meanwhile, I must be prepared to take responsibility for having prolonged what may be a truly unendurable existence. If the error is made in the other direction, no opportunity for correction may be possible.

This same principle regarding ambivalence applies to a suicide prevention center, minister, social agency, or a hospital emergency room. The response of the helping agency may be far from fulfilling the needs of the person involved, but in my view, the ambivalence expressed is a clear indication for it to limit the exercise of his right to suicide. . . .

It seems inevitable to me that we must eventually establish procedures for the voluntary cessation of life, with the time, place, and manner largely controlled by the person concerned. It will necessarily involve a series of deliberate steps providing assurance that appropriate criteria are met, such as those proposed above, as we now observe specific criteria when a life is terminated by abortion or by capital punishment.

The critical word is "control." I would anticipate a decrease in the actual number of suicides when this procedure is established, due to the psychological power of this issue. If I know something is available to me and will remain available till I am moved to seize it, the chances of my seizing it now are thereby much reduced. It is only by holding off that I maintain the option of changing my mind. During this period of delay the opportunity for therapeutic effort—and the therapy of time itself—may be used to advantage.

Finally, we have to make sure we are not speaking only to the strong. It is too easy to formulate a way of dealing with a troublesome problem in such a manner, that if the person in question could approach it as we suggest, he would not be a person who would have the problem in the first place.

When we discuss—in the abstract—the right to suicide, we tend to gloss over the intricacies of words like "freedom," "quality of life," "choice," or even "help," to say nothing of "rational" and "realistic." Each of these concepts deserves a full inquiry in itself, though in practice we use them on the tacit assumption that general agreement exists as to their meaning.

Therefore it is we who, in trying to be of service to someone else, have the task of determining what is rational for us, and what our perception of reality is. And we must recognize that in the final analysis it will be not only the suicidal person but we who have exercised a choice, by doing what we do to resolve our feelings about this difficult human problem.

From "Apologia for Suicide"

Mary Rose Barrington

The root cause of the widespread aversion to suicide is almost certainly death itself rather than dislike of the means by which death is brought about. The leaf turns a mindless face to the sun for one summer before falling for ever into the mud; death, however it comes to pass, rubs our clever faces in the same mud, where we too join the leaves. The inconceivability of this transformation in status is partly shot through with an indirect illumination, due to the death of others. Yet bereavement is not death. Here to mourn, we are still here, and the imagination boggles at the notion that things could ever be otherwise. Not only does the imagination boggle, as to some extent it must, but the mind unfortunately averts. The averted mind acknowledges, in a theoretical way, that death does indeed happen to people here and there and now and then, but to some extent the attitude to death resembles the attitude of the heavy smoker to lung cancer; he reckons that if he is lucky it will not happen to *him*, at least not yet, and perhaps not ever. This confused sort of faith in the immortality of the body must underlie many a triumphal call from the hospital ward or theatre, that the patient's life has been saved—and he will therefore die next week instead of this week, and in rather greater discomfort. People who insist that life must always be better than death often sound as if they are choosing eternal life in contrast to eternal death, when the fact is that they have no choice in the matter; it is death now, or death later. Once this fact is fully grasped it is possible for the question to arise as to whether death now would not be preferable.

Opponents of suicide will sometimes throw dust in the eyes of the

Reprinted with permission from *Euthanasia and the Right to Die*, ed. A. B. Downing (New York: Humanities Press; London: Peter Owen Ltd., 1970) pp. 152–70.

uncommitted by asking at some point why one should ever choose to go on living if one once questions the value of life; for as we all know, adversity is usually round the corner, if not at our heels. Here, it seems to me, a special case must be made out for people suffering from the sort of adversity with which the proponents of euthanasia are concerned: namely, an apparently irremediable state of physical debility that makes life unbearable to the sufferer. Some adversities come and go; in the words of the Anglo-Saxon poet reviewing all the disasters known to Norse mythology, "That passed away, so may this." Some things that do not pass away include inoperable cancers in the region of the throat that choke their victims slowly to death. Not only do they not pass away, but like many extremely unpleasant conditions they cannot be alleviated by pain-killing drugs. Pain itself can be controlled, provided the doctor in charge is prepared to put the relief of pain before the prolongation of life; but analgesics will not help a patient to live with total incontinence, reduced to the status of a helpless baby after a life of independent adulthood. And for the person who manages to avoid these grave afflictions there remains the spectre of senile decay, a physical and mental crumbling into a travesty of the normal person. Could anything be more reasonable than for a person faced with these living deaths to weigh up the pros and cons of living out his life until his heart finally fails, and going instead to meet death half-way?

It is true, of course, that, all things being equal, people do want to go on living. If we are enjoying life, there seems no obvious reason to stop doing so and be mourned by our families and forgotten by our friends. If we are not enjoying it, then it seems a miserable end to die in a trough of depression, and better to wait for things to become more favourable. Most people, moreover, have a moral obligation to continue living, owed to their parents while they are still alive, their children while they are dependent, and their spouses all the time. Trained professional workers may even feel that they have a duty to society to continue giving their services. Whatever the grounds, it is both natural and reasonable that without some special cause nobody ever wants to die *yet.* But must these truisms be taken to embody the whole truth about the attitude of thinking people to life and death? A psychiatrist has been quoted as saying: "I don't think you can consider anyone normal who tries to take his own life."[1] The abnormality of the suicide is taken for granted, and the possibility that he might have been doing something sensible (for him) is not presented to the mind for even momentary consideration. It might as well be argued that no one can be considered normal who does not want to procreate as many children as possible, and this was no doubt urged by the wise men of yesterday; today the tune is very different, and in this essay we are concerned with what they may be singing tomorrow. . . .

It may be worth pausing here to consider whether the words "natural end," in the sense usually ascribed to the term, have much bearing on reality. Very little is "natural" about our present-day existence, and least natural of all is the prolonged period of dying that is suffered by so many

---

[1]Reported in *The Observer* (June 26, 1967).

incurable patients solicitously kept alive to be killed by their disease. The sufferings of animals (other than man) are heart-rending enough, but a dying process spread over weeks, months or years seems to be one form of suffering that animals are normally spared. When severe illness strikes them they tend to stop eating, sleep and die. The whole weight of Western society forces attention on the natural right to live, but throws a blanket of silence over the natural right to die. If I seem to be suggesting that in a civilized society suicide ought to be considered a quite proper way for a well-brought-up person to end his life (unless he has the good luck to die suddenly and without warning), that is indeed the tenor of my argument; if it is received with astonishment and incredulity, the reader is referred to the reception of recommendations made earlier in the century that birth control should be practiced and encouraged. The idea is no more extraordinary, and would be equally calculated to diminish the sum total of suffering among humankind. . . .

. . . It is frequently said that hard-hearted people would be encouraged to make their elderly relatives feel that they had outlived their welcome and ought to remove themselves, even if they happened to be enjoying life. No one can say categorically that nothing of the sort would happen, but the sensibility of even hard-hearted people to the possible consequences of their own unkindness seems just as likely. A relation who had stood down from life in a spirit of magnanimity and family affection would, after an inevitable period of heart-searching and self-recrimination, leave behind a pleasant memory; a victim of callous treatment hanging like an accusing albatross around the neck of the living would suggest another and rather ugly story. Needless to say, whoever was responsible would not in any event be the sort of person to show consideration to an aged person in decline.

Whether or not some undesirable fringe results would stem from a free acceptance of suicide in our society, the problem of three or four contemporaneous generations peopling a world that hitherto has had to support only two or three is with us here and now, and will be neither generated nor exacerbated by a fresh attitude to life and death. The disabled, aged parent, loved or unloved, abnegating or demanding, is placed in one of the tragic dilemmas inherent in human existence, and one that becomes more acute as standards of living rise. One more in the mud-hut is not a problem in the same way as one more in a small, overcrowded urban dwelling; and the British temperament demands a privacy incompatible with the more sociable Mediterranean custom of packing a grandmother and an aunt or two in the attic. Mere existence presents a mild problem; disabled existence presents a chronic problem. The old person may have no talent for being a patient, and the young one may find it intolerable to be a nurse. A physical decline threatens to be accompanied by an inevitable decline in the quality of important human relationships—human relationships, it is worth repeating, not superhuman ones. Given superhuman love, patience, fortitude and all other sweet-natured qualities in a plenitude not normally present in ordinary people, there would be no problem. But the problem is there, and voluntary termination of life offers a possible solution that may be better than none at all. The young have been urged from time immemorial to have valiant hearts, to lay down their lives for their loved ones when their lives have hardly started; it may be that in time to come the disabled aged will be glad to live in a society that approves an honourable death met willingly, perhaps in the company of another "old soldier" of the same generation, and with justifiable pride. Death taken in one's own time, and with a sense of purpose, may in fact be far more bearable than the process of waiting to be arbitrarily extinguished.[2] A patient near the end of his life who arranged his death so as, for example, to permit an immediate transfer of a vital organ to a younger person, might well feel that he was converting his death into a creative act instead of waiting passively to be suppressed.

A lot of kindly people may feel that this is lacking in respect for the honourable estate of old age; but to insist on the obligation of old people to live through a period of decline and helplessness seems to me to be lacking in a feeling for the demands of human *self*-respect. They may reply that this shows a false notion of what constitutes self-respect, and that great spiritual qualities may be brought out by dependence and infirmity, and the response to such a state. It is tempting in a world dominated by suffering to find all misery purposeful, and indeed in some situations the "cross-to-bear" and the willing bearer may feel that they are contributing a poignant note to some cosmic symphony that is richer for their patience and self-sacrifice. Since we are talking of options and not of compulsions, people who felt like this would no doubt continue to play their chosen parts; but what a truly ruthless thing to impose those parts on people who feel that they are meaningless and discordant, and better written out.

What should be clear is that with so many men and so many opinions there is no room here for rules of life, or ready-made solutions by formula, least of all by the blanket injunction that, rather than allow any of these questions to be faced, life must be lived out to the bitter end, in sickness and in health, for better or for worse, until death brings release. It is true that the embargo on suicide relieves the ailing dependent of a choice, and some would no doubt be glad of the relief, having no mind for self-sacrifice. But in order to protect the mildly disabled from the burden of choice, the severely sick and suffering patient who urgently wants to die is subjected to the same compulsion to live. The willingness of many people to accept this sheltering of the stronger at the expense of the crying needs of the incomparably weaker may be because the slightly ailing are more visible and therefore make a more immediate claim on sympathy. Everyone knows aged and dependent people who might find themselves morally bound to consider the advisability of continuing to live if an option were truly available; the seriously afflicted lie hidden behind hospital windows, or secluded from sight on the upper floors of private houses. *They* are threatened not with delicate moral considerations, but with the harder realities of pain, disease and degeneration. Not only are they largely invisible, but their guardians are

---

[2]It will be noted that reference is made here in all cases to the aged. In a longer exposition I would argue that very different considerations apply to the young disabled who have not yet enjoyed a full lifespan, and who should be given far greater public assistance to enable them to enjoy life as best they can.

much given to the issuing of soothing reports about, for example, the hundred thousand or more patients who die of cancer every year, reports in which words like "happiness" and "dignity" are used liberally, and words like "pain" and "humiliation" tactfully suppressed. Let us not be misled by the reassuring face so often assumed by doctors who would have us believe that terminal suffering is just a bad fairy tale put out by alarmist bogey-men. One can only hope that the pathetic human wrecks who lie vomiting and gasping their lives out are as sanguine and cheerful about their lamentable condition as the smiling doctor who on their behalf assures us that no one (including the members of the Euthanasia Society) really wants euthanasia.

That voluntary euthanasia is in fact assisted suicide is no doubt clear to most people, but curiously enough many who would support the moral right of an incurably sick person to commit suicide will oppose his having the right to seek assistance from doctors if he is to effect his wish. The argument has so far been concentrated upon the person who clearly sees the writing on the wall (perhaps because he has a doctor who is prepared to decipher it) and has the moral courage, whether or not encouraged by a sympathetic society, to anticipate the dying period. Further, this hypothetical person has access to the means of suicide and knows how to make use of those means. How he has acquired the means and the knowledge is obscure, but a determined person will make sure that he is equipped with both as a standby for the future. Yet the average patient desperately in need of help to cut short his suffering could well be a person unaccustomed to holding his own against authority, enfeebled by illness, dependent on pain-killing drugs, having no access to the means of suicide and not knowing how to make use of the means even if they were available; an entirely helpless person, in no way in a position to compass his own death. To acknowledge the right of a person to end his own life to avoid a period of suffering is a mere sham unless the right for him to call on expert assistance is also acknowledged. . . .

Hostile sections of the medical profession will continue to assert that it is their business to cure and not to kill, and that in any case a patient who is in a miserable state from having his body invaded with cancers (or whatever) is in no state to make a decision about life and death. A patient who is in so pitiable a condition that he says he wishes to die is *ipso facto* not in a fit condition to make a reliable statement about his wishes. Arguments of this ilk seem at times to pass from black comedy to black farce. With the same sort of metaphysical reasoning it will be maintained that a patient who requested, and was given, euthanasia on Monday evening might, had he lived until Tuesday morning, have changed his mind. It has even been suggested that patients would, if voluntary euthanasia were available for incurable patients, feel themselves reluctantly obliged to ask for it to spare the nursing staff. And, as was remarked earlier, although laying down one's life in battle is generally considered praiseworthy, to lay down your life to spare yourself pointless suffering, to release medical staff so that they can tend people who would have some chance of living enjoyable lives given greater attention and assistance, to release your family and friends from anxiety and anguish, *these* motives are considered shocking. More accurately, a mere contemplation of these motives shocks the conditioned mind so severely that no rational comment can fight its way through to the surface; it is forced back by the death taboo.

Here again it must be made clear that what is needed is the fostering of a new attitude to death that should ultimately grow from within, and not be imposed from without upon people psychologically unable to rethink their ingrained views. The suffering and dying patients of today have been brought up to feel that it is natural and inevitable, and even some sort of a duty, to live out their terminal period, and it would do them no service to try to persuade them into adopting an attitude that to most of them would seem oppressive, as aimed against them rather than for their benefit. If people have an ineradicable instinct, or fundamental conviction, that binds them to cling to life when their body is anticipating death by falling into a state of irrevocable decay, they clearly must be given treatment and encouragement consistent with their emotional and spiritual needs, and kindness *for them* will consist of assurances that not only is their suffering a matter of the greatest concern, but that so also is their continued existence. It is future generations, faced perhaps with a lifespan of eighty or ninety years, of which nearly half will have to be dependent on the earning power of the other half, who will have to decide how much of their useful, active life is to be devoted to supporting themselves through a terminal period "*sans* everything," prolonged into a dreaded ordeal by ever-increasing medical skill directed to the preservation of life. It may well be that, as in the case of family planning, economic reality will open up a spring, the waters of which will filter down to deeper levels, and that then the new way of death will take root. The opponents of euthanasia conjure up a favourite vision of a nightmare future in which anxious patients will be obsessed with the fear that their relatives and doctors may make surreptitious plans to kill them; the anxiety of the twenty-first century patient may, on the contrary, be that they are neglecting to make such plans.

From "Euthanasia Legislation: Some Non-Religious Objections"

Yale Kamisar

A book by Glanville Williams, *The Sanctity of Life and the Criminal Law,* once again brought to the fore the controversial topic of euthanasia, more popularly known as "mercy-killing." In keeping with the trend of the euthanasia movement over the past generation, Williams concentrates his efforts for reform on the *voluntary* type of euthanasia, for example the cancer victim begging for death, as opposed to the *involuntary* variety—that is, the case of the congenital idiot, the permanently insane or the senile. . . .

The existing law on euthanasia is hardly perfect. But if it is not too good, neither, as I have suggested, is it much worse than the rest of the criminal law. At any rate, the imperfections of existing law are not cured by Williams's proposal. Indeed, I believe adoption of his views would add more difficulties than it would remove.

Williams strongly suggests that "euthanasia can be condemned only according to a religious opinion."[1] He tends to view the opposing camps as Roman Catholics versus Liberals. Although this has a certain initial appeal to me, a non-Catholic and self-styled liberal, I deny that this is the only way the battle lines can, or should, be drawn. I leave the religious arguments to the theologians. I share the view that "those who hold the faith may follow its precepts without requiring those who do not hold it to act as if they did." But I do find substantial utilitarian obstacles on the high road to euthanasia. I am not enamoured of the *status quo* on mercy-killing. But while I am not prepared to defend it against all comers, I am prepared to defend it against the proposals for change which have come forth to date.

As an ultimate philosophical proposition, the case for voluntary euthanasia is strong. Whatever may be said for and against suicide generally, the appeal of death is immeasurably greater when it is sought not for a poor reason or just any reason, but for "good cause", so to speak; when it is invoked not on behalf of a "socially useful" person, but on behalf of, for example, the pain-racked "hopelessly incurable" cancer victim. *If* a person is *in fact* (1) presently incurable, (2) beyond the aid of any respite which may come along in his life expectancy, suffering (3) intolerable and (4) unmitigable pain and of a (5) fixed and (6) rational desire to die, I would hate to have

---

Reprinted with permission from *Euthanasia and the Right to Die,* ed. A. B. Downing (New York: Humanities Press; London: Peter Owen Ltd., 1970) pp. 85–133.

[1]Williams, p. 278. This seems to be the position taken by Bertrand Russell in reviewing Williams's book: 'The central theme of the book is the conflict in the criminal law between the two divergent systems of ethics which may be called respectively utilitarian and taboo morality. . . . Utilitarian morality in the wide sense in which I am using the word, judges actions by their effects. . . . In taboo morality . . . forbidden actions are sin, and they do not cease to be so when their consequences are such as we should all welcome.' (*Stanford Law Review,* 10 [1958], 382) I trust Russell would agree, should he read this article, that the issue is not quite so simple. At any rate, I trust he would agree that I stay within the system of utilitarian ethics.

to argue that the hand of death should be stayed. But abstract propositions and carefully formed hypotheticals are one thing; specific proposals designed to cover everyday situations are something else again.

In essence, Williams's specific proposal is that death be authorized for a person in the above situation "by giving the medical practitioner a wide discretion and trusting to his good sense."[2] This, I submit, raises too great a risk of abuse and mistake to warrant a change in the existing law. That a proposal entails risk of mistake is hardly a conclusive reason against it. But neither is it irrelevant. Under any euthanasia programme the consequences of mistake, of course, are always fatal. As I shall endeavour to show, the incidence of mistake of one kind or another is likely to be quite appreciable. If this indeed be the case, unless the need for the authorized conduct is compelling enough to override it, I take it the risk of mistake *is* a conclusive reason against such authorization. I submit, too, that the possible radiations from the proposed legislation—for example, involuntary euthanasia of idiots and imbeciles (the typical "mercy-killings" reported by the press)—and the emergence of the legal precedent that there are lives not "worth living," give additional cause for reflection.

I see the issue, then, as the need for voluntary euthanasia versus (1) the incidence of mistake and abuse; and (2) the danger that legal machinery initially designed to kill those who are a nuisance to themselves may some day engulf those who are a nuisance to others.

The "freedom to choose a merciful death by euthanasia" may well be regarded as a special area of civil liberties. This is definitely a part of Professor Williams's approach:

> If the law were to remove its ban on euthanasia, the effect would merely be to leave this subject to the individual conscience. This proposal would . . . be easy to defend, as restoring personal liberty in a field in which men differ on the question of conscience. . . . On a question like this there is surely everything to be said for the liberty of the individual.[3]

I am perfectly willing to accept civil liberties as the battlefield, but issues of "liberty" and "freedom" mean little until we begin to pin down *whose* "liberty" and "freedom" and for *what* need and at *what* price. Williams champions the "personal liberty" of the dying to die painlessly. I am more concerned about the life and liberty of those who would needlessly be killed in the process or who would irrationally choose to partake of the process. Williams's price on behalf of those who are *in fact* "hopeless incurables" and *in fact* of a fixed and rational desire to die is the sacrifice of (1) some few, who, though they know it not, because their physicians know it not, need not and should not die; (2) others, probably not so few, who, though they go through the motions of "volunteering," are casualties of strain, pain or narcotics to such an extent that they really know not what they do. My price on behalf of those who, despite appearances to the contrary,

[2]Id., p. 302.
[3]Id., pp. 304, 309.

have some relatively normal and reasonably useful life left in them, or who are incapable of making the choice, is the lingering on for awhile of those who, if you will, *in fact* have no desire and no reason to linger on. . . .

Nothing rouses Professor Glanville Williams's ire more than the fact that opponents of the euthanasia movement argue that euthanasia proposals offer either inadequate protection or over-elaborate safeguards. Williams appears to meet this dilemma with the insinuation that because arguments are made in the antithesis *they must each be invalid, each be obstructionist, and each be made in bad faith.*

It just may be, however, that each alternative argument is quite valid, that the trouble lies with the euthanasiasts themselves in seeking a goal which is *inherently inconsistent:* a procedure for death which *both* (1) provides ample safeguards against abuse and mistake, and (2) is "quick" and "easy" in operation. Professor Williams meets the problem with more than bitter comments about the tactics of the opposition. He makes a brave try to break through the dilemma:

> The reformers might be well advised, in their next proposal, to abandon all their cumbrous safeguards and to do as their opponents wish, giving the medical practitioner a wide discretion and trusting to his good sense.
>
> The sense of the bill would then be simple. It would provide that no medical practitioner should be guilty of an offence in respect of an act done intentionally to accelerate the death of a patient who is seriously ill, unless it is proved that the act was not done in good faith with the consent of the patient and for the purpose of saving him from severe pain in an illness believed to be of an incurable and fatal character. Under this formula it would be for the physician, if charged, to show that the patient was seriously ill, but for the prosecution to prove that the physician acted from some motive other than the humanitarian one allowed to him by law.[4]

[4]Id., pp. 302 ff. The desire to give doctors a free hand is expressed *passim* numerous times, e.g.: '[T]here should be no formalities and . . . everything should be left to the discretion of the doctor.' (p. 303) '. . . the bill would merely leave this question to the discretion and conscience of the individual medical practitioner'. (p. 304) 'It would be the purpose of the proposed legislation to set doctors free from the fear of the law so that they can think only of the relief of their patients.' (p. 305) 'It would bring the whole subject within ordinary medical practice.' (Ibid.) Williams suggests that the pertinent provisions might be worded as follows:

'I. For the avoidance of doubt, it is hereby declared that it shall be lawful for a physician whose patient is seriously ill . . . 'b. to refrain from taking steps to prolong the patient's life by medical means; . . . unless it is proved that . . . the omission was not made, in good faith for the purpose of saving the patient from severe pain in an illness believed to be of an incurable and fatal character.

'2. It shall be lawful for a physician, after consultation with another physician, to accelerate by any merciful means the death of a patient who is seriously ill, unless it is proved that the act was not done in good faith with the consent of the patient and for the purpose of saving him from severe pain in an illness believed to be of an incurable and fatal character.' (p. 308)

The completely unrestricted authorization to kill by omission may well be based on Williams's belief that, under existing law, ' "mercy-killing" by omission to prolong life is probably lawful' since the physician is 'probably exempted' from the duty to use reasonable care to conserve his patient's life 'if life has become a burden'. (p. 291) And he adds—as if this settles the legal question—that 'the morality of an omission in these circumstances is conceded

Evidently, the presumption is that the general practitioner is a sufficient buffer between the patient and the restless spouse, or overwrought
or overreaching relative, as well as a depository of enough general scientific

---

by Catholics'. (Ibid.) If Williams means, as he seems to, *that once a doctor has undertaken treatment
and the patient is entrusted solely to his care* he may sit by the bedside of the patient whose life has
'become a burden' and let him die—e.g. by not replacing the oxygen bottle—I submit that he
is quite mistaken.

The outer limits of criminal liability for inaction are hardly free from doubt, but it seems
fairly clear under existing law that the special and traditional relationship of physician and
patient imposes a 'legal duty to act', particularly where the patient is helpless and completely
dependent on the physician, and that the physician who withholds life-preserving medical
means of the type described above commits criminal homicide by omission. In this regard, see
Burdick, *Crimes*, 2 (1946), § 466c; Hall, *Principles of Criminal Law* (1947), pp. 272–8; Kenny,
Outlines of Criminal Law (16th edn: Turner, 1952), pp. 14–15, 107–9; Perkins, *Criminal Law*
(1957), pp. 513–27; Russell, *Crime*, I (10th edn: Turner, 1950), pp. 449–66; Hughes, 'Criminal
Omissions', *Yale Law Journal*, 67 (1958), 590, 599–600, 621–6, 630 *n.* 142; Kirchheimer,
'Criminal Omissions', *Harvard Law Review*, 55 (1942), 615, 625–8; Wechsler and Michael, op.
cit. (*n.* 6 above), 724–5. Nor am I at all certain that the Catholics do 'concede' this point.
Williams's reference is to Sullivan, op. cit. (*n.* II above), p. 64. But Sullivan considers therein
what might be viewed as relatively removed and indirect omissions, e.g. whether to call in a
very expensive specialist, whether to undergo a very painful or very drastic operation.

The Catholic approach raises nice questions and draws fine lines, e.g. how many limbs
must be amputated before an operation is to be regarded as non-obligatory 'extraordinary',
as opposed to 'ordinary', means; but they will not be dwelt upon herein. Suffice to say that
apparently there has never been an indictment, let alone a conviction, for a 'mercy-killing' by
omission, not even one which directly and immediately produces death. This, of course, is not
to say that no such negative 'mercy-killings' have ever occurred. There is reason to think that
not too infrequently this is the fate of the defective newborn infant. Williams simply asserts
that the 'beneficient tendency of nature [in that 'monsters' usually die quickly after birth] is
assisted, in Britain at any rate, by the practice of doctors and nurses, who, when an infant is
born seriously malformed, do not "strive officiously to keep alive" '. (p. 32) Fletcher makes a
similar and likewise undocumented observation that 'it has always been a quite common
practice of midwives and, in modern times doctors, simply to fail to respirate monstrous babies
at birth'. (op. cit [*n.* 2 above], p. 207 *n.* 54) A supposition to the same effect was made twenty
years earlier in Gregg, 'The Right to Kill', *N. American Review*, 237 (1934), 239, 242. A noted
obstetrician and gynaecologist, Dr. Frederick Loomis, has told of occasions where expectant
fathers have, in effect, asked him to destroy the child, if born abnormal. (Loomis, *Consultation
Room* [1946], p. 53)

It is difficult to discuss the consultation feature of Williams's proposal for affirmative
'mercy-killing', because Williams himself never discusses it. This fact, plus the fact that Williams's recurrent theme is to give the general practitioner a free hand, indicates that he himself
does not regard consultation as a significant feature of his plan. The attending physician need
only consult another general practitioner and there is no requirement that there be any
concurrence in his diagnosis. There is no requirement of a written report. There is no indication as to what point in time there need be consultation. Probably consultation would be
thought necessary only in regard to diagnosis of the disease and from that point in respect of
the extent and mitigatory nature of the pain, the firmness and rationality of the desire to die
to be judged solely by the attending physician. For the view that even under rather elaborate
consultation requirements, in many thinly staffed communities the consultant doctor would
merely reflect the view of the attending physician, see 'Life and Death', *Time Magazine* (March
13, 1950), p. 50. After reviewing eleven case-histories of patients wrongly diagnosed as having
advanced cancer—diagnoses that stood uncorrected over long periods of time and after several
admissions at leading hospitals—Drs Laszlo, Colmer, Silver and Standard conclude: '[I]t
became increasingly clear that the original error was one easily made, but that the continuation
of that error was due to an acceptance of the original data without exploring their verity and
completeness.' (Errors in Diagnosis and Management of Cancer', *Annals of Internal Medicine*, 33
[1950], 670)

know-how and enough information about current research developments
and trends, to assure a minimum of error in diagnosis and anticipation of
new measures of relief. Whether or not the general practitioner will accept
the responsibility Williams would confer on him is itself a problem of major
proportions. Putting that question aside, the soundness of the underlying
premises of Williams's "legislative suggestion" will be examined in the
course of the discussion of various aspects of the euthanasia problem.

Under current proposals to establish legal machinery, elaborate or
otherwise, for the administration of a quick and easy death, it is not enough
that those authorized to pass on the question decide that the patient, in
effect, is "better off dead." The patient must concur in this opinion. Much
of the appeal in the current proposal lies in this so-called "voluntary"
attribute.

But is the adult patient really in a position to concur? Is he truly able
to make euthanasia a "voluntary" act? . . .

By hypothesis, voluntary euthanasia is not to be resorted to until
narcotics have long since been administered and the patient has developed
a tolerance to them. *When*, then, does the patient make the choice? While
heavily drugged? Or is narcotic relief to be withdrawn for the time of
decision? But if heavy dosage no longer deadens pain, indeed, no longer
makes it bearable, how overwhelming is it when whatever relief narcotics
offer is taken away too?

"Hypersensitivity to pain after analgesia has worn off is nearly always
noted."[5] Moreover, "the mental side-effects of narcotics, unfortunately for
anyone wishing to suspend them temporarily without unduly tormenting
the patient, appear to outlast the analgesic effect" and "by many hours."[6]
The situation is further complicated by the fact that "a person in terminal
stages of cancer who had been given morphine steadily for a matter of weeks
would certainly be dependent upon it physically and would probably be
addicted to it and react with the addict's responses."[7]

The narcotics problem aside, Dr. Benjamin Miller, who probably has
personally experienced more pain than any other commentator on the euthanasia scene, observes:

[5]Goodman and Gilman, *The Pharmacological Basis of Therapeutics* (2nd edn, 1955), p. 235.
To the same effect is Seevers and Pfeiffer, 'A Study of the Analgesia, Subjective Depression
and Euphoria Produced by Morphine, Heroin, Dilaudid and Codeine in the Normal Human
Subject', *Journal of Pharmacological and Experimental Therapy*, 56 (1936), 166, 182, 187.

[6]Sharpe, 'Medication as a Threat to Testamentary Capacity', *N. Carolina Law Review*, 35
(1957), 380, 392, and medical authorities cited therein. In the case of ACTH or cortisone
therapy, the situation is complicated by the fact that 'a frequent pattern of recovery' from
psychoses induced by such therapy is 'by the occurrence of lucid intervals of increasing frequency and duration, punctuated by relapses in psychotic behavior'. (Clark *et al.*, 'Further
Observations on Mental Disturbances Associated with Cortisone and ACTH Therapy', *New
England Journal of Medicine*, 249 [1953], 178, 183)

[7]Sharpe, op. cit., 384. Goodman and Gilman observe that while 'different individuals
require varying periods of time before the repeated administration of morphine results in
tolerance . . . as a rule . . . after about two to three weeks of continued use of the same dose
of alkaloid the usual depressant effects fail to appear', whereupon 'phenomenally large doses
may be taken'. (Op. cit. [*n*. 24 above], p. 234) For a discussion of 'the nature of addiction', see
Maurer and Vogel, *Narcotics and Narcotic Addiction* (1954), pp. 20–31.

Anyone who has been severely ill knows how distorted his judgment became during the worst moments of the illness. Pain and the toxic effect of disease, or the violent reaction to certain surgical procedures may change our capacity for rational and courageous thought.[8]

Undoubtedly, some euthanasia candidates will have their lucid moments. How they are to be distinguished from fellow-sufferers who do not, or how these instances are to be distinguished from others when the patient is exercising an irrational judgment, is not an easy matter. Particularly is this so under Williams's proposal, where no specially qualified persons, psychiatrically trained or otherwise, are to assist in the process.

Assuming, for purposes of argument, that the occasion when a euthanasia candidate possesses a sufficiently clear mind can be ascertained and that a request for euthanasia is then made, there remain other problems. The mind of the pain-racked may occasionally be clear, but is it not also likely to be uncertain and variable? This point was pressed hard by the great physician, Lord Horder, in the House of Lords debates:

> During the morning depression he [the patient] will be found to favour the application under this Bill, later in the day he will think quite differently, or will have forgotten all about it. The mental clarity with which noble Lords who present this Bill are able to think and to speak must not be thought to have any counterpart in the alternating moods and confused judgments of the sick man.[9]

The concept of "voluntary" in voluntary euthanasia would have a great deal more substance to it if, as is the case with voluntary admission statutes for the mentally ill, the patient retained the right to reverse the process within a specified number of days after he gives written notice of his desire to do so—but unfortunately this cannot be. The choice here, of course, is an irrevocable one. . . .

If consent is given at a time when the patient's condition has so degenerated that he has become a fit candidate for euthanasia, when, if ever, will it be "clear and incontrovertible"? Is the suggested alternative of consent in advance a satisfactory solution? Can such a consent be deemed an informed one? Is this much different from holding a man to a prior statement of intent that if such and such an employment opportunity would present itself he would accept it, or if such and such a young woman were to come along he would marry her? Need one marshal authority for the proposition that many an "iffy" inclination is disregarded when the actual facts are at hand?

Professor Williams states that where a pre-pain desire for "ultimate

---

[8]'Why I Oppose Mercy Killings', *Woman's Home Companion* (June 1950), pp. 38, 103.

[9]*House of Lords Debates*, 103, 5th series (1936), cols 466, 492–3. To the same effect is Lord Horder's speech in the 1950 debates (op. cit., 169, 5th series [1950], cols 551, 569). See also Gumpert, 'A False Mercy', *The Nation*, 170 (1950), 80: 'Even the incapacitated, agonized patient in despair most of the time, may still get some joy from existence. His moood will change between longing for death and fear of death. Who would want to decide what should be done on such unsafe ground?'

euthanasia" is "reaffirmed" under pain, "there is the best possible proof of full consent." Perhaps. But what if it is alternately renounced and reaffirmed under pain? What if it is neither affirmed or renounced? What if it is only renounced? Will a physician be free to go ahead on the ground that the prior desire was "rational," but the present desire "irrational"? Under Williams's plan, will not the physician frequently "be walking in the margin of the law" —just as he is now? Do we really accomplish much more under this proposal than to put the euthanasia principle on the books?

Even if the patient's choice could be said to be "clear and incontrovertible," do not other difficulties remain? Is this the kind of choice, assuming that it can be made in a fixed and rational manner, that we want to offer a gravely ill person? Will we not sweep up, in the process, some who are not really tired of life, but think others are tired of them; some who do not really want to die, but who feel they should not live on, because to do so when there looms the legal alternative of euthanasia is to do a selfish or a cowardly act? Will not some feel an obligation to have themselves "eliminated" in order that funds allocated for their terminal care might be better used by their families or, financial worries aside, in order to relieve their families of the emotional strain involved?

It would not be surprising for the gravely ill person to seek to inquire of those close to him whether he should avail himself of the legal alternative of euthanasia. Certainly, he is likely to wonder about their attitude in the matter. It is quite possible, is it not, that he will not exactly be gratified by any inclination on their part—however noble their motives may be in fact —that he resort to the new procedure? At this stage, the patient-family relationship may well be a good deal less than it ought to be.

And what of the relatives? If their views will not always influence the patient, will they not at least influence the attending physician? Will a physician assume the risks to his reputation, if not his pocketbook, by administering the *coup de grâce* over the objection—however irrational—of a close relative. Do not the relatives, then, also have a "choice"? Is not the decision on their part to do nothing and say nothing *itself* a "choice"? In many families there will be some, will there not, who will consider a stand against euthanasia the only proof of love, devotion and gratitude for past events? What of the stress and strife if close relatives differ over the desirability of euthanatizing the patient?

At such a time, members of the family are not likely to be in the best state of mind, either, to make this kind of decision. Financial stress and conscious or unconscious competition for the family's estate aside,

> the chronic illness and persistent pain in terminal carcinoma may place strong and excessive stresses upon the family's emotional ties with the patient. The family members who have strong emotional attachment to start with are most likely to take the patient's fears, pains and fate personally. Panic often strikes them. Whatever guilt feelings they may have toward the patient emerge to plague them.
>
> If the patient is maintained at home, many frustrations and physical demands may be imposed on the family by the advanced illness. There may develop

extreme weakness, incontinence and bad odors. The pressure of caring for the individual under these circumstances is likely to arouse a resentment and, in turn, guilt feelings on the part of those who have to do the nursing. . . .[10]

Putting aside the problem of whether the good sense of the general practitioner warrants dispensing with other personnel, there still remain the problems posed by *any* voluntary euthanasia programme: the aforementioned considerable pressures on the patient and his family. Are these the kind of pressures we want to inflict on any person, let alone a very sick person? Are these the kind of pressures we want to impose on any family, let alone an emotionally shattered family? And if so, why are they not also proper considerations for the crippled, the paralyzed, the quadruple amputee, the iron-lung occupant and their families? . . . One cannot help but think of how fallible the *average* general practitioner must be, how fallible the *young doctor just starting practice* must be—and this, of course, is all that some small communities have in the way of medical care—how fallible the *worst* practitioner, young or old, must be. If the range of skill and judgment among licensed physicians approaches the wide gap between the very best and the very worst members of the bar—and I have no reason to think it does not—then the minimally competent physician is hardly the man to be given the responsibility for ending another's life.[11] Yet, under Williams's proposal at least, the marginal physician, as well as his more distinguished brethren, would have legal authorization to make just such decisions. Under Williams's proposal, euthanatizing a patient or two would all be part of the routine day's work.

Perhaps it is not amiss to add as a final note, that no less a euthanasiast than Dr. C. Killick Millard had such little faith in the average general practitioner that as regards the *mere administering of the coup de grâce, he observed:*

> In order to prevent any likelihood of bungling, it would be very necessary that only medical practitioners who had been specially licensed to euthanize (after acquiring special knowledge and skill) should be allowed to administer euthanasia. Quite possibly, the work would largely be left in the hands of the official euthanizors who would have to be appointed specially for each area.[12]

True, the percentage of correct diagnosis is particularly high in cancer. The short answer, however, is that euthanasiasts most emphatically do not propose to restrict mercy-killing to cancer cases. Dr Millard has maintained that "there are very many diseases besides cancer which tend to kill 'by inches', and where death, when it does at last come to the rescue, is brought

---

[10]Zarling, 'Psychological Aspects of Pain in Terminal Malignancies', *Management of Pain in Cancer* (Schiffrin edn, 1956), pp. 211–12.

[11]As to how bad the bad physician can be, see generally, even with a grain of salt, Belli, *Modern Trials*, 3 (1954), §§ 327–53. See also Regan, *Doctor and Patient and the Law* (3rd edn, 1956), pp. 17–40.

[12]'The Case for Euthanasia', *Fortnightly Review*, 136 (1931), 701–717. Under his proposed safeguards (two independent doctors, followed by a 'medical referee') Dr. Millard viewed error in diagnosis as a non-deterrable 'remote possibility'. (Ibid.)

about by pain and exhaustion".[13] Furthermore, even if mercy-killings were to be limited to cancer, however relatively accurate the diagnosis in these cases, here, too, "incurability of a disease is never more than an estimate based upon experience, and how fallacious experience may be in medicine only those who have a great deal of experience fully realize." . . .[14]

Faulty diagnosis is only one ground for error. Even if the diagnosis is correct, a second ground for error lies in the possibility that some measure of relief, if not a full cure, may come to the fore within the life expectancy of the patient. Since Glanville Williams does not deign this objection to euthanasia worth more than a passing reference, it is necessary to turn elsewhere to ascertain how it has been met. One answer is: "It must be little comfort to a man slowly coming apart from multiple sclerosis to think that fifteen years from now, death might not be his only hope."[15]

To state the problem this way is of course, to avoid it entirely. How do we know that fifteen *days* or fifteen *hours* from now, "death might not be [the incurable's] only hope"?

A second answer is: "No cure for cancer which might be found 'tomorrow' would be of any value to a man or woman 'so far advanced in cancerous toxemia as to be an applicant for euthanasia.' "[16]

As I shall endeavour to show, this approach is a good deal easier to formulate than it is to apply. For one thing, it presumes that we know today *what* cures will be found tomorrow. For another, it overlooks that if such cases can be said to exist, the patient is likely to be *so far* advanced in cancerous toxemia as to be no longer capable of understanding the step he is taking and hence *beyond* the stage when euthanasia ought to be administered.

Thirty-six years ago, Dr Haven Emerson, then President of the American Public Health Association, made the point that "no one can say today what will be incurable tomorrow. No one can predict what disease will be fatal or permanently incurable until medicine becomes stationary and sterile." Dr Emerson went so far as to say that "to be at all accurate we must drop altogether the term "incurables" and substitute for it some such term as 'chronic illness.' "[17]

---

[13]Op. cit., 702.

[14]Frohman, 'Vexing Problems in Forensic Medicine: A Physician's View' *N.Y.U. Law Review* 31 (1956), 1215, 1216. Dr Frohman added: 'We practice our art with the tools and information yielded by laboratory and research scientists, but an ill patient is not subject to experimental control, nor are his reactions always predictable. A good physician employs his scientific tools whenever they are useful, but many are the times when intuition, change, and faith are his most successful techniques.'

[15]'Pro & Con: Shall We Legalize "Mercy Killing"? ', *Reader's Digest* (Nov. 1938), pp. 94, 96.

[16]James, 'Euthanasia—Right or Wrong?', *Survey Graphic* (May 1948), pp. 241, 243; Wolbarst, 'The Doctor Looks at Euthanasia', *Medical Record,* 149 (1939), 354, 355.

[17]Emerson, 'Who Is Incurable? A Query and a Reply', *New York Times* (Oct. 22, 1933), § 8, p. 5 col. I.

At that time Dr Emerson did not have to go back more than a decade to document his contention. Before Banting and Best's insulin discovery, many a diabetic had been doomed. Before the Whipple-Minot-Murphy liver treatment made it a relatively minor malady, many a pernicious anaemia sufferer had been branded "hopeless." Before the uses of sulphanilomide were disclosed, a patient with widespread streptococcal blood-poisoning was a condemned man.

Today, we may take even that most resolute disease, cancer, and we need look back no further than the last two decades of research in this field to document the same contention. True, many types of cancer still run their course virtually unhampered by man's arduous efforts to inhibit them. But the number of cancers coming under some control is ever increasing. With medicine attacking on so many fronts with so many weapons, who would bet a man's life on when and how the next type of cancer will yield, if only just a bit? Of course, we would not be betting much of a life. For even in those areas where gains have been registered, the life is not "saved," death is only postponed. In a sense this is the case with every 'cure' for every ailment. But it may be urged that, after all, there is a great deal of difference between the typical "cure" which achieves an indefinite postponement, more or less, and the cancer respite which results in only a brief intermission, so to speak, of rarely more than six months or a year. Is this really long enough to warrant all the bother?

Well, how long *is* long enough? In many recent cases of cancer respite, the patient, though experiencing only temporary relief, underwent sufficient improvement to retake his place in society. Six or twelve or eighteen months is long enough to do most of the things which socially justify our existence, is it not? Long enough for a nurse to care for more patients, a teacher to impart learning to more classes, a judge to write a great opinion, a novelist to write a stimulating book, a scientist to make an important discovery and, after all, for a factory-hand to put the wheels on another year's Cadillac.
. . .

. . . Professor Williams's view is:

> It may be allowed that mistakes are always possible, but this is so in any of the affairs of life. And it is just as possible to make a mistake by doing nothing as by acting. All that can be expected of any moral agent is that he should do his best on the facts as they appear to him.[18]

That mistakes are always possible, that mistakes are always made, does not, it is true, deter society from pursuing a particular line of conduct—if the line of conduct is *compelled* by needs which override the risk of mistake. A thousand *Convicting the Innocent*'s or *Not Guilty*'s may stir us, may spur us to improve the administration of the criminal law, but they cannot and should not bring the business of deterring and incapacitating dangerous criminals or would-be dangerous criminals to an abrupt and complete halt.

[18]Williams, p. 283.

A relevant question, then, is what is the need for euthanasia which leads us to tolerate the mistakes, the very fatal mistakes, which will inevitably occur? What is the compelling force which requires us to tinker with deeply entrenched and almost universal precepts of criminal law?

Let us first examine the qualitative need for euthanasia.

Proponents of euthanasia like to present for consideration the case of the surgical operation, particularly a highly dangerous one: risk of death is substantial, perhaps even more probable than not; in addition, there is always the risk that the doctors have misjudged the situation and that no operation was needed at all. Yet it is not unlawful to perform the operation.

The short answer is the witticism that whatever the incidence of death in connection with different types of operations, "no doubt, it is in all cases below 100 per cent, which is the incidence rate for euthanasia."[19] But this may not be the full answer. There are occasions where the law permits action involving about a 100 per cent incidence of death—for example, self-defence. There may well be other instances where the law should condone such action—for example, the "necessity" cases illustrated by the over-crowded lifeboat, the starving survivors of a shipwreck and—perhaps best of all—by Professor Lon Fuller's penetrating and fascinating tale of the trapped cave explorers.

In all these situations, death for some may well be excused, if not justified, yet the prospect that some deaths will be unnecessary is a real one. He who kills in self-defence may have misjudged the facts. They who throw passengers overboard to lighten the load may no sooner do so than see "masts and sails of rescue . . . emerge out of the fog."[20] But no human being will ever find himself in a situation where he knows for an absolute certainty that one or several must die that he or others may live. "Modern legal systems . . . do not require divine knowledge of human beings."[21]

[19]Rudd, 'Euthanasia', *Journal of Clinical & Experimental Psychopathology,* 14 (1953), I, 4.

[20]Cardozo, 'What Medicine Can Do for Law', *Law and Literature* (1931), p. 113.

[21]Hall, *General Principles of Criminal Law* (1947), p. 399. Cardozo, on the other hand, seems to say that without such certainty it is wrong for those in a 'necessity' situation to escape their plight by sacrificing any life. (Loc. cit. [*n.* 20 above]) On this point, as on the whole question of 'necessity', his reasoning, it is submitted, is paled by the careful, intensive analyses found in Hall, op. cit., pp. 377–426, and Williams, *Criminal Law: The General Part* (Wm Stevens, 1953; 2nd edn, 1961), pp. 737–44. See also Cahn, *The Moral Decision* (1955). Although he takes the position that in the Holmes' situation, 'if none sacrifice themselves of free will to spare the others—they must all wait and die together', Cahn rejects Cardozo's view as one which 'seems to deny that we can ever reach enough certainty as to our factual beliefs to be morally justified in the action we take'. (Ibid., pp. 70–71)

Section 3.02 of the *Model Penal Code* (Tent. Draft No. 8, 1958) provides (unless the legislature has otherwise spoken) that certain 'necessity' killings shall be deemed justifiable so long as the actor was not 'reckless or negligent in bringing about the situation requiring a choice of evils or in appraising the necessity for his conduct'. The section only applies to a situation where 'the evil sought to be avoided by such conduct is greater than that sought to be prevented by the law', e.g. killing one that several may live. The defence would not be available, e.g. 'to one who acted to save himself at the expense of another, as by seizing a raft when men are shipwrecked'. (Ibid., *Comment* to Section 3.02, p. 8) For 'in all ordinary circumstances lives in being must be assumed . . . to be of equal value, equally deserving of the law'. (Ibid.)

Reasonable mistakes, then, may be tolerated if, as in the above circumstances and as in the case of the surgical operation, these mistakes are the inevitable by-products of efforts to save one or more human lives.

The need the euthanasiast advances, however, is a good deal less compelling. It is only to ease pain.

Let us next examine the quantitative need for euthanasia.

No figures are available, so far as I can determine, as to the number of, say, cancer victims, who undergo intolerable or overwhelming pain. That an appreciable number do suffer such pain, I have no doubt. But that anything approaching this number whatever it is, need suffer such pain, I have—viewing the many sundry palliative measures now available—considerable doubt. The whole field of severe pain and its management in the terminal stage of cancer is, according to an eminent physician, "a subject neglected far too much by the medical profession."[22] Other well-qualified commentators have recently noted the "obvious lack of interest in the literature about the problem of cancer pain"[23] and have scored "the deplorable attitude of defeatism and therapeutic inactivity found in some quarters."[24]

The picture of the advanced cancer victim beyond the relief of morphine and like drugs is a poignant one, but apparently no small number of these situations may have been brought about by premature or excessive application of these drugs. Psychotherapy "unfortunately . . . has barely been explored[25] in this area, although a survey conducted on approximately three hundred patients with advanced cancer disclosed that "over 50 per cent of patients who had received analgesics for long periods of time could be adequately controlled by placebo medication."[26] Nor should it be overlooked that nowadays drugs are only one of many ways—and by no means always the most effective way—of attacking the pain problem. Radiation, Röntgen and X-ray therapy; the administration of various endocrine substances; intrathecal alcohol injections and other types of nerve blocking; and various neurosurgical operations such as spinothalmic chordotomy and spinothalmic tractomy, have all furnished striking relief in many cases.

---

[22]Foreword by Dr Warren H. Cole in *Management of Pain in Cancer* (Schiffrin edn, 1956).

[23]Bonica and Backup, 'Control of Cancer Pain,' *New Medicine*, 54 (1955), 22.

[24]Ibid.

[25]'The opinion appears to prevail in the medical profession that severe pain requiring potent analgesics and narcotics frequently occurs in advanced cancer. Fortunately, this does not appear to be the case. Fear and anxiety, the patient's need for more attention from the family or from the physician, are frequently mistaken for expressions of pain. Reassurance and an unhesitating approach in presenting a plan of management to the patient are well known patient "remedies", and probably the clue to success of many medical quackeries. Since superficial psychotherapy as practiced by physicians without psychiatric training is often helpful, actual psychiatric treatment is expected to be of more value. Unfortunately, the potential therapeutic usefulness of this tool has barely been explored.' (Laszlo and Spencer, 'Medical Problems in the Management of Cancer', *Medical Clinics of N. America*, 37 [1953], 869, 875)

[26]Ibid. 'Placebo' medication is medication having no pharmacologic effect given for the purpose of pleasing or humouring the patient. The survey was conducted on patients in Montefiore Hospital, New York City. One clear implication is that 'analgesics should be prescribed only after an adequate trial of placebos'.

These various formidable non-narcotic measures, it should be added, are conspicuously absent from the prolific writings of the euthanasiasts.

That of those who do suffer and must necessarily suffer the requisite pain, many *really* desire death, I have considerable doubt. Further, that of those who may desire death at a given moment, many have a fixed and rational desire for death, I likewise have considerable doubt. Finally, taking those who may have such a desire, again I must register a strong note of scepticism that many cannot do the job themselves. It is not that I condone suicide. It is simply that I find it easier to prefer a *laissez-faire* approach in such matters over an approach aided and sanctioned by the state.

The need is only one variable. The incidence of mistake is another. Can it not be said that although the need is not very great it is great enough to outweigh the few mistakes which are likely to occur? I think not. The incidence of error may be small in euthanasia, but as I have endeavoured to show, and as Professor Williams has not taken pains to deny, under our present state of knowledge appreciable error is inevitable.

Even if the need for voluntary euthanasia could be said to outweigh the risk of mistake, this is not the end of the matter. That "all that can be expected of any moral agent is that he should do his best on the facts as they appear to him"[27] may be true as far as it goes, but it would seem that where the consequence of error is so irreparable it is not too much to expect of society that there be *a good deal more than one moral agent* "to do his best on the facts as they appear to him."

From "The Adolescent Patient's Decision to Die"

John E. Schowalter, Julian B. Ferholt, and Nancy M. Mann

Those who are treating a severely ill patient who decides to die are faced with an agonizing dilemma. The problem is magnified when life can be sustained for a significant period if the patient accepts dependence on a drug, a procedure, or a machine. A patient may, however, refuse further transfusions, another course of a cytotoxic drug, further cancer surgery or radiation, an organ transplant, renal dialysis or an artificial organ or pacemaker. New techniques to prolong life make this problem increasingly common in situations where death is not imminent, but the quality of life is greatly impaired. In pediatrics the problem of a patient's decision to die is complicated even more by special developmental ethical, legal, and family considerations. . . . The basic question to be faced is should a physician

[27]Williams, p. 283.

Reprinted with permission from *Pediatrics* 51:1, 97–103, January 1973. Copyright 1973 by the American Academy of Pediatrics.

always oppose a patient's request to end his life and, if not, under what conditions should he respect or even support a patient in his decision to die? These are situations of conflict between our commitment to relieve suffering and our commitment to prolong life. Sometimes it is evident to everyone that death is imminent, the suffering severe, and that efforts to prolong life will only prolong suffering, while at other times it is clear that the wish to die is irrationally out of proportion to the suffering. There is also, however, a very difficult middle ground. Especially in these cases patients may disagree with their parents, patient and family may disagree with the medical staff, various members of the medical staff may disagree with each other.

On the Adolescent Ward of Yale-New Haven Hospital, the authors recently helped to treat an adolescent who chose to die. This paper is an outcome of our considerations prior to and following her death.

Case Report

Karen was a 16-year-old Catholic girl, the second oldest of seven siblings. She was first hospitalized in September 1968, after a three-week course of nephrotic syndrome. She did not respond to medical management. A renal biopsy in April 1969 revealed "chronic, active glomerulonephritis," and by spring of 1970 a rapid decrease in renal function prompted the decision to plan for dialysis and transplantation. A bilateral nephrectomy was performed in August 1970, and Karen received a transplant of her father's kidney the following month. The transplant functioned quite well initially, but several months later proteinuria became increasingly severe, and suddenly in March 1971 the kidney completely ceased to function. Prior to surgery and following the transplant's failure, thrice-weekly hemodialysis was performed. Karen tolerated dialysis poorly, routinely having chills, nausea, vomiting, severe headaches, and weakness.

In April 1970 and prior to transplantation, a child psychiatrist (J.F.) was asked to evaluate the family. Karen was found to have a reactive depression, but this was considered appropriate. The father responded to his daughter's illness by immersing himself in his profession. The mother evidenced a suspiciousness of Karen's medical management that contained circumferential speech, loosening of thought associations, and an inappropriate lability of affect. Referral of the mother for psychiatric outpatient treatment was recommended but never accomplished.

The child psychiatrist was again consulted in July 1970. Karen and her parents met regularly with the social worker (N.M.) and the child psychiatrist (J.F.) prior to and after the transplant. The family did well psychologically during the immediate posttransplant period, but as Karen's new kidney failed, she became moderately depressed and the parents became increasingly distraught. Marital difficulties developed as the family could not deal directly with their disappointment at the transplant failing. The marital problems lessened with open discussion of the parents' feelings about the possible failure of the transplant.

In early April 1971, after it was clear that the kidney would never function, Karen and her parents expressed the wish to stop medical treatment and let "nature take its course." The medical staff was upset and they could not agree on the proper course of action. The social worker and psychiatrist attempted to have the girl and her family explore their decision in the hope that with further understanding of the decision, they would reject it. Most other staff members conveyed to the family that such wishes were unheard of and unacceptable, and that a decision to stop treatment could never be an alternative. The family did decide to continue dialysis, medication, and diet therapy. Karen's renal incapacity returned to pretransplant levels and she returned to a socially isolated life, diet restriction, chronic discomfort, and fatigue.

On May 10, Karen was hospitalized following ten days of high fever. Three days later the transplant was removed. Its pathology resembled that of the original kidneys, and the possibility of a similar reaction forming in subsequent transplants was established.

On May 21, the arteriovenous shunt placed in Karen's arm for hemodialysis was found to be infected, and part of the vein wall was excised and the shunt revised. During this portion of the hospitalization, Karen and the parents grudgingly went along with the medical recommendations, but they continued to ponder the possibility of stopping treatment. The child psychiatrist was out of town from the end of April, and the social worker was now counseling Karen as well as her parents. On May 24, the shunt clotted closed. Karen, with her parents' agreement, refused shunt revision and any further dialysis.

Those connected with Karen's treatment were stunned by frustration and anger. They felt that the decision was immoral and unsound medically. The idea of a 16-year-old patient deciding her own fate was anathema. Karen had occasionally spoken to her parish priest. Following her decision she stopped seeing him but continued talking with the hospital chaplain. She came to the personal conclusion that there was no such place as hell and even if there was not a heaven, nothingness would be far better than the suffering which would continue if she lived. On May 26, the child psychiatry consultant for the ward (J.S.), who was familiar with the situation from the time of the transplant, was asked to evaluate the girl. He found no evidence of psychotic thinking and was convinced that Karen had carefully thought out her decision and had grasped its implications.

The child psychiatrist and the attending ward physician (who happened to be a nephrologist) decided independently that Karen's decision was made as rationally as any such decision could be. They believed the staff had little choice but to comply with her request, making her dying as comfortable as possible and providing the opportunity through daily counseling for her to change her mind at any time. At first no other staff member agreed with this decision. Nurses, house officers, and consultants spent sleepless nights; faces were haggard, tempers short, and the ward morale, which usually ran high, was undermined. Almost daily staff meetings were held to discuss the policy toward Karen. Alternative suggestions ranged from having the courts take custody of the child and force treatment to demanding the parents take the girl home to die so as not to taint the hospital or staff with the voluntary death. Some staff members felt they were being forced to act as accomplices to what they believed was a suicide. Much anger was expressed at the parents for participating in Karen's decision ("It's on their heads not ours"), and many voiced a belief that if the parents gave Karen back to "Medicine" that all would be well.

The attitude of the ward staff changed, however, as the bleak medical alternatives were discussed in the ward meetings and when Karen's appetite and spirits improved after she made her decision. By May 30, when a nurse from the dialysis unit visited Karen and upset her by insisting that she return to dialysis, a majority of the staff agreed with the family that this strident approach was undesirable, and the nurse was asked not to visit. Those that knew Karen the best found it easier to acquiesce to her decision than those, especially the house officers, who recently came onto the floor. This reaction was consistent with a previous finding that those who directly witness a dying patient's suffering are less eager than more remote physicians to prolong the life of the child in extremis.

Karen died on June 2, with both parents at her bedside. The relative speed and peacefulness of her dying were unusual for a uremic death. Shortly prior to her death she thanked the staff for what she said she knew had been a hard time for them and she told her parents she hoped they would be happy. We later learned that before her death she had written a will and picked a burial spot near her home and near her favorite horseback riding trail. In the final days she supported her parents as they faltered in their decision; she told her father, "Daddy, I will be happy there (in the ground) if there is no machine and they don't work on me any more." Six months later the family is proceeding through a quite normal grief sequence with a minimum of psychiatric (J.F.) and pastoral assistance.

It is clear in this case that issues of morality are entangled for the staff with feelings of omnipotence, impotence, control, and altruism. For the family also the motivations are complex and multidetermined. However, it is not our intent to discuss this case further but to use it to illustrate the dilemma facing those who care for an ill child who chooses to die. We will present a brief review of the literature and a summary of our approach to these difficult problems.

DEVELOPMENTAL CONSIDERATIONS

Although Freud stated that probably no one can ever fully comprehend his own death, a crucial consideration in evaluating a patient's wish to die is whether or not he can understand the concept of death. The school of Piagetian psychology suggests that the grasping of the possibilities and limitations of one's self in relation to a finite future develop within the stage of formal operations, occurring during adolescence. Other psychologists as well as pediatric clinicians concur. So, it is generally agreed that by age 14 or 15 most adolescents can understand the meaning of death.

It is rare for children who have not yet reached adolescence to decide to die. When this does occur, it is likely that the child does not comprehend the meaning of death, and the real meaning of his wish must be investigated and responded to. When an adolescent decides to die, his understanding of death's meaning and permanence must also be assessed.

On the one hand it must be kept in mind that the cognitive understanding of death can exist without the emotional maturity necessary to make final decisions regarding one's own life. On the other hand, older adolescents, like our patient, can appreciate their suffering and fatigue and can comprehend when it is likely that life will never offer any more than continued disability, doubt, and suffering.

PSYCHOLOGICAL REACTIONS OF STAFF

A patient's wish for death forces staff members to confront their personal mortality and sometimes a latent self-destructive wish. This experience can be very uncomfortable, and some people must react with denial. Studies have shown that physicians and medical students are often individuals with especially strong feelings about death and with strong wishes to avoid facing death. Our society reinforces the tendency to deny death and condemn suicide. Suicide is punished by everything from life insurance nonpayment to the threat of criminal prosecution and from incarceration in a mental hospital to religious damnation. In addition, for a physician the choosing of death by a patient represents defeat and a rebuff of his role as healer.

So if, as Kasper suggests, the physician considers his own fears about death, puts them as intellectual questions and tries to answer them for other people, a patient's decision to die can threaten the physician on both personal and professional grounds.

McKegney and Lange reported on four adults in dialysis who chose to die. These authors stress the importance of the staff recognizing the possibility of a patient wishing to die and aiding the patient to bring forth and discuss this wish before it becomes crystallized into a firm conviction. In these reported cases the dialysis staff members continued to operate on the assumption that life was always preferable to death. When the patients did not share this value judgment, the staff became angry, accusing them of not living up to their part of the bargain. This staff reaction, which we also noted, is understandable, especially since dialysis staff seem to especially demand that patients do well in return for devoted care.

As a result of these psychological stresses, staff often react with anger, irritability, or depression which may trigger an attempt to seek a rapid conclusion of events without proper exploration. A staff member may deny the obvious fact that a patient wishes to die and even transmit to the family that such thoughts are not acceptable. On the other hand, he may avoid strong feelings by a too easy compliance with the wishes of the patient. If unnoticed, these psychological reactions may interfere with the professional's ability to determine and serve the best interests of his patient.

PSYCHOLOGICAL REACTIONS OF PATIENTS WITH CHRONIC RENAL DISEASE

Patients with chronic renal disease are the best studied group in terms of their reacting to a very uncomfortable, usually fatal disorder. Suicidal behavior has been one focus of this literature. In the study of one group of 14 patients, the fear of living the unsatisfactory life of the chronically ill and handicapped seemed almost as intolerable as the fear of imminent death; while in another study of 25 patients, the main concern was not in dying or living as much as "that it would be decided one way or the other quickly." Other studies emphasize the patient's concern about the quality of his life. Abram *et al.*, in a questionnaire study including 127 centers and involving

3,478 renal dialysis patients, found that if suicides were considered as those patients who died suddenly by their own hand as well as those who died following voluntary withdrawal from the program or following refusal to adhere to the treatment regimen, that the suicide rate was 400 times that of the general population. If only outright suicides and deaths following withdrawal from treatment were included, this "suicide" rate was 100 times that in the general population. Although the accuracy of the percentages from such a questionnaire study is suspect, the fact that many patients with chronic renal disease do choose death over prolonged dying does seem substantiated.

Although most reports of reactions of patients with chronic kidney disease have been in adults, cases of nonpsychotic children on dialysis who exhibited self-destructive behavior, including trying to remove their shunt, have been reported and discussed. Reinhart's experience in Pittsburgh led him to the extreme position of seriously questioning the value of chronic dialysis or renal transplantation for children at all at this time.

Many reports question the quality of life on chronic dialysis for some patients and their families. Perhaps this is an area where in our enthusiasm for a new procedure we frequently underestimate the psychological suffering of patients. In our opinion, psychological services to these patients are essential, and indications for the procedure must include psychosocial factors. No matter how useful it is to have the statistics of other patients' experiences with a disease, every evaluation must consider the patient's specific handicaps in relation to the personal values of each family, the developmental stage of each patient, and the services in the community available to support and improve the quality of the patient's life.

MORAL AND LEGAL CONSIDERATIONS

. . . Honoring a child's wish to die can be viewed as committing a homicide, abetting a suicide, or administering euthanasia, depending on the circumstances and one's philosophy. Euthanasia is commonly understood to only mean actively causing a patient's death rather than passively allowing it to occur, and suicide is commonly understood to mean taking one's own life rather than allowing death to occur by "natural" causes. Fletcher, however, categorizes euthanasia as voluntary (depending on the patient's knowledge and wishes) and as active or passive (depending on whether death is hastened by action or inaction). Karen's death would be considered passive, voluntary euthanasia. That is, the physicians chose to honor an informed rational choice to die by inaction based on the judgment that the child accurately perceived her own best interests.

Most physicians' ethics oppose actively causing death. In Williams' questionnaire study of 333 members of the Association of Professors of Medicine and the Association of American Physicians, 87% voted in favor of passive euthanasia and 80% have practiced it, while 85% of the physicians opposed active euthanasia. In a study of 418 physicians in Seattle, 59% favored passive euthanasia (after having obtained a signed request from

relatives), and 31% favored active euthanasia. Morison and Kass have recently debated whether or not it is correct to distinguish ethically between intent and means. Intent in all euthanasia is the same, but the means differ.
. . .

Passive, voluntary and even active, nonvoluntary euthanasia are occasionally performed in the terminally ill child or the monstrously deformed newborn. Voluntary euthanasia in a child who is chronically but not terminally ill is rare but may become increasingly common with the increasing number of patients' lives being sustained by artificial and often uncomfortable and expensive means. Karen, for example, was not terminal at the time of the decision, because dialysis could have prolonged her life for a considerable period of time.

Those against legalized euthanasia emphasize its possible misuses and associate it with totalitarian eugenics. They stress that approval of euthanasia would contradict the physician's commitment to heal and undermine the confidence of all patients in their physicians. The possibility of a mistaken diagnosis or of a cure being discovered during the patient's prolonged dying are also cited as objections to the practice of euthanasia. Religious opposition to all forms of euthanasia rests on belief in the divine nature of suffering or the exclusive right of God to determine the time of death. . . .

Those who accept limited euthanasia try to define guidelines. Catholic moral theology makes the useful distinction between ordinary and extraordinary means of actions. Pope Pius XII stated that "it is not obligatory for physicians to use extraordinary means to prolong life indefinitely in hopeless cases." Gerald Kelly, the Catholic Theologian, wrote that "extraordinary means of preserving life are all medicines, treatments and operations which cannot be obtained or used without excessive expense, pain, or other inconvenience for the patient or for others or which, if used, would not offer reasonable hope of benefit to the patient." Gustafson points out one difficulty with the definition of "extraordinary"; the same procedure may be ordinary for one patient but extraordinary for another, depending on the extent of the problems the patient has.

A second difficulty in using the ordinary-extraordinary distinction as a guideline is the interpretation of the word hopeless. An assessment of hopelessness includes the patient's nearness to death and the amount of his suffering, as well as the physician's attitudes toward physical suffering, psychological suffering, and the relative importance of quality to quantity of life. Gustafson warns that in assessing the quality of life no single quality can be allowed to be considered determinative. We need to encompass the variety, complexity, and interplay of the qualities we value. Major considerations might include self-determination, happiness, satisfaction in fulfilling even limited goals, and providing occasion for meaningful experiences for others, both distressing and joyful. . . .

DISCUSSION AND CONCLUSION

We believe there are instances when a physician should honor an adolescent patient's wish to die. Until the courts, hospitals, and medical societies take a stand on the issue of passive, voluntary euthanasia, the decision is left to the physician. Many considerations must be brought to bear on each case, and the use of a team of consulting specialists, including colleagues in pediatrics, psychiatry, theology, and the law is optimal. Whether the ultimate responsibility for the decision to allow passive euthanasia should rest with the responsible physician or be diffused onto a small team is a question that warrants much further debate.

As when approaching any dying patient, it is wise to arrive unencumbered with formulas for the occasion, since it will not be covered by rote. It must first be determined whether or not the child has made his decision in a rational and informed manner. Such a decision cannot be obtained in the presence of definable mental illness or persuading outside pressures. The child's cognitive ability to understand death must also be assessed. This ability would be unusual before age 14 or 15. From the physician's personal point of view, he will undoubtedly be influenced by the amount of the child's suffering, the likelihood of improvement in the quality of life now judged unsatisfactory, the closeness of death, the extent of his participation in "causing" the death, as well as his philosophy regarding the dignity of life and the importance of quality as well as length of life.

The purpose of this paper is to draw attention to the dilemma of the medical team and the individual physician who are caring for an adolescent who chooses to die. We have outlined the general areas which we think must be considered in each case. Perhaps uniform criteria to weigh these considerations are not sensible at this time, but a body of medical literature on individual cases would be helpful by providing precedents which could be studied and debated. Karen's case was the stimulant for this paper, and the need for further thought in this area remains our most compelling conclusion.

MORAL PROBLEMS ON A SOCIAL SCALE

Chapter 4

INTRODUCTION

In some areas of human enterprise, inequalities are easy to accept, especially if the system creating them is basically just. But when social inequalities place life and death at stake, it is difficult to maintain that justice is being done. Vital to the conception of a just society is that risks and harms, as well as benefits, be fairly distributed. Certain categories in society, such as black males 18 to 22 years of age, suffer a greater burden of accidents and illnesses than do others. Life and health are things that money often can buy; social stresses and consequent ill health are unequally shared. Because unequal distribution of morbidity and mortality is partly due to general social inequalities, one might argue that a fair health-care system must tend to equalize as well as to maximize the distribution of good health. Instead, the health-care system tends to reflect and hence aggravate the existing social inequalities. Given this situation, a number of basic questions arise about the justice of our methods of delivering health care. Is it unjust that some people get better care than others because of differences in ability to pay? If the present system is unjust, what would a system of care meeting the requirements of justice be like? Can a just system be achieved without sacrificing other important goals, such as quality of care?

Before we can discuss the issue of justice in substantive areas of medical care, we need to see clearly how the issue of justice arises in this context. We need to step back and bring into focus our views on justice in society generally.

The terms "just" and "unjust" can be used to describe social arrangements, sets of laws, formal or informal social practices, the acts of institutions, or the attitudes and actions of individuals. The terms are not associated with any particular social arrangements or actions. Depending on circumstances, a wide variety of social rules or individual actions might be counted as just or unjust. To say that the rules of a society are just is to make a claim entailing that its members should follow those rules. Appropriate responses to just actions of individuals include obedience, cooperation, and praise. Injustice, on the other hand, is grounds for noncooperation, resistance, and condemnation.

Although "just" is sometimes used as a general term of approval, a more specific conception is sought when we talk of social or distributive justice. For example, when inmates of Alabama mental hospitals argued that they were unjustly deprived of treatment programs, they argued that they had a *claim* to treatment on the grounds that it was *unfair* to incarcerate them without treatment. This provided their argument with a stronger basis than if they had simply said that it would be *better* if they received treatment. Moreover, a society focusing all of its health services on a privileged segment of the population distributes health care unjustly even though it may provide more health care overall than under more equitable arrangements. Justice differs from the maximization of overall benefits. To appeal to justice is to use a special sort of argument; injustice is a special sort of wrong.

Basic to various conceptions of justice are such notions as the harmony and balance of human affairs, the dignity of human beings, personal liberty, participation in collective decision-making, equality among persons with regard to needs and aspirations, fairness, and give-and-take. Any complete conception of justice will combine several of these notions. Disagreement often rests on which is the root conception and which the branches.

This chapter begins with two philosophical developments of the conception of justice. Each arranges in a different manner the elements of justice cited above. Each attempts to characterize these elements more exactly and to relate justice to other moral concepts.

John Rawls attempts to represent the inexact ordinary conception of justice by means of a more exact conception suited to moral theory. He calls this process the formation of an "analytic construction" of justice. In so doing, he works at a higher level of abstraction than William Frankena. Rawls mentions no particular goods or liberties, nor particular human qualities to which standards of justice may apply. Instead, he offers a framework into which, he argues, any complete theory of justice must fit.

For Rawls, justice and fairness are related concepts, the former applying to major social institutions and societies as a whole. These concepts, he suggests, have in common the concept of reciprocity. Reciprocity, however, is not simply give-and-take. Basically, it is equal and mutual decision-making in which each person has a voice and vote to express personal interests. In his view, justice is generated by conflicts of interests among individuals at a grass-roots level. Rawls' notion contrasts with Frankena's and some classical notions of justice. The latter notions treat justice as a good generated by society as a whole or as handed down by a central executive. Rawls' conception of justice also differs from utilitarian conceptions. Justice is concerned with the well-being of each, not the aggregate happiness of all. Moreover, the utilitarian conception of good counts in favor of an institution all its good consequences irrespective of the relationships among persons. In contrast, Rawls claims that happiness produced unjustly should not be counted in favor of an institution or practice.

Rawls thinks of the principles of justice as super-ordinate laws generated by a group of self-interested people getting together to negotiate constraints on the establishment of future social institutions. Because these laws are to govern the design of future institutions, the participants cannot tell what social position they will have under these laws. As a result, the principles of justice must assure each participant that her or his self-interest will never be ignored in the future, no matter what her or his position.

Rawls argues that two basic principles would be generated by reciprocal self-interest in a context of such negotiation. The first principle is one of equality—each shall have maximum liberty compatible with a like liberty for all. Liberty is a formula to cover as much as possible—the use of goods, access to positions and procedures, and liberty of personal tastes and expression. The second principle asserts that differences in what is distributed to persons are justifiable only if it can be reasonably expected that such differences will work out for the benefit of all—and then only if the privileges and offices in question are open to all.

William Frankena places the equality of distribution of goods at the root of his account of justice. A just society presumes equality among people, and treats persons equally except as unequal treatment is required by considerations of substantial weight. Frankena calls these considerations "justicizing" considerations to distinguish the narrower arguments concerning social justice from arguments "justifying" more general positions.

Frankena's first task is to characterize differences between people justifying or justicizing different treatment. In the field of health care, for example, having a heart attack clearly justicizes treatment different from that for a broken leg. Difference in social position is clearly not generally relevant to the moral importance of one's medical need. Yet medicine is costly. Do differences in ability to pay justicize differences in medical treatment? Frankena makes a list of qualities which are generally taken to justicize different treatment by society—capacity, need, merit, making of agreements, and others.

Frankena's next task is to say what these justicizing differences have in common. He argues that differences in treatment are justified only to equalize the good life for each person. Differences are justified only to further equality of happiness in the long run. He concludes that a just state makes a minimum standard contribution to the happiness of each, supplemented by the same relative contribution to the happiness of each. By appealing to the equal happiness of each rather than to overall happiness, Frankena, like Rawls, rejects utilitarianism. The equal happiness of each as a condition of a just society, Frankena believes, is rooted in human dignity.

Three sections of this chapter—"Allocation of Scarce Medical Resources," "The Right to Health Care," and "Medical Resources as Commodities"—raise substantive medical issues inviting considerations of justice. The allocation of scarce resources raises the issue of justice in an acute form. Scarcity forces upon medical personnel decisions that make vital distinctions among persons, however unwelcome these distinctions may be. If many are ill and few can be treated, any form of selection will cause suffering or even death even when medical ideology says that all who need it deserve treatment. The ideal solution to some of these decision problems is to eliminate the scarcity. For example, government funds have helped to reduce the scarcity of hemodialysis, discussed in the section on the allocation of scarce resources. In the short run, however, decisions must often be made before the scarcity can be eliminated. And the newest treatments will likely always be scarce. How can currently scarce resources be distributed so that no one suffers unjustly?

Scarcity of health-care resources raises at least three basically different kinds of decision problems. First, because overall national resources are limited and labor and capital can be distributed with some flexibility into various areas, to what extent should there be national investment in medicine as opposed to investment in other areas such as housing, recreation, or transportation? A variety of difficult questions lurk here. For example, is it unjust that there is considerable expenditure for recreation, consumer goods, and luxuries although some persons are perishing for lack of adequate medical resources? Or, for example, funds may be available either for the care of the unemployably mentally retarded or for unemployment benefits. The retarded have a claim for funds based on greater medical need; the unemployed have a claim based on their prior greater social contribution. Which distinctions among people better serve the ends of justice when adopted as bases for differences in distribution of social benefits?

Second, within the aggregate of medical expenditures there must be allocation of the medical resources. Paul Freund raises some of these questions in his article. Should medical funds be spent on more basic research or on better distribution of known treatments? Should money be spent on the treatment of minor and widespread ailments in such a way that many people will receive some small benefit, or should money be spent on expensive treatment for rare but serious diseases?

The third issue, tackled by Nicholas Rescher, is the question of who in particular should receive exotic life-saving therapy, such as artificial and natural implanted organs or the use of expensive machinery, when there are more medically qualified candidates than can be accommodated. Answers suggested run from using social worth as the ultimate determinant—a view perhaps based on maximizing social utility or perhaps reward for personal merit—to random selection— a view based on a feeling of universal equality in the face of death.

Often raised is the question of who should make these kinds of decisions. This question arises partly from a wish to ensure justice by means of the right procedure in decision-making, and partly from despair of finding any incontrovertible set of principles on the basis of which to make such decisions. Responses to the "Who's to say?" question vary from placing responsibility for such decisions on single medical person to having lay committees determine social worth.

Health itself, like health care, is limited. Some of us enjoy it to a greater degree than others. Like other goods, health and disease are in some ways transferable. A social order may distribute resources in such a way as to distribute health more or less equally throughout its population, or to reduce the health of some groups and enhance the health of others. Poverty, for example, reduces health. Even the conception of normal health will be affected by the composite health conditions of different social groups in a society.

Justice in health goes beyond the provision of medical treatment, to the ultimate aims of health care and to the social conditions under which we live. For example, are we unjustly deprived of good mental and physical health by overcrowding, stress, and pollution in industrial society, or do the enormous productive facilities of modern industry, making possible the support of so many of us, compensate for these costs to our health? And, are these social classes unjustly deprived of health by social conditions to such an extent that provision of medical treatment for damage already done is inadequate compensation?

In the public debate on health care, it is often claimed, and often denied, that people have a right to health and to health care. As polemic on behalf of those who suffer for lack of health care, the claim that health care is a right is invaluable. The truth or falsity of the claim is difficult to determine, however. Rights are among the more mysterious inhabitants of the ethical domain. The identification and attribution of rights poses difficult methodological problems. Some philosophers are inclined to deny the existence of rights and to claim that "rights" talk is unnecessary and obfuscatory. Others, such as Joel Feinberg, writing in the section on "The Right to Health Care," think that talk of rights and their preservation is necessary to the evolution and survival of just societies.

Confusion is generated partly by the fact that we can justifiably claim to possess a right even though that claim is currently unprotected by law or social custom. Claims of a right to early term abortion at parental discretion, for example, preceded legal establishment of that right. To reduce confusion, one might distinguish between realized and unrealized rights. Or, one could distinguish between realized rights and morally valid claims that there should exist certain realized rights. Thomas Szasz refers to unrealized rights as "claims."

Another source of confusion is that some feel that it is incoherent to claim a right to what society cannot provide or guarantee due to the limitations of nature—for example, health or life. Yet a claim to possess a right may be simply a claim on society to do what it can within natural limitations. What is possible, moreover, may depend on what rights are recognized. For example, it would be possible for a society that takes the right to health care seriously to provide more health care than one that sees other needs as more pressing.

The validity of a claim to possess rights depends in part on what rights are. Rights are commonly translated into obligations, a slightly easier concept to handle. It is typically held that "*S* has a right to do *A*" means that "Whenever *S* wants to engage in action *A*, others have an obligation not to interfere with *S*." This translation implies that a right to health care would place obligations on others not to keep those seeking health care from getting it, or more strongly, to provide health care to those who want it. Feinberg argues that this account paints an incomplete picture of rights. Missing from the account, he says, is our ability to make claims on one another. To have a right to do *A* is basically to have a valid claim to do it.

Feinberg explains what he means by "claim" by connecting the concept with such activities as "claiming that. . . ." According to his account, at the root of rights is a justifiable need to be heard and to have one's needs recognized by others:

> To think of oneself as the holder of rights is . . . to have that minimal self-respect that is necessary to be worthy of the love and esteem of others. Indeed, respect for persons . . . may simply be respect for their rights, so that there cannot be one without the other; and what is called "human dignity" may simply be the recognizable capacity to assert claims.

Some of the issues Feinberg raises are related to Michael Tooley's arguments in Chapter 3 on the necessary qualities of being capable of claiming rights.

Missing from Feinberg's account is an account of how rights fit into a theory of justice. In a society with an inegalitarian conception of justice, the pattern of rights and duties protects differences in treatment between classes. In an egalitarian system of justice, equal rights are conferred on all. A particular scheme of rights thus protects a particular scheme of justice, making it possible for members of a society to make claims on others for cooperation even where these claims conflict with the self-interest of others.

Do we have a right to health, health care, or treatment? On a Rawlsian view, a claim to a right to health care would assert that all are entitled to equal access to health care, and that the only justifiable differences in treatment are those increasing the welfare of all in the long run. Is this a defensible claim? Szasz rightly points out that the concept of treatment is too vague to permit a defense of the right to treatment. It seems conceivable, however, to set minimal standards of adequate health care so that a specific objective could be claimed by a right to health care.

As both the Illich and Millis articles suggest, the right to *health* and the right to *health care* differ. The latter entails only an apparatus to treat existing disease. Consistent with a right to health care is a sickly population. An implication of the claim that persons have a right to health is that the social causes of disease—pollution, poverty, and stress for example—violate a human right. A right to health, however, makes no claims on particular institutions to remedy these social ills. Some think that the right to health care is based on the right to health. Others would argue that there is no right to health, but that there exists only a right to health care resting on the concept of a beneficent and libertarian society providing services that people want and need. Sigerist, in "Socialized Medicine," agrees that there is a right to health care, and claims that a new system of providing such care is needed. His article, written in 1938, seems as timely today as when it first appeared.

Those who oppose the right to health care are disturbed primarily by the fact that rights imply obligations. If people have a right to health care, then particular people, perhaps physicians, health-care workers, and hospital personnel, have an obligation to provide it. R. M. Sade argues that physicians have no such obligation because people are entitled to disburse their skills in any way they see fit. Szasz presents a more sophisticated argument to the same effect. However, Szasz notes that these obligations focus on the profession in part because of some of the privileges sought by the profession. Licensure, which protects medical practice, also tends to focus the obligation to provide medical care on license-holders. Taking another approach, L. E. Bellin claims that all professionals, by virtue of the social value of their skills, have an obligation to serve the people at least some of the time. Whatever is said about the rights of health-care workers, the right to health care can be independently defended, for there is nothing logically out of place in supposing that there exists conflict between the rights of the population to health care and the right of physicians to practise as they please.

Even among those who agree that inhabitants of modern industrial societies possess a right to health care, there is much disagreement on what social mechanisms are capable of realizing or protecting that right. Socialized medicine, national health insurance, and the market system have their defenders. Either a government that provides medical services directly or one that guarantees them through some other institution may satisfy a right to medical services, so that we cannot move directly from a claim that health care is a right to a particular form of service. It is necessary to appeal to additional premises about human nature and to general theories about the role of the State in society. Medicine provides merely one example of the problems modern societies encounter in meeting human needs. In spite of its limitations, the claim that health care is a right can still be used as grounds for criticizing inadequate and inequitable health delivery systems.

The section "Medical Resources as Commodities" compares types of socioeconomic structures designed to meet health needs. It focuses on the acquisition of blood for medical use by means of purchase and donorship. Richard Titmuss compares the systems of blood distribution in the United States and Britain, characterizing the American system as a market system and the British system as a donorship system. He claims that the British system is superior morally and also on economic grounds of cost, quality, and efficiency. He uses this contrast to raise issues of altruism and self-interest as motive forces in the distribution of goods.

Representing the medical system in microcosm, blood can be viewed as a model for the health-care system as a whole. Blood is a symbol of human unity and of the hopes and fears invested in medicine. Blood is transferable, so that it is possible to modify or even to rectify partially the existing distribution of health by the transfer of blood from the healthy to the unhealthy. Unlike kidneys, blood can be regenerated by the donor, so that blood represents a renewable source of altruism rather than an outright human sacrifice.

Titmuss' main charge against the market system is that it poisons the well of altruism. If others are selling their blood, the donor receives less pleasure in giving blood. The market system thus reduces the liberty to act altruistically. Blood for money tends to drive out blood for love. Money blood, furthermore, tends to be of poorer quality than gift blood—a self-interested hepatitis carrier might sell blood for money, but would have no altruistic motive to spread bad blood. The market system, he argues, also strengthens inequalities of health when it might be more just for a system of blood distribution to correct social health inequalities. The wealthy buy blood from the poor, who risk their health for limited monetary gain. In contrast, Titmuss sees the donor system as economically sound partly because blood is distributed only to meet health needs and not to satisfy the vagaries of the blood market.

Because blood, like money, is a transferable and regenerating resource, it would be possible to redistribute blood by taxation as well as by gift or sale, as Freund suggests in this chapter. Most would feel threatened, however, by a blood tax. Critics of socialized medicine sometimes see it as a coercive system taxing health resources, but the British system of blood donorship under socialism indicates that health care might be provided in a noncoercive fashion by government. Society may be able to rely on those who have the motivation to provide health care, instead of drafting physicians into public service (provided, if Titmuss is right, that there is no coexisting system of health care for profit).

Titmuss' critics writing in this subsection point out that his empirical observations comparing U.S. and British blood distribution may be attributed to factors other than those he cites. The observed differences could result from altruism strengthened in Britain by a cultural unity greater than that in the United States. Or, the highly organized British health service through which blood is distributed may be the cause of more efficient use than is possible in the diverse and fragmented American system. R. M. Solow, moreover, points out that Titmuss tends to set up a false opposition between altruism and economics, when there is an economics of altruism as well as one of self-interest, even though the former is often neglected. Other critics of Titmuss, not represented here, have held that the failings of the American blood distribution system result from its undercommercialization, arguing that a commercial, profit-making, national system regulated like a public utility might well be the optimal system.

Titmuss' discussion of altruism in distribution of resources suggests re-examination of the concepts of justice presented here. The concepts presented here are, for the most part, rooted in self-interest. Is altruism a part of the concept of justice, or does it stand outside justice and introduce social virtues of another kind? Or, is to recognize the dignity and equality of human beings precisely to take an altruistic stance? If it is true that justice is simply a balancing of competing self-interests, the failure of an institution to meet the demands of justice is not a failure to meet an ideal. It is, rather, a failure to meet the minimum standards necessary to justify associations among human beings.

A.J.

THE NATURE OF SOCIAL JUSTICE

From "The Concept of Social Justice"

William K. Frankena

PRELIMINARIES

I propose to take social justice, not as a property of individuals and their actions, but as a predicate of societies—particularly such societies as are called nations—and of their acts and institutions. The terms "justice" and "injustice" may also refer to the actions of individuals, but our concern is with their social application—with justice and injustice writ large, to use Plato's phrase—that is, with their manifestation by a society in its dealings with its individual members and subsocieties.

Although social justice will be considered as a property or virtue of national societies, it is not simply a property or virtue of such a society in its *formal,* or legal aspect—what is called the state. That is political justice, a part of social justice. But society does not consist merely of the law or the state: it has also a more *informal* aspect, comprised of its cultural institutions, conventions, moral rules, and moral sanctions. In order for a society to be fully just, it must be just in its informal as well as in its formal aspect.

Niebuhr and many other theologians usually associate justice with love. They assert, on the one hand, that justice is a function or political application of the law of love, and, on the other, that love is the fulfillment of justice. Now, it is true that in a society of love all of the demands of justice would be fulfilled. But, to use medieval terminology, they would be fulfilled *eminently,* not *formally*—that is, they would be overfulfilled rather than literally fulfilled. Such a society would not be called unjust, of course, but it would hardly be correct to describe it as just. It seems more accurate to contrast love and justice than to link them, even the theologians referred to like to say there is a "tension" between them. I shall, therefore, here adopt the view that social justice cannot be defined in terms of love. This view is represented by Emil Brunner.[1]

> The sphere in which there are just claims, rights, debits and credits, and in which justice is therefore the supreme principle, and the sphere in which the gift of love is supreme, where there are no deserts, where love, without acknowledging any claim, gives all—these two spheres lie as far apart as heaven from hell. . . . If ever we are to get clear a conception of the nature of justice, we must also get a clear idea of it as differentiated from and contrasted with love.

Reprinted with permission of author and publisher from *Social Justice,* ed. R. B. Brandt, (Englewood Cliffs, N.J.: Prentice-Hall, Inc.) pp. 1–6, 9–23. Copyright © 1962 by Prentice-Hall, Inc.

[1] *Justice and the Social Order* (London: Lutterworth Press, 1945), pp. 104, 114.

That is a bit strong, as theological pronouncements sometimes are, but it is on the right track. Also it implies what is the last of my preliminary points: that social justice is not the only feature of an ideal society. Societies can be loving, efficient, prosperous, or good, as well as just, but they may well be just without being notably benevolent, efficient, prosperous, or good. Our problem is to define the concept of a just society, not that of an ideal society.

AN ANCIENT FORMULA FOR JUSTICE

To define the concept of social justice we must answer two questions which it is important to distinguish from one another. First, what are the criteria or principles of social justice? In other words, what features make or render a society just or unjust? Second, what are we doing or saying when we say of a society that it is just or unjust? Let us begin with the former. As is stated in an ancient formula, a society is just if it renders to its various members what is due them. But what is it that is due them? To reply that that is due them which is justly theirs or to which they have a right, is to add nothing. For we must still determine what it is that is their due or their right. To specify that their due or their right is what is accorded to them by the laws of the state may, speaking legally, suffice. The laws of the state, however, may be themselves unjust, and if so, it follows that social justice cannot consist wholly in their observance. Since social justice includes moral as well as legal justice, one might say that a society is just if its laws and actions conform to its moral standards. But even the prevailing moral principles of a society may be unjust or oppressive.

It may be said that a man's due or right is that which is his by virtue not merely of the law or of prevailing moral rules, but of valid moral principles, and that a society is just if it accords its members what it is required to accord them by valid moral principles. According to this view, social justice consists in the apportionment of goods and evils, rewards and punishments, jobs and privileges, in accordance with moral standards which can be shown to be valid. In other words, social justice is any system of distribution and retribution which is governed by valid moral principles. This view, if true, still leaves unsolved the very difficult question of which moral principles are valid, but at least simplifies matters by telling us that the answer to this question will provide the definition of justice. The concept of justice, it says, involves no special problems; all we have to do is to find out what is right.

This view is indeed plausible, for what could be more obvious than that a society is just if it treats its members as it ought to? And yet can justice be so simply equated with acting rightly? It does not seem to me that it can. Not all right acts—for example, acts of benevolence, mercy, or returning good for evil—can be properly described as just. Nor are all wrong acts unjust. As R. B. Brandt points out, incest may be wrong but the terms "just" and "unjust" simply do not apply.[2] Not all moral principles are "principles

---

[2] *Ethical Theory* (Englewood Cliffs, N.J.: Prentice-Hall, Inc., 1959), p. 409. Cf. also J. Hospers, *Human Conduct* (New York: Harcourt, Brace and World, Inc., 1961), pp. 416f.

of justice" even if they are valid—for example, the principles J. S. Mill calls generosity and beneficence are not. Justice, then, is acting in accordance with the principles of justice; it is not simply acting in accordance with valid moral principles.

This point may be emphasized in another way. Whether justice can be defined as a process of distributing and retributing in accordance with valid moral principles seems to depend on which moral principles turn out to be valid. Suppose the so-called principle of utility is understood, as some utilitarians seem to understand it, to mean that the right course of action is simply that which produces the greatest quantitative balance of something good (say, pleasure) over something evil (say, pain) regardless of how this quantity is distributed. Suppose, furthermore, that this principle of utility turns out to be the only valid principle of morality. Then distributing and retributing in accordance with valid moral principles will not coincide with what is called justice, though it may yield what is called beneficence. Justice is not simply the greatest possible balance of pleasure over pain or of good over evil. Justice has to do, not so much with the quantity of good or evil, as with the manner in which it is distributed. Two courses of action may produce the same relative quantities of good and evil, yet one course may be just and the other unjust because of the ways in which they apportion these quantities.

Therefore, unless we depart from our ordinary understanding of the term "justice," social justice cannot be defined merely by saying that a society is just which acts, distributes, and so on, in accordance with valid moral principles. If this is correct, however, then right-making characteristics or justifying considerations must be distinguished from just-making or justicizing considerations. Just-making considerations are only one species of right-making considerations. And, theoretically at least, a consideration of one kind may overrule a consideration of the other. In particular, a just-making consideration may be overruled by a right-making one which is not included under justice. As Portia says to Shylock,

> . . . earthly power doth then show likest God's
> When mercy seasons justice.

Furthermore, an inequality may sometimes be justified by its utility; the action or policy that promotes the inequality would then be right—but it might not be, strictly speaking, just.

It is true, as Brandt has pointed out,[3] that in such a case we should not call the action or policy unjust—that we hesitate to speak of something as unjust if we cannot also correctly speak of it as wrong. And this seems to imply that justice can be defined in terms of right-dealing after all. The answer may perhaps lie in an interesting passage in Mill. He writes that in order to save a life, "it may not only be allowable, but a duty" to do something which is contrary to the principles of justice—for example, "to

[3] *Op. cit.*, pp. 409f. But cf Hospers, *op. cit.*, pp. 417, 421f; G. Vlastos, "Justice," *Revue internationale de philosophie*, 41 (1937), p. 17.

steal or take by force the necessary food or medicine, or to kidnap and compel to officiate the only qualified medical practitioner." He continues:[4]

> In such cases, as we do not call anything justice which is not a virtue, we usually say, not that justice must give way to some other moral principle, but that what is just in ordinary cases is, by reason of that other principle, not just in the particular case. By this useful accommodation of language, the character of indefeasibility attributed to justice is kept up, and we are saved from the necessity of maintaining that there can be laudable injustice.

The point is that "just" and "unjust" seem to play a double role. On the one hand, they refer to certain sorts of right-making considerations as against others; on the other hand, they have much the same force as do the more general terms "right" and "wrong," so much so that one can hardly conjoin "just" and "wrong," or "right" and "unjust." It is the first of these roles which is especially important in defining the criteria of social justice, and which is neglected by the view we have been discussing. . . .

EQUALITY AND JUSTICE

Justice, whether social or not, seems to have at its center the notion of an allotment of something to persons—duties, goods, offices, opportunities, penalties, punishments, privileges, roles, status, and so on. Moreover, at least in the case of distributive justice, it seems centrally to involve the notion of *comparative* allotment. In the paradigm case, two things, A and B, are being allotted to two individuals, C and D, A to C and B to D. Whether justice is done depends on how A's being given to C compares with B's being given to D. In this sense Aristotle was right in saying that justice involves a proportion in which A is to B as C is to D. It is a requirement both of reason and of common thinking about justice that similar cases be treated similarly. This means that if C and D are similar, then A and B must be similar. But, if this is so, then it would appear that justice also demands that if C and D are dissimilar, then A and B must be dissimilar. That is to say, justice is comparative.

Actually, of course, justice does not require that all similarities and dissimilarities be respected in this way. We do not regard it as unjust to treat similar blocks of wood dissimilarly or dissimilar ones similarly: we are concerned only about human beings (and possibly animals). Even in the case of human beings, however, justice does not call for similar treatment of every similarity or for dissimilar treatment of every dissimilarity. We do not think it is necessarily unjust, even if other things are equal, to deal similarly with people of different colors or dissimilarly with people of the same color. In fact, the historical quest for social justice has consisted largely of attempts to eliminate certain dissimilarities as bases for difference of treatment and certain similarities as bases for sameness of treatment. That is, it seems to

[4]All references to Mill are to *Utilitarianism.* Ch. V. Here see, e.g., Oskar Piest's ed. (New York: Liberal Arts Press, 1949), pp. 68f.

be part of the concept of justice that not all similarities justify (or justicize) similar treatment or all differences different treatment. The point of the quest for social justice has not been merely that similarities and differences in people have too often been arbitrarily ignored; it has been mainly that the wrong similarities and differences have been taken as a basis for action. Similarities and differences should form the basis for action if it is to be just, but not all of them are relevant. The question is "Which of them are just- or unjust-making? Which of them are relevant? And is there a relation between them?"

It is important to remember that not all morally justifying considerations are just-making or justicizing. "Relevant" considerations in matters of justice cannot therefore be identified with "moral" ones, as D. D. Raphael does.[5] And it will not do to say, as Brandt does, that justice consists in treating people equally except as unequal treatment is justified by *moral* considerations of substantial weight in the circumstances.[6] If I am right, this description should be revised: justice is treating persons equally, except as unequal treatment is required by *just-making* considerations (i.e., by principles of *justice,* not merely *moral* principles) of substantial weight in the circumstances. With this emendation, the description seems to me to be correct, both in theory and as a reflection of the ordinary notion of justice. The only question then is whether there are any principles of *justice* which overrule the principle of equality, what they are, and whether they are such as to render the principle of equality otiose or not.

So far treating people equally has been equated with treating them similarly or in the same way. But suppose that society is allotting musical instruments to C and D, and that C prefers a banjo and D a guitar. If society gives C a banjo and D a guitar it is treating them *differently* yet *equally.* If justice is equal treatment of all men, then it is treatment which is equal in this sense and not simply identical. Surely neither morality nor justice, however stuffy and universalizing they may be in the eyes of Nietzsche and the existentialists, can require such monotony as identical treatment would involve. It is hard to believe that even the most egalitarian theory of justice calls for complete uniformity and not merely for substantial equality. I shall, therefore, speak in terms of equality, except when it does not matter or when it is necessary to speak in terms of similarity of treatment.

What considerations, and especially what similarities and dissimilarities in people, are just- (or unjust-) making? It is agreed that justice prescribes equals to equals and unequals to unequals, but what are the relevant respects in which people must be equal or unequal for treatment of them to be just or unjust? I have anticipated an at least partially egalitarian answer to this question, but the classical reply of Plato, Aristotle, and their many followers was different. According to them, social justice does not involve any kind of equal allotment to all men. Justice is not linked with any quality in which men are all necessarily similar or which they all share by virtue of being men. It is tied to some property which men may or may not have, and

[5]"Equality and Equity," *Philosophy,* XXI (1946), p. 5.
[6]*Op. cit.,* p. 410.

which, in fact, they have in varying amounts or degrees or not at all. Justice simply is the apportionment of what is to be apportioned in accordance with the amount or degree in which the recipients possess some required feature —personal ability, desert, merit, rank, or wealth.

This position has lately been maintained by Sir David Ross and, inconsistently, I think, by Brunner.[7] According to W. B. Gallie, it is characteristic of "liberal" as against "socialist" morality.[8] It is, however, not necessarily inegalitarian in substance; how inegalitarian it turns out to be depends on how unequal it finds men to be in the respect which it takes as basic. If it found them to be equal in this respect it would in practice have to be egalitarian, but, of course, it would not be taking equality of treatment for all men, or indeed any pair of men, as a basic requirement of justice. In this respect it may represent the classical concept of social justice, but, as Gallie and Vlastos have pointed out,[9] it hardly does justice to the modern concept in which, as Mill's list[10] shows, equality of treatment (not merely the equal treatment of equals, but the equal treatment of all human beings as such) is one of the basic principles of justice. It is, however, true, as Gallie, Vlastos, and Mill recognize, that the modern concept of social justice is complex and includes a meritarian as well as an egalitarian element. It recognizes the demand to respect differences between persons as well as the demand to respect personality as such.[11]

Views which accept the principle of equality as a basic and at least *prima facie* requirement of justice may, of course, take less complex forms. It might be held, for example, that justice calls for a strict equality in the treatment of C and D, no matter who C and D are, and that no inequality is ever justified. Or it might be maintained that, although inequalities are sometimes justified and right, they are never just. Every departure from complete equality would then be regarded as beyond the pale of justice, though not beyond that of the morally right or obligatory. Such theories are possible and have an apparent simplicity, but they limit the usual scope of justice. Not every departure from equality is ordinarily regarded as a departure from justice, let alone from morality. For one thing, such departures are allowed on the ground of differences in ability, merit, or desert. Certain other departures from a direct or simple equality, called for by differences in need, or involved in carrying out agreements, covenants, contracts, and promises, are also recognized as just, and not merely as justified or right.

[7]W. D. Ross, *The Right and the Good* (Oxford: The Clarendon Press, 1930), pp. 26f.; Brunner, *op. cit.*, pp. 29ff.

[8]"Liberal Morality and Socialist Morality," *Philosophy, Politics and Society*, ed. Peter Laslett (Oxford: Basil Blackwell, 1956), p. 123.

[9]Gallie, *op. cit.*, pp. 122, 129; Vlastos, *op. cit.*, p. 9.

[10]I.e., his list of what he calls "the various modes of action and arrangements of human affairs which are classed, by universal or widely spread opinion, as just or as unjust." Cf. *Utilitarianism*, Ch. V, pp. 47ff.—Ed.

[11]This complexity may, perhaps have the following justification. The formal rule of reason which we took to be central to justice, insofar as it is comparative, has two parts: to treat similars similarly and to treat dissimilars dissimilarly. The egalitarian principle may be regarded as a way of specifying the first part, and the meritarian as a way of specifying the second.

Much more reasonable, as well as closer to ordinary thinking, is the conception of social justice as the equal treatment of all persons, except as inequality is required by relevant—that is, just-making—considerations or principles. This is the view which I accepted as an emendation of Brandt's. It takes equality of treatment to be a basic *prima facie* requirement of justice, but allows that it may on occasion be overruled by other principles of justice (or by some other kind of moral principle). This view, however, is not necessarily very egalitarian. It does hold that all men are to be treated equally and that inequalities must be justified. But it also allows that inequalities may be justified, and everything depends on the ease and the kinds of considerations by which they may be justified. In fact, it tells us very little until it gives us answers to the following questions: What is meant by equal or similar treatment? What considerations are relevant to the justification of inequalities or dissimilarities? Are there any respects in which men are actually to be treated equally or similarly, or is this requirement always overruled by other considerations? Are there not always differences in personality, need, desert, merit, which completely nullify the *prima facie* rule of equality?

OTHER PRINCIPLES OF JUSTICE AND THEIR RELATION TO EQUALITY

The concept of social justice which prevails in our culture has now been partly defined. According to this concept, a society is without justice insofar as it is without rules (statutes or precedents, written or unwritten rules, legal and moral rules); it must, in both its formal and informal aspects, treat similar cases similarly. It must also treat human beings equally, or it must show why—a requirement which governs its rules as well as its acts and institutions. That is, the primary similarity to be respected is that which all men, as such, have. But a just society must also respect some though not all differences. In particular it must respect differences in capacities and needs, and in contribution, desert, or merit. Such differences may often make it just to treat people unequally in certain respects, thus at least qualifying the *prima facie* requirements of equality. But many other differences—for example, differences in blood and color—are not just-making. The recognition of capacity and need and the recognition of contribution and desert are not, however, the only principles of justice which may qualify the principle of equality. There is also the principle that agreements should be kept.

Are there any other principles of social justice besides the principle of equality, that of recognizing capacity and need, and that of keeping agreements? I have argued that the principle of beneficence or utility is not a principle of justice, though it is a moral principle. That is, a society is not unjust if it is not by its own direct action bringing about the greatest possible balance of good over evil. It is still, however, an old and familiar view (which I accept) that it is unjust for society or the state to injure a citizen, to withhold a good from him, or to interfere with his liberty (except to prevent him from committing a crime, to punish him for committing one, or to procure the money and other means of carrying out its just functions), and that this is unjust even if society or the state deals similarly with all its citizens. It seems to me also that a society is unjust if, by its actions, laws, and mores, it unnecessarily impoverishes the lives of its members materially, aesthetically, or otherwise, by holding them to a level below that which some members at least might well attain by their own efforts. If such views are correct, we must add to the principles of social justice those of non-injury, non-interference, and non-impoverishment.

These additions make it harder to discover what it is, if anything, that relates these principles of justice. It has sometimes been argued, however, that they are linked in that they all involve and ultimately depend on a recognition of the equality or equal intrinsic value of every human personality—or at least that they do so insofar as they are principles of justice. If this could be established, the area of justice could then be described as the area of moral reasoning in which the final appeal is to the ideal of the equality of all men. There is much to be said for this suggestion. Raphael, for instance, has very plausibly contended that differences in treatment on grounds of special need may be construed as attempts to restore inequalities due to natural or extraneous causes.[12] This would account for the justice of giving special attention to people—for example, those who are disabled or mentally backward—who are, for no fault of their own, at a disadvantage with respect to others.

More generally, it seems as if much, if not all, of the justice of recognizing differences in capacity, need, and so on, might be accounted for in terms of the ideal of equality, as follows. One of the chief considerations which not only justifies but also establishes as *just* differences in the treatment of human beings is the fact that the good life (not in the sense of the morally good life but in the sense, roughly, of the happy life) and its conditions are not the same for all, due to their differences in needs and potentialities. I am inclined to think that it is this fact, rather than that of differences in ability, merit, and the like, which primarily justifies differences in the handling of individuals. It is what justifies, for example, giving C a banjo, D a guitar, and E a skindiving outfit. Although C, D, and E are treated differently, they are not dealt with unequally, since their differing needs and capacities so far as these relate to the good life are equally considered and equally well cared for. The ideal of equality itself may require certain differences of treatment, including for example, differences in education and training. The principle involved in this claim is independent of the principle of recognizing differences in merit, but also of the principle of utility. For the differences in treatment involved are not justified simply by arguing that they are conducive to the general good life (though they may also be justified in this way), but by arguing that they are required for the good lives of the individuals concerned. It is not as if one must first look to see how the

[12] *Op. cit.*, p. 9.

general good is best subserved and only then can tell what treatment of individuals is just. Justice entails the presence of equal *prima facie* rights prior to any consideration of *general* utility.

Yet inequalities and differences in treatment are often said to be justified by their general utility. I do not deny this, but I do doubt that they can be shown to be *just* merely by an appeal to general utility. They can, however, often be shown to be just by an argument which is easily confused with that from the principle of utility: that initial inequalities in the distribution of offices, rewards, and so on, are required for the promotion of equality in the long run. In fact, much of what still needs to be done consists not so much of building up the biggest possible balance of welfare over illfare as in promoting the conditions for its equal distribution. It therefore seems plausible that much, if not all, of the justification of differences of function, as well as the recognition of ability, contribution, merit, and need—at least insofar as these may be denominated "just"—is based on such an indirect appeal to the ideal of equality. It also seems plausible that the introduction of incentives into economic and social systems, the redistribution of wealth through progressive taxation, and the reformation of the law may be *justicized,* if at all, only by such a line of argument, even if they may also be *justified* on other grounds.

If the duty to keep faith is assumed to be a requirement of justice, can it be justified in terms of the principle of equality? It does seem as if the practice of keeping promises and fulfilling contracts may be at least partly justified—and justicized—by such an indirect appeal to the promotion of equality. But perhaps the breaking of a promise can also be called unjust on the ground that it entails a direct violation of equality. The man who makes a promise and then breaks it, presumably for his own interest, is not only violating a useful practice but also favoring his good life over that of the others involved in the practice—in short, he is not treating persons as equals.

Retributive justice—for example, punishment—must also be considered. Aristotle and others have brought it under the principle of equality between the offender and the injured which had been disturbed. It might also be contended that, having violated the principle of equality, the criminal may justly be regarded as having forfeited his claim to a good life on equal terms with others, and even his claim not to be pained. Critics of the retributive theory of punishment might prefer to argue that punishment is made just, and perhaps also obligatory, by the fact that it tends to promote the most equality in the long run by preventing people from infringing on the claims of others. This is a non-utilitarian line of reasoning which looks not to the past, but to the future—not to future welfare, but to future equality.

There is, then, a good deal to be said for the suggestion that the principles of justice are distinguished from other principles of morality by being governed by the ideal of equality. Certainly the *prima facie* duty of treating people as equals is not rendered otiose because it so often permits inequalities of one sort or another. Nevertheless, G. F. Hourani may not be wholly right when he says that justice is equality "evident or disguised."[13] The claims of special desert may remain at least partially recalcitrant to such an interpretation. But even if Raphael's conclusion that the unequal treatment called for by special desert is a "real deviation from equality,"[14] is false, there still remain the principles of non-injury, non-interference, and non-punishment. Although the rule that a just society must provide a certain minimum level of welfare for everyone may be construed as an offshoot of the rule of equality, violations of these negative principles are unjust but do not necessarily entail any inequality of treatment, direct or indirect. If a ruler were to boil his subjects in oil, jumping in afterward himself, it would be an injustice, but there would be no inequality of treatment.

It might be argued that the injustice involved depends on an inequality after all because the rule did not permit his subjects to participate in the decision to commit national suicide. And perhaps it might be further argued that whenever society or the state injures, interferes, or impoverishes unjustly, the injustice consists in the fact that it does not provide the individuals victimized an equal share in the process of decision-making. Then, excepting possibly the principle of recognizing desert, the principles of justice might all be claimed to rest, directly or indirectly, on the ideal of equality. I should myself welcome this conclusion, but it seems that a so-called primitive society might be so bound by tradition that although all its members had a substantially equal voice in all decisions its rules might nevertheless be unnecessarily restrictive or injurious, and therefore unjust.

If not all of these principles can be subsumed under equality, it might be argued that the recalcitrant ones should not be regarded as principles of justice, however valid they may be as moral principles. This strikes me as a rather drastic bit of conceptual legislation. Though such a departure from our ordinary understanding of social justice may be desirable in the interests of neatness, and not objectionable in principle, I am inclined to think that there is a less radical alternative.

BASIC THEORY OF JUSTICE

What we need at this point is a plausible line of thought that will explain both the role of equality in the concept of justice and those principles of justice which are not derivable from the ideal of equality. With the rule of non-interference with liberty particularly in mind, H. L. A. Hart has maintained that the sphere of justice and rights coincides not with that of equality, but with that in which the final appeal is to the claim of equal liberty for all.[15] Using a more positive conception of liberty, Raphael contends similarly that the essential points of justice and liberty are the same. The claims of desert and equality are both subsumed under the one concept of justice, he thinks, because both are concerned with protecting the interests of the

[13]*Ethical Value* (Ann Arbor: University of Michigan Press, 1955), p. 86.
[14]*Op. cit.*, p. 10.
[15]"Are There Any Natural Rights?" *Philosophical Review*, LXIV (1955), pp. 177ff.

individual, and so their concern is basically that of liberty.[16] Following a somewhat different line of thought, S. M. Brown argues that justice requires of society only that it provide institutions protecting the moral interests, persons, and estates of its members.[17] By restating what I take to be a familiar position, I shall not so much question as supplement these conclusions. In doing so I propose to argue that the principles of the family of justice, insofar as they go beyond the requirements of equality, direct or indirect, go beyond them only because they express a certain limited concern for the good lives of individual persons as such.

In opposition to the classical meritarian view of social justice, I accepted as part of my own view the principle that all men are to be treated as equals, not because they are equal in any respect but simply because they are human. They are human because they have emotions and desires, and are able to think, and hence are capable of enjoying a good life in a sense in which other animals are not. They are human because their lives may be "significant" in the manner which William James made so graphic in his essays "On a Certain Blindness in Human Beings" and "What Makes a Life Significant?":

> Whenever a process of life communicates an eagerness to him who lives it, there the life becomes genuinely significant. Sometimes the eagerness is more knit up with the motor activities, sometimes with the perceptions, sometimes with the imagination, sometimes with reflective thought. But, wherever it is found ... there *is* importance in the only real and positive sense in which importance ever anywhere can be.[18]

By the good life is meant not so much the morally good life as the happy or satisfactory life. As I see it, it is the fact that all men are similarly capable of enjoying a good life in this sense that justifies the *prima facie* requirement that they be treated as equals. To quote James again, "The practical consequence of such a philosophy [as is expressed in the passage just cited] is the well-known democratic respect for the sacredness of individuality. . . ."[19] It seems plausible to claim, however, that this insight (which Royce calls "moral" and James "religious") into the "sacredness" of human beings justifies not only their equal treatment but also a real, even if limited, concern for the goodness of their lives. It justifies treating them not only as equals but also, at least in certain ways, as ends.

A just society, then, is one which respects the good lives of its members and respects them equally. A just society must therefore promote equality; it may ignore certain differences and similarities but must consider others; and it must avoid unnecessary injury, interference, or impoverishment—all without reference to beneficence or general utility. The demand for equal-

---

[16] *Moral Judgment* (London: Allen & Unwin Ltd., 1955), pp. 67, 94.

[17] "Inalienable Rights," *Philosophical Review*, LXIV (1955) pp. 192–211.

[18] *Talks to Teachers on Psychology, and to Students on Some of Life's Ideals* (New York: Holt, Rinehart and Winston, Inc., 1899), pp. 264f.

[19] *Ibid.*, pp. vi.

ity is built into the very concept of justice. The just society, then, must consider and protect the good life of each man equally with that of any other, no matter how different these men may be, and so it must allow them equal consideration, equal opportunity, and equality before the law. The equal concern for the good lives of its members also requires society to treat them differently, for no matter how much one believes in a common human nature, individual needs and capacities differ, and what constitutes the good life for one individual may not do so for another. It is the society's very concern for the good lives of its members that determines which differences and which similarities it must respect (and which are relevant to justice). A society need not respect those differences which have only an *ad hoc* bearing or none at all, on the good lives of their possessors—for example, color of skin. But it must respect differences like preferring one religion to another, which do have a bearing on the individual good life.

None of this implies that society may impose or presuppose any fixed conception of the good life. As James says, "The pretension to dogmatize about [this] is the root of most human injustices and cruelties. . . ."[20] Nor does it mean that society must seek to make the life of one man as good as that of any other, for men may well be so different that the best life of which one is capable is not as good as that of which another is capable. The good lives open to men may not be equally good—even if they are called incommensurable they may still not be equally good. Nevertheless, they must be equally respected and protected. That is why I reject Rashdall's formula for justice, that "every man's good [is] to count as equal to the *like good* of every other man,"[21] for this suggests that two people are to be treated as equals only if they are capable of equally good lives. It is more accurate, in my opinion, to say that the just society must insofar as possible make *the same relative contribution* to the good life of every individual—except, of course, in cases of reward and punishment, and provided that a certain minimum standard has been achieved by all. This is what I understand as the recognition of equal intrinsic value of individual human beings.

But the regard which the just society must have for the good lives of its members involves more than equal treatment. If I am right, it does not involve direct action on the part of society to promote the good life of its members, whether this be conceived of as pleasure, happiness, self-realization, or some indefinable quality. Such direct action is beneficence, not justice. Nevertheless, a just society must be concerned for the goodness of its members' lives, and not merely for their equality, though in a more limited way than beneficence implies. A just society must protect each member from being injured or interfered with by others, and it must not, by omission or commission, itself inflict evil upon any of them, deprive them of goods which they might otherwise gain by their own efforts, or restrict their liberty—except so far as is necessary for their protection or the achievement of equality. Although we are speaking of the *just* society, and

---

[20] *Ibid.*, p. 265.

[21] H. Rashdall, *The Theory of Good and Evil* (London: Oxford University Press, 1907); 1, p. 240.

not of the *good* society, its concern with the goodness of the lives of its members need not be considered merely negative and protective. It seems reasonable to assign to the just society a more positive interest (though one which falls short of beneficence) by saying that it must, so far as possible, provide equally the conditions under which its members can by their own efforts (alone or in voluntary associations) achieve the best lives of which they are capable. This means that the society must at least maintain some minimum standard of living, education, and security for all its members.

Social justice then does not, as Ross thinks, consist *simply* in the apportionment of happiness or good life in accordance with the recipient's degree of moral goodness. In fact, society must for the most part allow virtue to be its own reward, else it is not virtue.[22] In the poem, "Easter," Arthur Clough complains that the world

> . . . visits still
> With equalest apportionment of ill
> Both good and bad alike, and brings to one same dust
> The just and the unjust.

Society, however, must be wary of taking on the whole enterprise of cosmic or poetic justice.[23] It must honor first of all the so-called intrinsic dignity of man, which is not the same as his moral worth. Still, it is difficult to deny that the recognition of differences in desert, merit, and service, in the form of reward and punishment and unequal apportionment, is one of the principles of social justice. It remains, therefore, to see how this principle—insofar as it is a requirement of justice and not merely of utility—can be provided for by our basic theory. It has already been suggested that recognition of this principle is required for the promotion of equality in the long run. It seems to be required also for protection, one of the duties of a just society. Punishments have often been plausibly justicized on this ground, but so may rewards and privileges of various kinds. The good life of one member of society is not independent of what other members do or do not do. Certain forms of reward may in themselves show respect for individual freedom and goodness of life, by protecting one member against the acts or failures to act on the part of others, or by guaranteeing that individual talents shall not be lost or squandered.

More might be said on this point, but it is clear that a recognition of desert, contribution, or merit can be justicized without appealing either to an ultimate principle of retribution or to the principle of beneficence. This theory of social justice lies between those of the classical liberals and those of the more extreme welfare theorists. The one group includes too little under justice, the other too much. Both tend to equate just-making or justicizing considerations with right-making or justifying ones, but classical liberals greatly restrict the range of *justified* social action while the welfare theorists unduly extend that of *justicized* social action. I hold that justice

[22]Cf. Rashdall, *op. cit.*, pp. 256ff.
[23]Cf. Hospers, *op. cit.*, pp. 462ff.

includes a more positive concern for equality and goodness of life than the classical liberals allow, and that the area of right social action may extend even further in a welfare direction. I am not so much concerned to deny the conclusions the welfare theorists draw about what society and the state may or should do—I mean to leave this an open question—as to argue that they cannot plausibly defend them all as requirements of justice.

A just society is, strictly speaking, not simply a loving one. It must in its actions and institutions fulfil certain formal requirements dictated by reason rather than love; it must be rule-governed in the sense that similars are treated similarly and dissimilars dissimilarly. But only certain similarities and differences are relevant: those relating to the good life, merit, and so on. To a considerable extent, the recognition of these differences and similarities is required by the very ideal of equality, which is part of the concept of justice. But there are other principles of justice as well. Social justice is the equal (though not always similar) treatment of all persons, at least in the long run. This equal treatment must be qualified in the light of certain principles: the recognition of contribution and desert, the keeping of agreements, non-injury, non-interference, non-impoverishment, protection, and perhaps the provision and improvement of opportunity. These principles seem to go beyond the requirements of equality, even in the long run—but, insofar as they are principles of justice, they may be roughly unified under a conception of social justice as involving a somewhat vaguely defined but still limited concern for the goodness of people's lives, as well as for their equality. This double concern is often referred to as respect for the intrinsic dignity or value of the human individual. This is not the position of the extreme egalitarian but it is essentially egalitarian in spirit; in any case it is not the position of the meritarian, although it does seek to accommodate his principles.

From "Justice as Reciprocity"

John Rawls

I

It might seem at first sight that the concepts of justice and fairness are the same, and that there is no reason to distinguish between them. To be sure, there may be occasions in ordinary speech when the phrases expressing these notions are not readily interchangeable, but it may appear that this is a matter of style and not a sign of important conceptual differences. I think that this impression is mistaken, yet there is, at the same time, some foundation for it. Justice and fairness are, indeed, different concepts, but they share a fundamental element in common, which I shall call the concept of reci-

Reprinted with permission of the author. Originally published version in *Utilitarianism: Text and Commentary* ed. S. Gorovitz (Indianapolis. Bobbs-Merrill, 1971) pp. 242–68.

procity. They represent this concept as applied to two distinct cases: very roughly, justice to a practice in which there is no option whether to engage in it or not, and one must play; fairness to a practice in which there is such an option, and one may decline the invitation. In this paper I shall present an analytic construction of the concept of justice from this point of view, and I shall refer to this analysis as the analysis of justice as reciprocity.

Throughout I consider justice as a virtue of social institutions only, or of what I have called practices.[1] Justice as a virtue of particular actions or of persons comes in at but one place, where I discuss the prima facie duty of fair play. Further, the concept of justice is to be understood in its customary way as representing but one of the many virtues of social institutions; for these institutions may be antiquated, inefficient, or degrading, or any number of other things, without being unjust. Justice is not to be confused with an all-inclusive vision of a good society, or thought of as identical with the concept of right. It is only one part of any such conception, and it is but one species of right. I shall focus attention, then, on the usual sense of justice in which it means essentially the elimination of arbitrary distinctions and the establishment within the structure of a practice of a proper share, balance, or equilibrium between competing claims. The principles of justice serve to specify the application of "arbitrary" and "proper," and they do this by formulating restrictions as to how practices may define positions and offices, and assign thereto powers and liabilities, rights and duties. While the definition of the sense of justice is sufficient to distinguish justice as a virtue of institutions from other such virtues as efficiency and humanity, it does not provide a complete conception of justice. For this the associated principles are needed. The major problem in the analysis of the concept of justice is how these principles are derived and connected with this moral concept, and what is their logical basis; and further, what principles, if any, have a special place and may properly be called the principles of justice? The argument is designed to lay the groundwork for answering these questions. . . .

II

The conception of justice which I want to consider has two principles associated with it. Both of them, and so the conception itself, are extremely familiar; and, indeed, this is as it should be, since one would hope eventually to make a case for regarding them as the principles of justice. It is unlikely that novel principles could be candidates for this position. It may be possible, however, by using the concept of reciprocity as a framework, to assemble these principles against a different background and to look at them in a new way. I shall now state them and then provide a brief commentary to clarify their meaning.

First, each person participating in a practice, or affected by it, has an

[1] I use the word "practice" throughout as a sort of technical term meaning any form of activity specified by a system of rules which defines offices and roles, rights and duties, penalties and defenses, and so on, and which gives the activity its structure. As examples one may think of games and rituals, trials and parliaments, markets and systems of property.

equal right to the most extensive liberty compatible with a like liberty for all; and second, inequalities are arbitrary unless it is reasonable to expect that they will work out to everyone's advantage, and provided that the positions and offices to which they attach, or from which they may be gained, are open to all. These principles express justice as a complex of three ideas: liberty, equality, and reward for services contributing to the common good. . . .[2]

A word about the term "person." This expression is to be construed variously depending on the circumstances. On some occasions it will mean human individuals, but in others it may refer to nations, provinces, business firms, churches, teams, and so on. The principles of justice apply to conflicting claims made by persons of all of these separate kinds. There is, perhaps, a certain logical priority to the case of human individuals: it may be possible to analyze the actions of so-called artificial persons as logical constructions of the actions of human persons, and it is plausible to maintain that the worth of institutions is derived solely from the benefits they bring to human individuals. Nevertheless an analysis of justice should not begin by making either of these assumptions, or by restricting itself to the case of human persons; and it can gain considerably from not doing so. As I shall use the term "person," then, it will be ambiguous in the manner indicated.

The first principle holds, of course, only if other things are equal: that is, while there must always be a justification for departing from the initial position of equal liberty (liberty being defined by reference to the pattern of rights and duties, powers and liabilities, established by a practice), and the burden of proof is placed on him who would depart from it, nevertheless, there can be, and often there is, a justification for doing so. Now, that similar particular cases, as defined by a practice, should be treated similarly as they arise, is part of the very concept of a practice; in accordance with the analysis of justice as regularity, it is involved in the notion of an activity in accordance with rules, and expresses the concept of equality in one of its forms: that is, equality as the impartial and equitable administration and application of the rules whatever they are, which define a practice. The first

[2]These principles are, of course, well known in one form or another. They are commonly appealed to in daily life to support judgments regarding social arrangements and they appear in many analyses of justice even where the writers differ widely on other matters. Thus if the principle of equal liberty is commonly associated with Kant (see *The Philosophy of Law*, W. Hastie, trans. [Edinburgh, 1887], pp. 561), it can also be found in works so different as J. S. Mill's *On Liberty* (1859) and Herbert Spencer's *Justice* (pt. IV of *Principles of Ethics*) (London, 1891). Recently H. L. A. Hart has argued for something like it in his paper "Are There Any Natural Rights?" *Philosophical Review*, 64 (1955), 175–191. The injustice of inequalities which are not won in return for a contribution to the common advantage is, of course, a frequent topic in political writings of all sorts. If the conception of justice developed here is distinctive at all, it is only in selecting these two principles in this form; but for another similar analysis, see W. D. Lamont, *The Principles of Moral Judgment;* (Oxford: Clarendon Press, 1946), ch. V. Moreover, the essential elements could, I think, be found in St. Thomas Aquinas and other medieval writers, even though they failed to draw out the implicit equalitarianism of their premises. See Ewart Lewis, *Medieval Political Ideas* (London: Routledge and Paul, 1954), vol. I, the introduction to ch. IV, especially pp. 220f. Obviously the important thing is not simply the announcement of these principles, but their interpretation and application, and the way they are related to one's conception of justice as a whole.

principle expresses the concept of equality in another form, namely, as applied to the definition and initial specification of the structure of practices themselves. It holds, for example, that there is a presumption against the distinctions and classifications made by legal systems and other practices to the extent that they infringe on the original and equal liberty of the persons participating in them, or affected by them. The second principle defines how this presumption may be rebutted.

It might be argued at this point that justice requires only that there be an equal liberty. If, however, a more extensive liberty were possible for all without loss or conflict, then it would be irrational to settle upon a lesser liberty. There is no reason for circumscribing rights unless their exercise would be incompatible, or would render the practice defining them less effective. Where such a limitation of liberty seems to have occurred, there must be some special explanation. It may have arisen from a mistake or misapprehension; or perhaps it persists from a time past when it had a rational basis, but does so no longer. Otherwise, such a limitation would be inexplicable; the acceptance of it would conflict with the premise that the persons engaged in the practice want the things which a more extensive liberty would make possible. Therefore no serious distortion of the concept of justice is likely to follow from associating with it a principle requiring the greatest equal liberty. This association is necessary once it is supposed, as I shall suppose, that the persons engaged in the practices to which the principles of justice apply are rational.

The second principle defines what sorts of inequalities are permissible; it specifies how the presumption laid down by the first principle may be put aside. Now by inequalities it is best to understand not any differences between offices and positions, but differences in the benefits and burdens attached to them either directly or indirectly, such as prestige and wealth, or liability to taxation and compulsory services. Players in a game do not protest against there being different positions, such as that of batter, pitcher, catcher, and the like, nor to there being various privileges and powers specified by the rules. Nor do citizens of a country object to there being the different offices of government such as that of president, senator, governor, judge, and so on, each with its special rights and duties. It is not differences of this kind that are normally thought of as inequalities, but differences in the resulting distribution established by a practice, or made possible by it, of the things men strive to attain or to avoid. Thus they may complain about the pattern of honors and rewards set up by a practice (e.g., the privileges and salaries of government officials) or they may object to the distribution of power and wealth which results from the various ways in which men avail themselves of the opportunities allowed by it (e.g., the concentration of wealth which may develop in a free price system allowing large entrepreneurial or speculative gains).

It should be noted that the second principle holds an inequality is allowed only if there is a reason to believe that the practice with the inequality, or resulting in it, will work for the advantage of *every* person engaging in it. Here it is important to stress that every person must gain from the inequality. Since the principle applies to practices, it implies then that the representative man in every office or position defined by a practice, when he views it as a going concern, must find it reasonable to prefer his condition and prospects with the inequality to what they would be under the practice without it. The principles exclude, therefore, the justification of inequalities on the grounds that the disadvantages of those in one position are outweighed by the greater advantages of those in another position. This rather simple restriction is the main modification I wish to make in the utilitarian principle as usually understood. When coupled with the notion of a practice, it is a restriction of consequence, and one which some utilitarians, notably Hume and Mill, have used in their discussions of justice without realizing apparently its significance, or at least without calling attention to it.[3]

Further, it is also necessary that the various offices to which special benefits or burdens attach are open to all. It may be, for example, to the common advantage, as just defined, to attach special benefits to certain offices. Perhaps by doing so the requisite talent can be attracted to them and encouraged to give its best efforts. But any offices having special benefits must be won in a fair competition in which contestants are judged on their merits. If some offices were not open, those excluded would normally be justified in feeling unjustly treated, even if they benefited from the greater efforts of those who were allowed to compete for them. Moreover, they would be justified in their complaint not only because they were excluded from certain external emoluments of office, but because they were barred from attaining the great intrinsic goods which the skillful and devoted exercise of some offices represents, and so they would be deprived, from the start, of one of the leading ways to achieve a full human life.

Now if one can assume that offices are open, it is necessary only to consider the design and structure of practices themselves and how they jointly, as a system, work together. It will be a mistake to focus attention on the varying relative positions of particular persons, who may be known to us by their proper names, and to require that each such change, as a once and for all transaction viewed in isolation, must be in itself just. It is the practice, or the system of practices, which is to be judged, and judged from a general point of view: unless one is prepared to criticize it from the standpoint of a representative man holding some particular office, one has no complaint against it. Thus, as one watches players in a game and is moved by the changing fortunes of the teams one may be downcast by the final outcome; one may say to oneself that the losing team deserved to win on

[3]It might seem as if J. S. Mill, in paragraph 36 of chapter V of *Utilitarianism,* expressed the utilitarian principle in this form, but in the remaining two paragraphs of the chapter, and elsewhere in the essay, he would appear not to grasp the significance of the change. Hume often emphasizes that every man must benefit. For example, in discussing the utility of general rules, he holds that they are requisite to the "well-being" of every individual; from a stable system of property "every individual person must find himself a gainer in balancing the account. . . ." "Every member of society is sensible of this interest; everyone expresses this sense to his fellows along with the resolution he has taken of squaring his actions by it, on the condition that others will do the same." (*A Treatise of Human Nature,* bk. III, pt. II, sect. II, par. 22.) Since in the discussion of the common good, I draw upon another aspect of Hume's account of justice, the logical importance of general rules, the conception of justice which I set out is perhaps closer to Hume's view than to any other.

the basis of its skill, endurance, and pluck under adverse circumstances. But it will not follow from this that one thinks the game itself, as defined by its rules, is unfair. Again, as one observes the course of a free price system over time one witnesses the rise of one particular group of firms and the decline of another. Some entrepreneurs make profits, others have to take losses; and these profits and losses are not always correlated with their foresight and ability, or with their efforts to turn out worthwhile products. The fate of entrepreneurs is often the outcome of chance, or determined by changes in tastes and demand which no one could have foreseen; it is not always, by any means, founded on their deserts. But it does not follow from this that such an economic system is unjust. That the relative positions of particular entrepreneurs should be determined in this way is a consequence of the rules of the capitalist game. If one wishes to challenge it, one must do so, not from the changing relative positions of this or that entrepreneur, in this or that particular turn of fortune, but from the standpoint of the representative entrepreneur and his legitimate expectations in the system as a working institution, also, of course, keeping in mind the relation of this institution to the other practices of society.

Nothing is more natural than for those who suffer from the particular changes taking place in accordance with a practice to resent it as unjust, especially when there is no obvious correlation between these changes and ordinary conceptions of merit. This is as natural as that those who gain from inequities should overlook them, and even in time come to regard them as their due. Yet since the principles apply to the form and structure of practices as such, and not to particular transactions, the conception of justice they express requires one to appraise a practice from a general point of view, and thus from that of a representative man holding the various offices and positions defined by it. One is required to take a reasonably long view, and to ascertain how the practice will work out when regarded as a continuing system. At a later point I shall argue that unless persons are prepared to take up this standpoint in their social criticism, agreement on questions of justice is hardly possible; and that once they are prepared to do so, an argument can be given for taking these principles as the principles of justice.

III

Given these principles one might try to derive them from a priori principles of reason, or claim that they were known by intuition. These are familiar enough steps and, at least in the case of the first principle, might be made with some success. Of all principles of justice that of equality in its several forms is undoubtedly the one most susceptible to a priori argument. But it is obvious that the second principle, while certainly a common one, cannot be claimed as acceptable on these grounds. Indeed, to many persons it will surely seem overly restrictive; to others it may seem too weak. Some will want to hold that there are cases where it is just to balance the gains of some against the losses of others, and that the principle as stated contains an exaggerated bias in the direction of equality; while there are bound to be those to whom it will seem an insufficient basis upon which to found an account of justice. These opinions are certainly of considerable force, and it is only by a study of the background of the principle and by an examination of its intended applications that one can hope to establish its merits. In any case, a priori and intuitive arguments, made at this point, are unconvincing. They are not likely to lead to an understanding of the basis of the principles of justice, not at least as principles of justice: for what one wants to know is the way in which these principles complete the sense of justice, and why they are associated with this moral concept, and not with some other. I wish, therefore, to look at the principles in a different way; I want to bring out how they are generated by imposing the constraints of having a morality upon persons who confront one another on those occasions when questions of justice arise.

In order to do this, it seems simplest to present a conjectural account of the derivation of these principles as follows. Imagine a society of persons amongst whom a certain system of practices is already well established. Now suppose that by and large they are mutually self-interested; their allegiance to their established practices is normally founded on the prospect of their own advantage. One need not, and indeed ought not, to assume that, in all senses of the term "person," the persons in this society are mutually self-interested. If this characterization holds when the line of division is the family, it is nevertheless likely to be true that members of families are bound by ties of sentiment and affection and willingly acknowledge duties in contradiction to self-interest. Mutual self-interestedness in the relations between families, nations, churches, and the like, is commonly associated with loyalty and devotion on the part of individual members. If this were not so the conflicts between these forms of association would not be pursued with such intensity and would not have such tragic consequences. If Hobbes' description of relations between persons seems unreal as applied to human individuals, it is often true enough of the relations between artificial persons; and these relations may assume their Hobbesian character largely in consequence of that element which that description professedly leaves out, the loyalty and devotion of individuals. Therefore, one can form a more realistic conception of this society if one thinks of it as consisting of mutually self-interested families, or some other association. Taking the term "person" widely from the start prepares one for doing this. It is not necessary to suppose, however, that these persons are mutually self-interested under all circumstances, but only in the usual situations in which they participate in their common practices concerning which the question of justice aprises.

Now suppose further that these persons are rational: they know their own interests more or less accurately; they realize that the several ends they pursue may conflict with each other, and they are able to decide what level of attainment of one they are willing to sacrifice for a given level of attainment of another; they are capable of tracing out the likely consequences of adopting one practice rather than another, and of adhering to a course of action once they have decided upon it; they can resist present temptations and the enticements of immediate gain; and the bare knowledge or perception of the difference between their condition and that of others is not, within certain limits and in itself, a source of great dissatisfaction. Only the very last point adds anything to the standard definition of rationality as it appears say in the theory of price; and there is no need to question the propriety of this definition given the purposes for which it is customarily used. But the notion of rationality, if it is to play a part in the analysis of justice should allow, I think, that a rational man will resent or will be dejected by differences of condition between himself and others only where there is an accompanying explanation: that is, if they are thought to derive from injustice, or from some other fault of institutions, or to be the consequence of letting chance work itself out for no useful common purpose. At any rate, I shall include this trait of character in the notion of rationality for the purpose of analyzing the concept of justice. The legitimacy of doing so will, I think, become clear as the analysis proceeds. So if these persons strike us as unpleasantly egoistic in their relations with one another, they are at least free in some degree from the fault of envy.[4]

Finally, assume that these persons have roughly similar needs, interests, and capacities, or needs, interests, and capacities in various ways complementary, so that fruitful cooperation amongst them is possible; and suppose that they are sufficiently equal in power and the instruments thereof to guarantee that in normal circumstances none is able to dominate the others. This condition (as well as the other conditions) may seem excessively vague; but in view of the conception of justice to which the arguments leads, there seems to be no reason for making it more exact at this point.[5]

Since these persons are conceived as engaging in their common practices, which are already established, there is no question of our supposing them to come together to deliberate as to how they will set up these practices for the first time. Yet we can imagine that from time to time they discuss with one another whether any of them has a legitimate complaint against their established institutions. This is only natural in any normal society. Now suppose that they have settled on doing this in the following way. They first try to arrive at the principles by which complaints and so practices themselves are to be judged. That is, they do not begin by complaining; they begin instead by establishing the criteria by which a complaint is to be counted legitimate. Their procedure for this is to let each person propose the principles upon which he wishes his complaints to be tried with the understanding that, if acknowledged, the complaints of others will be simi-

---

[4]There is no need to discuss here this addition to the usual conception of rationality. The reason for it will become clear as the argument proceeds, for it is analogous to, and is connected with, the modification of the utilitarian principle which the argument as a whole is designed to explain and to justify. In the same way that the satisfaction of interests, the representative claims of which violate the principles of justice, is not a reason for having a practice, unfounded envy, within limits, need not be taken into account. One could, of course, have another reason for this addition, namely, to see what conception of justice results when it is made. This alone would not be without interest.

[5]In this description of the situation of the persons, I have drawn on Hume's account of the circumstances in which justice arises, see *A Treatise of Human Nature*, bk. III, pt. II, sec. II, and *An Enquiry Concerning the Principles of Morals*, sec. III, pt. I. It is, in particular, the scarcity of good things and the lack of mutual benevolence that leads to conflicting claims, and which gives rise to the "cautious, jealous virtue of justice," a phrase from the *Enquiry*, ibid., par. 3.

larly tried; and moreover, that no complaints will be heard at all until everyone is roughly of one mind as to how complaints are to be judged. Thus while each person has a chance to propose the standards he wishes, these standards must prove acceptable to the others before his charges can be given a hearing. They all understand further that the principles proposed and acknowledged on this occasion are binding on future occasions. So each will be wary of proposing a principle which would give him a peculiar advantage in his present circumstances, supposing it to be accepted (which is, perhaps, in most cases unlikely). Each person knows that he will be bound by it in future circumstances the peculiarities of which cannot be known, and which might well be such that the principle is then to his disadvantage. The basic idea in this procedure is that everyone should be required to make in advance a firm commitment to acknowledge certain principles as applying to his own case and such that others also may reasonably be expected to acknowledge them; and that no one be given the opportunity to tailor the canons of a legitimate complaint to fit his own special conditions, and then to discard them when they no longer suit his purpose.[6] Hence each person will propose principles of a general kind which will, to a large degree, gain their sense from the various applications to be made of them, the particular circumstances of these applications being as yet unknown. These principles will express the conditions in accordance with which each person is the least unwilling to have his interests limited in the design of practices, given the competing interests of the others, on the supposition that the interests of others will be limited likewise. The restriction which would so arise might be thought of as those a person would keep in mind if he were designing a practice in which his enemy were to assign him his place.

The elements of this conjectural account can be divided into two main parts so that each part has a definite significance. Thus the character and respective situations of the parties, that is, their rationality and mutual self-interestedness, and their being of roughly similar needs, interests and capacities, and their having needs, interests and capacities in various ways complementary, so that fruitful forms of cooperation are possible, can be taken to represent the typical circumstances in which questions of justice arise. For questions of justice are involved when conflicting claims are made upon the design of a practice and where it is taken for granted that each

---

[6]Thus everyone is, so far as possible, prevented from acting on the kind of advice which Aristotle summarizes in the *Rhetoric*, k. I, ch. 15. There he describes a number of ways in which a man may argue his case, and which are, he observes, especially characteristic of forensic oratory. For example, if the written law tells against his case, a man must appeal to the universal law and insist on its greater equity and justice; he must argue that the juror's oath "I will give my verdict according to my honest opinion" means that one will not simply follow the letter of the unwritten law. On the other hand, if the law supports his case, he must argue that not to apply the law is as bad as to have no laws at all, or that less harm comes from an occasional mistake than from the growing habit of disobedience; and he must contend that the juror's oath is not meant to make the judges give a verdict contrary to law, but to save them from the guilt of perjury if they do not understand what the law really means. Such tactics are, of course, common in arguments of all kinds; the notion of a considered judgment, and Adam Smith's and Hume's idea of an impartial spectator, is in part derived from the conception of a person so placed that he has no incentive to make these manoeuvers.

person will insist, so far as possible, on what he considers his rights. It is typical of cases of justice to involve persons who are pressing on one another their claims, between which a fair balance or equilibrium must be found. So much is expressed by the sense of the concept.

On the other hand, the procedure whereby principles are proposed and acknowledged can be taken to represent the constraints of having a morality; it is these constraints which require rational and mutually self-interested persons to act reasonably, in this case, to acknowledge familiar principles of justice. (The condition that the parties be sufficiently equal in power and the instruments thereof to guarantee that in normal circumstances none is able to dominate the others is to make the adoption of such a procedure seem more realistic; but the argument is not affected if we do without this condition, and imagine that the procedure is simply laid down.) Once the procedure is adopted and carried through each person is committed to acknowledge principles as impartially applying to his own conduct and claims as well as to another's, and he is committed moreover to principles which may constitute a constraint, or limitation, upon the pursuit of his own interests. Now a person's having a morality is analogous to having made a firm commitment in advance to acknowledge principles having these consequences for one's own conduct. A man whose moral judgments always coincided with his interests could be suspected of having no morality at all. There are, of course, other aspects to having a morality: the acknowledgment of moral principles must not only show itself in accepting a reference to them as reasons for limiting one's claims, but also in acknowledging the burden of providing a special explanation, or excuse, when one acts contrary to them, or else in showing shame and remorse (although not on purpose!), and (sincerely) indicating a desire to make amends, and so on. These aspects of having a morality and, more particularly, the place of moral feelings such as shame and remorse cannot be considered here. For the present it is sufficient to remark that the procedure of the conjectural account expresses an essential aspect of having a morality: namely, the acknowledgment of principles as impartially applying to one's own claims as well as to others, and the consequent constraint upon the pursuit of one's own interests.[7]

The two parts into which the foregoing account may be divided are intended, then, to represent the kinds of circumstances in which questions of justice arise (as expressed by the sense of the concept of justice) and the constraints which having a morality would impose upon persons so situated. By imposing these constraints on persons in the occasions of justice one can see how certain principles are generated, and one understands why these

---

[7]The idea that accepting a principle as a moral principle implies that one generally acts on it, failing a special explanation, has been stressed by R. M. Hare, *The Language of Morals* (Oxford: The University Press, 1952). His formulation of it needs to be modified, however, along the lines suggested by P. L. Gardiner, "On Assenting to a Moral Principle," *Proceedings on the Aristotelian Society*, n.s. 55 (1955), 23–44. See also C. K. Grant, "Akrasia and the Criteria of Assent to Practical Principles," *Mind* 65 (1956), 400–407, where the complexity of the criteria for assent is discussed. That having a morality at all involves acknowledging and acting on principles which may be contrary to one's self-interest is mentioned below, see section 5.

principles, and not others, come to be associated with the concept of justice; for given all the conditions as described in the conjectural account, it would be natural if the two principles of justice were to be jointly acknowledged. Since there is no way for anyone to win special advantages for himself, each would consider it reasonable to acknowledge equality as an initial principle. There is, however, no reason why they should regard this position as final. If there are inequalities which satisfy the conditions of the second principle, the immediate gain which equality would allow can be considered as intelligently invested in view of its future return. If, as is quite likely, these inequalities work as incentives to draw out better efforts, the members of this society may look upon them as concessions to human nature: they, like us, may think that people ideally should want to serve one another. But as they are mutually self-interested, their acceptance of these inequalities is merely the acceptance of the relations in which they actually stand, and a recognition of the motives which lead them to engage in their common practices. Being themselves self-interested, they have no title to complain of one another. And so provided the conditions of the principle are met, there is no reason why they should not allow such inequalities. Indeed, it would be short-sighted of them not to do so, and could result, in most cases, only from their being dejected by the bare knowledge, or perception, that others are better situated. Each person will, however, insist on an advantage to himself, and so on a common advantage, for none is willing to sacrifice anything for the others.[8]

These remarks are not offered as a rigorous proof that persons conceived and situated as the conjectural account supposes, and required to adopt the procedure described, would settle on the two principles of justice stated and commented upon in section 2. For this a much more elaborate and formal argument would have to be given. I shall not undertake a proof in this sense. In a weaker sense, however, the argument may be considered a proof, or as a sketch of a proof, although there still remain certain details to be filled in, and various alternatives to be ruled out. These I shall take up in later lectures. For the moment the essential point is simply that the proposition I seek to establish is a necessary one, or better, it is a kind of theorem: namely, that when mutually self-interested and rational persons confront one another in the typical circumstances of justice, and when they are required by a procedure expressing the constraints of having a morality to jointly acknowledge principles by which their claims on the design of their common practices are to be judged, they will settle upon these two principles as restrictions governing the assignment of rights and duties, and thereby accept them as limiting their rights against one another. It is this theorem which accounts for these principles as principles of justice, and explains how they come to be associated with this moral concept. Moreover it is analogous to theorems about human conduct in other branches of social thought. That is, a simplified situation is described in which rational per-

---

[8]A similar argument is given by F. Y. Edgeworth in "The Pure Theory of Taxation," *Economic Journal 7* (1897). Reprinted in *Classics in the Theory of Public Finance*, ed. Musgrave and Peacock (New York: St. Martin's, 1958), pp. 120f.

sons, pursuing certain ends and related to one another in a definite way, are required to act, subject to certain limitations. Then, given this situation, it is shown that they will act in a certain manner. The failure so to act would only mean that one or more of the conditions did not obtain. The proposition we are interested in is not, then, an empirical hypothesis. This is, of course, as it should be; for this proposition is to play a part in an analysis of the concept of justice. Its point is to bring out how the principles associated with the concept derive from its sense, and to show the basis for saying that the principles of justice may be regarded as those principles which arise when the constraints of having a morality are imposed upon persons in typical circumstances of justice.

THE RIGHT TO HEALTH CARE

The Nature and Value of Rights

Joel Feinberg

I

I would like to begin by conducting a thought experiment. Try to imagine Nowheresville—a world very much like our own except that no one, or hardly any one (the qualification is not important), has *rights*. If this flaw makes Nowheresville too ugly to hold very long in contemplation, we can make it as pretty as we wish in other moral respects. We can, for example, make the human beings in it as attractive and virtuous as possible without taxing our conceptions of the limits of human nature. In particular, let the virtues of moral sensibility flourish. Fill this imagined world with as much benevolence, compassion, sympathy, and pity as it will conveniently hold without strain. Now we can imagine men helping one another from compassionate motives merely, quite as much or even more than they do in our actual world from a variety of more complicated motives.

This picture, pleasant as it is in some respects, would hardly have satisfied Immanuel Kant. Benevolently motivated actions do good, Kant admitted, and therefore are better, *ceteris paribus,* than malevolently motivated actions; but no action can have supreme kind of worth—what Kant called "moral worth"—unless its whole motivating power derives from the thought that it is *required by duty.* Accordingly, let us try to make Nowheresville more appealing to Kant by introducing the idea of duty into it, and letting the sense of duty be a sufficient motive for many beneficent and

Reprinted with permission of author and publisher from *Journal of Value Inquiry* 4:4, 243–257, Winter 1970.

honorable actions. But doesn't this bring our original thought experiment to an abortive conclusion? If duties are permitted entry into Nowheresville, are not rights necessarily smuggled in along with them?

The question is well-asked, and requires here a brief digression so that we might consider the so-called "doctrine of the logical correlativity of rights and duties." This is the doctrine that (i) all duties entail other people's rights and (ii) all rights entail other people's duties. Only the first part of the doctrine, the alleged entailment from duties to rights, need concern us here. Is this part of the doctrine correct? It should not be surprising that my answer is: "In a sense yes and in a sense no." Etymologically, the word "duty" is associated with actions that are *due* someone else, the payments of debts to creditors, the keeping of agreements with promisees, the payment of club dues, or legal fees, or tariff levies to appropriate authorities or their representatives. In this original sense of "duty," all duties are correlated with the rights of those *to* whom the duty is owed. On the other hand, there seem to be numerous classes of duties, both of a legal and non-legal kind, that are *not* logically correlated with the rights of other persons. This seems to be a consequence of the fact that the word "duty" has come to be used for *any* action understood to be *required*, whether by the rights of others, or by law, or by higher authority, or by conscience, or whatever. When the notion of requirement is in clear focus it is likely to seem the only element in the idea of duty that is essential, and the other component notion—that a duty is something *due* someone else—drops off. Thus, in this widespread but derivative usage, "duty" tends to be used for any action we feel we *must* (for whatever reason) do. It comes, in short, to be a term of moral modality merely; and it is no wonder that the first thesis of the logical correlativity doctrine often fails.

Let us then introduce duties into Nowheresville, but only in the sense of actions that are, or are believed to be, morally mandatory, but not in the older sense of actions that are due others and can be claimed by others as their right. Nowheresville now can have duties of the sort imposed by positive law. A legal duty is not something we are implored and advised to do merely; it is something the law, or an authority under the law, *requires* us to do whether we want to or not, under pain of penalty. When traffic lights turn red, however, there is no determinate person who can plausibly be said to claim our stopping as his due, so that the motorist owes it to *him* to stop, in the way a debtor owes it to his creditor to pay. In our own actual world, of course, we sometimes owe it to our *fellow motorists* to stop; but that kind of right-correlated duty does not exist in Nowheresville. There, motorists "owe" obedience to the Law, but they owe nothing to one another. When they collide, no matter who is at fault, no one is morally accountable to anyone else, and no one has any sound grievance or "right to complain."

When we leave legal contexts to consider moral obligations and other extra-legal duties, a greater variety of duties-without-correlative-rights present themselves. Duties of charity, for example, require us to contribute to one or another of a large number of eligible recipients, no one of whom can claim our contribution from us as his due. Charitable contributions are more like gratuitous services, favors, and gifts than like repayments of debts or reparations; and yet we do have duties to be charitable. Many persons, moreover, in our actual world believe that they are required by their own consciences to do more than that "duty" that *can* be demanded of them by their prospective beneficiaries. I have quoted elsewhere the citation from H. B. Acton of a character in a Malraux novel who "gave all his supply of poison to his fellow prisoners to enable them by suicide to escape the burning alive which was to be their fate and his." This man, Acton adds, "probably did not think that [the others] had more of a right to the poison than he had, though he thought it his duty to give it to them."[1] I am sure that there are many actual examples, less dramatically heroic than this fictitious one, of persons who believe, rightly or wrongly, that they *must do* something (hence the word "duty") for another person in excess of what that person can appropriately demand of him (hence the absence of "right").

Now the digression is over and we can return to Nowheresville and summarize what we have put in it thus far. We now find spontaneous benevolence in somewhat larger degree than in our actual world, and also the acknowledged existence of duties of obedience, duties of charity, and duties imposed by exacting private consciences, and also, let us suppose, a degree of conscientiousness in respect to those duties somewhat in excess of what is to be found in our actual world. I doubt that Kant would be fully satisfied with Nowheresville even now that duty and respect for law and authority have been added to it; but I feel certain that he would regard their addition at least as an improvement. I will now introduce two further moral practices into Nowheresville that will make that world very little more appealing to Kant, but will make it appear more familiar to us. These are the practices connected with the notions of *personal desert* and what I call a *sovereign monopoly of rights.*

When a person is said to deserve something good from us what is meant in part is that there would be a certain propriety in our giving that good thing to him in virtue of the kind of person he is, perhaps, or more likely, in virtue of some specific thing he has done. The propriety involved here is a much weaker kind than that which derives from our having promised him the good thing or from his having qualified for it by satisfying the well-advertised conditions of some public rule. In the latter case he could be said not merely to deserve the good thing but also to have a *right* to it, that is to be in a position to demand it as his due; and of course he will not have that sort of thing in Nowheresville. That weaker kind of propriety which is mere desert is simply a kind of *fittingness* between one party's character or action and another party's favorable response, much like that between humor and laughter, or good performance and applause.

The following seems to be the origin of the idea of deserving good or bad treatment from others: A master or lord was under no obligation to reward his servant for especially good service; still a master might naturally feel that there would be a special fittingness in giving a gratuitous reward as a grateful response to the good service (or conversely imposing a penalty

---

[1]H. B. Acton, "Symposium on 'Rights,'" *Proceedings of the Aristotelian Society,* Supplementary Volume 24 (1950), pp. 107–8.

for bad service). Such an act while surely fitting and proper was entirely supererogatory. The fitting response in turn from the rewarded servant should be gratitude. If the deserved reward had not been given him he should have had no complaint, since he only *deserved* the reward, as opposed to having a *right* to it, or a ground for claiming it has his due.

The idea of desert has evolved a good bit away from its beginnings by now, but nevertheless, it seems clearly to be one of those words J. L. Austin said "never entirely forget their pasts."[2] Today servants qualify for their wages by doing their agreed upon chores, no more and no less. If their wages are not forthcoming, their contractual rights have been violated and they can make legal claim to the money that is their due. If they do less than they agreed to do, however, the employers may "dock" them, by paying them proportionately less than the agreed upon fee. This is all a matter of right. But if the servant does a splendid job, above and beyond his minimal contractual duties, the employer is under no further obligation to reward him, for this was not agreed upon, even tacitly, in advance. The additional service was all the servant's idea and done entirely on his own. Nevertheless, the morally sensitive employer may feel that it would be exceptionally appropriate for him to respond, freely on *his* own, to the servant's meritorious service, with a reward. The employee cannot demand it as his due, but he will happily accept it, with gratitude, as a fitting response to his desert.

In our age of organized labor, even this picture is now archaic; for almost every kind of exchange of service is governed by hard bargained contracts so that even bonuses can sometimes be demanded as a matter of right, and nothing is given for nothing on either side of the bargaining table. And perhaps that is a good thing; for consider an anachronistic instance of the earlier kind of practice that survives, at least as a matter of form, in the quaint old practice of "tipping." The tip was originally conceived as a reward that has to be earned by "zealous service." It is not something to be taken for granted as a standard response to *any* service. That is to say that its payment is a *"gratuity,"* not a discharge of obligation, but something given apart from, or in addition to, anything the recipient can expect as a matter of right. That is what tipping originally meant at any rate, and tips are still referred to as "gratuities" in the tax forms. But try to explain all that to a New York cab driver! If he has *earned* his gratuity, by God, he has it coming, and there had better be sufficient acknowledgement of his desert or he'll give you a piece of his mind! I'm not generally prone to defend New York cab drivers, but they do have a point here. There is the making of a paradox in the queerly unstable concept of an "earned gratuity." One can understand how "desert" in the weak sense of "propriety" or "mere fittingness" tends to generate a stronger sense in which desert is itself the ground for a claim of right.

In Nowheresville, nevertheless, we will have only the original weak kind of desert. Indeed, it will be impossible to keep this idea out if we allow such practices as teachers grading students, judges awarding prizes, and servants serving benevolent but class-conscious masters. Nowheresville is a

[2] J. L. Austin, "A Plea for Excuses," *Proceedings of the Aristotelian Society,* Vol. 57 (1956–57).

reasonably good world in many ways, and its teachers, judges, and masters will generally try to give students, contestants, and servants the grades, prizes, and rewards they deserve. For this the recipients will be grateful; but they will never think to complain, or even feel aggrieved, when expected responses to desert fail. The masters, judges, and teachers don't *have* to do good things, after all, for *anyone.* One should be happy that they *ever* treat us well, and not grumble over their occasional lapses. Their hoped for responses, after all, are *gratuities,* and there is no wrong in the omission of what is merely gratuitous. Such is the response of persons who have no concept of *rights,* even persons who are proud of their own deserts.[3]

Surely, one might ask, rights have to come in somewhere, if we are to have even moderately complex forms of social organization. Without rules that confer rights and impose obligations, how can we have ownership of property, bargains and deals, promises and contracts, appointments and loans, marriages and partnerships? Very well, let us introduce all of these social and economic practices into Nowheresville, but *with one big twist.* With them I should like to introduce the curious notion of a "sovereign right-monopoly." You will recall that the subjects in Hobbes's *Leviathan* had no rights whatever against their sovereign. He could do as he liked with them, even gratuitously harm them, but this gave them no valid grievance against him. The sovereign, to be sure, had a certain duty to treat his subjects well, but this duty was owed not to the subjects directly, but to God, just as we might have a duty to a person to treat his property well, but of course no duty to the property itself but only to its owner. Thus, while the sovereign was quite capable of *harming* his subjects, he could commit no wrong against them that they could complain about, since they had no prior claims against his conduct. The only party *wronged* by the sovereign's mistreatment of his subjects was God, the supreme lawmaker. Thus, in repenting cruelty to his subjects, the sovereign might say to God, as David did after killing Uriah, "to Thee only have I sinned."[4]

Even in the *Leviathan,* however, ordinary people had ordinary rights *against one another.* They played roles, occupied offices, made agreements, and signed contracts. In a genuine "sovereign right-monopoly," as I shall be using that phrase, they will do all those things too, and thus incur genuine obligations toward one another; but the obligations (here is the twist) will not be owed directly *to* promisees, creditors, parents, and the like, but rather to God alone, or to the members of some elite, or to a single sovereign under God. Hence, the rights correlative to the obligations that derive from these transactions are all owned by some "outside" authority.

As far as I know, no philosopher has ever suggested that even our role and contract obligations (in this, our actual world) are all owed directly to a divine intermediary; but some theologians have approached such extreme moral occasionalism. I have in mind the familiar phrase in certain widely

---

[3]For a fuller discussion of the concept of personal desert see my "Justice and Personal Desert," *Nomos I'l, Justice,* ed. by C. J. Friedrich and J. Chapman (New York: Atherton Press, 1963), pp. 69–97.

[4]II Sam. 11. Cited with approval by Thomas Hobbes in *The Leviathan,* Part II, Chap. 21.

distributed religious tracts that "it takes three to marry," which suggests that marital vows are not made between bride and groom directly but between each spouse and God, so that if one breaks his vow, the other cannot rightly complain of being wronged, since only God could have claimed performance of the marital duties as his *own* due; and hence God alone had a claim-right violated by nonperformance. If John breaks his vow to God, he might then properly repent in the words of David: "To Thee only have I sinned."

In our actual world, very few spouses conceive of their mutual obligations in this way; but their small children, at a certain stage in their moral upbringing, are likely to feel precisely this way toward *their* mutual obligations. If Billy kicks Bobby and is punished by Daddy, he may come to feel contrition for his naughtiness induced by his painful estrangement from the loved parent. He may then be happy to make amends and sincere apology *to Daddy;* but when Daddy insists that he apologize to his wronged brother, that is another story. A direct apology to Billy would be a tacit recognition of Billy's status as a right-holder against him, some one he can wrong as well as harm, and someone to whom he is directly accountable for his wrongs. This is a status Bobby will happily accord Daddy; but it would imply a respect for Billy that he does not presently feel, so he bitterly resents according it to him. On the "three-to-marry" model, the relations between each spouse and God would be like those between Bobby and Daddy; respect for the other spouse as an independent claimant would not even be necessary; and where present, of course, never sufficient.

The advocates of the "three to marry" model who conceive it either as a description of our actual institution of marriage or a recommendation of what marriage ought to be, may wish to escape this embarrassment by granting rights to spouses in capacities other than as promisees. They may wish to say, for example, that when John promises God that he will be faithful to Mary, a right is thus conferred not only on God as promisee but also on Mary herself as third-party beneficiary, just as when John contracts with an insurance company and names Mary as his intended beneficiary, she has a right to the accumulated funds after John's death, even though the insurance company made no promise to her. But this seems to be an unnecessarily cumbersome complication contributing nothing to our understanding of the marriage bond. The life insurance transaction is necessarily a three party relation, involving occupants of three distinct offices, no two of whom alone could do the whole job. The transaction, after all, is defined as the purchase by the customer (first office) from the vendor (second office) of protection for a beneficiary (third office) against the customer's untimely death. Marriage, on the other hand, in this our actual world, appears to be a binary relation between a husband and wife, and even though third parties such as children, neighbors, psychiatrists, and priests may sometimes be helpful and even causally necessary for the survival of the relation, they are not logically necessary to our *conception* of the relation, and indeed many married couples do quite well without them. Still, I am not now purporting to describe our actual world, but rather trying to contrast it with a counterpart world of the imagination. In *that* world, it takes three to make almost *any* moral relation and all rights are owned by God or some sovereign under God.

There will, of course, be delegated authorities in the imaginary world, empowered to give commands to their underlings and to punish them for their disobedience. But the commands are all given in the name of the right-monopoly who in turn are the only persons to whom obligations are owed. Hence, even intermediate superiors do not have claim-rights against their subordinates but only legal *powers* to create obligations in the subordinates *to* the monopolistic right-holders, and also the legal *privilege* to impose penalties in the name of that monopoly.

2

So much for the imaginary "world without rights." If some of the moral concepts and practices I have allowed into that world do not sit well with one another, no matter. Imagine Nowheresville with all of these practices if you can, or with any harmonious subset of them, if you prefer. The important thing is not what I've let into it, but what I have kept out. The remainder of this paper will be devoted to an analysis of what precisely a world is missing when it does not contain rights and why that absence is morally important.

The most conspicuous difference, I think, between the Nowheresvillians and ourselves has something to do with the activity of *claiming.* Nowheresvillians, even when they are discriminated against invidiously, or left without the things they need, or otherwise badly treated, do not think to leap to their feet and make righteous demands against one another, though they may not hesitate to resort to force and trickery to get what they want. They have no notion of rights, so they do not have a notion of what is their due; hence they do not claim before they take. The conceptual linkage between personal rights and claiming has long been noticed by legal writers and is reflected in the standard usage in which "claim-rights" are distinguished from the mere liberties, immunities, and powers, also sometimes called "rights," with which they are easily confused. When a person has a legal claim-right to X, it must be the case (i) that he is at liberty in respect to X, i.e., that he has no duty to refrain from or relinquish X, and also (ii) that his liberty is the ground of other people's *duties* to grant him X or not to interfere with him in respect to X. Thus, in the sense of claim-rights, it is true by definition that rights logically entail other people's duties. The paradigmatic examples of such rights are the creditor's right to be paid a debt by his debtor, and the landowner's right not to be interfered with by anyone in the exclusive occupancy of his land. The creditor's right against his debtor, for example, and the debtor's duty to his creditor, are precisely the same relation seen from two different vantage points, as inextricably linked as the two sides of the same coin.

And yet, this is not quite an accurate account of the matter, for it fails to do justice to the way claim-rights are somehow prior to, or more basic than, the duties with which they are necessarily correlated. If Nip has a claim-right against Tuck, it is because of this fact that Tuck has a duty to Nip. It is only because something from Tuck is *due* Nip (directional element) that there is something Tuck *must do* (modal element). This is a relation, moreover, in which Tuck is bound and Nip is free. Nip not only *has* a right, but he can choose whether or not to exercise it, whether to claim it, whether to register complaints upon its infringement, even whether to release Tuck from his duty, and forget the whole thing. If the personal claim-right is also backed up by criminal sanctions, however, Tuck may yet have a duty of obedience to the law from which no one, not even Nip, may release him. He would even have such duties if he lived in Nowheresville; but duties subject to acts of claiming, duties derivative from and contingent upon the personal rights of others, are unknown and undreamed of in Nowheresville.

Many philosophical writers have simply identified rights with claims. The dictionaries tend to define "claims," in turn, as "assertions of right," a dizzying piece of circularity that led one philosopher to complain—"We go in search of rights and are directed to claims, and then back again to rights in bureaucratic futility."[5] What then is the relation between a claim and a right?

As we shall see, a right *is* a kind of claim, and a claim is "an assertion of right," so that a formal definition of either notion in terms of the other will not get us very far. Thus if a "formal definition" of the usual philosophical sort is what we are after, the game is over before it has begun, and we can say that the concept of a right is a "simple, undefinable, unanalysable primitive." Here as elsewhere in philosophy this will have the effect of making the commonplace seem unnecessarily mysterious. We would be better advised, I think, not to attempt a formal definition of either "right" or "claim," but rather to use the idea of a claim in informal elucidation of the idea of a right. This is made possible by the fact that *claiming* is an elaborate sort of rule-governed *activity*. A claim is that which is claimed, the object of the act of claiming. There is, after all, a verb "to claim," but no verb "to right." If we concentrate on the whole activity of claiming, which is public, familiar, and open to our observation, rather than on its upshot alone, we may learn more about the generic nature of rights than we could ever hope to learn from a formal definition, even if one were possible. Moreover, certain facts about rights more easily, if not solely, expressible in the language of claims and claiming are essential to a full understanding not only of what rights are, but also why they are so vitally important.

Let us begin then by distinguishing between: (i) making claim to ..., (ii) claiming that ..., and (iii) having a claim. One sort of thing we may be doing when we claim is to *make claim to something*. This is "to petition or seek by virtue of supposed right; to demand as due." Sometimes this is done by an acknowledged right-holder when he serves notice that he now wants turned over to him that which has already been acknowledged to be his, something borrowed, say, or improperly taken from him. This is often done by turning in a chit, a receipt, an I.O.U., a check, an insurance policy, or a deed, that is, a *title* to something currently in the possession of someone

[5]H. B. Acton, *Op. cit.*

else. On other occasions, making claim is making application for titles or rights themselves, as when a mining prospector stakes a claim to mineral rights, or a householder to a tract of land in the public domain, or an inventor to his patent rights. In the one kind of case, to make claim is to exercise rights one already has by presenting title; in the other kind of case it is to apply for the title itself, by showing that one has satisfied the conditions specified by a rule for the ownership of title and therefore that one can demand it as one's due.

Generally speaking, only the person who has a title or who has qualified for it, or someone speaking in his name, can make claim to something as a matter of right. It is an important fact about rights (or claims), then, that they can be claimed only by those who have them. Anyone can claim, of course, *that* this umbrella is yours, but only you or your representative can actually claim the umbrella. If Smith owes Jones five dollars, only Jones can claim the five dollars as his own, though any bystander can *claim that* it belongs to Jones. One important difference then between *making legal claim to* and *claiming that* is that the former is a legal performance with direct legal consequences whereas the latter is often a mere piece of descriptive commentary with no legal force. Legally speaking, *making claim to* can itself make things happen. This sense of "claiming," then, might well be called "the performative sense." The legal power to claim (performatively) one's right or the things to which one has a right seems to be essential to the very notion of a right. A right to which one could not make claim (i.e., not even for recognition) would be a very "imperfect" right indeed!

Claiming that one has a right (what we can call "propositional claiming" as opposed to "performative claiming") is another sort of thing one can do with language, but it is not the sort of doing that characteristically has legal consequences. To claim that one has rights is to make an assertion that one has them, and to make it in such a manner as to demand or insist that they be recognized. In this sense of "claim" many things in addition to rights can be claimed, that is, many other kinds of proposition can be asserted in the claiming way. I can claim, for example, that you, he, or she has certain rights, or that Julius Caesar once had certain rights; or I can claim that certain statements are true, or that I have certain skills, or accomplishments, or virtually anything at all. I can claim that the earth is flat. What is essential to *claiming that* is the manner of assertion. One can assert without even caring very much whether any one is listening, but part of the point of propositional claiming is to *make sure* people listen. When I claim to others that I know something, for example, I am not merely asserting it, but rather "obtruding my putative knowledge upon their attention, demanding that it be recognized, that appropriate notice be taken of it by those concerned. . . ."[6] Not every truth is properly assertable, much less claimable, in

[6]This is the important difference between rights and mere claims. It is analogous to the difference between *evidence* of guilt (subject to degrees of cogency) and conviction of guilt (which is all or nothing). One can "have evidence" that it is not conclusive just as one can "have a claim" that is not valid. "Prima-facieness" is built into the sense of "claim," but the notion of a "prima-facie right" makes little sense. On the latter point see A. I. Melden, *Rights and Right Conduct* (Oxford: Basil Blackwell, 1959), pp. 18–20, and Herbert Morris, "Persons and Punishment," *The Monist,* Vol. 52 (1968), pp. 498–9.

every context. To claim that something is the case in circumstances that justify no more than calm assertion is to behave like a boor. (This kind of boorishness, I might add, is probably less common in Nowheresville.) But not to claim in the appropriate circumstances that one has a right is to be spiritless or foolish. A list of "appropriate circumstances" would include occasions when one is challenged, when one's possession is denied, or seems insufficiently acknowledged or appreciated; and of course even in these circumstances, the claiming should be done only with an appropriate degree of vehemence.

Even if there are conceivable circumstances in which one would admit rights diffidently, there is no doubt that their characteristic use and that for which they are distinctively well suited, is to be claimed, demanded, affirmed, insisted upon. They are especially sturdy objects to "stand upon," a most useful sort of moral furniture. Having rights, of course, makes claiming possible; but it is claiming that gives rights their special moral significance. This feature of rights is connected in a way with the customary rhetoric about what it is to be a human being. Having rights enables us to "stand up like men," to look others in the eye, and to feel in some fundamental way the equal of anyone. To think of oneself as the holder of rights is not to be unduly but properly proud, to have that minimal self-respect that is necessary to be worthy of the love and esteem of others. Indeed, respect for persons (this is an intriguing idea) may simply be respect for their rights, so that there cannot be the one without the other; and what is called "human dignity" may simply be the recognizable capacity to assert claims. To respect a person then, or to think of him as possessed of human dignity, simply *is* to think of him as a potential maker of claims. Not all of this can be packed into a definition of "rights"; but these are *facts* about the possession of rights that argue well their supreme moral importance. More than anything else I am going to say, these facts explain what is wrong with Nowheresville.

We come now to the third interesting employment of the claiming vocabulary, that involving not the verb "to claim" but the substantive "a claim." What is it to *have a claim* and how is this related to rights? I would like to suggest that *having a claim consists in being in a position to claim, that is, to make claim to* or *claim that.* If this suggestion is correct it shows the primacy of the verbal over the nominative forms. It links claims to a kind of activity and obviates the temptation to think of claims as *things,* on the model of coins, pencils, and other material possessions which we can carry in our hip pockets. To be sure, we often make or establish our claims by presenting titles, and these typically have the form of receipts, tickets, certificates, and other pieces of paper or parchment. The title, however, is not the same thing as the claim; rather it is the evidence that establishes the claim as valid. On this analysis, one might have a claim without ever claiming that to which one is entitled, or without even knowing that one has the claim; for one might simply be ignorant of the fact that one is in a position to claim; or one might be unwilling to exploit that position for one reason or another, including fear that the legal machinery is broken down or corrupt and will not enforce one's claim despite its validity.

Nearly all writers maintain that there is some intimate connection between having a claim and having a right. Some identify right and claim without qualification; some define "right" as justified or justifiable claim, others as recognized claim, still others as valid claim. My own preference is for the latter definition. Some writers, however, reject the identification of rights with valid claims on the ground that all claims as such are valid, so that the expression "valid claim" is redundant. These writers, therefore, would identify rights with claims *simpliciter*. But this is a very simple confusion. All claims, to be sure, are *put forward* as justified, whether they are justified in fact or not. A claim conceded even by its maker to have no validity is not a claim at all, but a mere demand. The highwayman, for example, *demands* his victim's money; but he hardly makes claim to it as rightfully his own.

But it does not follow from this sound point that it is redundant to qualify claims as justified (or as I prefer, valid) in the definition of a right; for it remains true that not all claims put forward as valid really are valid; and only the valid ones can be acknowledged as rights.

If having a valid claim is not redundant, i.e., if it is not redundant to pronounce *another's* claim valid, there must be such a thing as having a claim that is not valid. What would this be like? One might accumulate just enough evidence to argue with relevance and cogency that one has a right (or ought to be granted a right), although one's case might not be overwhelmingly conclusive. In such a case, one might have strong enough argument to be entitled to a hearing and given fair consideration. When one is in this position, it might be said that one "has a claim" that deserves to be weighed carefully. Nevertheless, the balance of reasons may turn out to militate against recognition of the claim, so that the claim, which one admittedly had, and perhaps still does, is not a valid claim or right. "Having a claim" in this sense is an expression very much like the legal phrase "having a *prima facie* case." A plaintiff establishes a *prima facie* case for the defendant's liability when he establishes grounds that will be sufficient for liability unless out-weighed by reasons of a different sort that may be offered by the defendant. Similarly, in the criminal law, a grand jury returns an indictment when it thinks that the prosecution has sufficient evidence to be taken seriously and given a fair hearing, whatever countervailing reasons may eventually be offered on the other side. That initial evidence, serious but not conclusive, it also sometimes called a *prima facie* case. In a parallel "*prima facie* sense" of "claim," having a claim to X is not (yet) the same as having a right to X, but is rather having a case of at least minimal plausibility that one has a right to X, a case that does establish a right, not to X, but to a fair hearing and consideration. Claims, so conceived, differ in degree: some are stronger than others. Rights, on the other hand, do not differ in degree; no one right is more of a right than another.

Another reason for not identifying rights with claims *simply* is that there is a well-established usage in international law that makes a theoreti-cally interesting distinction between claims and rights. Statesmen are some-times led to speak of "claims" when they are concerned with the natural needs of deprived human beings in conditions of scarcity. Young orphans *need* good upbringings, balanced diets, education, and technical training everywhere in the world; but unfortunately there are many places where these goods are in such short supply that it is impossible to provision all who need them. If we persist, nevertheless, in speaking of these needs as constituting rights and not merely claims, we are committed to the conception of a right which is an entitlement *to* some good, but not a valid claim *against* any particular individual; for in conditions of scarcity there may be no determinate individuals who can plausibly be said to have a duty to provide the missing goods to those in need. J. E. S. Fawcett therefore prefers to keep the distinction between claims and rights firmly in mind. "Claims," he writes, "are needs and demands in movement, and there is a continuous transformation, as a society advances [toward greater abundance] of economic and social claims into civil and political rights . . . and not all countries or all claims are by any means at the same stage in the process."[7] The manifesto writers on the other side who seem to identify needs, or at least basic needs, with what they call "human rights," are more properly described, I think, as urging upon the world community the moral principle that *all* basic human needs ought to be recognized as *claims* (in the customary *prima facie* sense) worthy of sympathy and serious consideration right now, even though, in many cases, they cannot yet plausibly be treated as *valid* claims, that is, as grounds of any other people's duties. This way of talking avoids the anomaly of ascribing to all human beings now, even those in pre-industrial societies, such "economic and social rights" as "periodic holidays with pay."[8]

Still, for all of that, I have a certain sympathy with the manifesto writers, and I am even willing to speak of a special "manifesto sense" of "right," in which a right need not be correlated with another's duty. Natural needs are real claims if only upon hypothetical future beings not yet in existence. I accept the moral principle that to have an unfulfilled need is to have a kind of claim against the world, even if against no one in particular. A natural need for some good as such, like a natural desert, is always a reason in support of a claim to that good. A person in need, then, is always "in a position" to make a claim, even when there is no one in the corresponding position to do anything about it. Such claims, based on need alone, are "permanent possibilities of rights," the natural seed from which rights grow. When manifesto writers speak of them as if already actual rights, they are easily forgiven, for this is but a powerful way of expressing the conviction that they ought to be recognized by states here and now as potential rights and consequently as determinants of *present* aspirations and guides to *present* policies. That usage, I think, is a valid exercise of rhetorical licence.

I prefer to characterize rights as valid claims rather than justified ones, because I suspect that justification is rather too broad a qualification. "Validity," as I understand it, is justification of a peculiar and narrow kind, namely justification within a system of rules. A man has a legal right when the official

[7] J. E. S. Fawcett, "The International Protection of Human Rights," in *Political Theory and the Rights of Man,* ed. by D. D. Raphael (Bloomington: Indiana University Press, 1967), pp. 125 and 128.

[8] As declared in Article 24 of *The Universal Declaration of Human Rights* adopted on December 10, 1948, by the General Assembly of the United Nations.

recognition of his claim (as valid) is called for by the governing rules. This definition, of course, hardly applies to moral rights, but that is not because the genus of which moral rights are a species is something other than *claims*. A man has a moral right when he has a claim the recognition of which is called for—not (necessarily) by legal rules—but by moral principles, or the principles of an enlightened conscience.

There is one final kind of attack on the generic identification of rights with claims, and it has been launched with great spirit in a recent article by H. J. McCloskey, who holds that rights are not essentially claims at all, but rather entitlements. The springboard of his argument is his insistence that rights in their essential character are always *rights to,* not *rights against:*

> My right to life is not a right against anyone. It is my right and by virtue of it, it is normally permissible for me to sustain my life in the face of obstacles. It does give rise to rights against others *in the sense* that others have or may come to have duties to refrain from killing me, but it is essentially a right of mine, not an infinite list of claims, hypothetical and actual, against an infinite number of actual, potential, and as yet nonexistent human beings. . . . Similarly, the right of the tennis club member to play on the club courts is a right to play, not a right against some vague group of potential or possible obstructors.[9]

The argument seems to be that since rights are essentially rights *to,* whereas claims are essentially claims *against,* rights cannot be claims, though they can be grounds for claims. The argument is doubly defective though. First of all, contrary to McCloskey, rights (at least legal claim-rights) *are* held *against* others. McCloskey admits this in the case of *in personam* rights (what he calls "special rights") but denies it in the case of *in rem* rights (which he calls "general rights"):

> Special rights are sometimes against specific individuals or institutions—e.g., rights created by promises, contracts, etc. . . . but these differ from . . . characteristic . . . general rights where the right is simply a right to . . .[10]

As far as I can tell, the only reason McCloskey gives for denying that *in rem* rights are against others is that those against whom they would have to hold make up an enormously multitudinous and "vague" group, including hypothetical people not yet even in existence. Many others have found this a paradoxical consequence of the notion of *in rem* rights, but I see nothing troublesome in it. If a general rule gives me a right of noninterference in a certain respect against everybody, then there are literally hundreds of milllions of people who have a duty toward me in that respect; and if the same general rule gives the same right to everyone else, then it imposes on me literally hundreds of millions of duties—or duties towards hundreds of millions of people. I see nothing paradoxical about this, however. The duties, after all, are negative; and I can discharge all of them at a stroke

[9]H. J. McCloskey, "Rights," *Philosophical Quarterly,* Vol. 15 (1965), p. 118.
[10]*Loc. cit.*

simply by minding my own business. And if all human beings make up one moral community and there are hundreds of millions of human beings, we should expect there to be hundreds of millions of moral relations holding between them.

McCloskey's other premise is even more obviously defective. There is no good reason to think that all *claims* are "essentially" *against*, rather than *to*. Indeed most of the discussion of claims above has been of claims *to*, and as we have seen, the law finds it useful to recognize claims *to* (or "mere claims") that are not yet qualified to be claims *against*, or rights (except in a "manifesto sense" of "rights").

Whether we are speaking of claims or rights, however, we must notice that they seem to have two dimensions, as indicated by the prepositions "to" and "against," and it is quite natural to wonder whether either of these dimensions is somehow more fundamental or essential than the other. All rights seem to merge *entitlements to* do, have, omit, or be something with *claims against* others to act or refrain from acting in certain ways. In some statements of rights the entitlement is perfectly determinate (e.g., *to* play tennis) and the claim vague (e.g., *against* "some vague group of potential or possible obstructors"); but in other cases the object of the claim is clear and determinate (e.g., *against* one's parents), and the entitlement general and indeterminate (e.g., to be given a proper upbringing.) If we mean by "entitlement" that *to* which one has a right and by "claim" something directed at those *against* whom the right holds (as McCloskey apparently does), then we can say that all claim-rights necessarily involve both, though in individual cases the one element or the other may be in sharper focus.

In brief conclusion: To have a right is to have a claim against someone whose recognition as valid is called for by some set of governing rules or moral principles. To have a *claim* in turn, is to have a case meriting consideration, that is, to have reasons or grounds that put one in a position to engage in performative and propositional claiming. The activity of claiming, finally, as much as any other thing, makes for self-respect and respect for others, gives a sense to the notion of personal dignity, and distinguishes this otherwise morally flawed world from the even worse world of Nowheresville.

From "Socialized Medicine"

Henry E. Sigerist

In a report published last year by the American Foundation, a professor of medicine in a grade A medical school in the Middle West, member of the Association of American Physicians, wrote: "I do not believe that a patient is entitled to free medical service any more than he is entitled to free

Reprinted with permission from *The Yale Review* 27:3, 463–81, Spring 1938. Copyright Yale University Press.

housing, free clothing, and free feeding." In other words: if a society is unable to provide work for all its members, it is perfectly normal for the unemployed to be evicted from his home and to run around naked, sick, and starving. Such a view is not only barbaric but it is utterly foolish. Nobody seriously believes that any group of unemployed American workers would sit down quietly and wait for death to relieve them. They would kick before they starved, and any government that shared the professor's view would be overthrown at the first major economic crisis.

If our professor's statement represented the general view of American society, there would be no reason for discussing our present system of medical care. Medical service then would be a commodity sold on the market to whoever could afford to purchase it. American society, however, like any other civilized society, feels differently in the matter. It has come to realize that a highly specialized modern industrial nation cannot function normally if its members are sick and that it is a wasteful burden to carry a large number of sick and half sick people. The propertied class, moreover, knows very well that a diseased working class is a menace to its own health. Tuberculosis to-day is largely confined to the low income groups, but venereal diseases have not yet learned to respect class barriers.

Most people agree that it is in the interest of society to fight disease and to provide medical care for the whole population regardless of the economic status of the individual. This is, to begin with, a purely practical and utilitarian consideration. Our attitude, however, is also influenced by humanitarian motives. After all, some of the humanitarian ideals of the nineteenth century are still alive. Every society has many thousands of perfectly useless members, mostly feeble-minded and mentally diseased people who will never be able to work and will never contribute anything to society. And yet we do not destroy them. We consider them unfortunate fellow citizens. We feed them, nurse them, try to provide tolerable living conditions for them, hoping that science, some day, will give us sufficient data to allow us to reduce their number.

There are people to-day—their number is increasing—who think that man has a right to health. The chief cause of disease is poverty. If we are unable to provide work for everybody and to guarantee a decent standard of living to every individual willing to work, whatever his intelligence may be, we are collectively responsible for the chief cause of disease. The least we can do is to make provisions for the protection and restoration of the people's health. They have an undeniable right to such provisions.

Once we accept the principle that medical care must be available to all, we must examine whether the people actually receive the services they need, under the present system. There are still doctors who pretend quite ingenuously that there is not one man in the United States who could not get medical care in case of illness if he took the trouble to ask for it. They point out proudly that our hospitals have charity wards and that the medical profession, conscious of its humanitarian traditions, has always been ready to help the poor without remuneration.

Nobody will deny the good will and idealism of the medical profession. It has made desperate efforts to remain a liberal profession and has refused steadily but in vain to be dragged into business, into a competitive world that is ruled by iron economic necessities. The doctors are not responsible for the fact that the social and economic structure of society has changed. They did the best they could and kept to the job under increasingly adverse conditions. Their good will and idealism are still wanted, more than ever before; not for charity services, however, but to enable them to face the present conditions with an open mind and courageously, and to cooperate in their readjustment.

Long before the depression, it was felt that medicine had infinitely more to give than the people actually received. At the height of prosperity, in 1928, the Committee on the Costs of Medical Care was appointed to survey conditions. Whoever looked around without prejudice saw people, many people, who had not sufficient medical care. We all knew families whose budget was wrecked by a sudden illness, and we all had friends who hesitated to enter a hospital or to undergo certain treatments because they could not afford them. The many reports of the Committee on the Costs of Medical Care gave us facts and figures for what we vaguely knew, and demonstrated unmistakably that large sections of our population lacked adequate medical care.

If any doubts are left, they will be dispelled by the results of the National Health Survey that was undertaken by the United States Public Health Service as a W.P.A. project. From preliminary reports we already know that the lower a family's income is, the higher is the incidence of disease and the smaller the volume of medical care received. We know that hundreds of thousands of cases of illness are needless and could have been prevented, that many thousands of people die prematurely; and we also know that one-third of the population of this wealthy country is not only ill-fed, ill-housed, and ill-clothed, but also ill-cared for in sickness.

The facts that have become known as a result of the various surveys are so overwhelming that even the American Medical Association could not ignore them and had to admit recently that "a varying number of people may at times be insufficiently supplied with medical service."

The present conditions are not only most depressing and harmful to society but also unnecessary and stupid in a country that has such splendid medical equipment. No country in the world has a better standard of physicians, public health officers, nurses, and social workers; no country has better hospital or laboratory facilities. It is almost a miracle how the United States in less than half a century caught up with European medicine and surpassed it in many respects. Accumulated wealth and the wisdom of a group of medical leaders made it possible. And yet, one-third of the population has no medical service or not enough, and great possibilities of preventive medicine have not even been considered yet.

The cause of this maladjustment is easy to guess. Medical service, as a result of the progress of medicine, has become increasingly expensive. A hundred years ago a man with an indefinite pain in his belly went to see a doctor who asked a few questions, palpated the abdomen, and prescribed a laxative. The procedure did not cost much. Most people could afford the fee, or if they were totally indigent they were given the advice free of charge.

In most such cases, the patient recovered as he probably would have done without consulting a doctor. In some cases, however, a tumor possibly developed from which the patient died.

The same type of patient consulting a doctor to-day has a series of X-ray pictures and a number of laboratory tests made which may lead to the early recognition of a disease at a time when successful treatment is still possible. It is obvious, however, that such an examination, not to mention the treatment, costs money, more than most people can afford to pay at the time.

In other words, it is not only difficult for the indigent to secure for himself adequate medical care, but for all families of moderate income, all those whose income does not exceed $3,000 or even more. This, however, means more than three quarters of the entire population. The fee-for-service system may have worked—I doubt if it ever did—as long as medicine had little to give. Today it is impossible to protect the people's health effectively under any such system because there is too wide a gap between the scientific status of medicine and the economic status of the population. Therefore, if we think that the people's health is a major concern of society, we must necessarily devise some other system.

From "The Right to Health"

Thomas S. Szasz

WHEN IS INEQUALITY INEQUITY?

In every society—whether it be tribal or industrial, theologic or secular, capitalist or communist—goods and services are distributed unequally. This is, in fact, what words such as "rich" and "poor" really mean; it is their operational definition: The rich "have," and the poor "have not." The "haves" eat more nutritious food, dwell in more comfortable and spacious homes, and travel by means of more luxurious transportation than do the "have nots." Similar differences exist between the same persons and groups with respect to medical care. When the rich man falls ill, he occupies a hospital bed in a single room or private suite and receives treatment from the best—or, at least, the most expensive—physicians in town. When the poor man falls ill, he occupies a bed in the charity ward (though it may no longer be called that) and receives treatment from young men who, though called "doctors," are only medical students: In short, while it is not a disgrace to be poor, it is not a great honor either.

Although it is self-evident that the poor will always have more needs than the rich, and the rich more satisfactions than the poor, this fact is now

Reprinted with permission of author and publisher from *Georgetown Law Journal* 57, 734–751, 1969.

repeatedly rediscovered and denounced by psychiatric epidemiologists. For example, Ernest Gruenberg has stated that there is in our society "a pattern in which the prevalence of illness is an inverse function of family income, while the volume of medical care received is a direct function of family income."[1] In plain English, this means that poverty begets sickness, while affluence begets medical attention. The same statement, of course, could be made about every other important human need and satisfaction. An example of this would be: To earn a living, a poor man has a greater need for transportation than does a rich man, who could stay at home and live off his investments; yet, the former must do with the inferior public transportation system provided by the community, whereas the latter enjoys a fleet of private cars, boats, and airplanes. Such considerations do not deter Gruenberg and the many other physicians addressing themselves to this subject from observing plaintively and, I think, rather naively that "one may doubt . . . [that] efforts to redistribute medical care have eliminated the paradox." But there is no paradox, except, that is, in the eyes of the utopian social reformer who views all social differences as contagious diseases waiting to be wiped out by his therapeutic efforts.

The concept that medical treatment is a right rather than a privilege has gained increasing acceptance during the past decade. Its advocates are no doubt motivated by good intentions; they wish to correct certain inequalities existent in the distribution of health services in American society. That such inequalities exist is not in dispute. What is in dispute, however, is how to distinguish between inequalities and inequities,[2] and how to determine which governmental policies are best suited to the securing of good medical care for the maximum number of persons.

The desire to improve the lot of less fortunate people is laudable; indeed, I share this desire. Still, unless all inequalities are considered inequities—a view clearly incompatible with social organization and human life as we now know it—two important questions remain. First, which inequalities should be considered inequities? Second, what are the most appropriate means for minimizing or abolishing the inequalities we deem "unjust"? Appeals to good intentions are of no help in answering these questions.

There are two groups of people whose conditions with respect to medical care the advocates of a right to treatment regard as especially unfair or unjust, and whose situations they seek to ameliorate. One is the poor, who need ordinary medical care; the other group is composed of the inmates of public mental hospitals presumably in need of psychiatric care. The proposition, however, that poor people ought to have access to more, bet-

[1]Gruenberg, Book Review, 161 *Science* 347 (1968).

[2]Since the French Revolution, and increasingly during the past century, virtually all Western governments have fostered the belief that not only great inequalities of wealth, but also inequalities of all kinds—ambition, talent, and, of course, health—*are* inequities. The result has been described with unmatched irony by C. S. Lewis: "Men are not angered by mere misfortune but by misfortune conceived as injury. And the sense of injury depends on the feeling that a legitimate claim has been denied. The more claims on life, therefore, that your patient can be induced to make, the more often he will feel injured and, as a result, ill-tempered." C. S. Lewis, *The Screwtape Letters & Screwtape Proposes a Toast* 106 (1961).

ter, or less expensive medical care than they now do and that people in public mental hospitals ought to receive better psychiatric care than they now do pose two quite different problems. I shall, therefore, deal with each separately.

The availability of medical services for a particular person, or group of persons, in a particular society depends principally upon the supply of the services desired and the prospective user's power to command these services. No government or organization—whether it be the United States Government, the American Medical Association, or the Communist Party of the Soviet Union—can provide medical care, except to the degree it has the power to control the education of physicians, their right to practice medicine, and the manner in which they dispose of their time and energies. In other words, only individuals can provide medical treatment for the sick; institutions, such as the Church and the State, can promote, permit, or prohibit certain therapeutic activities but cannot by themselves provide medical services.

Social groups wielding power are notoriously prone, of course, to prohibit the free exercise of certain human skills and the availability of certain drugs and devices. For example, during the declining Middle Ages and the early Renaissance Period, the Church repeatedly prohibited Jewish physicians from practicing medicine and non-Jewish patients from seeking the former's services. The same prohibition was imposed by the Government of Nazi Germany. In the modern democracies of the free West, the State continues to exercise its prerogative to prohibit individuals from engaging in certain kinds of therapeutic activities. This prohibition is, to be sure, not on religious grounds, but rather because they are untrained or inadequately trained as physicians. This situation is an inevitable consequence of the fact that the State's licensing powers fulfill two unrelated and mutually incompatible functions: (1) to protect the public, *i.e.*, the actual or potential patients, from incompetent medical practitioners by ensuring an adequate level of training and competence on the part of all physicians; and (2) to protect the members of a special vested interest group, the physicians, from competition from an excessive number of similarly trained practitioners and from healers of different persuasions and skills who might prove more useful to their would-be clients than those officially approved. The result is a complex and powerful alliance—first between the Church and medicine, and subsequently, between State and medicine—with physicians playing double roles, both as medical healers and as agents of social control. This restrictive function of the State with respect to medical practice has been, and continues to be, especially significant in the United States.

Without delving further into the intricacies of this large and complex subject, it should suffice to note that our present system of medical training and practice is far removed from that of laissez-faire capitalism for which many, especially its opponents, mistake it. In actuality, the American Medical Association is not only an immensely powerful lobby of medical-vested interests—a force that liberal societies generally oppose—but it is also a state-protected monopoly, in effect a covert arm of the government—a force that the same reformers ardently support. The result of this alliance between organized medicine and the American Government has been the creation of a system of education and licensure with strict controls over the production and distribution of health care, which leads to an artificially created chronic shortage of medical personnel. This result has been achieved by limiting the number of students to be trained in medicine through the regulation of medical education and by limiting the number of practitioners through the regulation of medical licensure.

A basic economic precept is that when the supply of a given service is smaller than the demand for it, we have a seller's market. This is obviously beneficial for the sellers—in this case, the medical profession. Conversely, when the supply is greater than the demand, we have a buyer's market. This is beneficial for the buyers—in this case, the potential patients. One way—and, according to the supporters of a free market economy, the best way—to help buyers get more of what they want at the lowest possible price is to increase the supply of the needed product or service. This would suggest that instead of government grants for special Neighborhood Healing Centers and Community Mental Health Centers, the medical needs of the less affluent members of American society could be better served simply by repealing laws governing medical licensure. As logical as this may seem, in medical and liberal circles this suggestion is regarded as "hairbrained," or worse.[3]

Since medical care in the United States is in short supply, its availability to the poor may be improved by redistributing the existing supply, by increasing the supply, or by both. Many individuals and groups clamoring for an improvement in our medical care system fail to scrutinize this artificially created shortage of medical personnel and to look to a free market economy for restoration of the balance between demand and supply. Instead, they seek to remedy the imbalance by redistributing the existing supply—in effect, robbing Peter to pay Paul. This proposal is in the tradition of other modern liberal social reforms, such as the redistribution of wealth by progressive taxation and a system of compulsory social security. No doubt, a political and economic system more socialistic in character than the one we now have could promote an equalization in the quality of the health care received by rich and poor. Whether this would result in the quality of the medical care of the poor approximating that of the rich, or vice versa,

---

[3]For an excellent discussion of the deleterious effects of professional licensure requirements, see M. Friedman, *Capitalism and Freedom* 137–60 (1962). Friedman correctly recognizes that the justification for enacting special licensure provisions, especially for regulating medical practice, "is always said to be the necessity of protecting the public interest. However, the pressure on the legislature to license an occupation rarely comes from the members of the public. . . . On the contrary, the pressure invariably comes from members of the occupation itself." *Id.* at 140.

Unless one believes in the unique altruism of physicians, for which, it may be noted, there is no evidence, the conclusion is inescapable that the actual aim of restrictive licensure laws—as compared to the certification of a special competence of persons, such as mathematicians or physicists, which carries no implication of legal restraints on others not so certified —is the very opposite of their ostensible or professed aim. Under the pretense of protecting the public from incompetent practitioners, licensing laws protect the medical profession from the competition of other vendors of desired services and from the scrutiny of the enlightened public.

would remain to be seen. Experience suggests the latter. For over a century, we have had our version of state-supported psychiatric care for all who need it: the state mental hospitals system. The results of this effort are available for all to see. . . .

As my foregoing remarks indicate, I see two fundamental defects in the concept of a right to treatment. The first is scientific and medical, stemming from unclarified issues concerning what constitutes an illness or treatment and who qualifies as a patient or physician. The other is political and moral, stemming from unclarified issues concerning the differences between rights and claims.

In the present state of medical practice and popular opinion, definitions of the terms "illness," "treatment," "physician," and "patient" are so imprecise that a concept of a right to treatment can only serve to further muddy an already very confused situation. One example will illustrate what I mean.

One can "treat," in the medical sense of this term, only a disease, or, more precisely, only a person, now called a "patient," suffering from a disease. But what is a disease? Certainly, cancer, stroke, and heart disease are. But is obesity a disease? How about smoking cigarettes? Using heroin or marijuana? Malingering to avoid the draft or collect insurance compensation? Homosexuality? Kleptomania? Grief? Each one of these conditions has been declared a disease by medical and psychiatric authorities who hold impeccable institutional credentials. Furthermore, innumerable other conditions, varying from bachelorhood and divorce to political and religious prejudices, have been so termed.

Similarly, what is treatment? Certainly, the surgical removal of a cancerous breast is. But is an organ transplant treatment? If it is, and if such treatment is a right, how can those charged with guaranteeing people the protection of their right to treatment discharge their duties without having access to the requisite number of transplantable organs? On a simpler level, if ordinary obesity, due to eating too much, is a disease, how can a doctor treat it when its treatment depends on the patient eating less? What does it mean, then, that a patient has a right to be treated for obesity? I have already alluded to the facility with which this kind of right becomes equated with a societal and medical obligation to deprive the patient of his freedom —to eat, to drink, to take drugs, and so forth.

Who is a patient? Is he one who has a demonstrable bodily illness or injury, such as cancer or a fracture? A person who complains of bodily symptoms, but has no demonstrable illness, like the so-called "hypochondriac"? The person who feels perfectly well but is said to be ill by others, for example, the paranoid schizophrenic? Or is he a person, such as Senator Barry Goldwater, who professes political views differing from those of the psychiatrist who brands him insane?

Finally, who is a physician? Is he a person licensed to practice medicine? One certified to have completed a specified educational curriculum? One possessing certain medical skills as demonstrated by public performance? Or is he one claiming to possess such skills?

It seems to me that improvement in the health care of poor people and those now said to be mentally ill depends less on declarations about their rights to treatment and more on certain reforms in the language and conduct of those professing a desire to help them. In particular, such reforms must entail refinements in the use of medical concepts, such as illness and treatment, and a recognition of the basic differences between medical intervention as a service, which the individual is free to seek or reject, and medical intervention as a method of social control, which is imposed on him by force or fraud.

I can perhaps best illustrate this unsolved dilemma by citing some actual cases. As recently as 1965, a Connecticut statute made it a crime for any person to artificially prevent conception. Accordingly, a mother of ten requesting contraceptive help from a physician in a public hospital in Connecticut would have been refused this assistance. Did what she seek constitute "treatment"? Not according to the legislators who defined the prescription of birth control devices as immoral and illegal acts, rather than as interventions aimed at preserving health.

Today, a similar situation exists with respect to a woman's unwanted pregnancy and her wish for an abortion. Is being pregnant, when one does not want to be, an illness? Is an abortion a treatment? Or is it murder of the fetus? If it is murder, why is no "abortionist" ever prosecuted for murder? How can the preservation of a pregnant woman's mental health justify such murder, now called "therapeutic abortion"?

On the other hand, should a wholly secular, utilitarian point of view prevail, and the use of birth control devices and abortion be considered treatments, what would it mean for a woman to have a right to such interventions? Clearly, it would result in her having unhampered access to physicians willing to both prescribe birth control devices and perform abortions. Where would such a medico-legal posture leave a Roman Catholic obstetrician? By refusing to abort a woman wishing a termination of her pregnancy, he would be interfering with her right to treatment in a way that might be analogized to a white barber's refusing to cut the hair of a black customer, or vice versa, thus, interfering with his customer's civil rights.

As still another example, consider the situation of an unhappily married couple. Are they sick? If they define themselves as having a "neurotic marriage" and consult a psychiatrist, they would be considered sick and their insurance coverage might even pay for their treatment. But if they seek the solution of the problem in divorce and consult an attorney, they would not be considered sick. Thus, although unhappily married people are often considered "ill," divorce is never considered a treatment. If it were, it too would have to be a right. Where would that leave our present divorce laws?

One could go on and on. I shall cite, however, only one more instance —the practice of involuntary mental hospitalization—to show how deeply confused and confusing is our present situation with respect to the concept of treatment; and hence how very mischievous any extension of this concept, as a right secured by the government, is bound to be.

In most jurisdictions, persons said to be mentally ill and dangerous to themselves or others may be committed to a mental hospital. Such incarceration in a building called a "hospital" is considered a form of psychiatric, and hence medical, treatment. But who, in fact, is the patient? Who is being treated? Ostensibly, the person treated is the one who is incarcerated. But since he did not seek medical assistance, whereas those who secured his confinement did, one might argue that involuntary mental hospitalization is treatment for those who seek commitment, rather than for those who are committed. This would be analogous to arguing that a "therapeutic abortion" is a treatment for the pregnant woman, not for the aborted fetus—an assertion few would deny. If this argument is accepted, then, in any conflict, an injury to one party could be defined as a treatment to his opponent. The following recent statement on the psychiatric treatment of "acting-out adolescents" is illustrative: "The move toward 'freedom, love, peace' has encouraged anti-social acting out, including the increasing use of marijuana and psychedelic drugs. Consequently, emotionally disturbed young men who are acting in a way that directly conflicts with their parents' standards are being hospitalized in increasing numbers."[4] In this sort of situation, whose right to treatment do the advocates of this concept wish to guarantee —that of the parent to commit his rebellious son as mentally ill or that of the child to defy his parents without being subjected to quasi-medical penalties?

THE DISTINCTION BETWEEN "RIGHTS" AND "CLAIMS"

The second difficulty which the concept of a right to treatment poses is of a political and moral nature. It stems from confusing "rights" with "claims," and protection from injuries with provision for goods or services.

For a definition of right, I can do no better than to quote John Stuart Mill: "I have treated the idea of a right as *residing in the injured person and violated by the injury. . . .* When we call anything a person's right, we mean that he has a valid claim on society to protect him in the possession of it, either by force of law, or by that of education and opinion. . . . To have a right, then, is, I conceive, to have something which *society ought to defend me in the possession of.*"[5]

This helps us distinguish rights from claims. Rights, Mill says, are "possessions"; they are things people have by nature, like liberty; acquire by dint of hard work, like property; create by inventiveness, like a new machine; or inherit, like money. Characteristically, possessions are what a person *has,* and of which others, including the State, can therefore deprive him. Mill's point is the classic libertarian one: The State should protect the individual in his rights. This is what the Declaration of Independence means when it refers to the inalienable rights to life, liberty and the pursuit of happiness. It is important to note that, in political theory, no less than in everyday practice, this requires that the State be strong and resolute enough to protect the rights of the individual from infringement by others and that it be decentralized and restrained enough, typically through federalism and a constitution, to insure that it will not itself violate the rights of its people.

In the sense specified above, then, there can be no such thing as a right

[4]Krinsky & Jennings, *The Management and Treatment of Acting-Out Adolescents in a Separate Unit,* 19 *Hosp. & Community Psychiatry* 72 (1968).

[5]J. S. Mill, *Utilitarianism* 78–79 (1863) (emphasis added).

to treatment. Conceiving of a person's body as his possession—like his automobile or watch (though, no doubt, more valuable)—it is just as nonsensical to speak of his right to have his body repaired as it would be to speak of his right to have his automobile or watch repaired.

It is thus evident that in its current usage and especially in the phrase "right to treatment" the term "right" actually means claim. More specifically, "right" here means the recognition of the claims of one party, considered to be *in the right,* and the repudiation of the claims of another, opposing party, considered to be *in the wrong*—the "rightful" party having allied himself with the interests of the community and having enlisted the coercive powers of the State on his behalf. Let us analyze this situation in the case of medical treatment for an ordinary bodily disease. The patient, having lost some of his health, tries to regain it by means of medical attention and drugs. The medical attention he needs is, however, the property of his physician, and the drug he needs is the property of the manufacturer who produced it. The patient's right to treatment thus conflicts with the physician's right to liberty, *i.e.,* to sell his services freely, and the pharmaceutical manufacturer's rights in his own property, *i.e.,* to sell his products as he chooses. The advocates of a right to treatment for the patient are less than candid regarding their proposals for reconciling this proposed right with the right of the physician to liberty and that of the pharmaceutical manufacturer to property.

Nor is it clear how the right to treatment concept can be reconciled with the traditional Western concept of the patient's right to choose his physician. If the patient has a right to choose the doctor by whom he wishes to be treated, and if he *also* has a right to treatment, then, in effect, the doctor is the patient's slave. Obviously, the patient's right to choose his physician cannot be wrenched from its context and survive; its corollary is the physician's right to accept or reject a patient, except for rare cases of emergency treatment. No one, of course, envisions the absurdity of physicians being at the personal beck and call of individual patients, becoming literally their medical slaves, as some had been in ancient Greece and Rome.

The concept of a right to treatment has a different, much less absurd but far more ominous, implication. For just as the corollary of the individual's freedom to choose his physician is the physician's freedom to refuse to treat any particular patient, so the corollary of the individual's right to treatment is the denial of the physician's right to reject, as a patient, anyone officially so designated. This transformation removes, in one fell swoop, the individual's right to define himself as sick and to seek medical care as he sees fit, and the physician's right to define whom he considers sick and wishes to treat; it places these decisions instead in the hands of the State's medical bureaucracy. To see how this works in the United States on a less-than-total scale and coexisting with a flourishing system of private medical practice, one need only to look at our state mental hospitals. Every patient admitted to such a hospital has a right to treatment, and every physician serving in this hospital system has an obligation to treat each patient assigned to him by his superiors or committed to his care by the courts. Missing from this system, and similar systems, are the patient's traditional economic and legal controls over the medical relationship and the physician's traditional economic dependence on, and legal obligations to, the individual he has accepted for treatment.

As a result, bureaucratic care, as contrasted with its entrepreneurial counterpart, ceases to be a system of healing the sick and instead becomes a system of controlling the deviant. Although this outcome seems to be inevitable in the case of psychiatry (in view of the fact that ascription of the label "mental illness" so often functions as a quasi-medical rhetoric concealing social conflicts), it need not be inevitable for nonpsychiatric medical services. However, in every situation where medical care is provided bureaucratically, as in communist societies, the physician's role as agent of the sick patient is necessarily alloyed with, and often seriously compromised by, his role as agent of the State. Thus, the doctor becomes a kind of medical policeman—at times helping the individual, and at times harming him.

Returning to Mill's definition of a "right," one could say, further, that just as a man has a right to life and liberty, so, too, has he a right to health and, hence, a claim on the State to protect his health. It is important to note here that the right to health differs from the right to treatment in the same way as the right to property differs from the right to theft. Recognition of a right to health would obligate the State to prevent individuals from depriving each other of their health, just as recognition of the two other rights now prevents each individual from depriving every other individual of liberty and property. It would also obligate the State to respect the health of the individual and to deprive him of that asset only in accordance with due process of law, just as it now respects the individual's liberty and property and deprives him of them only in accordance with due process of law.

As matters now stand, the State not only fails to protect the individual's health, but it actually hinders him in his efforts to safeguard his own health, as in the case of its permitting industries to befoul the waters we drink and the air we breathe. The State similarly prohibits individuals from obtaining medical care from certain officially "unqualified," experts and from buying and ingesting certain, officially "dangerous," drugs. Sometimes, the State even deliberately deprives the individual of treatment under the very guise of providing treatment.[6]

[6]The following is an illustrative example. In June 1968, the Santa Monica Synanon center was raided by agents of the California Narcotic Authority. Two of the residents were removed for tests to determine if they were "clean." This interference with their voluntary effort to break the narcotics habit in accordance with the Synanon principles was lawful inasmuch as the persons arrested were parolees from California's Narcotic Rehabilitation Center at Corona, and as such, subject to periodic surprise testing by state authorities. On the advice of Synanon lawyers, the defendants refused to take the test. Their paroles were thereupon revoked, and they were recommitted to the Corona facility to serve out the full terms of their "psychiatric sentence." TIME, July 12, 1968, at 74.

The relapse rate of addicts treated at rehabilitation centers such as Corona is approximately 90%, whereas for those treated at Synanon, it is 20%. It can hardly be said, then, that the two patients, over whose abstinence from narcotics the State of California appears to have shown such touching solicitude, were being guaranteed their right to treatment at Corona, though such no doubt would be the official interpretation of their fate. In a larger sense, this is also an instance of the bureaucratic perversion of language which Orwell so eloquently described. To his lexicon of Newspeak, in which "war" means "peace" and "slavery" means "freedom," we may add "punishment" to mean "treatment." G. ORWELL. 1984, at 6 (1949).

To be sure, there are good reasons, in an age in which the powerful, centralized State is idolized as the source of all benefits, why the concept of a right to treatment is considered progressive and is popular, and why the concept of a right to health has, so far as I know, never even been articulated, much less recognized by legislators and the courts. On the one hand, recognition of a right to health, rather than to treatment, would impose greater obligations on the State to insure domestic peace, especially the protection of an individual's health as a type of private property; on the other hand, it would impose greater restraints on its own powers vis-à-vis the citizen, especially on its jurisdiction over the licensure of physicians and the dispensing of drugs. These would require a government to shoulder greater responsibilities for its duties as policeman, while limiting its alleged responsibilities for dispensing services—in short, the very antithesis of the type of State which modern liberal social reformers consider desirable and necessary for the attainment of their goals. Instead of fostering the independent judgment of the individual, such reformers encourage his submission to an ostensibly competent and benevolent authority; hence, they project the image of the medical therapist unto the State, while casting the citizen in the complementary role of sick patient. This, of course, places the individual in precisely that inferior and submissive role vis-à-vis the government from which the founding fathers sought, by means of the Constitution, to rescue him. Politically, the right to treatment is thus simply the right to submit to authority—a right which has always been dear both to those in power and those incapable of managing their own lives.

The State can protect and promote the interests of its sick, or potentially sick, citizens in one of only two ways: either by coercing physicians, and other medical and paramedical personnel, to serve patients—as State-owned slaves in the last analysis[7]—or by creating economic, moral, and political circumstances favorable to a plentiful supply of competent physicians and effective drugs.

The former solution corresponds to and reflects efforts to solve human problems by recourse to the all-powerful State. The rights promised by such a state—exemplified by the right to treatment—are not opportunities for uncoerced choices by individuals, but rather are powers vested in the State for the subjection of the interests of one group to those of another.

The latter solution corresponds to, and reflects efforts to, solve human problems by recourse to individual initiative and voluntary associations without interference by the State. The rights exacted from such a State—exemplified by the rights to life, liberty, and health—are limitations on its own powers and sphere of action and provide the conditions necessary for,

[7]The position of the physician in Czechoslovakia is illustrative. "The constitution [of Czechoslovakia] declares that health care is a right of the people and that it is the duty of the state to satisfy that right." In practice, this "right" is assured through the "assignment [by the Communist State] of a low economic (productive) status to the health services. . . . A skilled factory worker may earn much more than a doctor through premium pay. Even a taxi driver may earn more than a doctor. . . . Almost universal was the comment: 'We are not attracting the best people into medicine.' " Cooper, *Czechoslovakia Reflects Regional Plan Problems,* Hospital Tribune, Sept. 9, 1968, at 1, col. 1.

but of course do not insure the proper exercise of, free and responsible individual choices.

In these two solutions we recognize the fundamental polarities of the great ideological conflicts of our age, perhaps of all ages and of the human condition itself, namely, individualism and capitalism on the one side, collectivism and communism on the other. *Tertium non datur:* There is no other choice.

From "Medical Care as a Right: A Refutation"

Robert M. Sade

The current debate on health care in the United States is of the first order of importance to the health professions, and of no less importance to the political future of the nation, for precedents are now being set that will be applied to the rest of American society in the future. In the enormous volume of verbiage that has poured forth, certain fundamental issues have been so often misrepresented that they have now become commonly accepted fallacies. This paper will be concerned with the most important of these misconceptions, that health care is a right, as well as a brief consideration of some of its corollary fallacies.

RIGHTS—MORALITY AND POLITICS

The concept of rights has its roots in the moral nature of man and its practical expression in the political system that he creates. Both morality and politics must be discussed before the relation between political rights and health care can be appreciated.

A "right" defines a freedom of action. For instance, a right to a material object is the uncoerced choice of the use to which that object will be put; a right to a specific action, such as free speech, is the freedom to engage in that activity without forceful repression. The moral foundation of the rights of man begins with the fact that he is a living creature: he has the right to his own life. All other rights are corollaries of this primary one; without the right to life, there can be no others, and the concept of rights itself becomes meaningless.

The freedom to live, however, does not automatically ensure life. For man, a specific course of action is required to sustain his life, a course of action that must be guided by reason and reality and has as its goal the

Reprinted with permission of author and publisher from *The New England Journal of Medicine* 285:23, 1288–92, December 2, 1971. Copyright, Massachusetts Medical Society.

creation or acquisition of material values, such as food and clothing, and intellectual values, such as self-esteem and integrity. His moral system is the means by which he is able to select the values that will support his life and achieve his happiness.

Man must maintain a rather delicate homeostasis in a highly demanding and threatening environment, but has at his disposal a unique and efficient mechanism for dealing with it: his mind. His mind is able to perceive, to identify percepts, to integrate them into concepts, and to use those concepts in choosing actions suitable to the maintenance of his life. The rational function of mind is volitional, however; a man must *choose* to think, to be aware, to evaluate, to make conscious decisions. The extent to which he is able to achieve his goals will be directly proportional to his commitment to reason in seeking them.

The right to life implies three corollaries: the right to select the values that one deems necessary to sustain one's own life; the right to exercise one's own judgment of the best course of action to achieve the chosen values; and the right to dispose of those values, once gained, in any way one chooses, without coercion by other men. The denial of any one of these corollaries severely compromises or destroys the right to life itself. A man who is not allowed to choose his own goals, is prevented from setting his own course in achieving those goals and is not free to dispose of the values he has earned is no less than a slave to those who usurp those rights. The right to private property, therefore, is essential and indispensable to maintaining free men in a free society.

Thus, it is the nature of man as a living, thinking being that determines his rights—his "natural rights." The concept of natural rights was slow in dawning on human civilization. The first political expression of that concept had its beginnings in 17th and 18th century England through such exponents as John Locke and Edmund Burke, but came to its brilliant debut as a form of government after the American Revolution. Under the leadership of such men as Thomas Paine and Thomas Jefferson, the concept of man as a being sovereign unto himself, rather than a subdivision of the sovereignty of a king, emperor or state, was incorporated into the formal structure of government for the first time. Protection of the lives and property of individual citizens was the salient characteristic of the Constitution of 1787. Ayn Rand has pointed out that the principle of protection of the individual against the coercive force of government made the United States the first moral society in history.

In a free society, man exercises his right to sustain his own life by producing economic values in the form of goods and services that he is, or should be, free to exchange with other men who are similarly free to trade with him or not. The economic values produced, however, are not given as gifts by nature, but exist only by virtue of the thought and effort of individual men. Goods and services are thus owned as a consequence of the right to sustain life by one's own physical and mental effort.

If the chain of natural rights is interrupted, and the right to a loaf of bread, for example, is proclaimed as primary (avoiding the necessity of earning it), every man owns a loaf of bread, regardless of who produced it.

Since ownership is the power of disposal,[1] every man may take his loaf from the baker and dispose of it as he wishes with or without the baker's permission. Another element has thus been introduced into the relation between men: the use of force. It is crucial to observe who has initiated the use of force: it is the man who demands unearned bread as a right, not the man who produced it. At the level of an unstructured society it is clear who is moral and who immoral. The man who acted rationally by producing food to support his own life is moral. The man who expropriated the bread by force is immoral.

To protect this basic right to provide for the support of one's own life, men band together for their mutual protection and form governments. This is the only proper function of government: to provide for the defense of individuals against those who would take their lives or property by force. The state is the repository for retaliatory force in a just society wherein the only actions prohibited to individuals are those of physical harm or the threat of physical harm to other men. The closest that man has ever come to achieving this ideal of government was in this country after its War of Independence.

When a government ignores the progression of natural rights arising from the right to life, and agrees with a man, a group of men, or even a majority of its citizens, that every man has a right to a loaf of bread, it must protect that right by the passage of laws ensuring that everyone gets his loaf —in the process depriving the baker of the freedom to dispose of his own product. If the baker disobeys the law, asserting the priority of his right to support himself by his own rational disposition of the fruits of his mental and physical labor, he will be taken to court by force or threat of force where he will have more property forcibly taken from him (by fine) or have his liberty taken away (by incarceration). Now the initiator of violence is the government itself. The degree to which a government exercises its monopoly on the retaliatory use of force by asserting a claim to the lives and property of its citizens is the degree to which it has eroded its own legitimacy. It is a frequently overlooked fact that behind every law is a policeman's gun or a soldier's bayonet. When that gun and bayonet are used to initiate violence, to take property or to restrict liberty by force, there are no longer any rights, for the lives of the citizens belong to the state. In a just society with a moral government, it is clear that the only "right" to the bread belongs to the baker, and that a claim by any other man to that right is unjustified and can be enforced only by violence or the threat of violence.

RIGHTS—POLITICS AND MEDICINE

The concept of medical care as the patient's right is immoral because it denies the most fundamental of all rights, that of a man to his own life and the freedom of action to support it. Medical care is neither a right nor a

[1]Rand A: Man's rights, Capitalism: The unknown ideal. New York, New American Library, Inc. 1967, pp. 320–329.

privilege: it is a service that is provided by doctors and others to people who wish to purchase it. It is the provision of this service that a doctor depends upon for his livelihood, and is his means of supporting his own life. If the right to health care belongs to the patient, he starts out owning the services of a doctor without the necessity of either earning them or receiving them as a gift from the only man who has the right to give them: the doctor himself. In the narrative above substitute "doctor" for "baker" and "medical service" for "bread." American medicine is now at the point in the story where the state has proclaimed the nonexistent "right" to medical care as a fact of public policy, and has begun to pass the laws to enforce it. The doctor finds himself less and less his own master and more and more controlled by forces outside of his own judgment. . . .

Any doctor who is forced by law to join a group or a hospital he does not choose, or is prevented by law from prescribing a drug he thinks is best for his patient, or is compelled by law to make any decision he would not otherwise have made, is being forced to act against his own mind, which means forced to act against his own life. He is also being forced to violate his most fundamental professional commitment, that of using his own best judgment at all times for the greatest benefit of his patient. It is remarkable that this principle has never been identified by a public voice in the medical profession, and that the vast majority of doctors in this country are being led down the path to civil servitude, never knowing that their feelings of uneasy foreboding have a profoundly moral origin, and never recognizing that the main issues at stake are not those being formulated in Washington, but are their own honor, integrity and freedom, and their own survival as sovereign human beings.

SOME COROLLARIES

The basic fallacy that health care is a right has led to several corollary fallacies, among them the following:

That health is primarily a community or social rather than an individual concern.[2] A simple calculation from American mortality statistics[3] quickly corrects that false concept: 67 per cent of deaths in 1967 were due to diseases known to be caused or exacerbated by alcohol, tobacco smoking or overeating, or were due to accidents. Each of those factors is either largely or wholly correctable by individual action. Although no statistics are available, it is likely that morbidity, with the exception of common respiratory infections, has a relation like that of mortality to personal habits and excesses.

That state medicine has worked better in other countries than free enterprise has worked here. There is no evidence to support that contention, other than anecdotal testimonials and the spurious citation of infant mortality and

[2]Millis JS: Wisdom? Health? Can society guarantee them? N Engl J Med 283:260–261, 1970. [See below pp. 485–6.]

[3]Department of Health, Education, and Welfare, Public Health Service: Vital Statistics of the United States 1967. Vol II, Mortality. Part A. Washington, DC, Government Printing Office, 1969, p. 1–7.

longevity statistics. There is, on the other hand, a good deal of evidence to the contrary.[4,5]

That the provision of medical care somehow lies outside the laws of supply and demand, and that government-controlled health care will be free care. In fact, no service or commodity lies outside the economic laws. Regarding health care, market demand, individual want, and medical need are entirely different things, and have a very complex relation with the cost and the total supply of available care, as recently discussed and clarified by Jeffers et al.[6] They point out that " 'health is purchaseable', meaning that somebody has to pay for it, individually or collectively, at the expense of foregoing the current or future consumption of other things." The question is whether the decision of how to allocate the consumer's dollar should belong to the consumer or to the state. It has already been shown that the choice of how a doctor's services should be rendered belongs only to the doctor: in the same way the choice of whether to buy a doctor's service rather than some other commodity or service belongs to the consumer as a logical consequence of the right to his own life.

That opposition to national health legislation is tantamount to opposition to progress in health care. Progress is made by the free interaction of free minds developing new ideas in an atmosphere conducive to experimentation and trial. If group practice really is better than solo, we will find out because the success of groups will result in more groups (which has, in fact, been happening); if prepaid comprehensive care really is the best form of practice, it will succeed and the health industry will swell with new Kaiser–Permanente plans. But let one of these or any other form of practice become the law, and the system is in a straightjacket that will stifle progress. Progress requires freedom of action, and that is precisely what national health legislation aims at restricting.

That doctors should help design the legislation for a national health system, since they must live with and within whatever legislation is enacted. To accept this concept is to concede to the opposition its philosophic premises, and thus to lose the battle. The means by which nonproducers and hangers-on throughout history have been able to expropriate material and intellectual values from the producers has been identified only relatively recently: the sanction of the victim.[7] Historically, few people have lost their freedom and their rights without some degree of complicity in the plunder. If the American medical profession accepts the concept of health care as the right of the patient, it will have earned the Kennedy–Griffiths bill by default. The alternative for any health professional is to withhold his sanction and make clear who is being victimized. Any physician can say to those who would

[4]Financing Medical Care: An appraisal of foreign programs. Edited by H Shoeck. Caldwell, Idaho, Caxton Printers, Inc. 1962.

[5]Lynch MJ, Raphael SS: Medicine and the State. Springfield, Illinois, Charles C Thomas, 1963.

[6]Jeffers JR, Bognanno MF, Bartlett JC: On the demand versus need for medical services and the concept of "shortage." Am J Publ Health 61:46–63, 1971.

[7]Rand A: Atlas Shrugged. New York, Random House, 1957, p 1066.

shackle his judgment and control his profession: I do not recognize your right to my life and my mind, which belong to me and me alone; I will not participate in any legislated solution to any health problem.

In the face of the raw power that lies behind government programs, nonparticipation is the only way in which personal values can be maintained. And it is only with the attainment of the highest of those values—integrity, honesty and self-esteem—that the physician can achieve his most important professional value, the absolute priority of the welfare of his patients.

The preceding discussion should not be interpreted as proposing that there are no problems in the delivery of medical care. Problems such as high cost, few doctors, low quantity of available care in economically depressed areas may be real, but it is naïve to believe that governmental solutions through coercive legislation can be anything but shortsighted and formulated on the basis of political expediency. The only long-range plan that can hope to provide for the day after tomorrow is a "nonsystem"—that is, a system that proscribes the imposition by force (legislation) of any one group's conception of the best forms of medical care. We must identify our problems and seek to solve them by experimentation and trial in an atmosphere of freedom from compulsion. Our sanction of anything less will mean the loss of our personal values, the death of our profession, and a heavy blow to political liberty.

Wisdom? Health?
Can Society Guarantee Them?

John S. Millis

For many years the American people have accepted the concept that education is a necessity and that, therefore, it is to be regarded as a basic human right. Today, there are many voices advancing the idea that health is necessary to "life, liberty, and the pursuit of happiness," and that, therefore, health should also be regarded as a basic human right. There is a close analogy between education and health. The examination of experience with education may give useful guidance in the formation of public policy in health matters.

We, in America, have gone far to make universal educational opportunity a reality. We have a larger proportion of our youth in secondary and higher education than ever before in our history or in that of any other nation. Yet it is evident that we have produced disappointingly little rationality, civility, self-discipline and wisdom. Far too many people hold the idea

Reprinted from *The New England Journal of Medicine*, 283, 260–61, July 30, 1970. Copyright Massachusetts Medical Society.

that education consists of being taught. Teaching is surely a *necessary* element of education, but it is not *sufficient.* Learning must also be involved, and learning is a personal responsibility that no society, no laws, no guaranties can lift from the individual. Learning requires a positive decision on the part of the individual and a series of continuing acts of will. Thus, we must be content to guarantee educational opportunity, for we cannot guarantee wisdom.

Far too many people regard health as being "doctored." They therefore hope that with universal access to physicians and hospitals, they will all be healthy. Surely "doctoring" is a *necessary* element in health, but it is not *sufficient.* The provision of health service to all citizens will result in some improvement in our national figures on morbidity and mortality. However, that improvement may be disappointingly small, for the same stubborn fact of human behavior operates in both education and health. The fact is that there are large contributors to morbidity and mortality about which physicians and hospitals can do little. Accidents are the greatest cause of both morbidity and mortality for Americans between the ages of one and 37 years. Other important causes for all age groups are obesity, smoking, abuse of alcohol, abuse of drugs, environmental pollution and a life style that leads to organic and psychosomatic disease and disability. With the exception of environmental pollution, there is very little that society can do to control these causes except through intolerable restrictions on personal liberty. Rather, the control can come only through the behavior of the individual. Only his decisions and his actions can eliminate these causes of disability and death.

My conclusion is that we accept the concept that health is a necessity, but realize that we, as a society, can guarantee access to health service but not health itself. Personal health must remain a personal responsibility. Thus, as we work to provide for more health professionals and a more efficient system for the delivery of health service, we must also convince people that the achievement of health demands responsibility and action on the part of every individual.

Quality and Equality in Health Care—
What Can We Do About It?

Lowell E. Bellin

Before addressing this question, I pass along the following four aphorisms —unoriginal in content, but routinely ignored by critics of America's health-industrial complex:

Presented as a lecture at Case Western Reserve University. Published with the permission of the author.

1.   Motivation is *not* the relevant measure of the validity of a health program. Individual and organizational spokesmen may be *for* or *against* a specific method or program for *right* or for *wrong* reasons. This has *little* to do with whether the specific health program is right or wrong.

2.   It is time to stop romanticizing or villainizing providers or recipients of health services. The patient—and indeed the poor patient—is neither automatically deserving nor avaricious. The physician or any other practitioner is automatically neither the incarnation of Marcus Welby, nor an obtuse reactionary swine.

3.   The apocalyptic rhetoric of the 1960s, whatever its usefulness may have been during the 1960s, is tactically absurd now during the 1970s.

4.   In general, most statistics indicate that things are incrementally improving in the technology and delivery of health services. Nostalgia buffs who believe otherwise should stick to collecting Glen Miller records and stop mooning about the hyperidealized past. Anybody who yearns for the alleged good old days of health care during or before pre-antibiotic summer of '42 must be under 30 and was yet to be biologically conceived at that time.

Now to the question:

QUALITY AND EQUALITY IN HEALTH CARE—WHAT CAN WE DO ABOUT IT?

I suppose I am expected to proclaim to you today that, indeed, we *can* achieve quality and equality in health care and, then, go on to show how to perform this feat.

I must disappoint you. The answer I bring you from the bloody front of health administration is that pending the arrival of the End of Days, we *cannot* conceivably achieve both quality *and* equality in health care. Those who tell you otherwise prefer narcotizing delusions to acknowledging reality.

In order to proceed intelligently with today's question, we must first painfully refine the question.

Consider the word "quality." "Quality" often connotes the top of some kind of hierarchy of "how-ness"—i.e., *high* quality, as distinguished from *mediocre* or *low* quality. What the question means to say, presumably, is not "Can we achieve *quality*?" but rather "Can we achieve *acceptable* quality?" Acceptable quality is a moving target. What was acceptable quality yesterday is no longer acceptable quality today. Acceptable quality, then, is always culturally defined. Now consider the word "equality." *Equality* of what? For example, how about equality of geographic accessibility to superb technical services? Hardly. Improved communication and transportation cannot wipe out this permanent inequality. Optimally, only the unlikely establishment of a superior medical center within 10 minutes' travel time of every inhabitant in the land could do so. Recall, moreover, that even the best hospitals in the United States possess no homogeneity of quality of care.

Some departments are better than others. Within the same service of the same hospital, some physicians, some nurses, some paraprofessionals, some shifts of personnel are, and always will be better than others. Another truism: The wealthier and/or socially more manipulative will always be able to obtain amenities in health services beyond those received by others less endowed. So let us abandon forthwith all this cant about "equality."

A significant degree of inequality *must* remain the irreducible constant of human organization as it reflects the inadequacy of the human condition within our bureaucratized society.

What the question means to say presumably is *not* "Can we achieve equality?" but rather, "Can we achieve *less* inequality than we experience at present?" This is no quibble. The term "equality" is routinely used as a debater's ploy to cow the opposition, for who dares even *seem* to be in favor of inequality, much less advocate it in America?

So, the new question now recast for discussion is: Acceptable quality and less inequality in health care—what can we do about it?

The question in its new form provokes a lesser flow of adrenaline in the audience. Nevertheless it is useful to exchange the customary eschato-logical rhetoric of the health field for some semantic precision.

Expectations continue to evade the ability of most systems to satisfy them—certainly in the health care system where the ultimate expectation in the secular world can be no less than the technologic means to a comfortable physical immortality. But, can we satisfy even lesser, more realistic expecta-tions in an era when the tragic mortality from acute infectious and relatively inexpensive disease has been replaced by the morbidity and suffering of chronic and costly disease?

Actually the two goals—(a) culturally acceptable quality and (b) less inequality—can no more be separated from one another than the dancer from the dance.

How shall we raise the level of acceptable quality and get less inequal-ity in health care?

First of all, let's begin by inculcating more reality into our analysis of how programs work. Consider recent history. The Medicaid and Medicare experience since 1966 has demonstrated once more that most people—providers and recipients of health services alike—are motivated primarily by perceived self-interest. Given the durability of this human constant, then administration of publicly funded health care programs becomes viable only when such self-interest is acknowledged, rather than righteously con-demned, when the energies of such self-interest are tapped to help achieve programmatic objectives. Even in the here and now world of health care administration, we have been compelled to relearn that the energies of altruism are ephemeral—that specific social concerns, whether they be ser-vices for the masses, or marsh lands ecologically hospitable to water birds —are often faddish and have not generally lent themselves even in the short run to spans of attention of effective intensity. The implication is plain. Just because their overt goals are so explicitly altruistic, social planners must stop insisting that the motivations and the means to achieve these goals must be analogously altruistic. The picture of the underpaid teacher, preacher, or social worker should be deemed the sentimental anachronism it is. Similarly out of date is the conventional indignation toward the MD or DDS who is "overpaid" because, after all, according to the rhetoric, it is wrong for him to "profit" from the suffering of the sick. The political conservative has tended to be more realistic about the energies and demons that drive the bulk of mankind. My Master Plan follows in digest form:

THE MASTER PLAN

Double and Triple the Present Supply of Physicians and Dentists

It is false that substantial proliferation of clinicians will have no impact on the paucity of health professionals in undermanned areas because (as the argument goes) physicians and dentists will obstinately continue to open practices in affluent suburbia. Ultimately the market place will compel physicians who like to eat to settle in the less desirable urban and rural areas. For example: I would have preferred myself to settle in Boston or its environs when I completed my fellowship in cardiology there, but, instead, I reluctantly abandoned Medical Academe and the Boston Symphony Orchestra and moved to Springfield, Massachusetts where I practiced internal medicine for the next four years. Why? Because during my Boston postgraduate training, I was dismayed to see many able predecessors of mine, five to ten years out of their residencies, barely surviving economically in Boston by doing physical exams for life insurance companies. There is some point, then, at which the demand for more and more MDs in the desirable areas simply becomes exhausted. A locale's absorptive capacity is not infinite. The PhD space physicists, the engineers, the teachers and lately even the nurses have been forced to acknowledge this bitter truth in recent years.

A related phenomenon: In New York City, the Health Insurance Plan of Greater New York (HIP)—that well-known prepaid group practice of about 1000 physicians providing comprehensive care to about 800,000 subscribers—was able to recruit physicians and begin functioning after World War II because returning physicians were scared. Could they really start a postwar private practice on their own? The ideology of prepaid group practice was clearly not the only operative force that emboldened physicians in New York City to join HIP and thereby defy the taunts and professional persecution of their colleagues. The fear of financial insecurity helped.

Of course this is not the case today. In health care, the perniciousness of the sellers' market has been increasingly with us since the 1950s. Therefore, to achieve acceptable quality and less inequality in health care, we must behave rationally and deliberately convert the sellers' market of health practitioners into a buyers' market. Until we do this many of the so-called innovative plans about delivery of health services are simply pipe dreams. No one can start and maintain any enterprise on this earth with no bargaining position vis-à-vis personnel.

But how to double and triple the present supply of physicians and dentists?

So long as medical and dental school faculties perceive no imminent personal advantage to increase their pedagogical productivity, they will consistently maintain that increased class size and teaching load are synonyms for deterioration of academic standards. But there is more safe elasticity here than most institutions and faculty care to admit or even explore. The very idea of night medical and dental schools on a part-time or full-time basis provokes horror. At the same time space constraints in lecture halls and laboratories are cited as the fundamental obstacle to significant expansion, although buildings and laboratories remain empty after 5 P.M. This paper cannot detail the numerous potential methods that might be applied to increase the number of physicians and dentists. But if there were to be a serious commitment to increase the supply of physicians and dentists in the country, then one method to erode faculty resistance (which masquerades as "institutional" resistance) would be to pay specific financial incentives to medical and dental school teachers for each physician and dentist they ultimately graduate. Many of the insuperable obstacles to educational expansion of medical and dental schools would then vanish with gratifying rapidity as teachers would begin to apply their ingenuity to problems conventionally viewed as insoluble.

It is fashionable today to suggest that proliferation of paraprofessionals in health care will solve the problem. Paraprofessionals will alleviate the problem and will increase the productivity of physicians and dentists who will act increasingly in a supervisory rather than in a strictly technical capacity. But to rely on nurse clinicians, physicians assistants, etc. as the solution to providing care to the inner city and to rural America is a type of copout that deserves its own in-depth analysis. Some spokesmen for the poor are already questioning the sincerity and consistency of people who advocate paraprofessionals for the poor (under adequate supervision, of course), but traditional professionals for suburbia and for their own families.

Compel Practitioners to Serve in Undesirable Areas for 2 Years

Without governmental subsidy via Medicaid the current underdistribution of clinicians to poverty areas would be even worse than it is today. During my senior year in medical school, our class in public health was once addressed by a physician who told us that our future clinical skills were needed more in rural Mississippi than in suburbia. We listened, but none of my classmates to my knowledge ever was sufficiently motivated to move to rural Mississippi. Today, doctors practice in perfectly horrible areas of the City of New York. Where pietistic exhortation failed, Medicaid money has succeeded somewhat. Critics of Medicaid routinely condemn such physicians as money-grubbing and poorly qualified. When I presented some of these facts to a medical school class recently, one medical student commented, "Better no care at all, than to provide care of such bad quality."

Well, evidence is lacking to support this rhetorical anodyne. The medical student can indulge his absolutism and his doctrinaire smugness, but the working health administrator has no such option. He must address the dilemma: (1) Is it better to expel a poor practitioner forthwith from the program, or (2) Is it better to retain the poor practitioner, since expulsion would substantially diminish the accessibility of the population in question to any care whatsoever? So we are back once more to the consequences of the sellers' market. But, in the absence of adequate financial incentives and in the absence of a buyers' market to redistribute clinicians more rationally, what must we do in the meanwhile?

To deal immediately with the maldistribution of clinicians, those physicians and dentists now completing their postgraduate training should compulsorily be assigned to less desired areas for a specific period—say two years. The moral justification? The education of the MD and DDS has been subsidized by the taxpayer. The student's tuition pays for one-fourth or less of actual costs of the professional education.

But such justification is conventional and superfluous. If tomorrow all direct public subsidy to schools and to students were to vanish, the possession of one's citizenry alone would remain justification enough for particularistic obligatory service to one's nation. In time of war or near war military service is categorized as an obligation of citizenry. In time of social crisis— which is now and probably forever in view of the ever-widening definition of social crisis—peacetime compulsory service can be similarly categorized. Nor will these practitioners be working for a pittance. They can prosper on Medicaid and Medicare. A minimum income can be guaranteed. Even in peacetime it is pleasanter to work as an MD or DDS in the Bedford-Stuyvesant area of Brooklyn or in rural New Mexico than in Southeast Asia or in an Air Force base at Thule.

Incidentally, for analogous reasons I would certainly not limit such work assignment to physicians and dentists. All would have to put in their time in less desirable places—lawyers, pharmacists, architects, sociologists, etc.

A parenthetical comment. When I was quoted in the local press as favoring this compulsory approach, I was accused by the leadership of the local medical society as favoring the imposition of a tyranny reminiscent of Soviet labor camps.

Those who view such compulsory redistribution of health professionals as tyranny normatively oppose significant proliferation of medical and dental schools, although they favor generous financial incentives, publicly funded of course, to attract practitioners to poorly favored areas.

Implement Accountability of Health Professionals

Arms-length evaluation of the quality of care is an indispensable ingredient in any health care program. By all means, let professional peers judge practicing professionals—but let these professional peer judges be on the payroll of government. Intermediate-level peer review on the part of fiscal intermediaries or of professional societies is desirable, but only a Rip Van Winkle who has been asleep ever since the promulgation of Medicare and Medicaid can advocate ultimate accountability that is not operational accountability to government.

SALARY VS. FEE-FOR-SERVICE—
WHICH IS "THE" ANSWER?

Aficionados of articles and speeches about alleviating the health care crisis in America will have noted by now a curious omission: In such discussions it is *de riguer* to revile the "no system" of health care, the so-called "cottage industry" method of health care delivery, and the iniquities of the fee-for-service system. My critique of these will be more temperate than most.

Among the sancta of the American mystique is that for every social problem potentially susceptible to governmental intervention there exists a specific administrative gimmick to deal with it. The gimmick in health services is supposed to be salary rather than fee-for-service for practitioners. Now, in the main, there are but two ways to reimburse health practitioners for their work, just as there are but two ways to recompense anyone for any work performed: (1) piecework—in health services called "fee-for-service"; and (2) salary—in health services paid either by a hospital or group practice and sometimes in group practice associated with capitation payment, i.e., an overall payment by and for each enrolled patient for total care. The strengths and weaknesses of either method of compensation are remarkably similar to the strengths and weaknesses of either in other settings—and for similar reasons.

Fee-For-Service

The clinician performs a service and is paid for it.

Pro

1. This encourages productivity. With clinicians in short supply and badly distributed, it is prudent to use proven means to encourage productivity.

2. In the unsentimental exchange of money that characterizes the transaction called fee-for-service the clinician is motivated to satisfy the consumer.

Con

1. Fee-for-service encourages not only high productivity, but costly over-productivity—i.e., overutilization—services justified neither for preventive nor for therapeutic reasons. Piecework is demoralizing and dehumanizing to the worker. Unions have traditionally been opposed to piecework because the boss often cuts back on the rate of payment per piece as productivity increases. The unions aren't wrong about what bosses sometimes do. In Medicaid, New York State government cut fees across the board by 20%—in an effort to constrain expenditure. What happened was a further speed-up of productivity plus additional attenuation of quality of care. So even the AMA was not wrong, then, in its warnings that governmental subsidy can mean mediocritization. Union-haters and AMA-haters, please take note.

2. There is no objective rationale for the relative value of fee-for-service. Is a complete blood count costing $10 really five times as diagnostically important as a urinalysis costing $2?

Salary

When I was an Air Force doctor, a few MDs on our base were perennial goof-offs. There was no financial initiative for them to work hard, and they knew the Colonel wouldn't impose military sanctions. Fixed salary can promote low productivity and underutilization. The attraction of salary, particularly to planners, is that it more easily predicts personnel costs, thereby facilitating rational planning via pooling of risk in a health insurance mechanism. Salary obviously lends itself more easily than fee-for-service to cost control.

It is wise to be wary of inflated claims about any method of reimbursing either practitioners or institutions, particularly when such method promises to achieve desirable social objectives in the absence of controls and controllers. Every method of payment needs a type of control and controller suited specifically to that method. In the United States today ripoffs in quality and cost of health services occur both under fee-for-service *and* under prepaid capitation. Let no one convince you otherwise.

A comment about paying clinicians: Whatever the method of payment, practitioners must be encouraged to prosper. In a sellers' market social reformers have no choice but to constrain their egalitarian instincts. Leveling incomes below reasonable prosperity results only in driving good practitioners from the program, leaving bad practitioners who provide inadequate care and prosper anyway, since they are skilled at milking the system.

What about the current entrepreneurship system of solo practice? Will it give way to comprehensive prepaid group practice? I doubt it—at least until the sellers' market becomes a buyers' market. So again we are back to the old problem. I predict that so-called comprehensive prepaid group practice will be based in hospitals and neighborhood family care centers and will serve primarily the poor in the catchment areas of these institutions. I note that the middle class stubbornly continues to refuse to read the *American Journal of Public Health.* The fact is that enrollment in prepaid group practice in percentage of population served has not kept pace, much less exceeded, the growth in American population.

Whatever "revamping" of the system of delivery of health services occurs will occur gradually. In the sellers' market of providers—and given a tepid governmental commitment to radical restructuring of health care delivery—we are obliged to act with a good deal more cunning with respect to the system we inherited. Let us acknowledge that much of the talk about radical restructuring is just talk and a form of socially sanctioned escapism.

THE JOB OF RESEARCHERS

Let me give some advice to researchers in fields within or functionally contiguous to health administration. Part of the title of this talk is "What can *we* do about it?" Researchers are part of that "we."

Practitioners need additional knowledge that innovative administrative research can provide. We need that knowledge to try to order today's chaos and begin to predict tomorrow's reality. By research I do not mean the safe research that constitutes so much of current academic boondoggling. You know the type I mean—the topics that provoke quiet groans at professional conferences—"No, not that subject again."

For example, we need no more rehashes of the last dozen studies about the determinants of broken appointments in OPD clinics. We could use instead an analysis of the determinants that prevent administrators from acting to counteract the factors that promote such broken appointments. Manifestly, this type of research is dangerous research, but it's the kind of quality research and implementative research that we'd better get more of soon.

SUMMARY

What do we need from people who profess to help us move toward our goal of achieving acceptable quality and less inequality in health care?

We need both a sense and an application of reality. The theme of this paper is hostility to mythology in the field of health.

Two Watersheds:
The American Public Health System

Ivan Illich

The year 1913 marks a watershed in the history of modern medicine. Around that year a patient began to have more than a fifty-fifty chance that a graduate of a medical school would provide him with a specifically effective treatment (if, of course, he was suffering from one of the standard diseases recognized by the medical science of the time). Many shamans and herb doctors familiar with local diseases and remedies and trusted by their clients had always had equal or better results.

Since then medicine has gone on to define what constitutes disease and its treatment. The Westernized public learned to demand effective medical practice as defined by the progress of medical science. For the first time in history doctors could measure their efficiency against scales that they themselves had devised. This progress was due to new knowledge about the origins of some ancient scourges; water could be purified and infant mortality lowered; rat control could disarm the plague; treponemas could be made visible under the microscope and Salvarsan could eliminate them with statistically defined risks of poisoning the patient; syphilis could be avoided, or recognized and cured by rather simple procedures; diabetes could be diagnosed and self-treatment with insulin could prolong the life of the patient. Paradoxically the simpler the tools became, the more the medical profession insisted on a monopoly of their application, the longer became the training

Reprinted with permission of the author from *Social Policy* 4, 46–50, vol 4. March-April 1973.

demanded before a medicine man was initiated into the legitimate use of the simplest tool, and the more the entire population felt dependent on the doctor. Hygiene changed from being a virtue into a professionally organized ritual at the altar of a science.

Infant mortality was lowered, common forms of infection were prevented or treated, some forms of crisis intervention became quite effective. The spectacular decline in mortality and morbidity was due to changes in sanitation, agriculture, marketing, and general attitudes toward life. But although these changes were sometimes influenced by the attention that engineers paid to new facts discovered by medical science, they could only occasionally be ascribed to the intervention of doctors.

Indirectly industrialization profited from the new effectiveness attributed to medicine; work attendance was raised, and with it the claim to efficiency on the job. The destructiveness of new tools was hidden from public view by new techniques of providing spectacular treatments for those who fell victims to industrial violence such as the speed of cars, tension on the job, and poisons in the environment.

The sickening side effects of modern medicine became obvious after World War II, but doctors needed time to diagnose drug-resistant microbes of genetic damage caused by prenatal x rays as new epidemics. The claim made by George Bernard Shaw a generation earlier, that doctors had ceased to be healers and were assuming control over the patient's entire life, could still be regarded as a caricature. Only in the mid-1950s did it become evident that medicine had passed a second watershed and had itself created new kinds of disease.

Foremost among iatrogenic (doctor-induced) diseases was the pretense of doctors that they provided their clients with superior health. First, social planners and doctors became its victims. Soon this epidemic aberration spread to society at large. Then during the last fifteen years professional medicine became a major threat to health. Huge amounts of money were spent to stem immeasurable damage caused by medical treatments. The cost of healing was dwarfed by the cost of extending sick life. More people survived months longer with their lives hanging on a plastic tube, imprisoned in iron lungs, or hooked onto kidney machines. New sickness was defined and institutionalized; the cost of enabling people to survive in unhealthy cities and in sickening jobs skyrocketed. The monopoly of the medical profession was extended over an increasing range of everyday occurrences in every man's life.

The exclusion of mothers, aunts, and other nonprofessionals from the care of their pregnant, abnormal, hurt, sick, or dying relatives and friends resulted in new demands for medical services at a much faster rate than the medical establishment could deliver. As the value of *services* rose, it became almost impossible for people to *care*. Simultaneously more conditions were defined as needing treatment by creating new specializations or paraprofessions to keep the tools under the control of the guild.

At the time of the second watershed, preservation of the sick life of medically dependent people in an unhealthy environment became the principal business of the medical profession. Costly prevention and costly treatment became increasingly the privilege of those individuals who through previous consumption of medical services had established a claim to more of it. Access to specialists, prestige hospitals, and life machines goes preferentially to those people who live in large cities, where the cost of basic disease prevention, as of water treatment and pollution control, is already exceptionally high. The higher the per capita cost of prevention, the higher, paradoxically, became the per capita cost of treatment. The prior consumption of costly prevention and treatment establishes a claim for even more extraordinary care. Like the modern school system, hospital-based health care fits the principle that those who have will receive even more and those who have not will be taken for the little that they have. In schooling this means that high consumers of education will get postdoctoral grants, while dropouts learn that they have failed. In medicine the same principle assures that suffering will increase with increased medical care; the rich will be given more treatment for iatrogenic diseases and the poor will just suffer from them.

After this second turning point the unwanted hygienic by-products of medicine began to affect entire populations rather than just individual men. In rich countries medicine began to sustain the middle-aged until they became decrepit and needed more doctors and increasingly complex medical tools. In poor countries, thanks to modern medicine, a larger percentage of children began to survive into adolescence and more women survived more pregnancies. Populations increased beyond the capacities of their environments and the restraints and efficiencies of their cultures to nurture them. Western doctors abused drugs for the treatment of diseases with which native populations had learned to live. As a result they bred new strains of disease with which modern treatment, natural immunity, and traditional culture could not cope. On a worldwide scale, but particularly in the United States, medical care concentrated on breeding a human stock that was fit only for domesticated life within an increasingly more costly, man-made, scientifically controlled environment. One of the main speakers at the 1970 American Medical Association convention exhorted her pediatric colleagues to consider each newborn baby as a *patient* until the child could be certified as healthy. Hospital-born, formula-fed, antibiotic-stuffed children thus grow into adults who can breathe the air, eat the food, and survive the lifelessness of a modern city, who will breed and raise at almost any cost a generation even more dependent on medicine.

Bureaucratic medicine spread over the entire world. In 1968, after twenty years of Mao's regime, the Medical College of Shanghai had to conclude that it was engaged in the training of "so-called first-rate doctors . . . who ignore five million peasants and serve only minorities in cities. . . . They create large expenses for routine laboratory examinations . . . prescribe huge amounts of antibiotics unnecessarily . . . and in the absence of hospital or laboratory facilities have to limit themselves to explaining the mechanisms of the disease to people for whom they cannot do anything, and to whom this explanation is irrelevant." In China this recognition led to a major institutional inversion. Today the same college reports that one million health workers have reached acceptable levels of competence. These health workers are laymen who in periods of low agricultural manpower needs have attended short courses, starting with the dissection of pigs, gone on to the performance of routine lab tests, the study of the elements of bacteriology, pathology, clinical medicine, hygiene, and acupuncture, and continued in apprenticeship with doctors or previously trained colleagues. These "barefoot doctors" remain at their work places but are excused occasionally when fellow workers require their assistance. They have responsibility for environmental sanitation, for health education, immunization, first aid, primary medical care, post illness follow-up, as well as for gynecological assistance, birth control, and abortion education. Ten years after the second watershed of Western medicine had been acknowledged, China intends to have one fully competent health worker for every hundred people. China has proved that a sudden inversion of a major institution is possible. It remains to be seen if this deprofessionalization can be sustained against the overweening ideology of unlimited progress and pressures from classical doctors to incorporate their barefoot homonym as part-time professionals on the bottom rung of a medical hierarchy.

In the West during the 1960s dissatisfaction with medicine grew in proportion to its cost, reaching the greatest intensity in the United States. Rich foreigners flocked to the medical centers of Boston, Houston, and Denver to seek exotic repair jobs, while the infant mortality of the U.S. poor remained comparable to that in some tropical countries of Africa and Asia. Only the very rich in the United States can now afford what all people in poor countries have: personal attention around the deathbed. An American can now spend in two days of private nursing the median yearly cash income of the world's population.

Instead of exposing the systemic disorder, however, only the symptoms of "sick" medicine are now publicly indicted in the United States. Spokesmen for the poor object to the capitalist prejudices of the AMA and the income of doctors. Community leaders object to the lack of community control over the delivery systems of professional health maintenance or of sick care, believing that laymen on hospital boards can harness professional medics. Black spokesmen object to the concentration of research grants on the types of disease that tend to strike the white, elderly, overfed foundation official who approves them. They ask for research on sickle-cell anemia, which strikes only the Black. The general voter hopes that the end of the war in Vietnam will make more funds available for an increase of medical production. This general concern with symptoms, however, distracts attention from the malignant expansion of *institutional* health care, which is at the root of the rising costs and demands and the decline in well-being.

The crisis of medicine lies on a much deeper level than its symptoms reveal and is consistent with the present crisis of all industrial institutions. It results from the development of a professional complex supported and exhorted by society to provide increasingly better health, and from the willingness of clients to serve as guinea pigs in this vain experiment. People have lost the right to declare themselves sick; society now accepts their claims to sickness only after certification by medical bureaucrats.

It is not strictly necessary to this argument to accept 1913 and 1955 as the two watershed years in order to understand that early in the century medical practice emerged into an era of scientific verification of its results. And that later medical science itself became an alibi for the obvious damage often caused by the medical professional. At the first watershed the desirable effects of new scientific discoveries were easily measured and verified. Germ-free water reduced infant mortality related to diarrhea, aspirin reduced the pain of rheumatism, and malaria could be controlled by quinine. Some traditional cures were recognized as quackery, but, more importantly, the use of some simple habits and tools spread widely. People began to understand the relationship between health and a balanced diet, fresh air, calisthenics, pure water and soap. New devices ranging from toothbrushes to Band-Aids and condoms became widely available. The positive contribution of modern medicine to individual health during the early part of the twentieth century can hardly be questioned.

But then medicine began to approach the second watershed. Every year medical science reported a new breakthrough. Practitioners of new specialties rehabilitated some individuals suffering from rare diseases. The practice of medicine became centered on the performance of hospital-based staffs. Trust in miracle cures obliterated good sense and traditional wisdom on healing and health care. The irresponsible use of drugs spread from doctors to the general public. The second watershed was approached when the marginal utility of further professionalization declined, at least insofar as it can be expressed in terms of the physical well-being of the largest number of people. The second watershed was superseded when the marginal *dis*utility increased as further monopoly by the medical establishment became an indicator of more suffering for larger numbers of people. After the passage of this second watershed, medicine still claimed continued progress, as measured by the new land-marks doctors set for themselves and then reached: both predictable discoveries and costs. For instance, a few patients survived longer with transplants of various organs. On the other hand, the total social cost exacted by medicine ceased to be measurable in conventional terms. Society possessed no standards by which to add up the negative value of illusion, social control, prolonged suffering, loneliness, genetic deterioration, and frustration produced by medical treatment.

Other industrial institutions have passed through the same two watersheds. This is certainly true for the major social agencies that have been reorganized according to scientific criteria during the last 150 years. Education, the mails, social work, transportation, and even civil engineering have followed this evolution. At first new knowledge is applied to the solution of a clearly stated problem, and scientific measuring sticks are applied to account for the new efficiency. But at a second point the progress demonstrated in a previous achievement is used as a rationale for the exploitation of society as a whole in the service of a value that is determined and constantly revised by an element of society, by one of its self certifying professional elites.

In the case of transportation it has taken almost a century to pass from an era served by motorized vehicles to an era in which society has been reduced to virtual enslavement to the car. During the American Civil War steam power on wheels became effective. The new economy in transportation enabled many people to travel by rail at the speed of a royal coach, and to do so with a comfort kings had not dared dream of. Gradually desirable locomotion was associated and finally identified with high vehicular speeds. But when transportation had passed through its second watershed, vehicles had created more distances than they helped to bridge; more time was used by the entire society for the sake of traffic than was "saved."

It is sufficient to recognize the existence of these two watersheds in order to gain a fresh perspective on our present social crisis. In one decade several major institutions have moved jointly over their second watershed. Schools are losing their claim to be effective tools to provide education; cars have ceased to be effective tools for mass transportation; the assembly line has ceased to be an acceptable mode of production.

The characteristic reaction of the 1960s to the growing frustration was further technological and bureaucratic escalation. Self-defeating escalation of power became the core ritual practiced in highly industrialized nations. In this context the Vietnam War is both revealing and concealing. It makes this ritual visible for the entire world in a narrow theater of war, yet it also distracts attention from the same ritual being played out in many so-called peaceful arenas. The conduct of the war proves that a convivial army limited to bicycle speeds is served by the opponent's escalation of anonymous power. And yet many Americans argue that the resources squandered on the war in the Far East could be used effectively to overwhelm poverty at home. Others are anxious to use the $20 billion the war now costs for increasing international development assistance from its present low of $2 billion. They fail to grasp the underlying institutional structure common to a peaceful war on poverty and a bloody war on dissidence. Both escalate what they are meant to eliminate.

Although evidence shows that more of the same leads to utter defeat, nothing less than more and more seems worthwhile in a society infected by the growth mania. The desperate plea is not only for more bombs and more police, more medical examinations and more teachers, but also for more information and research. The editor-in-chief of the *Bulletin of Atomic Scientists* claims that most of our present problems are the result of recently acquired knowledge badly applied, and concludes that the only remedy for the mass created by this information is more of it. It has become fashionable to say that where science and technology have created problems, it is only more scientific understanding and better technology that can carry us past them. The cure for bad management is more management. The cure for specialized research is more costly interdisciplinary research, just as the cure for polluted rivers is more costly nonpolluting detergents. The pooling of stores of information, the building up of a knowledge stock, the attempt to overwhelm present problems by the production of more science is the ultimate attempt to solve a crisis by escalation.

MEDICAL RESOURCES AS COMMODITIES

Why Give To Strangers?

Richard M. Titmuss

In Alexander Solzhenitsyn's novel *Cancer Ward* Shulubin is talking to Kostoglotov:

> "We have to show the world a society in which all relationships, fundamental principles and laws flow directly from moral ethics, and from them *alone*. Ethical demands would determine all calculations: how to bring up children, what to prepare them for, to what purpose the work of grown-ups should be directed, and how their leisure should be occupied. As for scientific research, it should only be conducted where it doesn't damage ethical morality, in the first instance where it doesn't damage the researchers themselves."

> Kostoglotov then raises questions. "There has to be an economy after all doesn't there? That comes before everything else." "Does it?" said Shulubin. "That depends. For example, Vladimir Solovyov argues rather convincingly that an economy could and should be built on an ethical basis."

> "What's this? Ethics first and economics afterwards?" Kostoglotov looked bewildered.

The questions raised by Solzhenitsyn could as well be directed at social policy institutions. What, for example, are the connections between what we in Britain conventionally call the social services and the role of altruism in modern industrial societies? And have we a convenient model for studying such relationships? Blood as a living tissue and as a bond that links all men and women so closely that differences of colour, religious belief, and cultural heritage are insignificant beside it, may now constitute in Western societies one of the ultimate tests of where the "social" begins and the "economic" ends.

THE WORLD DEMAND FOR BLOOD

The transfer of blood and blood derivatives from one human being to another represents one of the greatest therapeutic instruments in the hands of modern medicine. But these developments have set in train social, economic, and ethical consequences which present society with issues of profound importance.

The demand for blood and blood products is increasing all over the world. In high-income countries, in particular, the rate of growth in demand has been rising so rapidly that shortages have begun to appear. In all Western countries, demand is growing faster than rates of growth in the population aged 18–65 from whom donors are drawn. And, despite a mas-

Reprinted with permission from *The Lancet,* 123–125, January 16, 1971.

sive research effort in the United States to find alternatives, there is often no substitute for human blood.

Many factors are responsible for this increase in demand. Some surgical procedures call for massive transfusions of blood (as many as 60 donations may be needed for a single open-heart operation, and in one American heart-transplant case over 300 pints of blood were used); artificial kidneys require substantial volumes of blood; and developments in organ transplants could create immense additional demands. Furthermore, more routine surgery is now used more frequently and is made available to a larger proportion of the population than formerly. A more violent or accident-prone world insistently demands more blood for road casualties and for war injuries (in 1968 more than 300,000 pints of blood were shipped from the U.S.A. and elsewhere to treat victims of the Vietnam war).

There seems to be no predictable limit to the demand for blood supplies, especially when one remembers the as-yet unmet needs for surgical and medical treatment.

SUPPLY OF BLOOD

On the biological, technical, and administrative side, three factors limit the supply of blood.

Only about half of a population is medically eligible to donate blood. Furthermore, the amount any one person can give in a year is restricted—two donations in the British National Blood Transfusion Service (probably the lowest limit and the most rigorous standard in the world); five in the United States, a minimum often exceeded by paid donors, commercial blood-banks, and pharmaceutical companies using techniques such as plasmapheresis; in Japan, where 90% of blood is bought and sold, the standard is even lower. These differences can be analysed as a process of redistribution of life chances in terms of age, sex, social class, income, ethnic group, and so on.

Human blood deteriorates after three weeks in the refrigerator, and this perishability presents great technical and administrative problems to those running transfusion services. But it does mean that, by measuring wastage (i.e., the amount of blood that has to be thrown away) the efficiencies of different blood collection and distribution systems can be compared.

Blood can be more deadly than any drug. Quite apart from the problems of cross-matching, storage, labelling, and so on, there are serious risks of disease transmission and other hazards. In Western countries a major hazard is serum hepatitis transmitted from carrier donor to susceptible patient. Since carriers cannot yet be reliably detected, the patient becomes the laboratory for testing "the gift." Donors, therefore, have to be screened every time they come to give blood, and the donor's truthfulness in answering questions about health, medical history, and drug habits becomes vital. Upon the honesty of the donor depends the life of the recipient of his blood. In this context we need to ask what conditions and arrangements permit and encourage maximum truthfulness on the part of the donors. Can honesty be pursued regardless of the donor's motives for giving blood? What systems, structures, and social policies encourage honesty or discourage and destroy voluntary and truthful gift relationships?

TYPES OF DONOR

To give or not to give, to lend, repay, or even to buy and sell blood are choices which lead us, if we are to understand these transactions in the context of any society, to the fundamentals of social and economic life.

The forms and functions of giving embody moral, social, psychological, religious, legal, and aesthetic ideas. They may reflect, sustain, strengthen, or loosen the cultural bonds of the group, large or small. They may inspire the worst excesses of war and tribalism or the tolerances of community.

Customs and practices of non-economic giving—unilateral and multilateral social transfers—thus may tell us much, as Marcel Mauss so sensitively demonstrated in his book *The Gift,* about the texture of personal and group relationships in different cultures. In some societies, past and present, gifts to men aim to buy peace; to express affection, regard, or loyalty; to unify the group; to fulfil a contractual set of obligations and rights; to function as acts of penitence, shame, or degradation; and to symbolise many other human sentiments. When one reads the work of anthropologists and sociologists such as Mauss and Lévi-Strauss, who have studied the social functions of giving, a number of themes relevant to any attempt to delineate a typology of blood-donors may be discerned.

From these readings and from statistics for different countries a spectrum of blood-donor types can be constructed. At one extreme is the paid donor who sells his blood for what the market will bear: some are semi-salaried, some are long-term prisoner volunteers, some are organised in blood trade-unions. As a market transaction, information that might have a bearing on the quality of the blood is withheld if possible from the buyer, since such information could affect the sale of the blood. Thus in the United States blood-group identification cards are loaned, at a price, to other sellers, and blood is illegally mislabelled and updated, and other devices are used which make it very difficult to screen out drug addicts, alcoholics and hepatitis carriers, and so on.

At the other extreme is the voluntary, unpaid donor. This type is the closest approximation in social reality to the abstract idea of a "free human gift." There are no tangible immediate rewards, monetary or non-monetary; there are no penalties; and donors know that their gifts are for unnamed strangers without distinction of age, sex, medical illness, income, class, religion, or ethnic group. No donor type can be characterised by complete disinterested spontaneous altruism. There must be some sense of obligation, approval, and interest; some awareness of the need for the gift; some expectation that a return gift may be needed and received at some future date. But the unpaid donation of blood is an act of free-will: there is no formal contract, legal bond, power situation; no sense of shame or guilt; no money and no explicit guarantee of or wish for reward or return gift.

Almost all the 1½ million registered donors in Britain and donors in some systems in European countries fall into this category. An analysis of blood-donor motives suggests that the main reason people give blood is most commonly a general desire to help people; almost a third of the British donors studied said that their gift was in response to an appeal for blood; 7% said it was to repay a transfusion given to someone they knew.

By contrast, in the United States less than 10% of supplies come from the voluntary community donor. Proportionately more and more blood is being supplied by the poor, the unskilled, the unemployed, Negroes, and other low-income groups, and with the rise in plasmapheresis there is emerging a new class of exploited high blood yielders. Redistribution in terms of "the gift of blood and blood products" from the poor to the rich seems to be one of the dominant effects of the American blood-banking system.

WHICH SYSTEM?

When we compare the commercial blood-bank, such as that found in the United States, with the voluntary system functioning as an integral part of the National Health Service in Britain we find that the commercial blood-bank fails on each of four counts—economic efficiency, administrative efficiency, price, and quality. Commercial blood-bank systems waste blood, and shortages, acute and chronic, characterise the demand-and-supply position. Administratively, there is more paperwork and greater computing and accounting overheads. The cost varies between £10 and £20 per unit in the United States, compared with £1 16s, (£2 if processing costs are included) in Britain. And, as judged by statistics for post-transfusion hepatitis, the risk of transfusing contaminated blood is greater if the blood is obtained from a commercial source.

Paradoxically—or so it may seem to some—the more commercialised blood-distribution becomes (and hence more wasteful, inefficient, and dangerous) the more will the gross national product be inflated. In part, and quite simply, this is the consequence of statistically "transferring" an unpaid service (voluntary donors, voluntary workers in the service, unpaid time), with much lower external costs, to a monetary and measurable paid activity involving costlier externalities. Similar effects on the gross national product would ensue if housewives were paid for housework or childless married couples were financially rewarded for adopting children or if hospital patients cooperating for teaching purposes charged medical students. The gross national product is also inflated when commercial markets accelerate "blood obsolescence"; the waste is counted because someone has paid for it.

What *The Economist* described in its 1969 survey of the American economy as the great "efficiency gap" between that country and Britain clearly does not apply to the distribution of human blood. The voluntary, socialised system in Britain is economically, professionally, administratively, and qualitatively more efficient than the mixed, commercialised, and individualistic American system.

Another myth, the Paretian myth of consumer sovereignty, has also to be shattered. In the commercial blood market the consumer is not king. He has less freedom of choice to live unharmed; little choice in determining price; is more subject to scarcity; is less free from bureaucratisation; has fewer opportunities to express altruism; and exercises fewer checks and controls in relation to consumption, quality, and external costs. Far from being sovereign, he is often exploited.

What also emerges from this case-study is the significance of the externalities (the values and disvalues external to but created by blood-distribution systems treated as entities) and the multiplier effects of such externalities on what we can only call "the quality of life." At one end of the spectrum of externalities is the individual affected by hepatitis; at the other end, the market behaviour of economically rich societies seeking to import blood from other societies who are thought to be too poor and economically decadent to pay their own blood-donors.

CONCLUSION

We started with blood as a model for examining how altruism and social policy might work together in a modern industrial society. We might equally have chosen eye banks, patients as teaching material, fostering, or even the whole concept of the community-based distribution of welfare to those in need. All these involve in some degree a gift relationship. The example chosen suggests, firstly, that gift exchange of a non-quantifiable nature has more important functions in a complex society than the writings of Lévi-Strauss and others might indicate. Secondly, the application of scientific and technological developments in such societies is further accelerating the spread of such complexity, and has increased rather than decreased the scientific as well as the social need for such relationships. Thirdly, for these and many other reasons, modern societies require more rather than less freedom of choice for the expression of altruism in the daily life of all social groups. This requirement can be argued for on social and ethical grounds, but, as we have seen for blood donors, it can also be argued for on scientific and economic criteria.

I believe that it is a responsibility of government, acting, for example, through social policy, to weaken market forces which put men in positions where they have little opportunity to make moral choices or to behave altruistically if they wish to do so. The voluntary blood-donor system is a practical example of a fellowship relationship operating on an institutional basis, in this instance the National Health Service. It shows how social policy decisions can foster such relationships between free and equal individuals. If we accept that man has a social and biological need to help then he should not be denied the chance to express this need by entering into a gift relationship.

Letter: Ethics And Economics In Blood Supply

A. J. Culyer

Sir,-Professor Titmuss, in his discussion of the role of giving in blood-supplies, is likely to mislead many of your readers (a) by suggesting a distinction between "economic" and "social" man and (b) by asserting that payment for blood causes higher social costs, acute and chronic shortages of blood, and a high risk of infection of recipients through viral hepatitis and other diseases, compared with donation. Although I do not "urge" and have not "urged" the introduction of payment to blood suppliers in Britain, as Titmuss asserts, the case for payment (if there is or ever will be one) does not stand or fall on these claims.

(*a*)   Man is a social animal with economic problems that are a subset of "social problems." They are not mutually incompatible categories. As a science, economics is the study of the *means* of achieving ends and only the ends can ever justify any specific means. In this sense nobody will dispute that "ethics" comes before "economics." So far as I know nobody (except Titmuss) has ever suggested otherwise.

(*b*)   The problem of post-transfusion hepatitis was barely discussed in my original study with M. H. Cooper of the role of "price," and I should like briefly to indicate some of the economic possibilities here. It is clearly not "price" *per se* that causes the disease but the social condition of those who are frequently drawn by "price" to supply blood. A variety of possibilities suggest themselves once this fallacy has been identified:
A.   Assume there is no clinical test by which hepatitis carriers can be identified before donation. One could (1) collect all blood, including infected blood, and distribute as usual on the grounds that it is better to incur a risk (of less than unity) that recipients contract hepatitis than to suffer even greater shortage. This seems a wrong policy since better choices are available. It is a valid criticism of Americans that they have largely adopted this policy; (2) offer a sufficiently high price that an excess supply is produced from amongst which those individuals with obviously undesired characteristics may be rejected—this is costly; (3) offer a "price" *in kind* of a sort to appeal to the appropriate social class (e.g., theatre tickets, free parking, Wine Society membership)—this is costly; (4) discriminate at the point of collection by offering "prices" only to certain prechosen categories of population (e.g., university students, teachers, residents of well-to-do districts)—this too will be costly.
B.   Retain donation only and encourage donation by advertising, jogging consciences, public lectures on ethics, offsetting costs of attendance (e.g., provide baby-sitting services), etc. In short, vary the non-price determinants of supply. This will be costly.
C.   It seems highly likely that in the near future a clinical test for detecting viral hepatitis will become generally available. It could be used to screen both donors and paid suppliers to remove the problem (almost) entirely. This would be costly.

Reprinted with permission from *The Lancet*, 1, 602–3, March 20, 1971.

These are some possibilities (by no means an exhaustive list) suggested by the economics of blood supply and demand whereby supplies could be increased if it were felt desirable to do so. It seems to me wrong to be complacent about the adequacy of current supplies in Britain. Apart from the postponement of operations, which occurs in all countries with an unknown relative frequency, one would wish to know how frequently patients are transfused with imperfectly matched blood; how often blood is used for purposes in which it is less useful than other purposes; how often a current or expected shortage affects *future* demand via the planned amounts of complementary inputs to be made available in the future; and other questions of a similar type. We are so ignorant about such things that complacency is irresponsible in implying that we ought not to bother to find out.

Regarding Titmuss's views on the wider role of altruism in the blood market, I have little to say. His assertions, however, strike me as lacking both the theory to predict and the facts to sustain the extraordinary view that *supplementing* (not replacing) donation with compensation in some form will have serious long-term disruptive effects on society. But even if that is on the cards, the choice is not for Titmuss, or me, or doctors, to make, but for the whole of society, since it affects the whole of society. In the limit, adherence to giving and giving alone would countenance the death of patients should suppliers turn out to be less philanthropic than he hopes, and I doubt if society would hesitate much between choosing between these conflicting ends. I doubt also whether the Americans would be much impressed by Titmuss's ideas as the solution to their problem. By contrast, the electicism of the economic approach may be useful to them.

Fundamentally, Titmuss does not understand economics. This leads him falsely to assert that the American system exploits the poor and redistributes real income to the relatively rich, whereas whatever the faults of the American system this is most unlikely to be one of them! It leads him to present totally misleading comparative cost statistics (ignoring costs not revealed in cash; the fact that cost is not independent of supply; the irrelevance of *unit* compared with *incremental* cost in policy decisions). It leads him falsely to be concerned about "inflating" G.N.P. (of all things). Finally, it leads him falsely to identify "Paretian" improvements in social welfare with "consumer sovereignty," whereas the latter is wholly inconsistent with the former.

All this is to sacrifice truth for the sake of special pleading. This dispassionate analyst must recognise that payment for blood, if suitably engineered, can be effective and may be desirable, but actual choice of donation-only/payment-only/donation-with-payment ought to be dependent upon the relative social costs of different methods in getting a given increase in supply. At the moment we have neither this information nor enough knowledge about present or future demand and adequacy to decide. Without this knowledge (which *economics* suggests is needed) a-priori reasoning cannot dictate policy, Professor Titmuss notwithstanding.

A. J. Culyer

From "Altruism and Commerce:
A Defense of Titmuss Against Arrow"

Peter Singer

Kenneth Arrow's discussion[1] of *The Gift Relationship* by Richard Titmuss[2] is to be welcomed because it draws attention to this remarkable book. Ostensibly, the book is a comparison of voluntary and commercial means of obtaining blood for medical purposes, but by means of this comparison Titmuss succeeds, as Arrow says, in raising "the largest descriptive and normative questions about the social order in a highly specific and richly factual context" (p. 362). Although Arrow praises the endeavor, he is not very keen on what Titmuss actually says about these issues. I wish to defend Titmuss against some of Arrow's criticisms. . . .

The overall picture . . . is that where payment for blood is unknown, the number of voluntary donors has risen and kept pace with the increased demand; whereas when the opportunity to give freely exists alongside the buying and selling of blood, the number of volunteers falls sharply and can only with difficulty, if at all, be made good by increases in the amount of blood bought. This suggests that to pay some people for their blood does discourage others from giving it altruistically; or alternatively, that a purely voluntary system encourages altruism in a way that a mixed commercial-voluntary system does not.

Arrow demands not merely evidence, but (p. 351) "at least a minimum of theoretical analysis. *Why* should it be that the creation of a market for blood would decrease the altruism embodied in giving blood?" The second kind of evidence to be found in *The Gift Relationship* is concerned with the motivation of voluntary donors in Britain. As such, it may help us to understand the connection between altruism and the voluntary system while at the same time supporting the claim that there is such a connection.

This evidence comes from a questionnaire survey of blood donors in England taken by Titmuss and his associates.[3] One question asked was: "Could you say why you *first* decided to become a blood donor?" Statistically, all that can be said is that nearly 80 percent of the 3,800 answers Titmuss collected indicate that the respondent was motivated by a high sense of social responsibility toward the needs of others. It is true that these people might have continued to give blood unpaid, and for the same reasons, even if a commercial system existed along with the voluntary one; but it is worth noting (although no statistical significance is being claimed here)

Reprinted with permission of author and publisher from *Philosophy and Public Affairs* 2:3, 312–319. Copyright © 1972 by Princeton University Press.

[1]Kenneth J. Arrow, "Gifts and Exchanges," *Philosophy and Public Affairs*, 1:4, 343–362, Summer 1972.

[2]Richard M. Titmuss, *The Gift Relationship: From Human Blood to Social Policy* (Great Britain: George Allen & Unwin, 1971).

[3]*Ibid.*, pp. 226–235, 276–320.

that at least some of the answers do suggest a connection between the special status of blood under the voluntary system, and the motivation of the donors. For instance, a young married woman, a machine operator earning £15 to £20 per week, replied:

> You can't get blood from supermarkets and chaine stores. People themselves must come forword, sick people cant get out of bed to ask you for a pint to save thier life so I came forword in hope to help somebody who needs blood.

Despite her obvious lack of education, this woman expressed the essential point Titmuss is making: in Britain the supply of blood is outside the otherwise pervasive supermarket society. No matter how much money you have, you can't buy yourself a pint of blood. You must rely on the altruism and good will of others to provide it for you. Hence commercial blood supplies are introduced, even though the voluntary system may continue to operate as well, this situation has been altered. Provided you have money, you do not then need the altruism of your fellow men and women, since you can buy the blood you need. So commerce replaces fellow-feeling. Marx was well aware of this effect of commerce, and described it vividly:

> The extent of the power of money is the extent of my power. Money's properties are my properties and essential powers—the properties and powers of its possessor. Thus what I am and am capable of is by no means determined by my individuality. I am ugly, but I can buy for myself the most beautiful of women. Therefore I am not ugly for the effect of ugliness—its deterrent power —is nullified by money. . . . That which I am unable to do as a *man* . . . I am able to do by means of *money.* . . . Money, then, appears as this overturning power both against the individual and against the bonds of society. . . . Assume *man* to be *man* and his relationship to the world to be a human one: then you can exchange love only for love, trust for trust, etc.[4]

We do not, however, need to go into the Marxist theory of money as an alienating force in order to understand how a voluntary blood supply system—or more generally, a system of free medicine like the British National Health Service—may strengthen feelings of community and mutual interdependence. I think it is clear that the woman whose reply has been quoted would have been less likely to give her blood if blood were a marketable commodity. Some of the other responses to Titmuss's questionnaire indicate this in different, though equally direct, ways:

> I get my surgical shoes thro' the N.H.S. This is some slight return and I want to help people (an insurance agent).
> To try and repay in some small way some unknown person whose blood

---

[4]Karl Marx, *The Economic and Philosophic Manuscripts of 1844*, trans. M. Milligan, ed. D. J. Struik (New York, 1967), pp. 167–169. (For more on the same theme, see also the section entitled "The Power of Money in Bourgeois Society.") I think this quotation shows that Titmuss himself is unfair to Marx when he relates the commercially minded attitude to blood supplies in the Soviet Union to Marx's theory of the commodity (*The Gift Relationship*, p. 195).

helped me recover from two operations and enable me to be with my family, thats why I bring them along also as they become old enough (a farmer's wife).

No man is an island (a maintenance fitter).[5]

The nature of these replies—not the mere fact that the donors were altruistically motivated, but their attitudes toward the National Health Service in general and the Blood Transfusion Service in particular—is evidence that at least for some people the possibility of others buying and selling blood would destroy the inspiring force behind their own donations. At the same time, these replies enable us to understand *why* the existence of a commercial system could be expected to make a difference. The idea that others are depending on one's generosity and concern, that one may oneself, in an emergency, need the assistance of a stranger, the feeling that there is still at least this vital area in which we must rely on the good will of others rather than the profit motive—all these vague ideas and feelings are incompatible with the existence of a market in blood. Do we really need any further "theoretical analysis"?

Arrow is critical of Titmuss for favoring the voluntary system on broad grounds of principle, unsupported by adequate statistical evidence. Yet Arrow has his own opposite preferences, at least equally unsupported. Arrow frankly admits that:

> . . . like many economists, I do not want to rely too heavily on substituting ethics for self-interest. I think it best on the whole that the requirement of ethical behavior be confined to those circumstances where the price system breaks down. . . . Wholesale usage of ethical standards is apt to have undesirable consequences. We do not wish to use up recklessly the scarce resources of altruistic motivation. . . . (pp. 354–355)

Arrow offers no evidence or theory for the view that altruism resembles, say, oil in being a scarce resource, the more of which we use the less we have. Why should we not assume that altruism is more like sexual potency—much used, it constantly renews itself, but if rarely called upon, it will begin to atrophy and will not be available when needed? It is this latter

---

[5] *The Gift Relationship*, pp. 227–228. In discussing the percentage of British donors who are fully voluntary, Arrow notes that in the case of 28 percent of British donors either they or their family have received blood transfusions (p. 347). Since this remark follows immediately on the comment that Titmuss has not classified British donors in a manner comparable to his classification of United States donors, it implies that Arrow would put these British donors into the same category as those in the United States who are replacing blood received by themselves or their relatives, and whom Titmuss does not count as fully voluntary. This seems to be another oversight on Arrow's part. Titmuss does classify British donors in exactly the same terms as United States donors, and concludes that 99 percent—all but the donations of prisoners, who may be under some external pressure—are fully voluntary (*The Gift Relationship*, p. 130). The point is that in Britain people who need blood get it irrespective of whether they have given blood, or undertake to give it in the future; in the United States various schemes exist under which unpaid donations either replace blood received that would otherwise have to be paid for, or are a form of credit in case one needs blood in the future. This is why "reciprocal" donations in the United States could have a purely self-interested motivation, whereas in Britain they are a sign of community feeling.

simile which consideration of my own feelings leads me to favor. I find it hardest to act with consideration for others when the norm in the circle of people I move in is to act egoistically. When altruism is expected of me, however, I find it much easier to be genuinely altruistic.

Indeed, there is experimental evidence for the view that altruism fosters increased altruism. Psychologists have found that if they set up situations calling for an altruistic response—for example, a woman looking helpless beside a broken-down car—more people will respond with offers of help if they have recently witnessed someone else behaving altruistically in a similar situation (i.e., because the experimenters put a man helping a woman to change a tire back down the road) than if they had not witnessed an altruistic act.[6] These results, hardly surprising results really, give some support to Titmuss's view that the opportunity for altruism promotes further altruism, and count against the idea that altruism is a finite resource.

From "Blood and Thunder"

Robert M. Solow

The Gift Relationship: From Human Blood to Social Policy. By Richard M. Titmuss. *New York: Pantheon Books,* 1971.

The subtitle of this extraordinarily interesting book gives a fair indication of its ambitions. Most of it is a detailed comparison of two alternative ways of organizing the collection and allocation of human blood for transfusion and similar purposes. On this level, it appears to be—and probably is—a devastating and unanswerable indictment of the American system as inferior to the British in efficiency, morality, and attractiveness. From this secure beachhead, Professor Titmuss launches a broad attack on the market as a mechanism for the mobilization and allocation of scarce resources, and, even more generally, on the whole economizing mode of thought which— as he might have said if he were a different sort of man—knows the price of everything and the value of nothing. On this broader front he scores some important points but is ultimately confused. I hope to show that what arouses Titmuss's anger and scorn is usually not, as he thinks, the use of economic reasoning but its misuse. There is a lesson here for everyone interested in social policy, because some economists do have a way of drifting into sharp propositions that cannot be fully supported even on narrowly economic grounds. But blood first, thunder afterward.

[6]A summary of this and other experiments along similar lines may be found in D. Wright, *The Psychology of Moral Behavior* (London and Baltimore, 1971) pp. 133–139.

Reprinted by permission of the author, the Yale Law Journal Company and Fred B. Rothman & Company from *The Yale Law Journal* 80, 1696–1711, 1971.

I

In Great Britain, the collection and allocation of blood is entirely in the hands of the National Blood Transfusion Service as an integral part of the National Health Service. (The actual functioning is decentralized through Regional Transfusion Centres corresponding roughly to the Regional Hospital Boards.) Essentially all blood is collected from voluntary donors who receive no reward but a cup of tea. Blood is allocated from the Regional Centres to hospitals by negotiated quota; there is provision for renegotiation of quotas, for special allocation of emergency supplies, and for national pooling of rare blood types. Hospitals do not have to pay for the blood they use, nor do the patients who ultimately receive transfused blood. (Even private patients who have contracted out of the National Health Service receive blood free from the Service.) There is apparently no explicit or implied obligation to replace blood used by oneself or one's family, or to earn insurance credits by supplying blood in advance. In fact, in a sample survey slightly over a quarter of donors report that they or a member of their immediate family have received blood in the past. Since it seems unlikely that as many as a quarter of all immediate families have members who have received transfusions, the receipt of blood is probably a motive for subsequent giving by the recipient or his relatives. But there is no accounting system for such gifts, and presumably no unpleasant pressure to pay back.

Donors appear to be broadly, though not exactly, representative of the population at large: males and the young are over-represented for obvious reasons; "professional, etc." occupations are over-represented and semi-skilled and unskilled occupations are under-represented, though it is impossible to say how much of this social-class bias represents differences in past and present health and therefore in eligibility.[1]

Blood is thus completely removed from the marketplace. It is supplied at zero fee and used at zero price. Recipients do not even know whom to thank.

In the United States, by contrast, there is no unified system for the collection and distribution of blood, but rather a variety of differentiated institutions. One of the consequences is that it is impossible to assemble comprehensive statistical information on any sort of uniform basis. There is a large element of guesswork, therefore, in any picture of how the apparatus actually works.

Titmuss classifies blood banks into five classes. (1) Red Cross Regional Blood Centers, based on 1700 local chapters, contribute about forty per cent of the total supply. (2) About one hundred non-profit community blood banks are believed to account for fifteen to twenty per cent of the total. (3) Some 6000 hospital blood banks are responsible for twenty to thirty per cent. (4) An unknown number of profit-making commercial blood banks, generally getting blood from paid donors, processing it, and selling it to hospitals, were believed in the early 1960s to account for some ten to fifteen

---

[1] *See generally* R. Titmuss, *The Gift Relationship: From Human Blood to Social Policy* 124–41 (1971) [hereinafter cited to page number only].

per cent of the total supply; but Titmuss and others believe their role has increased since then. (5) An unknown number of commercial blood banks directly operated by pharmaceutical firms supply plasma, plasma protein components and platelets obtained from paid donors by a new method called plasmapheresis.[2] (In plasmapheresis, the red cells are separated immediately from the plasma and injected back into the donor. It is claimed by some authorities that a single donor can safely give blood several times a week by this method, provided his health is good and his diet appropriate; but the technique is new, and apparently there remains some uncertainty about long-run effects on donors.)

It is even more difficult to arrive at any estimate of the sources of blood by type of donor. A knowledgeable person could no doubt quarrel with Titmuss's guesses, but it is unlikely that he is so far off as to render his general picture false. He distinguishes eight types of donors, but some of these are minor variations on others. The figures are for 1965–67 and may be changing. About a third of all blood comes from paid donors, some of whom sell their blood occasionally, some regularly. This fraction includes a small amount from donors who receive a cash payment, but whose main reason for "volunteering" may be group pressure from a trade union or other organization with a quota it would like to fill. A little over half of all blood comes from those who are in effect exchanging blood for blood. Some of them are making "insurance deposits"; for instance, a donation of one pint a year by some member of a family insures all members of the immediate family for their blood needs for that year. (There are also policies which, in exchange for cash premiums, insure against the cash costs of blood, but these, of course, are not sources of blood to the system.) Other people give blood in exchange for blood already received. Hospitals levy a cash charge per unit of blood delivered to patients; in the 1960s a typical charge was $30–$100 a pint, and for some types of surgery many pints are required. As an alternative to cash payment, the patient is urged to replace the blood he has used with his own blood or with that from one or more friends, relatives, hired donors, or members of a "blood plan group" to which the patient belongs for just such contingencies. Many hospitals require the patient to supply two units of blood for each unit used, and set cash fees accordingly.[3]

About five per cent of all blood comes from "captive voluntary donors," mostly servicemen and prisoners. Some prisoners receive a small cash payment. In some states there appears to be formal remission of sentences as a reward for donation of blood; one presumes that generally parole boards look more kindly on prisoners whose records show a history of blood donation. (In Britain, according to Titmuss, prisoners are treated like other members of the community and allowed to volunteer. There is no formal reward of any kind, but it is difficult, as he says, to know how the prisoners themselves see the situation.) The remaining ten per cent of all blood supplied in the United States comes from the voluntary donor, who is the source of essentially all blood in Great Britain.[4]

[2] Pp. 90–93.
[3] Pp. 75–88.
[4] Pp. 84–89.

These figures exclude blood components collected in plasmapheresis programs. Such programs draw entirely on paid donors, some "walk-in," some essentially salaried. When they are added in, about half of all blood is bought for cash, about forty per cent is exchanged for other blood, about seven per cent is voluntarily given, and the residue comes from the captive voluntary donor.[5]

Only the most fragmentary information exists on the demographic and socio-economic classification of blood donors. One blood bank, drawing mainly on replacement and individual and group credit donors, found that its donors were predominantly male, and somewhat younger and of higher socio-economic status than the community at large. Presumably this reflects the middle-class character of most tied programs. Data from blood banks, whether profit-making or not, which draw mainly on paid donors exhibit the expected heavy dependence on the low-paid occupational groups and, especially, on the unemployed. The Skid Row donor is real, but there are, no doubt, some who sell blood for bread, not booze.

II

Which system works better? Even leaving aside moral and aesthetic considerations, there are several criteria against which one could judge. On all of them, the British seem to do as well or better, usually much better.

Both systems manage to collect about the same amount of blood in total, with due allowance for the different size of the two countries. The statistics do not permit any precise comparison. Nevertheless, the official figures for England and Wales show that in the late 1960s the number of donations was about three per hundred of population; the fragmentary data for the United States suggest something similar. Plasmapheresis adds something to the American collections.

On the other hand, a much larger fraction of the available blood is wasted in the United States (Blood can be safely stored only for about twenty days; outdated blood can, however, be converted to dried plasma and other products which last for much longer.) If conversion to plasma is not counted as waste, only a tiny fraction of blood collected in England and Wales is wasted—something like one to two per cent. On this question the American statistics are particularly unsatisfactory, with differential under-reporting of collections and transfusions, and no clear measure of the amount of outdated blood converted to plasma. In some years the apparent gap between collections and transfusions is as much as a third of collections. Actual waste must be less, because of conversion. If the rate of conversion is extrapolated from British data, and other similar guesses are made, it appears that the wastage rate in the United States is no lower than ten per cent of collections and may be higher than that. One may say, then, that the American system wastes about ten times as much blood as the British, proportionately, despite the fact that blood is expensive in the United States and "free" in Great Britain.[6]

[5]P. 96.
[6]Pp. 22–23, 56–58.

This waste results from defects in planning and administration, from failures to match demand and supply properly, from the over-ordering and hoarding of blood by hospitals and blood banks, from incorrect estimates of the demand for blood by type, from transportation delays, and other such factors in the system. A different kind of waste is the medically unnecessary use of blood, but of course it is intrinsically impossible to have complete data on this. One survey in London suggested that six and one-half per cent of the blood use was medically unnecessary. One is tempted to say that the figure must be lower in a system in which hospitals and patients pay for blood, but it is precisely Titmuss's point that one ought not to say that, and the figures on administrative waste suggest that he is right. In any case, unnecessary surgery and unnecessary transfusions are certainly not unknown in the United States, but Titmuss quotes no figure comparable with the one just given for London. He mentions one survey of five common operations on two million patients in 1959–1962 which estimated a waste of 160,000 pints of blood, but gives no survey figure for the total use of blood, which could, but need not, exceed 2,000,000 pints.[7]

Waste of blood is not logically incompatible with the existence of occasional and local shortages of blood; supreme inefficiency might permit waste and near-chronic shortage to co-exist. Here again, Titmuss argues that the British system has proved superior. He claims that there have not been any significant or prolonged shortages of blood in England and Wales since 1948. In contrast, he is able to cite a number of statements by American students and medical men asserting that many hospitals and areas are chronically short of blood, and that elective surgery is frequently postponed or cancelled because the required blood is unavailable. He concludes: "Among the large urban and metropolitan areas only a minority of places . . . appear to have no chronic shortages of fresh blood. Generally, throughout the United States, there are widespread reports from many areas and by numerous experts of actual and potential demand exceeding the available supply of blood."[8]

This is not quite the same thing as data. Some mildly contradictory evidence is contained in a small mail survey of consultants to the National Blood Transfusion Service conducted by two English economists.[9] It is a very small sample, with a response rate of only about a half. But thirty-six per cent of the surgeons who replied reported that they had "sometimes" postponed operations for lack of blood supply. (Another one per cent replied that they had "often" done so.) Some twenty-two per cent had "sometimes" experienced undue delay in obtaining emergency supplies through the NBTS (plus two per cent who had "often" experienced such delays). Nevertheless, in the full sample of physicians and surgeons, fifty-five per

[7]Pp. 196–97.

[8]P. 65.

[9]M. Cooper & A. Culyer, *The Price of Blood* 18–19 (1968). It should be noted that Cooper and Culyer are diametrically at odds with Titmuss's attitudes; their pamphlet is indeed an attempt to make the case for the buying and selling of blood in Britain. I shall come back to it later.

cent characterized the blood supplies to their hospitals as "excellent," forty-one per cent as "adequate," and only four per cent as "poor." It is very difficult to weigh this sort of evidence against a culling of alarmist statements about the situation in the United States. It is hard to escape the conclusion, however, that the British have it at least an order of magnitude better.

There is one other standard against which one can compare the two systems for supplying blood: the quality of the product. The main risk is serum hepatitis, incurred by transfusion recipients from contaminated blood. There are reports that three and six-tenths per cent of all transfused hospital patients in the United States later contracted the disease. Serum hepatitis has been said by the *Journal of the American Medical Association* to cause death in about one of 150 transfusions in persons older than forty (who receive much of the blood).[10] In Great Britain, no study (there have only been a few) shows the incidence of hepatitis following transfusions to be greater than one per cent, and the most recent study estimates the risk to be negligible.[11]

There appears to be no practical way to test donated blood for hepatitis. The only protection against contaminated blood is the willingness of the prospective donor to report that he has had or been exposed to hepatitis, if he knows it. It is evident that in any system in which blood is sold for money by donors who need the money, the donor has a motive to conceal his history of hepatitis if he has one and knows it. Further, since sellers of blood will come predominantly from the poor—not to mention the Skid Row syndrome—prospective donors can be expected to have a higher incidence of hepatitis than the population at large, and less knowledge of it. It is hardly a surprise, then, that "many studies in different parts of the United States have incriminated the paid donor (and blood obtained from commercial blood banks) as the major source of infection."[12]

Moreover, hepatitis can be transmitted in plasma as well as in whole blood. Since plasma is often pooled from the blood of several hundred donors, one or two of whom can infect the whole lot, the risk from large-pool plasma is very high, though it is cheap and easy to process. In Britain, the risk is recognized and small-pool plasma (from fewer than ten donors) became the rule in 1945.[13]

By all these measures—and remember that I have not yet mentioned the morality of a system in which poor people sell their blood for the use of rich people who buy it—the British system seems to be far more efficient—more economical, one might say—than the American. There is a certain paradox, then, in the fact that in England blood is free, whereas here blood is dear.

[10]P. 145.
[11]Pp. 154–55.
[12]Pp. 147–48.
[13]Pp. 145–52.

III

Titmuss thinks he understands why this happens, though I do not recall that he ever states clearly and concisely his view of the causal connection. I imagine it goes something like this.

Contrary to the view of "economists," it is precisely the element of commercialism that causes the American system to operate so badly, and precisely its absence that permits the British system to operate so well. There is in ordinary people a very large (inexhaustible?) fund of altruism, of feelings of solidarity, of willingness or need to enter into gift relationships.[14] The British system taps this and finds as much as it needs.

Even a small admixture of commercialism, however, is enough to poison the well. The altruistic impulse is diminished or destroyed by the realization that what one is offering as a gift others are selling as a commodity. The existence of a market sector thus contaminates the voluntary system. The attitude of personal caring disappears; perhaps this accounts for the greater waste in the American system. Titmuss goes so far as to argue that the buying and selling of some blood is a narrowing of the freedom of potential voluntary donors; it restricts the "freedom to give" because one can not give and get satisfaction from giving what is elsewhere entering the market.[15]

It is not a convincing argument. We can all agree on one point, that the use of paid donors must be responsible for the substantial and growing risk of hepatitis from transfusion. A history of hepatitis and the motive to conceal it are likely to coincide only in those who sell blood for money. But the rest of the story seems far-fetched. I know that on none of the many occasions on which I have failed to appear at the local Bloodmobile has my realization of the existence of a market in blood played the slightest part.

[14]Obviously the gift of blood is not like a birthday present. Usually the donor and recipient never meet, do not know each other, do not even know each other's name. Nor is there really much resemblance between giving blood and the Melanesian kula or the Pacific Northwest potlatch, as Titmuss suggests there is. See M. Mauss, *The Gift* (1. Gunnison transl. 1954) (originally published in 1925 as *Essai sur le don, Forme Archaïque de L'échange*). The latter customs are in large part formal ceremonies; there is also a much larger element of exchange, and a definite tinge of aggression (*Id.* at 35). One motive for giving blood is certainly the wish to help maintain a system of which one might sometime be a beneficiary. But more usually it seems closer to a contribution than to a gift, for example the donation of goods or money to the victims of a famine or a flood. It is an important element, I think, that the thing given has only slight value to the giver, but very great value to the recipient.

[15]At times one senses that Titmuss is going even further, to a claim that doing away with markets not only avoids pollution of altruism, but absolutely encourages more altruism. This line of argument is similar to the claim of anarchists, from Godwin to Kropotkin, that if only the whole panoply of harmful institutions could be disassembled, there would be found enough sense of one's responsibility for others, enough mutual aid, to provide for everyone's needs without compulsion. This claim is difficult enough to evaluate when made cleanly. But it is not Titmuss's claim. At least in this book, Titmuss seems to suggest that a fund of altruism can be released in one context at a time, without need for a transformation of society altogether. The selling of soap is commercial in Britain too. In any event, Titmuss has trouble enough advancing the position that markets are evil because they kill altruism. This review is directed at that narrower thesis.

Each reader of this review can ask himself the same question. Professor Nathan Glazer did ask some students on the occasion of a Harvard University blood drive; this consideration was never raised.[16] I would be tempted to guess that the historical connection was just the reverse: that the purchase-and-sale sector made headway in the United States only when the voluntary system proved inadequate to supply the medical needs for blood.

There are some tantalizing loose ends in Titmuss's work that might have yielded more light on this issue had they been followed up. In isolation, they merely cast doubt on Titmuss's hypothesis. We learn, for instance, that ". . . Seattle, which had one of the best organized and effective blood banking and cross-matching agencies in the country . . . , and which collected 35,000 units annually, reported in recent years an outdating proportion of less than 2 per cent."[17] One wonders why. Was there no access to paid donors in Seattle, or did hospitals there charge patients in some different and less commercial way? We are not told, though there is an indication that Seattle did have commercial blood banking, and even bought blood from derelicts. . . .[18]

IV

Even if Titmuss fails to produce a convincing explanation of the success of the British system and the failure of the American, the facts themselves pose more of a challenge to "economists" than to him. Dennis Robertson once gave a talk entitled "What Do Economists Economize?" His answer was "love"; he meant that altruism is a scarce resource, and the business of economists is to find institutional arrangements that will accomplish society's purposes without depending too much on disinterested kindness. That is what economists since Adam Smith have found so fascinating about the competitive market: that the unrestricted interaction of self-interested people under appropriate conditions[19] results in an outcome with certain socially desirable properties willed by none of them.

It is a routine observation that when a resource is made available at a price that does not adequately reflect its scarcity, it will be used wastefully, *i.e.*, in low-priority rather than in high-priority ways (perhaps including conservation). That is the standard case for tolls on congested roads and effluent charges on polluted rivers. Here we are presented with a case in which free blood is adequately supplied and carefully husbanded, while dear blood is wasted and contaminated. Is this reason to doubt the case for congestion tolls and effluent charges? I don't think so. But it is reason to

[16]Glazer, *Blood*, THE PUBLIC INTEREST. Summer 1971, at 89.

[17]P. 65.

[18]P. 113.

[19]The conditions are pretty stringent: they include the ready availability of knowledge about prices and products to all participants, the absence of monopoly, and the insignificance of those "externalities" that are now beginning to seem very significant indeed.

remember that economic reasoning applies only where economic motives predominate.

It is one thing to suggest that the supply of altruism is limited and quite another thing to pretend that no motive but greed ever operated, even "in our culture." It is fair comment, I fear, that some devoted marketeers do just that. There is a pretty example of this in Cooper and Culyer. They say, discussing waste of blood: "If the price (of blood) to hospitals is zero, there will be no incentive to conserve blood to the limit, and hence the amount that would be considered 'adequate' will be larger than the amount that would be considered 'adequate' if a price had to be paid."[20] It is a standard economic argument, and I have no doubt that it applies in those situations that are institutionalized as "economic." But it is certainly gratuitous to assert that doctors and hospital administrators respond, presumably necessarily respond, to *no other* stimulus but money. That assertion is not itself economics: it is psychology, and very likely bad psychology.

Over-enthusiastic marketeers sometimes fall into another bad habit. It is a kind of cultivated moral obtuseness. Here is an example from Cooper and Culyer. The text of their pamphlet nowhere mentions the hepatitis problem as a possible or even probable consequence of the introduction of a commercial market for blood. At the end, however, there are some suggested questions for discussion. One of them reads: "There is evidence to show that blood from 'professional' donors is more likely to carry disease. What difference does this make to the economic analysis of this Paper?" And the next question goes: "Is it right to subject patients to additional risks by transfusing them with inferior blood? Compare your answer with treatment by inferior surgeons, hospitals, etc. If inferiority is a reflection of the fundamental fact of scarcity, can anything be done to remove it?"[21]

I am afraid I can imagine what they would find an acceptable answer to these questions. It would presumably involve the labelling of some blood as "risky" and some as "safe." (Since blood cannot practically be tested for safety, presumably all blood from paid donors would have to be labelled as risky: perhaps one can imagine several grades according to the type of donor —alcoholic, penniless artist, poor but honest, little old lady. But the grade-labelling would have to be policed to avoid cheating, so there is danger of interference with economic liberty even here.) Risky blood would of course sell at a lower price than safe blood. Poor people would buy cheap blood; rich people could afford safe blood. If that strikes you as awful, reflect on the fundamental fact of scarcity. Upon reflection, it may not be clear to you that the mere fact of scarcity implies that the quality of blood a man receives should be correlated with his capacity to earn income.[22] You may even be troubled by the fact that the risky blood gets introduced into an otherwise reasonably satisfactory situation only through Cooper and Culyer's belief

---

[20] M. Cooper & A. Culyer, *supra* note 9, at 21.

[21] *Id.* at 46.

[22] Should the cut of meat a man eats be correlated with his capacity to earn income? It would carry me too far afield to discuss that question here. Perhaps most readers would agree that it is worse that poor people should be transfused with risky blood than that they should eat inferior meat.

that buying and selling blood is a useful practice. Suppose that the introduction of a commercial market would in fact result in some marginal improvement in efficiency (though Titmuss's story suggests it wouldn't). The judgment that such an improvement could justify the creation of differentials in quality of blood received by income class does strike me as morally obtuse.

This leads to a deeper and more important point. In their enthusiasm for market allocations, many economists seem to drift into assertions that go beyond what economic analysis will support. The nice thing about free competitive markets is that—under the right conditions, some of which I mentioned earlier—they lead to outcomes that are Pareto-efficient or Pareto-optimal, to use the technical term. That means that the final situation is such that no physically feasible shift of resources could make everyone better off (or at least make some people better off without making anyone worse off). "Better off" means better off in one's own estimation.

Inefficient situations are clearly bad in the sense that some physically feasible efficient situation can be found in which everyone is better off. It would be better to be in that efficient situation. Any efficient situation is certainly better than certain inefficient situations, namely, those in which everyone is worse off. But it is definitely not true that any efficient situation is better than any inefficient situation. A may be an efficient situation and B an inefficient one; but some people may be better off in B than they would be in A, though others must be better off in A. We would say that the distribution of income differs between A and B. The economist has no technical right to recommend a move from B to A. He can recommend a move from B to one of the efficient situations that is clearly superior to B, say C; or, which comes to the same thing, he could recommend a move from B to A accompanied by a redistribution of income that would be, in effect, a move from A to C. Without the redistribution, there is no sense in which A is economically better than B.

This is old stuff in welfare economics, but it is sometimes forgotten in the heat of advocacy. Suppose some scarce resource is being distributed free or at some artificially low (or high) price that does not adequately reflect the cost of making it available. If economic motives predominate, the resource will be over-used (or under-used) in the sense that everyone could be made better off if less (or more) of this resource were produced and consumed and the production and consumption of other things were increased (or decreased). This is Cooper and Culyer's case for pricing blood, except that they merely assume that only economic motives can matter. Going over to rational pricing will almost always have distributional effects as well as efficiency effects; in fact there is usually a sense in which the distributional effects are first-order and the efficiency effects second-order. Suppose I protest that the introduction of rational pricing will hurt the poor or the innocent or the worthy and help the rich or the slick or the unworthy. The marketeer's response is that the right way to help the poor is directly through transfers of purchasing power; there is no virtue in generating wasteful misallocation of resources in order to bring about a desirable distribution of income when direct non-distorting methods are available. He is right about that. Well, then, he goes on, you think about what to do next, and in the meanwhile let's have rational pricing of whatever-it-is and get rid of the inefficiency. But there he is wrong. An improvement in efficiency accompanied by adverse distributional effects is not a good thing pending corrective redistribution. It is a good thing only when it is accompanied by corrective redistribution.

This proposition cuts both ways. I have alluded to the unattractiveness of a system in which the poor sell their blood to the rich. The marketeer replies: to eliminate that possibility will do harm to the poor as well as to the rich, perhaps more harm to the poor than to the rich. Leaving aside addicts, alcoholics, and other incompetents, those who sell blood receive something in exchange of greater value to them, else they wouldn't do as they do. Now it is my turn to say that there are better ways of increasing the income of the poor to the point where they would cease supplying blood for money even if the opportunity remained. But it is not enough to say that there are better ways. Unless they are actually effective, to cut off the option of selling blood is to satisfy my moral judgments at the expense of those who would voluntarily choose that option.

In summary, some of Titmuss's complaints about the enthusiasts of the market are valid. But they are valid complaints about invalid overextensions of economic reasoning, not about economic reasoning itself. The dichotomy between efficiency and distribution is a necessary analytical distinction, not a justification for regressive policy measures.

V

There is another side to the coin. Efficiency in the use of scarce resources is a worthwhile goal. If you believe that, and if you believe, in addition, that autonomy of the individual decision-making person is a good thing, then you ought to find the free competitive market an attractive way to organize a lot of activities, *provided the distribution of income is fair.* In a society of equals or near-equals, one might even look more kindly on the sale of blood, though I can easily understand and share the feeling that might make one wish to prevent it as one would wish to prevent people from selling their eyes or kidneys or votes or selling themselves into slavery.

Titmuss, on the contrary, is rather down on buying and selling, sometimes for defensible reasons, sometimes for poor reasons, sometimes for reasons of taste on which right-thinking people need not agree. For example, there are some things or services that are best kept from the market, not because it would be technically difficult or inefficient to market them, but because the "social" consequences would be bad even if the narrowly "economic" consequences were good. I would rather say that if, in total, the social consequences are bad then the economic consequences are bad too, and only appear to be good because the accounting is incomplete. But that is a quibble about words; the point is that it may well be socially destructive to admit the routine exchangeability of certain things. We would prefer to maintain that they are beyond price (although this sometimes means only that we would prefer not to know what the price really is).

I have already mentioned Titmuss's argument that the economist's attempts to economize on altruism merely destroy more altruism than they save. There is no intellectual difficulty here; anyone, economist or other, would recognize that as false economy. But Titmuss makes a very weak case for this belief; it can hardly be regarded as established in general, or even in the specific instance of blood donation.

A less legitimate argument occasionally crops up in this book and elsewhere. It is an old thought that to put something in correspondence with "money" is to dirty or demean it. But there is a confusion here. Money itself is surely more or less irrelevant; a return to barter would not eliminate the moral problems connected with buying and selling. Whenever people must choose among alternatives, they must somehow reduce their preferences to some kind of common denominator, if only the intensity of desire itself: I want X more than Y and Y more than Z, so that if presented with a choice I will choose X. If people must exchange with one another, they will certainly have to represent and discuss the terms on which they are prepared to exchange units of X for Y and units of Y for Z. I can see no special moral problem that arises when relative prices are expressed in money terms. Quite the contrary, though it has become less fashionable to say so, there are real *moral* as well as economic advantages in having an impersonal, universalistic way for people to express and exhibit the strength of their preferences. Prescription by authority or ascription by custom and status are not always attractive alternatives to the market registration of the sum of individual wishes.

Allocation through a market will work only where autonomous individuals must exchange resources, each trying to do the best for himself according to his own preferences. Allocation through a market will seem morally right only in spheres in which self-interest is an approved motive and it is felt to be right that individual preferences should count. It would be a grim world if that covered everything. But it would be a very difficult world to organize in a decentralized way if that covered nothing. *Given rough equality,* I should think the free market provides a tolerable and even preferable way of organizing a fairly large area of economic activity. One of the reasons Professor Titmuss disagrees—if, as I think, he does disagree—is that he seems to attribute somewhat less importance to the notion that individual preferences should count. There is a slight, rather typically Fabian, authoritarian streak in Titmuss; he seems to believe that ordinary people ought to be happy to have many decisions made for them by professional experts who will, fortunately, often turn out to be moderately well-born Englishmen.

From "The Allocation of Exotic Medical Lifesaving Therapy"

Nicholas Rescher

THE PROBLEM

Technological progress has in recent years transformed the limits of the possible in medical therapy. However, the elevated state of sophistication of modern medical technology has brought the economists' classic problem of scarcity in its wake as an unfortunate side product. The enormously sophisticated and complex equipment and the highly trained teams of experts requisite for its utilization are scarce resources in relation to potential demand. The administrators of the great medical institutions that preside over these scarce resources thus come to be faced increasingly with the awesome choice: *Whose life to save?*

A (somewhat hypothetical) paradigm example of this problem may be sketched within the following set of definitive assumptions: We suppose that persons in some particular medically morbid condition are "mortally afflicted": It is virtually certain that they will die within a short time period (say ninety days). We assume that some very complex course of treatment (e.g., a heart transplant) represents a substantial probability of life prolongation for persons in this mortally afflicted condition. We assume that the facilities available in terms of human resources, mechanical instrumentalities, and requisite materials (e.g., hearts in the case of a heart transplant) make it possible to give a certain treatment—this "exotic (medical) lifesaving therapy," or ELT for short—to a certain, relatively small number of people. And finally we assume that a substantially greater pool of people in the mortally afflicted condition is at hand. The problem then may be formulated as follows: How is one to select within the pool of afflicted patients the ones to be given the ELT treatment in question; how to select those "whose lives are to be saved"? Faced with many candidates for an ELT process that can be made available to only a few, doctors and medical administrators confront the decision of who is to be given a chance at survival and who is, in effect, to be condemned to die.

As has already been implied, the "heroic" variety of spare-part surgery can pretty well be assimilated to this paradigm. One can foresee the time when heart transplantation, for example, will have become pretty much a routine medical procedure, albeit on a very limited basis, since a cardiac surgeon with the technical competence to transplant hearts can operate at best a rather small number of times each week and the elaborate facilities for such operations will most probably exist on a modest scale. Moreover, in "spare-part" surgery there is always the problem of availability of the "spare parts" themselves. A report in one British newspaper gives the following picture: "Of the 150,000 who die of heart disease each year [in the U.K.], Mr. Donald Longmore, research surgeon at the National Heart Hospital [in London] estimates that 22,000 might be eligible for heart surgery. Another 30,000 would need heart and lung transplants. But there are probably only between 7,000 and 14,000 potential donors a year."[1] Envisaging this situation in which at the very most something like one in four heart-malfunction victims can be saved, we clearly confront a problem in ELT allocation.

A perhaps even more drastic case in point is afforded by long-term haemodialysis, an ongoing process by which a complex device—an "artificial kidney machine"—is used periodically in cases of chronic renal failure to substitute for a non-functional kidney in "cleaning" potential poisons from the blood. Only a few major institutions have chronic haemodialysis units, whose complex operation is an extremely expensive proposition. For the present and the foreseeable future the situation is that "the number of places available for chronic haemodialysis is hopelessly inadequate."[2]

The traditional medical ethos has insulated the physician against facing the very existence of this problem. When swearing the Hippocratic Oath, he commits himself to work for the benefit of the sick in "whatsoever house I enter."[3] In taking this stance, the physician substantially renounces the explicit choice of saving certain lives rather than others. Of course, doctors have always in fact had to face such choices on the battlefield or in times of disaster, but there the issue had to be resolved hurriedly, under pressure, and in circumstances in which the very nature of the case effectively precluded calm deliberation by the decision maker as well as criticism by others. In sharp contrast, however, cases of the type we have postulated in the present discussion arise predictably, and represent choices to be made deliberately and "in cold blood."

It is, to begin with, appropriate to remark that this problem is not

[1] Christine Doyle, "Spare-Part Heart Surgeons Worried by Their Success," *Observer*, May 12, 1968.

[2] J. D. N. Nabarro, "Selection of Patients for Haemodialysis," *British Medical Journal* (March 11, 1967), p. 623. Although several thousand patients die in the U.K. each year from renal failure—there are about thirty new cases per million of population—only 10 per cent of these can for the forseeable future be accommodated with chronic haemodialysis. Kidney transplantation—itself a very tricky procedure—cannot make a more than minor contribution here. As this article goes to press, I learn that patients can be maintained in home dialysis at an operating cost about half that of maintaining them in a hospital dialysis unit (roughly an $8,000 minimum). In the United States, around 7,000 patients with terminal uremia who could benefit from haemodialysis evolve yearly. As of mid-1968, some 1,000 of these can be accommodated in existing hospital units. By June 1967, a world-wide total of some 120 patients were in treatment by home dialysis. (Data from a forthcoming paper, "Home Dialysis," by C. M. Conty and H. V. Murdaugh. See also R. A. Baillod *et al.*, "Overnight Haemodialysis in the Home," *Proceedings of the European Dialysis and Transplant Association*, VI [1965], 99 ff.).

[3] For the Hippocratic Oath see *Hippocrates: Works* (Loeb ed., London, 1959), I, p. 298.

fundamentally a medical problem. For when there are sufficiently many afflicted candidates for ELT then—so we may assume—there will also be more than enough for whom the purely medical grounds for ELT allocation are decisively strong in any individual case, and just about equally strong throughout the group. But in this circumstance a selection of some afflicted patients over and against others cannot *ex hypothesi* be made on the basis of purely medical considerations.

The selection problem, as we have said, is in substantial measure not a medical one. It is a problem *for* medical men, which must somehow be solved by them, but that does not make it a medical issue—any more than the problem of hospital building is a medical issue. As a problem it belongs to the category of philosophical problems—specifically a problem of moral philosophy or ethics. Structurally, it bears a substantial kinship with those issues in this field that revolve about the notorious whom-to-save-on-the-lifeboat and whom-to-throw-to-the-wolves-pursuing-the-sled questions. But whereas questions of this just-indicated sort are artificial, hypothetical, and far-fetched, the ELT issue poses a *genuine* policy question for the reasonable administrators in medical institutions, indeed a question that threatens to become commonplace in the foreseeable future.

Now what the medical administrator needs to have, and what the philosopher is presumably *ex officio* in a position to help in providing, is a body of *rational guidelines* for making choices in these literally life-or-death situations. This is an issue in which many interested parties have a substantial stake, including the responsible decision maker who wants to satisfy his conscience that he is acting in a reasonable way. Moreover, the family and associates of the man who is turned away—to say nothing of the man himself —have the right to an acceptable explanation. And indeed even the general public wants to know that what is being done is fitting and proper. All of these interested parties are entitled to insist that a reasonable code of operating principles provides a defensible rationale for making the life-and-death choices involved in ELT.

THE TWO TYPES OF CRITERIA

Two distinguishable types of criteria are bound up in the issue of making ELT choices. We shall call these *Criteria of Inclusion* and *Criteria of Comparison,* respectively. The distinction at issue here requires some explanation. We can think of the selection as being made by a two-stage process: (1) the selection from among all possible candidates (by a suitable screening process of a group to be taken under serious consideration as candidates for therapy, and then (2) the actual singling out within this group, of the particular individuals to whom therapy is to be given. Thus the first process narrows down the range of comparative choice by eliminating *en bloc* whole categories of potential candidates. The second process calls for a more refined, case-by-case comparison of those candidates that remain. By means of the first set of criteria one forms a selection group; by means of the second set, an actual selection is made within this group.

Thus what we shall call a "selection system" for the choice of patients to receive therapy of the ELT type will consist of criteria of these two kinds. Such a system will be acceptable only when the reasonableness of its component criteria can be established.

ESSENTIAL FEATURES
OF AN ACCEPTABLE ELT SELECTION SYSTEM

To qualify as reasonable, an ELT selection must meet two important "regulative" requirements: it must be *simple* enough to be readily intelligible, and it must be *plausible,* that is, patently reasonable in a way that can be apprehended easily and without involving ramified subtleties. Those medical administrators responsible for ELT choices must follow a modus operandi that virtually all the people involved can readily understand to be acceptable (at a reasonable level of generality, at any rate). Appearances are critically important here. It is not enough that the choice be made in a *justifiable* way; it must be possible for people—*plain* people—to "see" (i.e., understand without elaborate teaching or indoctrination) that *it is justified,* insofar as any mode of procedure can be justified in cases of this sort.

One "constitutive" requirement is obviously an essential feature of a reasonable selection system: all of its component criteria—those of inclusion and those of comparison alike—must be reasonable in the sense of being *rationally defensible.* The ramifications of this requirement call for detailed consideration. But one of its aspects should be noted without further ado: it must be *fair*—it must treat relevantly like cases alike, leaving no room for "influence" or favoritism, etc.

THE BASIC SCREENING STAGE: CRITERIA OF INCLUSION
(AND EXCLUSION)

Three sorts of considerations are prominent among the plausible criteria of inclusion/exclusion at the basic screening stage: the constituency factor, the progress-of-science factor, and the prospect-of-success factor.

The Constituency Factor

It is a "fact of life" that ELT can be available only in the institutional setting of a hospital or medical institute or the like. Such institutions generally have normal clientele boundaries. A veterans' hospital will not concern itself primarily with treating non-veterans, a children's hospital cannot be expected to accommodate the "senior citizen," an army hospital can regard college professors as outside its sphere. Sometimes the boundaries are geographic—a state hospital may admit only residents of a certain state. (There are, of course, indefensible constituency principles—say race or religion, party membership, or ability to pay; and there are cases of borderline legitimacy, e.g., sex.[4]) A medical institution is justified in considering for ELT only persons within its own constituency, provided this constituency is constituted upon a defensible basis. Thus the haemodialysis selection committee in Seattle "agreed to consider only those applications who were residents of the state of Washington. . . . They justified this stand on the grounds that since the basic research . . . had been done at . . . a state-supported institution—the people whose taxes had paid for the research should be its first beneficiaries."[5]

While thus insisting that constituency considerations represent a valid and legitimate factor in ELT selection, I do feel there is much to be said for minimizing their role in life-or-death cases. Indeed a refusal to recognize them at all is a significant part of medical tradition, going back to the very oath of Hippocrates. They represent a departure from the ideal arising with the institutionalization of medicine, moving it away from its original status as an art practiced by an individual practitioner.

The Progress-of-Science Factor

The needs of medical research can provide a second valid principle of inclusion. The research interests of the medical staff in relation to the specific nature of the cases at issue is a significant consideration. It may be important for the progress of medical science—and thus of potential benefit to many persons in the future—to determine how effective the ELT at issue is with diabetics or persons over sixty or with a negative RH factor. Considerations of this sort represent another type of legitimate factor in ELT selection.

A very definitely *borderline* case under this head would revolve around the question of a patient's willingness to pay, not in monetary terms, but in offering himself as an experimental subject, say by contracting to return at designated times for a series of tests substantially unrelated to his own health, but yielding data of importance to medical knowledge in general.

The Prospect-of-Success Factor

It may be that while the ELT at issue is not without *some* effectiveness in general, it has been established to be highly effective only with patients in certain specific categories (e.g., females under forty of a specific blood type). This difference in effectiveness—in the absolute or in the probability of success—is (we assume) so marked as to constitute virtually a difference in kind rather than in degree. In this case, it would be perfectly legitimate to adopt the general rule of making the ELT at issue available only or primarily to persons in this substantial-promise-of-success category. (It is on grounds of this sort that young children and persons over fifty are generally ruled out as candidates for haemodialysis.)

[4]Another example of borderline legitimacy is posed by an endowment "with strings attached," e.g., "In accepting this legacy the hospital agrees to admit and provide all needed treatment for any direct descendant of myself, its founder."

[5]Shana Alexander, "They Decide Who Lives, Who Dies," *Life,* LIII (November 9, 1962), 102–25 (see p. 107).

We have maintained that the three factors of constituency, progress of science, and prospect of success represent legitimate criteria of inclusion for ELT selection. But it remains to examine the considerations which legitimate them. The legitimating factors are in the final analysis practical or pragmatic in nature. From the practical angle it is advantageous—indeed to some extent necessary—that the arrangements governing medical institutions should embody certain constituency principles. It makes good pragmatic and utilitarian sense that progress-of-science considerations should be operative here. And, finally, the practical aspect is reinforced by a whole host of other considerations—including moral ones—in supporting the prospect-of-success criterion. The workings of each of these factors are of course conditioned by the ever-present element of limited availability. They are operative only in this context, that is, prospect of success is a legitimate consideration at all only because we are dealing with a situation of scarcity.

THE FINAL SELECTION STAGE: CRITERIA OF SELECTION

Five sorts of elements must, as we see it, figure primarily among the plausible criteria of selection that are to be brought to bear in further screening the group constituted after application of the criteria of inclusion: the relative-likelihood-of-success factor, the life-expectancy factor, the family role factor, the potential-contributions factor, and the services-rendered factor. The first two represent the *biomedical* aspect, the second three the *social* aspect.

The Relative-Likelihood-of-Success Factor

It is clear that the relative likelihood of success is a legitimate and appropriate factor in making a selection within the group of qualified patients that are to receive ELT. This is obviously one of the considerations that must count very significantly in a reasonable selection procedure.

The present criterion is, of course, closely related to item *C* of the preceding selection. There we were concerned with prospect-of-success considerations categorically and *en bloc*. Here at present they come into play in a particularized case-by-case comparison among individuals. If the therapy at issue is not a once-and-for-all proposition and requires ongoing treatment, cognate considerations must be brought in. Thus, for example, in the case of a chronic ELT procedure such as haemodialysis it would clearly make sense to give priority to patients with a potentially reversible condition (who would thus need treatment for only a fraction of their remaining lives).

The Life-Expectancy Factor

Even if the ELT is "successful" in the patient's case he may, considering his age and/or other aspects of his general medical condition, look forward to only a very short probable future life. This is obviously another factor that must be taken into account.

The Family Role Factor

A person's life is a thing of importance not only to himself but to others —friends, associates, neighbors, colleagues, etc. But his (or her) relationship to his immediate family is a thing of unique intimacy and significance. The nature of his relationship to his wife, children, and parents, and the issue of their financial and psychological dependence upon him, are obviously matters that deserve to be given weight in the ELT selection process. Other things being anything like equal, the mother of minor children must take priority over the middle-aged bachelor.

The Potential Future-Contributions Factor
(Prospective Service)

In "choosing to save" one life rather than another, "the society," through the mediation of the particular medical institution in question— which should certainly look upon itself as a trustee for the social interest— is clearly warranted in considering the likely pattern of future *services to be rendered* by the patient (adequate recovery assumed), considering his age, talent, training, and past record of performance. In its allocations of ELT, society "invests" a scarce resource in one person as against another and is thus entitled to look to the probable prospective "return" on its investment.

It may well be that a thoroughly egalitarian society is reluctant to put someone's social contribution into the scale in situations of the sort at issue. One popular article states that "the most difficult standard would be the candidate's value to society," and goes on to quote someone who said: "You can't just pick a brilliant painter over a laborer. The average citizen would be quickly eliminated."[6] But what if it were not a brilliant painter but a brilliant surgeon or medical researcher that was at issue? One wonders if the author of the *obiter dictum* that one "can't just pick" would still feel equally sure of his ground. In any case, the fact that the standard is difficult to apply is certainly no reason for not attempting to apply it. The problem of ELT selection is inevitably burdened with difficult standards.

Some might feel that in assessing a patient's value to society one should ask not only who if permitted to continue living can make the greatest contribution to society in some creative or constructive way, but also who by dying would leave behind the greatest burden on society in assuming the discharge of their residual responsibilities.[7] Certainly the philosophical utilitarian would give equal weight to both these considerations. Just here is where I would part ways with orthodox utilitarianism. For—though this is not the place to do so—I should be prepared to argue that a civilized society has an obligation to promote the furtherance of positive achievements in

[6]Lawrence Lader, "Who Has the Right to Live?" *Good Housekeeping* (January 1968), p. 144.

[7]This approach could thus be continued to embrace the previous factor, that of family role, the preceding item (*C*).

cultural and related areas even if this means the assumption of certain added burdens.[8]

The Past Services-Rendered Factor (Retrospective Service)

A person's services to another person or group have always been taken to constitute a valid basis for a claim upon this person or group—of course a moral and not necessarily a legal claim. Society's obligation for the recognition and reward of services rendered—an obligation whose discharge is also very possibly conducive to self-interest in the long run—is thus another factor to be taken into account. This should be viewed as a morally necessary correlative of the previously considered factor of *prospective* service. It would be morally indefensible of society in effect to say: "Never mind about services you rendered yesterday—it is only the services to be rendered tomorrow that will count with us today." We live in very future-oriented times, constantly preoccupied in a distinctly utilitarian way with future satisfactions. And this disinclines us to give much recognition to past services. But parity considerations of the sort just adduced indicate that such recognition should be given *on grounds of equity*. No doubt a justification for giving weight to services rendered can also be attempted along utilitarian lines. ("The reward of past services rendered spurs people on to greater future efforts and is thus socially advantageous in the long-run future.") In saying that past services should be counted "on grounds of equity"—rather than "on grounds of utility"—I take the view that even if this utilitarian defense could somehow be shown to be fallacious, I should still be prepared to maintain the propriety of taking services rendered into account. The position does not rest on a utilitarian basis and so would not collapse with the removal of such a basis.[9]

As we have said, these five factors fall into three groups: the biomedical factors *A* and *B*, the familial factor *C*, and the social factors *D* and *E*. With items *A* and *B* the need for a detailed analysis of the medical considerations comes to the fore. The age of the patient, his medical history, his physical and psychological condition, his specific disease, etc., will all need to be taken into exact account. These biomedical factors represent technical issues: They call for the physicians' expert judgment and the medical statisticians' hard data. And they are ethically uncontroversial factors—their legitimacy and appropriateness are evident from the very nature of the case.

[8]Moreover a doctrinaire utilitarian would presumably be willing to withdraw a continuing mode of ELT such as haemodialysis from a patient to make room for a more promising candidate who came to view at a later stage and who could not otherwise be accommodated. I should be unwilling to adopt this course, partly on grounds of utility (with a view to the demoralization of insecurity), partly on the non-utilitarian ground that a "moral commitment" has been made and must be honored.

[9]Of course the difficult question remains of the relative weight that should be given to prospective and retrospective service in cases where these factors conflict. There is good reason to treat them on a par.

Greater problems arise with the familial and social factors. They involve intangibles that are difficult to judge. How is one to develop subcriteria for weighing the relative social contributions of (say) an architect or a librarian or a mother of young children? And they involve highly problematic issues. (For example, should good moral character be rated a plus and bad a minus in judging services rendered?) And there is something strikingly unpleasant in grappling with issues of this sort for people brought up in times greatly inclined towards maxims of the type "Judge not!" and "Live and let live!" All the same, in the situation that concerns us here such distasteful problems must be faced, since a failure to choose to save some is tantamount to sentencing all. Unpleasant choices are intrinsic to the problem of ELT selection; they are of the very essence of the matter.[10]

But is reference to all these factors indeed inevitable? The justification for taking account of the medical factors is pretty obvious. But why should the social aspect of services rendered and to be rendered be taken into account at all? The answer is that they must be taken into account not from the *medical* but from the *ethical* point of view. Despite disagreement on many fundamental issues, moral philosophers of the present day are pretty well in consensus that the justification of human actions is to be sought largely and primarily—if not exclusively—in the principles of utility and of justice.[11] But utility requires reference of services to be rendered and justice calls for a recognition of services that have been rendered. Moral considerations would thus demand recognition of these two factors. (This, of course, still leaves open the question of whether the point of view provides a valid basis of action: Why base one's actions upon moral principles?—or, to put it bluntly—Why be moral? The present paper is, however, hardly the place to grapple with so fundamental an issue, which has been canvassed in the literature of philosophical ethics since Plato.)

MORE THAN MEDICAL ISSUES ARE INVOLVED

An active controversy has of late sprung up in medical circles over the question of whether non-physician laymen should be given a role in ELT selection (in the specific context of chronic haemodialysis). . . .

[10]This in the symposium on "Selection of Patients for Haemodialysis," *British Medical Journal* (March 11, 1967), pp. 622–24. F. M. Parsons writes: "But other forms of selecting patients [distinct from first come, first served] are suspect in my view if they imply evaluation of man by man. What criteria could be used? Who could justify a claim that the life of a mayor would be more valuable than that of the humblest citizen of his borough? Whatever we may think as individuals none of us is indispensable." But having just set out this hard-line view he immediately backs away from it: "On the other hand, to assume that there was little to choose between Alexander Fleming and Adolf Hitler . . . would be nonsense, and we should be naive if we were to pretend that we could not be influenced by their achievements and characters if we had to choose between the two of them. Whether we like it or not we cannot escape the fact that this kind of selection for long-term haemodialysis will be required until very large sums of money become available for equipment and services [so that *everyone* who needs treatment can be accommodated]."

[11]The relative fundamentality of these principles is, however, a substantially disputed issue.

But no amount of flag waving about the doctor's facing up to his responsibility—or prostrations before the idol of the doctor-patient relationship and reluctance to admit laymen into the sacred precincts of the conference chambers of medical consultations—can obscure the essential fact that ELT selection is not a wholly medical problem. When there are more than enough places in an ELT program to accommodate all who need it, then it will clearly be a medical question to decide who does have the need and which among these would successfully respond. But when an admitted gross insufficiency of places exists, when there are ten or fifty or one hundred highly eligible candidates for each place in the program, then it is unrealistic to take the view that purely medical criteria can furnish a sufficient basis for selection. The question of ELT selection becomes serious as a phenomenon of scale—because, as more candidates present themselves, strictly medical factors are increasingly less adequate as a selection criterion precisely because by numerical category crowding there will be more and more cases whose "status is much the same" so far as purely medical considerations go.

The ELT selection problem clearly raises issues that transcend the medical sphere because—in the nature of the case—many residual issues remain to be dealt with once *all* of the medical questions have been faced. Because of this there is good reason why laymen as well as physicians should be involved in the selection process. Once the medical considerations have been brought to bear, fundamental social issues remain to be resolved. The instrumentalities of ELT have been created through the social investment of scarce resources, and the interests of the society deserve to play a role in their utilization. As representatives of their social interests, lay opinions should function to complement and supplement medical views once the proper arena of medical considerations is left behind.[12] Those physicians who have urged the presence of lay members on selection panels can, from this point of view, be recognized as having seen the issue in proper perspective.

One physician has argued against lay representation on selection panels for haemodialysis as follows: "If the doctor advises dialysis and the lay panel refuses, the patient will regard this as a death sentence passed by an anonymous court from which he has no right of appeal."[13] But this drawback is not specific to the use of a lay panel. Rather, it is a feature inherent in every *selection* procedure, regardless of whether the selection is done by the head doctor of the unit, by a panel of physicians, etc. No matter who does the selecting among patients recommended for dialysis, the feelings of the patient who has been rejected (and knows it) can be expected to be much the same, provided that he recognizes the actual nature of the choice (and is not deceived by the possibly convenient but ultimately poisonous fiction that because the selection was made by physicians it was made entirely on medical grounds).

[12]To say this is of course not to deny that such questions of applied medical ethics will invariably involve a host of medical considerations—it is only to insist that extramedical considerations will also invariably be at issue.

[13]M. A. Wilson, "Selection of Patients for Haemodialysis," *op. cit.*, p. 624.

In summary, then, the question of ELT selection would appear to be one that is in its very nature heavily laden with issues of medical research, practice, and administration. But it will not be a question that can be resolved on solely medical grounds. Strictly social issues of justice and utility will invariably arise in this area—questions going outside the medical area in whose resolution medical laymen can and should play a substantial role.

THE INHERENT IMPERFECTION (NON-OPTIMALITY) OF ANY SELECTION SYSTEM

Our discussion to this point of the design of a selection system for ELT has left a gap that is a very fundamental and serious omission. We have argued that five factors must be taken into substantial and explicit account:

A. *Relative likelihood of success.* Is the chance of the treatment's being "successful" to be rated as high, good, average, etc.?[14]

B. *Expectancy of future life.* Assuming the "success" of the treatment, how much longer does the patient stand a good chance (75 per cent or better) of living—considering his age and general condition?

C. *Family role.* To what extent does the patient have responsibilities to others in his immediate family?

D. *Social contributions rendered.* Are the patient's past services to his society outstanding, substantial, average, etc.?

E. *Social contributions to be rendered.* Considering his age, talents, training, and past record of performance, is there a substantial probability that the patient will—*adequate recovery being assumed*—render in the future services to his society that can be characterized as outstanding, substantial, average, etc.?

This list is clearly insufficient for the construction of a reasonable selection system, since that would require not only *that these factors be taken into account* (somehow or other), but—going beyond this—would specify *a specific set of procedures for taking account of them.* The specific procedures that would constitute such a system would have to take account of the interrelationship of these factors (e.g., *B* and *E*), and to set out exact guidelines as to the relevant weight that is to be given to each of them. This is something our discussion has not as yet considered.

In fact, I should want to maintain that there is no such thing here as a single rationally superior selection system. The position of affairs seems to me to be something like this: (1) It is necessary (for reasons already canvassed) to *have* a system, and to have a system that is rationally defensible, and (2) to be rationally defensible, this system must take the factors *A–E* into substantial and explicit account. But (3) the exact manner in which a rationally defensible system takes account of these factors cannot be fixed

[14]In the case of an ongoing treatment involving complex procedure and dietary and other mode-of-life restrictions—and chronic haemodialysis definitely falls into this category—the patient's psychological makeup, his willpower to "stick with it" in the face of substantial discouragements—will obviously also be a substantial factor here. The man who gives up, takes not his life alone, but (figuratively speaking) also that of the person he replaced in the treatment schedule.

in any one specific way on the basis of general considerations. Any of the variety of ways that give *A–E* "their due" will be acceptable and viable. One cannot hope to find within this range of workable systems some one that is *optimal* in relation to the alternatives. There is no one system that does "the (uniquely) best"—only a variety of systems that do "as well as one can expect to do" in cases of this sort.

The situation is structurally very much akin to that of rules of partition of an estate among the relations of a decedent. It is important *that there be* such rules. And it is reasonable that spouse, children, parents, siblings, etc., be taken account of in these rules. But the question of the exact method of division—say that when the decedent has neither living spouse nor living children then his estate is to be divided, dividing 60 per cent between parents, 40 per cent between siblings versus dividing 90 per cent between parents, 10 per cent between siblings—cannot be settled on the basis of any general abstract considerations of reasonableness. Within broad limits, a *variety* of resolutions are all perfectly acceptable—so that no one procedure can justifiably be regarded as "the (uniquely) best" because it is superior to all others.[15]

A POSSIBLE BASIS FOR A REASONABLE SELECTION SYSTEM

Having said that there is no such thing as *the optimal* selection system for ELT, I want now to sketch out the broad features of what I would regard as *one acceptable* system.

The basis for the system would be a point rating. The scoring here at issue would give roughly equal weight to the medical considerations (*A* and *B*) in comparison with the extramedical considerations (*C* = family role, *D* = services rendered, and *E* = services to be rendered), also giving roughly equal weight to the three items involved here (*C*, *D*, and *E*). The result of such a scoring procedure would provide the essential *starting point* of our ELT selection mechanism. I deliberately say "starting point" because it seems to me that one should not follow the results of this scoring in an *automatic* way. I would propose that the actual selection should only be guided but not actually be dictated by this scoring procedure, along lines now to be explained.

THE DESIRABILITY OF INTRODUCING AN ELEMENT OF CHANCE

The detailed procedure I would propose—not of course as optimal (for reasons we have seen), but as eminently acceptable—would combine the scoring procedure just discussed with an element of chance. The resulting selection system would function as follows:

[15]To say that acceptable solutions can range over broad limits is *not* to say that there are no limits at all. It is an obviously intriguing and fundamental problem to raise the question of the factors that set these limits. This complex issue cannot be dealt with adequately here. Suffice it to say that considerations regarding precedent and people's expectations, factors of social utility, and matters of fairness and sense of justice all come into play.

1.   First the criteria of inclusion of Section IV above would be applied to constitute a *first phase selection group*—which (we shall suppose) is substantially larger than the number *n* of persons who can actually be accommodated with ELT.

2.   Next the criteria of selection of Section V are brought to bear via a scoring procedure of the type described in Section VIII. On this basis a *second phase selection group* is constituted which is only *somewhat* larger—say by a third or a half—than the critical number *n* at issue.

3.   If this second phase selection group is relatively homogeneous as regards rating by the scoring procedure—that is, if there are no really major disparities within this group (as would be likely if the initial group was significantly larger than *n*)—then the final selection is made by *random* selection of *n* persons from within this group.

This introduction of the element of chance—in what could be dramatized as a "lottery of life and death"—must be justified. The fact is that such a procedure would bring with it three substantial advantages.

First, as we have argued above (in Section VII), any acceptable selection system is inherently non-optimal. The introduction of the element of chance prevents the results that life-and-death choices are made by the automatic application of an admittedly imperfect selection method.

Second, a recourse to chance would doubtless make matters easier for the rejected patient and those who have a specific interest in him. It would surely be quite hard for them to accept his exclusion by relatively mechanical application of objective criteria in whose implementation subjective judgment is involved. But the circumstances of life have conditioned us to accept the workings of chance and to tolerate the element of luck (good or bad): human life is an inherently contingent process. Nobody, after all, has an absolute right to ELT—but most of us would feel that we have "every bit as much right" to it as anyone else in significantly similar circumstances. The introduction of the element of chance assures a like handling of like cases over the widest possible area that seems reasonable in the circumstances.

Third (and perhaps least), such a recourse to random selection does much to relieve the administrators of the selection system of the awesome burden of ultimate and absolute responsibility.

These three considerations would seem to build up a substantial case for introducing the element of chance into the mechanism of the system for ELT selection in a way limited and circumscribed by other weightier considerations, along some such lines as those set forth above.[16]

It should be recognized that this injection of *man-made* chance supplements the element of *natural* chance that is present inevitably and in any case (apart from the role of chance in singling out certain persons as victims for

---

[16]One writer has mooted the suggestion that: "Perhaps the right thing to do, difficult as it may be to accept, is to select [for haemodialysis] from among the medically and psychologically qualified patients on a strictly random basis" (S. Gorovitz, "Ethics and the Allocation of Medical Resources," *Medical Research Engineering,* V [1966], p. 7). Outright random selection would, however, seem indefensible because of its refusal to give weight to considerations which, under the circumstances, *deserve* to be given weight. The proposed procedure of superimposing a certain degree of randomness upon the rational-choice criteria would seem to combine the advantages of the two without importing the worst defects of either.

the affliction at issue). . . . As F. M. Parsons has observed: "any vacancies [in an ELT program—specifically haemodialysis] will be filled immediately by the first suitable patients, even though their claims for therapy may subsequently prove less than those of other patients refused later."[17] Life is a chancy business and even the most rational of human arrangements can cover this over to a very limited extent at best.

From "Organ Transplants: Ethical and Legal Problems"

Paul A. Freund

Until we secure an adequate supply of organs—natural or artificial—to meet the needs, there will be problems of allocation of these resources: from whom they should come and to whom they should be transferred. By what criteria should these decisions be made? The question implicates moral, legal, and medical considerations, which differ in the cases of removal after death and removal during life.

The moral and legal problems attending the taking of an organ from a cadaver appear to be well on the way to resolution. Although objection to the mutilation of a corpse has been traditional in Orthodox Judaism, as the life-saving potential of transplants has become clearer the resistance on religious grounds has weakened.[1] Legal obstacles have been more widespread. Under the principles of the common law a person could not in his lifetime determine by will or agreement how his bodily organs should be treated after death; and the authority of the next of kin was essentially limited to providing a decent burial. While more recent legal precedents could be construed to authorize the next of kin to donate organs, the

---

[17]"Selection of Patients for Haemodialysis," *op. cit.*, p. 623. The question of whether a patient for chronic treatment should ever be terminated from the program (say if he contracts cancer) poses a variety of difficult ethical problems with which we need not at present concern ourselves. But it does seem plausible to take the (somewhat antiutilitarian) view that a patient should not be terminated simply because a "better qualified" patient comes along later on. It would seem that a quasi-contractual relationship has been created through established expectations and reciprocal understandings, and that the situation is in this regard akin to that of the man who, having undertaken to sell his house to one buyer, cannot afterward unilaterally undo this arrangement to sell it to a higher bidder who "needs it worse" (thus maximizing the over-all utility).

Reprinted with permission of author and publisher from *Proceedings of the American Philosophical Society* 115:4, 276–81, August 1971.

[1]D. Daube, "Limitations on Self-Sacrifice in Jewish Law and Tradition," *Theology* 72 (1969): pp. 291, 299; Carroll, "The Ethics of Transplantation," *Amer. Bar Assn. Jour.* 56 (1970): pp. 137, 138. (The Chief Rabbi of Israel hailed the first heart transplant in that country; the rabbinate, at the same time, asserted that post mortem operations are prohibited by the Torah.)

authority was not beyond peradventure clear, and since the next of kin might be unknown, or unavailable, or hostile, the procedure for securing approval was at best unsatisfactory, especially in situations where the utmost promptness in removal was essential for the viability of the organ.[2]

The problem of obtaining the necessary consent has now been resolved from another direction. The Uniform Anatomical Gift Act, which has been adopted in forty-eight states, authorizes an individual to donate his body, or certain organs or tissues, for purpose of transplantation or other scientific use, by means of a relatively simple witnessed document, and there is a growing practice of using a card to signify his authorization. Many persons are now card-carrying potential donors of organs. Alternatively, the Act authorizes the next of kin (in order of priority, beginning with a surviving spouse) to grant authorization. The most serious problems that remain in the field of transplants from cadavers are thus the biological ones: the medical requirement that certain organs, notably the heart, be utilized in an oxygenated condition, precluding storage or even appreciable delay, and so necessitating early typing and matching of tissues.

Turning from the donation of organs after death to their donation for live transplants, we have to differentiate between paired and unpaired organs.

In the case of paired organs, like kidneys, the law is permissive, where the loss and the risk of further injury to the donor are moderate in relation to the anticipated benefit to the recipient. Indeed, a renal transplant has been authorized by a Massachusetts court even between minors who were twins, despite the rule that a child may not be made the subject of harm unless for his own benefit; the court reasoned, after interviewing the healthy twin, that he would suffer lasting psychic trauma if he were not allowed to contribute an organ to his brother so that they could continue to enjoy the blessings of life together.

From the ground of permitting the donation of a paired organ to save a life, should the law move to the position of requiring such contributions, through a process of random selection? In Kantian terms, would we will a universal rule imposing an obligation on others to save us, and in return accept an obligation to save others in the same way? Compulsory vaccination is of course a different matter, since an unvaccinated person may be a positive menace. The law has hesitated to equate a duty to come to the aid of another with a duty to refrain from doing harm. Why should this reluctance persist? Three possible reasons can be suggested. First, there is a practical calculus. Compulsory giving may range along a spectrum from taxation to enforced martyrdom. There is an intuitively felt difference between the taking of one's substance and of one's selfhood. In a situation of catastrophe one can imagine a conscription of blood, which is self-replenishing, more readily than a conscription of organs. The disproportion between risk to the donor and expected benefit to the donee would have to be greater

---

[2]". . . in the light of current medical advances . . . existing 'anatomical' statutes, such as [the law providing for surrender of unclaimed bodies for the advance of medical science] are inadequate, and the need for appropriate statutory provision to implement the desires of the dying to aid the living is increasingly urgent." *Holland v. Metalious*, 105 N. H. 290, 293, 198 Atl.2d 654, 656 (1964).

and surer to warrant compulsion than to support a voluntary sacrifice; otherwise we might be in the position of the traveler in the desert, carrying a canister of water sufficient for one person, who is obliged to share it with another and thereby causes two deaths. Secondly, there would be practical problems of selection among all possible donors, since randomness is not a self-defining concept. And finally, enforced giving would diminish the moral quality of the act, though this consideration would be less relevant if scope were also left for voluntary donations. . . .

There is one further question that ought to be raised in connection with the selection of donors: should a person be encouraged or permitted to sell his organs for purposes of transplant? In the case of donations of blood, where the risk to the donor is negligible, the question is relatively unimportant. We would not object on moral grounds to paying someone to stand in line for us at a ticket counter, though we would have the most serious moral qualms about paying for someone to take our place in a conscript army.[3] To save oneself by putting another in mortal danger through trading on his poverty strikes one as an immoral bargain. Is the case different if the bargain is struck not by the more affluent beneficiary but more impersonally by the state or a philanthropic institution? The question is analogous to that raised by a so-called volunteer army, using the inducement of higher pay for service, and the answer is equally debatable. The Uniform Anatomical Gift Act takes no position on the issue, leaving it to state law, although it can be said that the acceptability of compensation is strongest where the donation is to be made after death. In the case of an *inter vivos* transplant of serious nature, the allowance of a pecuniary motive is repugnant, as if society had a vested interest in maintaining an impoverished class of citizens to serve as risk-takers for others. If the need for organs is felt to be crucial, and if both payment and conscription are ruled out, a possibility remains of liberalizing the law concerning bodies at death, by enacting that post-mortem removal of organs may be effected unless the decedent or next of kin have affirmatively interposed an objection.[4] This is a step whose consideration ought to await evidence on the adequacy of the Uniform Act.

It is time to turn from the selection of donors to that of donees. Few decisions can be as harrowing as the choice of who shall live and who shall die, as any judge or governor can attest; and yet in those cases the law is dealing with persons whose guilt, at least in a legal sense, has been found, and where there is no constraint on sparing the lives of all. In our problem we are dealing with the constraints of scarcity and the consequent necessity of preferences for secular salvation and doom of innocent persons.

In 1943, when penicillin was in short supply for our forces in North Africa, two groups of soldiers could have benefited from its use: those who had contracted venereal disease, and those who suffered from infected

[3]Nevertheless it is to be recalled that in our early history it was customary to condition the exemption of conscientious objectors from military service on their providing a substitute or the money necessary to engage one. See J. Cardozo, in *Hamilton v. Regents*, 293 U.S. 245, 266–277 (1934).

[4]D. Sanders and J. Dukeminier, "Medical Advance and Legal Lag: Hemodialysis and Kidney Transplantation," *U. C. L. A. Law Rev.* 15 (1968): pp. 357, 410–413.

battle wounds. The consulting surgeon advised, on moral grounds, that the wounded be given priority, but the medical officer in charge ruled that preference be given to the other group. The latter, he reasoned, could be restored to active duty more quickly, and immediate manpower was needed; moreover, if untreated they could be a threat to others. For good or ill, life's values are seldom so one-dimensional as they are on the front lines in wartime. Nevertheless efforts have been made to assess the comparative worth of patients to society in the rationing of scarce medical resources, notably renal dialysis equipment. At the center in Seattle, after a medical and psychiatric screening to identify those patients who could benefit substantially from the treatment, they are evaluated by an anonymous but predominantly lay committee, operating under no more definite criteria than social worth, which in practice has been judged by such factors as the number and need of dependents and civic service performed, such as scout leadership, religious-social teaching, and Red Cross activities.[5] One less confident that one's middle-class values represent eternal verities or even the clear hope of the future might well find it impossible to serve on such a committee. More pointedly, where the facilities are operated by a public agency there is a real question whether some more articulated and warrantable standards must be formulated to satisfy the demands of the constitutional guarantees of due process of law and equal protection of the laws.[6] When mortals are called on to make ultimate choice for life or death among their innocent fellows, the only tolerable criterion may be equality of worth as a human being. Translated into practical terms this means a procedure for selection based on randomness within a group, or on objective factors like age or priority of application.

Scarcity of resources presents not only a problem of selection of donors and donees but of allocation of medical facilities and personnel between transplant and other undertakings. At a large teaching hospital in Boston the decision was made not to engage in heart transplant surgery at the present time. To have done so would have required a material inroad on the program of open-heart surgery, where the operative results have been favorable in eighty to ninety per cent of the cases. Meanwhile basic work on the biological aspects of transplantation continued. Not every institution that has undertaken heart transplants, it can be said, was ideally suited for the mission. Should the decision to engage or not to engage in this form of surgery be left to the individual institution, or should not an effort be made to ration this enterprise in order to achieve a minimum of dislocation and a maximum of scientific progress in the experimental stage of a promising therapeutic procedure?

The upshot of our whole discussion is that the choices enforced by a scarcity of resources, and the awesome moral questions raised by deliberate programs to increase the number of donors of viable organs, point to a

[5] *Idem* at pp. 366–380.

[6] See Note, "Patient Selection for Artificial and Transplant Organs," *Harv. Law Rev.* **82** (1969): pp. 1322, 1331–1337.

search for a solution that would by-pass these issues, so uncomfortable for human decision. It may not be thought an evasion, one hopes, to suggest that what is urgently needed is a program for the development of artificial organs, like teeth and limbs, to supersede the transplant of natural organs. The physical obstacles are admittedly formidable: how, for example, to provide a lasting and safe power supply for an implanted mechanical heart, and how to overcome the problem of clotting presented by a large foreign surface at the site of the heart. Yet the eventuality of biologists and engineers supplanting moralists and lawyers in the collaborative quest for bodily renewal is a consummation devoutly to be wished.

PEDAGOGICAL POSTSCRIPT

Appendix A

1. INSTITUTIONAL RESOURCES

The following institutions have been particularly prominent in the area of philosophy and medicine, and can provide a variety of resources to persons who wish to pursue the subject beyond the limitations of this book.

The Institute of Society, Ethics and the Life Sciences (The Hastings Center), 360 Broadway, Hastings-on-Hudson, New York 10706, offers many services to persons interested in philosophy and medicine. Individual membership in the Institute provides the Institute's publications, including the *Hastings Center Report* which contains articles on timely topics, bibliographical information, announcements, etc.

The Society for Health and Human Values, 723 Witherspoon Building, Philadelphia, Pennsylvania 19107, issues various publications such as a helpful annotated bibliography on Abortion and Euthanasia, a newsletter, etc. Members receive the publications, as well as information about the Society's many other activities such as the *Journal of Medicine and Philosophy*, annual meetings in conjunction with the American Association of Medical Colleges, and research and fellowship programs.

The American Philosophical Association's Committee on Philosophy and Medicine publishes a newsletter, provides information on curriculum development, and conducts symposia in conjunction with regular APA meetings and in other contexts. Information is available from The American Philosophical Association, University of Delaware, Newark, Delaware 19711.

The Joseph and Rose Kennedy Institute for the Study of Human Reproduction and Bioethics operates the Kennedy Center for Bioethics, Georgetown University, Washington, D.C. 20007, which engages in programs of research and training in bioethics. The Center is preparing the *Encyclopedia of Bioethics* under the general editorship of Warren Reich, and conducts various bibliographical projects (see below).

2. BIBLIOGRAPHIES

A number of bibliographies are of particular value in philosophy and medicine. The Hastings Center (see above) publishes an annual bibliography with some annotation, and with entries grouped under topical headings. The Department of Health, Education and Welfare has published *Ethical Issues in Health Services: A Report and Annotated Bibliography* compiled by Dr. James Carmody. This publication, DHEW number HSM 73-3008, published in 1970, is available from DHEW; it is also available from the National Technical Information Service, U.S. Department of Commerce, Springfield, Virginia 22151, as Report No. PB 195-732. Supplement 1, 1970–1973, also by Carmody, has publication number HRA 74-3123.

The Kennedy Center for Bioethics (see above) offers a comprehensive *Bibliography of Bioethics* compiled by Leroy Walters. The bibliography includes print and non-print reference materials (newspapers and journal articles, books, monographs, essays within books, court decisions, state and federal laws, films, video and audio tapes) and will be published yearly. Volume I (1975, 250 pp.) is available from the publisher, Gale Research Press, Book Tower, Detroit, Michigan 48226. The Kennedy Institute also has a subscription series for monthly listings of its new acquisitions. *New Title in Bioethics* is available at $6/year from the Center for Bioethics, Kennedy Institute, Georgetown University, Washington, D.C. 20057.

The Society for Health and Human Values (see above) has published a bibliography, *Abortion and Euthanasia: An Annotated Bibliography*, compiled by K. Danner Clouser and A. Zucker, which contains critical annotation.

3. QUESTIONS FOR DISCUSSION

There follow some questions that may be useful for class or group discussions, essay topics, or examinations.

1. It is sometimes assumed that the problems of medical ethics arise out of exotic cases involving unusual medical technology, severe retardation, terminal illness, and the like. But ordinary medical practice involves moral issues too. Give one or two examples, explaining what the moral issues are, and discussing those issues.

2. Nurses and physicians have a clear professional obligation to act in the interests of their patients. Yet, social pressures in the real world sometimes make it difficult for health care workers to act in the interest of a patient without personal risk (for example, of job loss, harrassment by other personnel, conflict with authorities, legal sanctions, loss of chance for promotion). So, sometimes a professional may seem to have a conflict between personal interest and the interest of the patient. How should one go about resolving such a conflict?

3. Discuss the following quotations:
(a) Mercy killing is merely a euphemistic term; easy death by lethal doses of drugs or other means to hasten the end of life is murder and against the Fifth Commandment, which states, "Thou shalt not kill." If legalized, it will be but

legal murder. Mercy killing is contrary to the natural law because it is against human nature and, consequently, against the duties of reason. Euthanasia is detrimental to the welfare of society because it destroys man's idea of sacrifice, loyalty, and courage in bearing pain.

—Knights of Columbus

(b) . . . the proponents of euthanasia now seek only the death of those who are a nuisance to themselves, but soon it will be broadened to include those who are a nuisance to others.

—G. K. Chesterton

(c) I have no sympathy with the man who would shorten the death agony of a dog but prolong that of a human being.

—Dr. R. E. Osgood

4.   An elderly patient asks that his death be speeded by medication. The physician, seeing that death is imminent and that the patient is in pain, consents to the request. She leaves orders for the nurse that the rate of medication be increased. The nurse follows the instructions, and the patient quickly and painlessly dies as a result of the medication. Do not worry, for the sake of the question, whether these acts were right or wrong. Discuss, instead, exactly who was responsible for what acts.

5.   Dying persons and severely handicapped persons face some similar challenges. Discuss the respects in which dying persons and severely handicapped persons should be treated similarly or differently.

6.   A staff meeting has been called in the pediatric intensive care ward to discuss a critical problem. A 2-week-old infant is in the unit born with Down's Syndrome and bilateral hydroureteronephrosis secondary to urethral valves, for the correction of which the family has refused surgery. The infant is becoming increasingly uremic and will eventually die without corrective surgery. The staff is in agreement that the parents should not be taken to court and surgery legally ordered. Moreover, the staff agrees that active euthanasia would be out of place. The question at issue is who should take care of the baby while it dies. Dr. Max argues that the baby should be taken home, because no life and death decision should be made by the parents without being fully confronted with the emotional impact of their grave decision. However, Dr. Moritz argues that the baby should be left in the hospital because the emotional turbulence of a dying baby in the home would so overwhelm the parents that a reasonable decision would be precluded.
Discuss the issues raised by this case.

7.   Who should survive? Everyone who can, or just some? Why?

8.   We prohibit the use of thalidomide because we believe that we have a responsibility to prevent future generations from being born with severe birth defects. In keeping with this commitment to the quality of future humans, we should prevent those with severe heritable diseases from reproducing. Discuss this issue, explaining what the nature and extent of our obligations to future generations are, and describing the consequences of your position for policy decisions about genetic matters.

9.   Some physicians believe that due to their expertise in medicine they alone are able to judge the best interest of their patients in medical decisions (in consultation, of course, with the patients). So, in counseling patients, these physicians attempt to direct their patients to the (medically) correct decision. Are physicians right to adopt such a policy?

10. "In a medical situation of any seriousness, the physician must make the final medical decision because the patient (assuming he is not a medical specialist himself) can neither fully understand nor be fully informed of the relevant facts upon which the decision must be based. Therefore, the patient, in his role as patient, necessarily relinquishes his autonomy and becomes subservient to the will of the physician." Discuss this claim, including a consideration of the processes of decision-making under risk and uncertainty, the notion of informed consent, and the concept of personal integrity.

11. Sometimes, people have such serious mental difficulties that they are not capable of voluntary choice. Commitment of such persons is not really involuntary commitment. It is more properly called "nonvoluntary" commitment. Nonvoluntary commitment, where needed, is as justifiable as restraining an uncontrolled child. Assess this position.

12. Are psychiatrists merely conducting moral indoctrination under the cloak of medical practice?

13. Discuss this argument: "There is no fundamental difference between treatment of mental illnesses by means of drugs and the treatment of mental illnesses by means of "talk" therapies (for example, psychoanalysis or transactional analysis). Either form of therapy can be conducted voluntarily or involuntarily. Both types involve the shaping of mental content by changing the physical constitution of the brain—in one case chemically, in the other by "re-programming" the neural network."

14. Assess the following argument: "Moral or ethical disagreements are fundamentally irresolvable. Either they come down to disagreements about matters of fact and so are not really ethical disagreements, or they come down to fundamental moral disagreements. In the case of fundamental moral disagreements, what seems right to me is right for me and what seems right to you is right for you. There is nothing more to be discussed."

15. "In a particular situation, if we have all the facts, we will then know the right thing to do." Discuss this position.

16. Different moral perspectives can give rise to different judgments about actions. Describe a medical situation in which different decisions might be made by a Kantian (or Rawlsian) on the one hand and a utilitarian on the other. Explain what the difference would be and how it would arise.

17. "In any morally troubling situation, there are at least two possible courses of action, each of which is favored by some of the values we hold. (If this were not the case, the situation would not be morally troubling.) Since people can reasonably differ about which values are more important in any given situation, and since it is not possible to prove one value more fundamental than another, disagreement about the right course of action is the inevitable result. But such disagreement is pointless. Since no value can be proven dominant in such situations, no choice is genuinely the right one in contrast to other choices. It makes no real moral difference what one does in such a situation." Discuss this position.

18. Some writers argue that the morality of an action is a function of its consequences, whereas others hold that the morality of an action depends solely on issues of other sorts. In light of what you know about rights, justice, social welfare, and other valuative considerations, discuss the morally relevant factors in making a decision in a morally troubling situation, and state and defend your position with respect to this disagreement.

19.   The most recent version (1972) of the American Medical Association's official statement of its Principles of Medical Ethics contains the following remark in the introduction:

Men of good conscience inherently know what is right or wrong, and what is to be done or to be avoided. Written documents attempt to express for the guidance of all what each knows to be true. Thus the Principles of Medical Ethics are truly guides to good conduct.

Discuss this position.

20.   Some argue that the practice of keeping confidence in the medical profession is designed to protect patients; others argue that its real, but not usually admitted, purpose is to protect medical practitioners. Which side are you on and why?

21.   Assess this position: Terminal patients should know their condition. Yet, it is not the role of the physician to communicate this to patients. For, the element of the Hippocratic Oath which says *primum non nocere* ("above all, do no harm") requires physicians not to cause unnecessary pain. So, if patients want to be told their condition, they must get the information from someone not bound by this oath.

22.   Assess the following position: If it makes one feel happier, it is best to deny that one is going to die someday. For, it is better to hold false beliefs that make one happy than to hold true beliefs that make one unhappy.

23.   Some have claimed that prisoners should never be used as experimental subjects. Others believe this practice is often morally acceptable. Both sides of the controversy accept the principle that it is ethically impermissible to experiment on a person without that person's consent. Both sides further agree that coerced participation in an experiment does not represent true consent. The central disagreement seems to be over what kinds and degrees of pressures on a person count as coercion. Develop a concept of coercion which clarifies the dispute and indicate how your understanding of coercion helps to resolve the basic issue—the use of prisoners as experimental subjects.

24.   It has been argued that the social consequences of certain kinds of medical research are potentially so dangerous that such research should be discontinued. Examples include cloning, test tube reproduction, etc. Should any research be discontinued or prohibited because of the possibility of its results being put to dangerous use? Discuss this issue, illustrating your discussion with a focus on some particular line of research and its potential justifications and risks.

25.   Discuss the following quotation from Victor Sidel:

. . . the constitution of WHO . . . says health is a state of complete physical, mental, and social well-being and not merely the absence of disease or infirmity. There is, unfortunately, relatively little, in my opinion, that can be accomplished to bring about social well-being when it is narrowly construed or constituted as a therapeutic art. And there are in fact many who would argue that the path to physical and mental well-being is also rarely within the scope of conventional medical care alone. Therefore, if the medical worker is to be a promotor of health rather than simply a reactor against established disease or disability, part of his work must go beyond traditional medical care into areas of social and political change . . .

26.   The federal government has a responsibility to provide access to good medical care for all its citizens. Some citizens live in areas that provide no access to good medical care, and in which physicians do not wish to practice. Physicians have a right to practice wherever they please. Therefore the federal government cannot possibly fulfill its responsibility. Discuss this argument in detail, and propose some method of resolving the apparent impasse.

27.   Discuss this position:

The basic fault in American health service is the discrepancy between our assertion of health care as a basic human right and our practice of treating it as a marketplace commodity . . . [Although we ought to do so,] we have not organized the provision or "delivery" of health services in the way that other services deemed essential to society have been organized, such as education or protection against fire.

28.   "Tay Sachs disease, a fatal degenerative neurological deficiency, can be diagnosed in utero via amniocentesis. It is also possible to identify those who, while lacking the disease themselves, will be possible transmitters of it. Fetuses determined to be victims of the disease should be aborted, but those who are merely carriers should not. Such individuals, however, should be sterilized at an appropriate age as a matter of state policy." Discuss this claim and the issues that it raises.

29.   Discuss these two issues that arise in connection with public health policy. (A) Should public health policy aim for normal health for everyone or optimal health for everyone? Address the issues that arise in attempting to characterize normal and optimal health. (B) Some argue that it is better to invest in advanced medical research that will ultimately improve the medical professions's ability to cure, than to invest in meeting the present health needs of those who receive inferior medical care. Address the issues that arise in attempting to resolve this priority dispute.

30.   Physicians are obliged to combat illness. Much illness is attributable to industrial and automotive pollutants, chemical food additives, pesticides, and other environmental problems. What then is the responsibility of the physician with respect to environmental issues? Is he not obliged to be particularly concerned with and active about environmental issues? Is he not as entitled as any other citizen to practice his profession and exercise his right to abstain from involvement in environmental issues?

4. OTHER RESOURCES

Some information that might be of use to persons planning courses in medical ethics may be obtained from the following sources:

(1)   *The Teaching of Medical Ethics,* ed. Veatch, Gaylin, and Morgan, the Hastings Center, 1973. Proceedings of a 1972 conference on the teaching of medical ethics.

(2)   An annotated bibliography of films and video-tapes for use in medical ethics courses, available from the Council for Philosophical Studies, Skinner

Hall 1131, University of Maryland, College Park, Maryland 20742. No charge.

(3)   The Education Program at the Hastings Center (see above) distributes reprints of many articles relating to ethics and the life sciences, both singly and in packets grouped by topic. For prices and a list of available reprints, contact the Hastings Center.

Several cases that raise moral issues have been described in various issues of the *Hastings Center Report.* By far the best location for case studies, however, is Robert Veatch's *Case Studies in Medical Ethics,* Harvard University Press, forthcoming.

APPENDIX B
MORAL PRECEPTS IN MEDICINE

The manuscript for this Appendix contained the following items:

Oath of Hippocrates;
World Medical Association, Hippocratic Oath;
American Medical Association, Principles of Medical Ethics;
World Health Organization, Principles;
American Hospital Association, Patients' Bill of Rights;
American Hospital Association, The Right of the Patient to
      Refuse Treatment;
The Nuremburg Code;
The Declaration of Helsinki;
A Living Will;
Excerpt from DHEW Policy on the Protection of Human Subjects.

Information on how this material may be obtained is available upon request. Write to Philosophy Editor, College Division, Prentice-Hall, Inc., Englewood Cliffs, New Jersey 07632, asking for Appendix B of *Moral Problems in Medicine.*

INDEX